DAVID J. MAGEE, Ph.D.

Faculty of Rehabilitative Medicine
Department of Physical Therapy
University of Alberta
Edmonton, Alberta, Canada

ORTHOPEDIC PHYSICAL ASSESSMENT

W. B. SAUNDERS COMPANY 1987

PHILADELPHIA   RIO DE JANEIRO
LONDON   SYDNEY
TORONTO   TOKYO
MEXICO CITY   HONG KONG

W. B. Saunders Company: West Washington Square
Philadelphia, PA   19105

Library of Congress Cataloging-in-Publication Data

Magee, David J.

Orthopedic physical assessment.

Includes index.

1. Orthopedia—Diagnosis.   2. Physical diagnosis.
   I. Title. [DNLM: 1. Bone Diseases—diagnosis.   2. Joint
   Diseases—diagnosis.   3. Orthopedics. WE 168 M191o]

RD734.M34 1987   617'.3   86–13855

ISBN 0–7216–1855–3

Editor: Harry Benson
Developmental Editor: Fran Mues
Designer: Karen O'Keefe
Production Manager: Bill Preston
Manuscript Editor: Carol Wolf
Illustrators: Phillip Ashley, Glenn Edelmayer, and Karen McGarry
Cover Illustrator: Karen McGarry
Illustration Coordinator: Peg Shaw
Page Layout Artist: Patti Maddaloni

Orthopedic Physical Assessment   ISBN   0–7216–1855–3

Last digit is the print number: 9   8   7   6   5   4   3   2

To my parents,
who taught me to pick a goal in life
and to take it seriously

Preface

This manuscript was originally developed as part of a manual for physical therapy students at the University of Alberta. That original manual covered conditions and treatment as well as assessment.

The text is the result of my interpretation of the teachings of recognized experts in the field of orthopedic assessment: James Cyriax, Hans Debrunner, Stanley Hoppenfeld, Freddy Kaltenborn, Geoff Maitland, Robin McKenzie, John Mennell, and Alan Stoddard, to name a few. It is my belief that a book such as this will be of benefit to paramedical and medical students throughout their training and into their practice as well as to other health professionals.

The aim of the book is to provide the reader with a systematic approach to carry out an orthopedic assessment and an understanding of the reason for the various aspects of the assessment. Initially, in each chapter, pertinent arthrology is reviewed. The reader is then taken through history, observation, and examination of each joint of the body. The examination is organized in a consistent fashion beginning with active, passive, and resisted isometric movements. The movements are followed by tests designed by different individuals to evaluate specific structures, and a quick assessment of sensory distribution and reflexes to differentiate between peripheral nerves and nerve root problems. Palpation is discussed next to help the examiner pinpoint the problem. The assessment is concluded by a review of different roentgenographic views and the possible findings that the examiner might see in these views.

At the end of each chapter is a précis for quick review prior to beginning an assessment and a list of references should the examiner wish to do further in-depth reading.

The text is liberally provided with artistic renderings and photos to illustrate different points and to provide visual examples of the conditions and anatomic variations referred to in the manuscript.

This book is my first attempt at a project of this magnitude. Any feedback from readers with constructive ideas of how to improve the text would be greatly appreciated.

DAVID J. MAGEE

Acknowledgments

To write a book such as this one, although undertaken by one person, is in reality a bringing together of ideas of colleagues, friends, and experts in the field of orthopedic assessment. In particular, I would like to thank:

Dr. David C. Reid, F.R.C.S.(C), for his teachings, contributions, and ideas in the preparation of this manuscript.

The physical therapy staffs of the Royal Alexandra Hospital, Glenrose Provincial Hospital, and the Workers' Compensation Board Clinic in Edmonton, Alberta, for their valued suggestions.

My graduate and undergraduate students, who helped collect many of the articles used as references in this book.

The many authors and publishers who have agreed to have some of their photographs, drawings, and tables appear in the text so that explanations to students can be clearer.

Alan Garard, Georgina Gray, Marney Dickey, Doug Gilroy, and Martin Parfitt, for being models for many of the photographs.

Dorothy Tomniuk, for her untiring and uncomplaining efforts of typing and retyping this manuscript until it met the author's standards.

Dr. Parkinson, Mrs. Keo, and the staff of Associated Radiologists, for providing x-ray film to be photographed in order to illustrate many of the physical conditions discussed in the book.

Martin Parfitt and Donna Ford, for taking the time and effort to review the manuscript.

Baxter Venable, Carol Wolf, and the staff of W. B. Saunders Company, for their suggestions in writing this text.

My teachers and colleagues, who encouraged me to pursue my chosen career.

To these people, and many others, I say thank you. Without your help and encouragement; this book would never have been written.

Contents

1

Principles and Concepts

In order to complete an orthopedic assessment of a patient, it is important to carry out a proper and thorough examination. A correct diagnosis depends upon a knowledge of functional anatomy, an accurate patient history, diligent observation and a thorough examination. It is only through a complete assessment involving the aforementioned factors that an accurate diagnosis can be made. The purpose of the assessment should be to fully and clearly understand the patient's problems and the physical basis for the symptoms that cause the patient to complain. As Cyriax has stated: "Diagnosis is only a matter of applying one's anatomy."[1]

Regardless of which system is selected for assessment, the examiner should establish a sequential method to ensure that nothing is overlooked. In addition, the examiner should focus attention on only one aspect of the assessment at a time.

This chapter presents the following features of a total assessment:

1. Patient history.
2. Observation.
3. Examination.
4. Special tests.
5. Reflexes and cutaneous distribution.
6. Joint play movements.
7. Palpation.
8. X-ray studies (roentgenograms).

At the end of each chapter, the reader is provided with a summary, or précis, of the assessment procedures for that chapter. This section is provided to enable the examiner to quickly review the pertinent steps of assessment for the joint or structures being assessed. If further information is required, the examiner can refer to the more detailed sections of the chapter.

Patient History

A complete medial history should be taken and written to ensure reliability. Naturally, emphasis should be placed on that portion of the assessment having the greatest clinical relevance. Often the examiner can make the diagnosis by simply listening to the patient. One should never skip over subject areas. Repetition helps the examiner to become familiar with the characteristic history of the patient's complaints so that unusual deviation, which often indicates problems, can be immediately noticed. Even if the diagnosis is obvious, the history will give valuable information about the disorder, its prognosis, and the appropriate treatment desired. The history also enables the examiner to determine the type of person the patient is, the treatment the patient has received, and the behavior of the injury. Not only should the history of the present illness or injury be included; relevant past history, treatment, and results should also be noted. Past medical history should include any major illnesses or surgery, accidents, or allergies. In some cases, it may be necessary to delve into the social and family histories of the patient when they appear relevant.

It is important that the examiner help to keep the patient to the point and discourage irrelevant information; this should be done politely but firmly.

The history is usually taken in an orderly sequence. The questions asked should be easy to understand and should not "lead" the patient. For example, the examiner should not say: "Does this increase your pain?" It would be better to say: "Does this alter your pain in any way?" The examiner should ask one question at a time and should receive an answer to a question before proceeding with another question. The examiner should pose these pertinent questions:

1. What is the patient's age? Many conditions occur within certain age ranges. For example, various growth disorders, such as Legg-Perthes disease or Scheuermann's disease, are seen in adolescents or teenagers. Degenerative conditions, such as osteoarthritis and osteoporosis, are more likely to be seen in an older population.

2. What is the patient's occupation? As an example, we would expect a laborer to have stronger muscles than a sedentary worker and possibly be less likely to suffer a muscle strain. In contrast, laborers would be more susceptible to injury because of the type of job they have. Sedentary workers, although they usually have no need for immediate muscle strength, may find that on weekends, for example, their muscles or joints become overstressed.

3. Was the onset of the problem slow or sudden? Did the condition start as an insidious mild ache and then progress to continuous pain? Does the pain get worse as the day progresses? Was it a sudden onset due to trauma, or was it sudden with locking? Knowledge of these facts helps the examiner determine the cause of the problem.

4. Has the condition occurred before? If so, what was the onset like? Where was the site of the original condition, and has there been any radiation (spread of pain)? If the person is feeling better, how long did it take to recover? Did any treatment help to relieve symptoms? Does the current problem appear to be the same as the previous problem, or is it different? Answers to these questions help the examiner to determine the location of the injury.

5. Was there any inciting trauma? Does the patient remember a specific episode in which the body part was injured, or did the problem slowly develop over a period of time? If there has been inciting trauma, it is often easier to determine where the problem is.

6. How long has the patient had the problem? What is the duration and frequency of the symptoms? Answers to these questions help the examiner to determine whether the condition is acute or chronic and to get an idea of the patient's tolerance to pain.

7. Is the intensity, duration, and/or frequency of pain increasing? These changes usually mean the condition is getting worse. Is the pain decreasing? This change usually means the condition is improving. Is the pain static? If so, how long has it been that way? This question may help the examiner to learn whether the condition is acute or chronic or how long it has been chronic. These factors may become important in treatment.

8. Is the pain constant, periodic, or occasional? Does the condition bother the patient at that exact moment? If the patient is not bothered, the pain is not constant. If the pain is periodic or occasional, the examiner should try to ascertain what the patient is doing or what position or posture irritates the problem. The examiner should be observing the patient at the same time. Does there appear to be constant pain? Does the patient appear to be lacking sleep because of pain? Does the patient move around a great deal in an attempt to find a comfortable position?

9. Where was the pain when the individual first had the complaint? Has the pain moved or spread? Ask the patient to point to exactly where the pain was and where it is now. Generally, pain enlarges or becomes more distal as the lesion worsens and vice versa. The more distal and superficial the problem, the more accurate the patient can determine where the pain is. In the case of referred pain, the patient will usually point out a general area; with a localized lesion, the patient will point to a specific location. Pain also may shift as the lesion shifts. For example, with an internal derangement of the knee, pain may occur in flexion one time and in extension another time if it is due to a loose body within the joint. What are the exact movements that cause pain? At this stage, the patient should not be asked to do the movements because they will be done in the examination. However, the examiner should remember which movements the patient says are painful so that when the examination is carried out these movements can be done last to avoid overflow of painful symptoms. Are there any other factors that aggravate or help to relieve the pain? Is there any alteration in intensity of the pain?

10. Is the pain associated with rest? Activity?

Certain postures? Visceral function? Time of day? For example, pain on activity that decreases with rest usually indicates a mechanical obstruction to movement, such as adhesions. Morning pain with stiffness that improves with activity usually indicates chronic inflammation and edema. Pain or aching as the day progresses usually indicates increased congestion in a joint. Pain that is not affected by rest or activity usually indicates bone pain. Chronic pain is often associated with multiple factors such as fatigue, posture, or activity. If the pain occurs at night, how does the patient lie in bed — supine, on the side, or prone? Does sleeping alter the pain, or does it wake the patient when changing position? What type of mattress and pillow are used? Foam pillows will often cause more problems for persons with cervical problems because these pillow have more "bounce" to them than do feather pillows. Too many pillows, pillows improperly positioned, or too soft a mattress may also cause problems.

11. What type of pain is exhibited? *Nerve pain* tends to be sharp, bright, and burning in quality and also tends to run in the distribution of specific nerves. *Bone pain* tends to be deep, boring, and very localized. *Vascular pain* tends to be diffuse, aching, and poorly localized and may be referred to other areas of the body. *Muscle pain* is usually hard to localize, is dull and aching, is often aggravated by injury, and may be referred to other areas.

12. What types of sensations does the patient feel? If the problem is in bone, there usually is very little radiation of pain. If pressure is applied to a nerve root, there will be pain caused by pressure on the dura mater, which is the outermost covering of the spinal cord. If there is pressure on the nerve trunk, no pain occurs but there is paresthesia or abnormal sensation such as a "pins and needles" feeling, or tingling. If the nerve itself is affected, regardless of where the irritation occurs along the nerve, the pain is perceived by the brain as coming from the periphery. This is an example of referred pain. Muscular, ligamentous, and bursal types of pain are indistinguishable.

13. Does a joint exhibit locking, unlocking, twinges, instability, giving way? Locking may just mean that the joint will not fully extend, as is the case with a meniscal tear, or it may mean that it will not extend one time or flex the next time in the case of a loose body moving around within the joint. Giving way is often due to reflex inhibition of the muscles so that the patient feels that the limb will buckle if weight is placed on it.

14. Are there any changes in color of the limb? Ischemic changes due to circulatory problems may include white, brittle skin; loss of hair; and abnormal nails on the foot or hand.

When taking the history the examiner should determine the following:

1. Has the patient had an x-ray examination? If so, x-ray overexposure may be avoided; if not, an x-ray examination may help yield a diagnosis.

2. Has the patient been receiving steroids or any other medication? If so, for how long? High dosages of steroids for long periods of time may, for example, lead to osteoporosis.

3. Has the patient been taking any other medication that is pertinent? Patients do not always regard every drug as "medication." An example is the birth control pill; if a person takes such medication over a long period of time, it may not seem as pertinent to them.

4. Does the patient have any bilateral cord symptoms, fainting, or "drop" attacks? Is bladder function normal? Is there any "saddle" involvement, or vertigo? These last questions are important to ask because these symptoms indicate severe neurologic problems that must be dealt with carefully.

5. Does the patient have a history of surgery? If so, when was the surgery performed, what was the site of operation, and what condition was being treated? Sometimes the condition the examiner will be asked to treat is the result of the surgery.

It is evident that the taking of an accurate, detailed history is very important. With experience, one is often able to make a "preliminary" diagnosis from the history alone.

Observation

In an assessment, observation is the "looking" phase. The examiner should note the patient's way of moving, along with the general posture, manner and attitude, and willingness to cooperate. The patient must be undressed adequately to be observed properly. Males should wear only shorts and females should wear bra and shorts. On entering the assessment area, the patient's gait should be observed. This initial gait assessment is only a cursory one. (If there appears to be a gait abnormality, the gait may be checked in greater detail once the patient is suitably undressed. Such problems as a Trendelenburg sign or drop foot are easily noticed even if the patient is dressed.)

Once the patient is in the examining room and suitably undressed, the examiner should observe the posture, noting the following:

1. Is there any obvious deformity? Examples might include torticollis, fractures, scoliosis, or kyphosis.

2. Are the bony contours of the body normal and symmetric, or is there an obvious deviation?

The examiner must remember that the body is not perfectly symmetric and deviation may mean nothing. For example, individuals will often have a lower shoulder on the dominant side or they may demonstrate a slight scoliosis of the spine adjacent to the heart. However, any deviation should be noted because it may contribute to a more accurate diagnosis.

3. Are the soft-tissue (e.g., muscle, skin) contours normal and symmetric? Is there any obvious muscle wasting?

4. Are the limb positions equal or symmetric? Compare limb size, shape, any atrophy, color, and temperature.

5. Are the color and texture of the skin normal? Does the appearance of the skin differ in the area of pain from other areas of the body, or are other areas of the body different in skin texture? For example, trophic changes in the skin resulting from peripheral nerve lesions include the loss of skin elasticity, the skin becomes shiny, there is hair loss on the skin, and the skin breaks down easily and heals slowly. The nails may become brittle and ridged.

6. Are there any scars that may indicate recent injury or surgery? Recent scars will be red because they are still healing and contain capillaries, and older scars are white and primarily avascular. Are there any sinuses that may indicate infection? If so, are the sinuses draining or dry?

7. Is there any crepitus or abnormal sound in the joints when the patient moves them?

8. Is there any heat, swelling, or redness in the area being observed? All of these signs are indications of inflammation or an active inflammatory condition.

9. What is the patient's facial expression? Is it evident that the patient appears to be in discomfort or is lacking sleep?

10. Is the patient willing to move? Are patterns of movement normal? If not, how are they abnormal? Any alteration should be noted and included in the observation section of the assessment.

The examiner should be positioned so that the dominant eye is used and should compare both sides of the patient simultaneously. During the observation stage the examiner is only looking at the patient and does not ask the patient to move; the examiner does not palpate, except possibly to learn whether an area is warm or hot.

Examination

In the examination portion of the assessment, a number of principles must be followed:

1. Unless bilateral movement is required, the normal side is tested first. This allows the exam-

iner to establish a baseline for normal movement and shows the patient what to expect, resulting in increased patient confidence.

2. *Active* movements are done before *passive* movements. Passive movements are followed by *resisted isometric* movements. (These movements are further detailed later in this section.)

3. Any movements that are painful are done last to prevent an overflow of painful symptoms to the next movement.

4. If active range of motion is not full, overpressure is applied only with extreme care.

5. When the patient is doing active movements, if the range of motion is full, overpressure may be applied to determine the end feel of the joint. This often negates the need to do passive movements.

6. Each active, passive, or resisted isometric movement is repeated several times to see whether symptoms increase or decrease, whether a different pattern of movement results, whether there is increased weakness, or whether there is possible vascular insufficiency.

7. Resisted isometric movements are done in a neutral or resting position.

8. When the examiner is doing passive range of motion or ligamentous tests, it is not only the degree of opening that is important but also the quality (i.e., *end feel*) of the opening.

9. When the examiner is doing ligamentous tests, the appropriate stress is applied gently and repeated several times; the stress is increased up to but not beyond the point of pain. By doing the test this way, maximum instability can be demonstrated without causing muscle spasm.

10. When *myotomes* (a group of muscles supplied by a single nerve root) are being tested, each contraction is held for a minimum of 5 seconds to see if weakness becomes evident. Myotomal weakness takes time to develop.

11. At the completion of an assessment, the examiner warns the patient that the movements may exacerbate symptoms.

The examination described in this chapter emphasizes the joints of the body. It is necessary to examine all appropriate tissues to delineate the affected area, which can then be examined in detail. Applying tension, stretch, or isometric contraction to specific tissues, in turn, produces either a normal or an appropriate abnormal response. This action enables the examiner to determine the nature and site of the present symptoms and the patient's response to these symptoms. The examination shows whether these activities provoke or change the patient's pain and, in this way, gives subjective information. Thus, the examiner focuses on the patient's feelings or opinions as well as objective observation. The patient must be clear about his (the subjective) side of the examination. For instance, the question "Does the movement make any difference to the pain? Or does it bring on or change the pain?" must not be confused with already existing pain. In addition, the examiner is attempting to see whether patient responses are measurably abnormal. Do the movements cause any abnormalities in function? For example, a loss of movement or weakness in muscles can be measured and therefore is an objective response. Thus, the examiner looks for two sets of data: (1) what the patient feels (subjective), and (2) responses that can be measured or are found by the examiner (objective).

The examination is therefore very extensive. In the upper part of the body, the examination begins with the cervical spine and includes the temporomandibular joints, the whole scapular area, the shoulder region, and the upper limb to the fingers. In the lower part of the body, the examination begins at the lumbar spine and continues to the toes. This phase, often called a *scanning* or *screening examination*, may not be essential if there is a definite history of trauma to a specific joint. However, if one has any doubt whatsoever where the injury is located, it is necessary to perform this scanning examination. The idea of the scanning examination was developed by Cyriax,[1] who, more than any other author, also originated the concepts of "contractile" and "inert" tissue, "end feel," and "capsular patterns." The medical and paramedical professions owe a great deal to this man for his development of a comprehensive and systematic physical examination of the moving parts of the body.

In the examination, there should be an unchanging pattern that varies only slightly to elaborate certain clues given by the history. For example, if the history is characteristic of a disc lesion, the examination should be a detailed one of all the tissues that might be affected by the disc and a brief one of all the other joints to exclude contradictory signs. If the history suggests arthritis of the hip, the examination should be a detailed one of the hip and a brief one of the other joints — again, to exclude contradictory signs. As the movements are tested, the examiner is sometimes looking for the patient's subjective responses and sometimes for objective findings. For example, if examination of the cervical spine shows clear signs of a disc problem, as the examination is continued down the arm, the examiner will be looking more for muscle weakness (objective) rather than expecting to elicit pain (subjective). In contrast, if the history suggests a muscle lesion, pain will likely be provoked when the arm is examined. In either case, the structures expected to be normal are not omitted from examination.

Nerve Root System

To further comprehend the value of the scanning examination, the examiner must understand peripheral nerve distribution and the nerve root system of the body (Fig. 1–1). A nerve root is the portion of the nerve that connects it to the spinal cord. Nerve roots are made up of anterior (ventral) and posterior (dorsal) parts that unite near or in the intervertebral foramen to form a single nerve root or *spinal nerve*. They are the most proximal parts of the peripheral nervous system.

Within the human body, there are 31 nerve roots: eight cervical, twelve thoracic, five lumbar, five sacral, and one coccygeal. Each nerve root has two components: (1) a *somatic* portion that innervates the skeletal muscles and provides sensory input from the skin, fascia, muscles and joints; and (2) a *visceral* component that is part of the autonomic nervous system.[2] The autonomic system supplies the blood vessels, dura mater, periosteum, ligaments, and intervertebral discs, to name a few of the structures. The spinal nerve roots may combine to form a plexus, such as the *brachial plexus*. Thus the nerve roots, by intermingling, form the peripheral nerves, such as the *median nerve*. For this reason, if pressure is applied to the nerve root, the distribution of the sensation or motor function will often be felt or exhibited in more than one peripheral nerve and will not demonstrate the same sensory distribution or altered motor function as the peripheral nerve (Table 1–1).

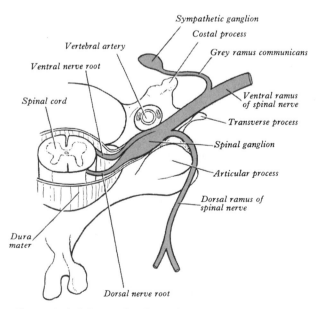

Figure 1–1. Scheme showing spinal cord, nerve root portions, and spinal nerve. (From Williams, P., and R. Warwick (eds.): Gray's Anatomy, 36th Br. ed. Philadelphia, W. B. Saunders Co., 1980, p. 1088.

Table 1–1. Nerve Root Dermatomes, Myotomes, Reflexes, and Paresthetic Areas

Root	Dermatome*	Muscle Weakness (Myotome)	Reflexes Affected	Paresthesias
	Vertex of skull			
C2	Temple, forehead, occiput			
C3	Entire neck, posterior cheek, temporal area, prolongation forward under mandible			Cheek, side of neck
C4	Shoulder area, clavicular area and upper scapular area			Horizontal band along clavicle and upper scapula
C5	Deltoid area, anterior aspect of whole arm to base of thumb	Supraspinatus, intraspinatus, deltoid, biceps	Biceps, brachioradialis	
C6	Anterior arm and radial side of hand to thumb and index finers	Bisceps, supinator, wrist extensors	Biceps	Thumb and index finger
C7	Lateral arm and lateral forearm to index, long and ring fingers	Triceps, wrist flexors (rarely wrist extensors)	Triceps	Index, long and ring fingers
C8	Medial arm and forearm to long ring and little fingers	Ulnar deviators, thumb extensors, thumb adductors (rarely, triceps)		Little finger alone or with two adjacent fingers; *not* ring or long fingers, alone or together (C7)
T1	Medial side of forearm to base of little finger	Disc lesions at upper two thoracic levels do not appear to give rise to root weakness. Weakness of intrinsic muscles of the hand is due to other pathology, e.g., thoracic outlet pressure, neoplasm of lung, and ulnar nerve lesion. Dural and nerve root stress has T1 elbow-flexion with arm horizontal. T1 and T2 scapulae forward and backward on chest wall. Neck flexion at any thoracic level.		
T2	Medial side of upper arm to medial elbow, pectoral and midscapular areas			
T3–12	T3–6, upper thorax; T5–7, costal margin; T8–12, abdomen and lumbar region	Articular and dural signs and root pain are common. Root signs (cutaneous analgesia) rare and with such indefinite area as to have little localizing value. Weakness is not detectable.		
L1	Back, over trochanter and groin	None	None	Groin; after holding posture, which causes pain
L2	Back, front of thigh to knee	Psoas, hip adductors	None	Occasionally anterior thigh
L3	Back, upper buttock, anterior thigh and knee, medial lower leg	Psoas, quadriceps, thigh atrophy	Knee jerk sluggish, PKB positive, pain on full SLR.	Medial knee, anterior lower leg
L4	Medial buttock, lateral thigh, medial leg, dorsum of foot, big toe	Tibialis anterior extensor hallucis	SLR limited neck flexion pain, weak or a bent knee jerk, side flexion limited	Medial aspect of calf and ankle
L5	Buttock, posterior and lateral thigh, lateral aspect of leg, dorsum of foot, medial half of sole and 1st, 2nd, and 3rd toes	Extensor hallucis peroneal, gluteus medius, dorsiflexor, hamstrings-calf atrophy	SLR limited one side, neck flexion painful, ankle decreased, crossed-leg raising—pain	Lateral aspect of leg, medial three toes
S1	Buttock thigh and leg posterior	Calf and hamstring wasting of gluteals, peroneals, plantar flexors	SLR limited	Lateral two toes, lateral foot, lateral leg to knee, plantar aspect of foot
S2	Same as S1	Same as S1 except peroneals	Same as S1	Lateral leg, knee, and heel
S3	Groin, medial thigh to knee	None	None	None
S4	Perineum, genitals, lower sacrum	Bladder, rectum	None	Saddle area, genitals, anus, impotence, massive posterior

*In any part of which pain may be felt.
Abbreviations: PKB = Prone knee bending; SLR = straignt leg raising.

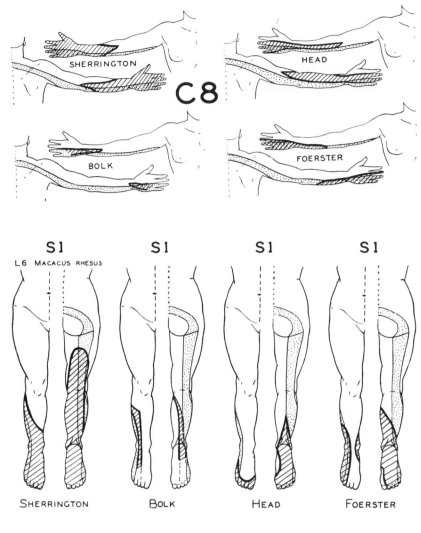

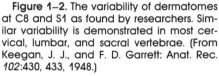

Figure 1–2. The variability of dermatomes at C8 and S1 as found by researchers. Similar variability is demonstrated in most cervical, lumbar, and sacral vertebrae. (From Keegan, J. J., and F. D. Garrett: Anat. Rec. *102*:430, 433, 1948.)

Dermatomes

The sensory distribution of each nerve root, or dermatome, varies from person to person, and there is often a great deal of overlap. A dermatome is defined as the area skin supplied by a single nerve root. One must be aware of the general distribution of these dermatomes and realize that there is a great deal of variability and overlap. Thus when dermatomes are described in the following chapters, they should be considered as examples only, since slight differences may occur. The variability in dermatomes was aptly demonstrated by Keegan and Garrett in 1948[3] (Fig. 1–2).

Peripheral Nerves

The examiner must also be aware of the sensory, motor, and sympathetic distribution of peripheral nerves to be able to differentiate between lesions of nerve roots and peripheral nerves. The effects of a mixed (motor, sensory, and sympathetic) peripheral nerve lesion include:

1. Flaccid paralysis (motor).
2. Loss of reflexes (motor).
3. Muscle wasting and atrophy (motor).
4. Loss of sensation (sensory).
5. Trophic changes in the skin (sensory).
6. Loss of secretions from sweat glands (sympathetic).
7. Loss of pilomotor response (sympathetic).

Pressure on a peripheral nerve resulting in a neuropraxia leads to temporary nonfunctioning of the nerve. With this type of injury, there is primarily motor involvement with little sensory or autonomic involvement. Pressure on a nerve root leads to loss of tone and muscle mass. Spinal nerve roots have a poorly developed *epineurium* and lack a *perineurium*. This makes the nerve root more susceptible to compressive forces, tensile deformation, chemical irritants (such as alcohol, lead, or arsenic), or metabolic abnormalities. For example, diabetes may cause a metabolic peripheral neuropathy of one or more nerves.

In peripheral nerves, the epineurium consists of a loose areolar connective tissue matrix surrounding the nerve fiber and allows changes in growth length of the bundled nerve fibers (funiculi) without allowing the bundles to be strained. The perineurium protects the nerve bundles by acting as a diffusion barrier to irritants and provides tensile strength and elasticity to the nerve.

Myotomes

As defined earlier, myotomes are a group of muscles supplied by a single nerve root. A lesion of a single nerve root is usually associated with *paresis* (incomplete paralysis) of the muscle (myotome) supplied by that nerve root. On the other hand, a lesion of a peripheral nerve leads to complete paralysis of the muscles supplied by that nerve, especially if the injury results in *axonotmesis* or *neurotmesis*. The difference in the amount of resulting paralysis is due to the fact that more than one myotome contributes to the formation of a muscle embryologically.

Sclerotomes

A sclerotome is an area of bone or fascia supplied by a single nerve root (Fig. 1–3). As with dermatomes, sclerotomes can show a great deal of variability among individuals.

Referred Pain

It is the nature of this makeup of dermatomes, myotomes, and sclerotomes that can lead to "referred" pain, which is felt in a part of the body that is usually a considerable distance from the tissues that have caused the pain and is explained as an error in perception on the part of the brain. Many theories of the mechanism of referred pain have been developed, but none has been proved conclusively. Generally, referred pain may involve one or more of the following mechanisms:

1. Misinterpretation by the brain as to the source of the painful impulses.

2. Inability of the brain to interpret a summation of noxious stimuli from various sources.

3. Disturbance of the internuncial pool by afferent nerve impulses.

Referral of pain is a common occurrence in problems associated with the musculoskeletal system. Pain is often felt at points remote from the site of the lesion. The reference of pain is an indicator of the segment that is at fault. For

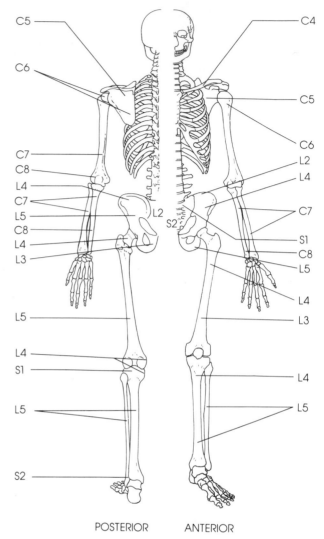

Figure 1–3. Sclerotomes of the body. Lines from nerve roots show area supplied by sclerotomes.

example, pain in the L5 dermatome could arise from irritation around the L5 nerve root, from an L5 disc, from facet involvement of L4-5, from any muscle supplied by the L5 nerve root, or from any visceral structures having L5 innervation.

MOVEMENTS

Because the assessment is an examination of the moving parts of the body, testing of the active, passive, and resisted isometric movements can yield information concerning the tissues that could be at fault.

Active Movements

Active movements can be "actively" performed by voluntary muscles and have their own special value; i.e., they combine tests of a patient's willingness to perform the movement, joint range, and muscle power. Both contractile and inert tissues are involved or moved during active movements. When active movements occur, one or more rigid structures (bones) move and such movement results in all structures attaching to that bone to move as well. The examiner should note which movements, if any, cause pain and the amount and quality of pain that results. For example, small, unguarded movements causing intense pain indicate an irritable joint.

Contractile tissues may have tension placed on them by stretching or contracting.[1] These structures include the muscles, their tendons, and their attachments into the bone. *Inert tissues* have tension put on them by stretching or by pinching.[1] They include all those structures that would not be considered contractile, such as joint capsules, ligaments, bursae, blood vessels, nerves and their sheaths, cartilage, dura mater, and so on.

If there is an organic lesion, some movements will be found to be abnormal or painful and others will not. Negative findings must balance positive ones, and the examination must be extensive enough to allow characteristic patterns to emerge. Determination of the problem is not made on the strength of the first positive finding; it is made only when it is clear that there are no other contradictory signs. Movements should be repeated several times quickly to rule out any problem such as vascular insufficiency. The active component is a functional test of the anatomic and dynamic aspects of the body and joints. When testing active movements, the examiner should note:

1. When and where in the movement the onset of pain occurs.

2. Whether the movement increases the intensity and quality of the pain.

3. The reaction of the patient to pain.

4. The amount of observable restriction.

5. The pattern of movement.

6. The movement of associated joints.

7. The willingness of the patient to move the part.

8. The quality of the movement.

9. Any limitation and its nature.

Passive Movements

In passive movement, the joint is put through a range of motion by the examiner while the patient is relaxed. The movement must proceed through as full a range of movement as possible. Although the movement must be gentle, the examiner must find out whether there is any limitation of range (hypomobility) or excess of range (hypermobility) and, if so, whether it is painful. The examiner should also attempt to determine the cause of the limitation (e.g., pain, spasm, adhesions, or compression) and the quality of the movement (e.g., lead pipe, cogwheel).

End Feel[1]

The examiner should determine the quality of end feel (the sensation the examiner "feels" in the joint as it reaches the end of the range of motion) of each passive movement. A proper evaluation of end feel can help the examiner to assess the type of pathology present to determine a prognosis for the condition, and to learn the severity or stage of the problem.

There are three classical *normal* end feels:

1. *Bone to bone*. This is a "hard," unyielding sensation that is also painless. An example of normal bone-to-bone end feel would be elbow extension.

2. *Soft-tissue approximation*. With this type of end feel, there is a yielding compression that stops further movement. Examples are elbow and knee flexion in which movement is stopped by the muscles. In a particularly slim individual with little muscle bulk, the end feel of the elbow flexion might be a bone-to-bone type.

3. *Tissue stretch*. There is a hard (springy) type of movement with a slight give. Toward the end of range of motion, there is a feeling of "springy" resistance. Tissue stretch is the most common type of normal end feel. Examples are lateral rotation of the shoulder and knee and metacarpophalangeal joint extension.

There are five classic *abnormal* end feels:[1]

1. *Muscle spasm*. Invoked by movement, with a sudden dramatic arrest of movement often accompanied by pain, the end feel is sudden and hard. Cyriax calls this a "vibrant twang."[1]

2. *Capsular*. Although this end feel is very similar to tissue stretch, it does not occur where one would expect. The range of movement is obviously reduced, and the capsule can be postulated to be at fault. Muscle spasm usually does not occur in conjunction with the capsular type of end feel.

3. *Bone to bone*. This abnormal end feel is similar to the normal bone-to-bone type, but the restriction or sensation of restriction occurs before the normal end of range of movement would normally occur or where one would not suspect to have a bone-to-bone end feel.

4. *Empty*. The empty end feel is detected when considerable pain is produced by movement. The movement is obviously impossible because of the pain, although no real mechanical resistance is being detected. Examples might be an acute bursitis (subacromial) or a neoplasm. Patients often have difficulty describing the empty end feel, and there is no muscle spasm involved.

5. *Springy block.* Similar to a tissue stretch, it occurs where one would not expect it to occur; it tends to be found in joints with menisci. There is a rebound effect, and it usually indicates an internal derangement within the joint. One might find a springy block end feel with a torn meniscus of a knee when it is locked or unable to go into full extension.

Capsular Pattern[1]

With passive movement, it must be remembered that a full range of motion must be carried out. A short, too-soft movement in the midrange does not achieve the proper results. In addition to looking at the end-feel, the examiner must look at the *pattern of limitation.* If the capsule of the joint is affected, it will be found that a pattern of proportional limitation is the feature that indicates the presence of a capsular pattern in the joint. It is the result of a total joint reaction with muscle spasm, capsular contraction, and generalized osteophyte formation being possible mechanisms at fault. Each joint has a characteristic pattern of proportional limitation. The presence of this capsular pattern does not indicate the type of joint involvement present; only an analysis of the end feel can do this. Only joints that are controlled by muscles have a capsular pattern. Thus, joints such as the sacroiliac and distal tibiofibular joints do not exhibit a capsular pattern. Table 1–2 illustrates some of the common capsular patterns seen in joints.

Noncapsular Patterns[1]

The examiner must also be aware of *noncapsular patterns,*which suggest a limitation of movement that does exist but does not correspond to the classic capsular pattern for that joint. In the shoulder, abduction might be restricted but there might be very little rotational restriction. Thus, a total capsular reaction is absent, but there are other possibilities, such as ligamentous adhesions, in which only part of a capsule or the accessory ligaments are involved. Thus, a local restriction in one direction, often accompanied by pain, is produced, and full pain-free range of movement in all other directions is obvious. A second possibility is *internal derangement of a joint.* Only certain joints, such as the knee and elbow, are commonly affected in this case. Intercapsular fragments may interfere with the normal sequence of motion. Movements causing impingement with the fragments will be limited, whereas other motions will be free. In the knee, for example, a torn meniscus may cause a blocking of

Table 1–2. Common Capsular Patterns of Joints

Joint(s)	Restriction*
Temporomandibular	Limitation of mouth opening
Occipitoatlanto	Extension, side flexion equally limited
Cervical spine	Side flexion and rotation equally limited, extension
Glenohumeral	Lateral rotation, abduction, medial rotation
Sternoclavicular	Pain at extreme of range of movement
Acromioclavicular	Pain at extreme of range of movement
Humeroulnar	Flexion, extension
Radiohumeral	Flexion, extension supination, pronation
Proximal radioulnar	Supination, pronation
Distal radioulnar	Full range of movement, pain at extremes of rotation
Wrist	Flexion and extension equally limited
Trapeziometacarpal	Abduction, extension
Metacarpophalangeal and interphalangeal	Flexion, extension
Thoracic spine	Side flexion and rotation equally limited, extension
Lumbar spine	Side flexion and rotation equally limited, extension
Sacroiliac, symphysis pubis, and sacro-coccygeal	Pain when joints are stressed
Hip†	Flexion, abduction, medial rotation (but is some cases medial rotation is most limited)
Knee	Flexion, extension
Tibiofibular	Pain when joint stressed
Talocrural	Plantar flexion, dorsiflexion
Talocalcaneal (subtalar)	Limitation of varus range of movement
Midtarsal	Dorsiflexion, plantar flexion, adduction and medial rotation
First metatarsophalangeal	Extension, flexion
Second to fifth metatarsophalangeal	Variable
Interphalangeal	Flexion, extension

*Movements are listed in order of restriction.
†For the hip, flexion, abduction, and medial rotation will always be the movements most limited in a capsular pattern. However, the order of restriction may vary.

extension, but flexion is usually free. Loose bodies cause limitation when they are caught between articular surfaces. A third possibility is *extra-articular lesions.* These lesions are revealed by disproportionate limitation, extra-articular adhesions, or an acutely inflamed structure limiting movement in a particular direction. For example, limited straight leg raising in the lumbar disc syndrome is referred to as a *constant length phenomenon*. This phenomenon results when the limitation of movement in one joint is dependent upon the position in which another joint is held. Thus, the restricted tissue (in this case, the sciatic nerve) must lie outside the joint or joints (in this case, hip and knee) being tested. Muscle adhesion causing restriction of motion is a further example of this phenomenon.

Inert Tissue[1]

Once the active and passive movements are completed, the examiner should be able to determine whether there are problems with any of the *inert tissues*. The examiner makes such a determination by judging the degree of pain and the limitation of movement within the joint. For lesions of inert tissue, the examiner may find that active and passive movements are painful in the same direction. Usually pain occurs as the limitation of motion approaches. Resisted isometric movements, which will be discussed shortly, are not usually painful unless there is some compression occurring.

Inert tissue refers to all tissue that is not considered contractile. Four classic patterns may be seen in lesions of inert tissue:

1. The first pattern is one of pain and limitation of movement in every direction. In this pattern, the entire joint is affected, indicating arthritis or capsulitis. As previously stated, each joint has its own capsular pattern and the amount of limitation is not usually the same in each direction. With capsular patterns, although there is a set "pattern" for each joint, other directions may also be affected. All movements of the joint may be affected, but it will be found that the motions described for capsular pattern are always in that particular order. In early capsular patterns, only one movement may be restricted; this movement is usually the one that has the potential for the greatest restriction. For example, in an early capsular pattern of the shoulder, only lateral rotation may be limited and the limitation may be slight.

2. A patient with a lesion of inert tissue may experience pain and limitation or excessive movement in some directions but not in others, such as in a ligament sprain or local capsular adhesion. Those movements that stretch or move the affected structure cause the pain. Internal derangement that results in a blocking of a joint may also be an example of a lesion of inert tissue where a variable pattern exists. Extra-articular limitation occurs when a lesion outside the joint affects the movement of that joint. Because these movements pinch or stretch the involved structure (e.g., bursitis in the buttock or acute subacromial bursitis), there will be pain and limitation of movement on stretch or compression of these structures. If a structure such as a ligament has been torn, the range of motion may increase if swelling is minimal, indicating instability of the joint. Swelling, because it stretches the tissues, often masks this instability.

3. There may be limited movement that is painless. The end feel for this type of condition is often the abnormal bone-to-bone type, and it usually indicates a symptomless osteoarthritis. If this situation is encountered, it should be left alone because it is not causing the patient any problem other than restricted range of motion and to deal with it could potentially lead to further problems.

4. If the range of movement is full and there is no pain, there is no lesion of the inert tissues being tested by that movement; however, there may be lesions of inert tissue in other directions or around the other joints.

Resisted Isometric Movements

Resisted isometric movements are tested last in examination of the joints. This type of movement consists of a strong, static (isometric) voluntary muscle contraction. If movement is allowed to occur at the joint, inert tissue around the joint will also move, and if pain is felt, it will not be clear whether it arises from contractile or inert tissues. The joint, therefore, is put in a neutral or resting position so that minimal tension is placed on the inert tissue. The patient is asked to contract the muscle strongly while the examiner resists to prevent any movement occurring and to ensure that the patient is using maximum effort. There is no question that movement cannot be completely eliminated, but by doing it in this fashion any movement will be minimized. Some compression of the inert tissues (cartilage and so on) will occur with the contraction; there may be some joint shear occurring as well, but it will be minimal if done as just described. To do the test properly, the examiner positions the joint in the resting position, asks the patient to hold the limb in that position, and applies resistance. In this way, the examiner can ensure the contraction is isometric.

If the contraction appears weak, the examiner must make sure that the weakness is not due to pain or the patient's fear or unwillingness. The examiner can often resolve such a finding by having the patient make a contraction on the good side first so that the movement normally will not cause pain. The movement must be as pure as sible. Although some inert tissue may be compressed during this action, compression will be minimal and a clear pattern of the problem will usually emerge.

Contractile Tissue[1]

With resisted isometric testing, the examiner checks for problems of *contractile tissue*, which consists of muscles, tendons, and their attachments. One would find that active movements, and resisted isometric testing would both be affected. Usually, passive movements are normal; in other words, passive movements are full and pain-free, although pain may be exhibited at the end of the range of motion when the muscle is stretched. If the muscles are tested as described, the examiner will find that not all movements are affected except in patients with psychogenic pain or sometimes with an acute joint lesion, when even a small amount of tension on the muscles about the joints provokes pain. However, if the joint lesion is severe, passive movements, when tested, will be markedly affected so that no confusion arises as to where the lesion lies. As with testing lesions of inert tissue, there are four classic patterns that may be seen with lesions of contractile tissue.[1] (In this case, however, we are dealing with pain and strength rather than pain and limited or excessive range of motion.)

1. If the movement is *strong and pain-free,* this indicates that there is no lesion of the muscles being tested, regardless of how tender the muscles may be when touched. The muscles function painlessly and are not the source of the patient's discomfort.

2. If the movement is *strong and painful,* this indicates a local lesion of the muscle or tendon. Such a lesion could be a first- or second-degree muscle strain. Typically, there is no primary limitation of passive movement, except, for example, in a gross muscle tear with hematoma and muscle spasm. In this case, the patient may develop secondary joint stiffness caused by disuse superimposed on the muscle lesion. This stiffness then takes precedence in the treatment.

3. If the movement is *weak and painful,* this indicates a severe lesion around that joint, such as a fracture. The weakness that results is usually due to reflex inhibition of the muscles around the joint.

4. If the movement is *weak and painless,* this indicates a rupture of a muscle (third-degree strain) or involvement of the nerve supplying that muscle.

If all movements appear painful, pain is often due to fatigue, emotional hypersensitivity, or emotional problems. It must be remembered that patients may equate effort with discomfort, and

Table 1–3. Muscle Test Grading

Grade	Value	Movement
5	Normal	Complete range of motion against gravity with maximal resistance
4	Good	Complete range of motion against gravity with some (moderate) resistance
3+	Fair +	Complete range of motion against gravity with minimal resistance
3	Fair	Complete range of motion against gravity
3−	Fair −	Some but no complete range of motion against gravity
2+	Poor +	Initiates motion against gravity
2	Poor	Complete range of motion with gravity eliminated
2−	Poor −	Initiates motion if gravity is eliminated
1	Trace	Evidence of slight contractility but there is no joint motion
0	Zero	No contraction palpated

they must be told that this is not necessarily the case.

Grading System

If the examiner desires, a grading system with a scale of 0 to 5 may be used (Table 1–3). However, because this grading system involves moving through a range of motion, it is more appropriate to observe the resisted isometric movements to determine which movements are painful and then observe the individual muscles using individual muscle tests[4] and the grading system to determine exactly which muscle is at fault.

Other Findings

When carrying out the examination of the joints, the examiner must be aware of other findings that may become evident that will help to determine the nature and location of the problem. For example, it should be noted whether there is excessive range of motion or *hypermobility* within the joints. When doing any examination, the examiner should compare both the normal and involved sides of the body. This comparison will give some idea as to whether the findings on the affected side would be considered normal. For example, the excessive range may just be a normal range of motion for that individual. It must also be remembered that joints on the non-dominant side tend to be more flexible than those on the dominant side.

It is also important to note whether there is a *painful arc* present; this indicates that an internal

Table 1–4. Laboratory Findings in Bone Disease*

Condition	Calcium	Inorganic Phosphorus	Alkaline Phosphatase	Calcium	Phosphorus
Hyperparathyroidism, primary	↑	↓	↑	↑	↑
Hyperparathyroidism, secondary	N-↓	↑	R ↑	↑	↑
Hyperthyroidism, marked	N	N	↑	↑	↑
Hypothyroidism	N	N	N	N	N
Senile osteoporosis	N	N-O ↓	N	N	N
Rickets (child)	↓	↓	↑	N	N
Osteomalacia (adult)	N-↓	↓	↑	N	N
Paget's disease	R ↑	R↓	↑	N	N
Multiple myeloma	↑	N-↑	R ↑	↑	↑

*Adapted from Quinn, J.: In Meschan, I.: Synopsis of Roentgen Signs. Philadelphia, W. B. Saunders Co., 1962.
Key: N = normal; O = occasionally; R = rarely; ↑ = increased; ↓ = decreased.

structure is being squeezed. *Sounds* such as crepitus, clicking, or snapping should be noted because they are often due to structures slipping over one another (e.g., tendons slipping over bone). *Pain at the extreme of range of motion* may be due to squeezing or stretching in which a particular joint may be affected.

Special Tests

Once the examiner has completed the history, observation, and examination, special tests may be performed for the involved joint. Many special tests can be used for each joint to determine whether a particular type of disease, condition, or injury is present. These tests are strongly suggestive of a particular problem and must be viewed as such. In addition, these tests, strongly suggestive of disease when they yield positive results, do not necessarily rule out the disease when they yield negative results. For each joint examination described herein, specific tests are mentioned for specific conditions. Whether to do these special tests is up to the individual examiner. Often, many tests will show the same results. These different methods will be shown, and the examiner should pick the ones that give the best results.

For example, for years, the *anterior drawer sign* had been the test to determine whether there was a problem with the anterior cruciate ligament of the knee. Literature in the last few years has indicated that the *Lachman test* is much more effective.

In addition to physical tests, the examiner may also make use of *laboratory tests* for specific conditions. With osteomyelitis, for example, a

positive blood culture is likely to be obtained and the white blood cell (WBC) count will be elevated, along with an increased erythrocyte sedimentation rate (ESR). The examiner, if a physician, may decide to draw fluid out of a joint with a hypodermic needle to view the synovial fluid. Tables 1–4 and 1–5 present a classification of synovial fluid and laboratory findings in bone disease as examples of laboratory tests.

Reflexes and Cutaneous Distribution

Following the special tests, the examiner can test the reflexes to obtain an indication of the state of the nerve or nerve roots supplying that reflex. With a loss or abnormality of conduction, there will be a diminution (hyporeflexia) or loss (aflexia) of the stretch reflex. With upper motor

Table 1–5. Classification of Synovial Fluid*

Type	Appearance	Significance
Group 1	Clear yellow	Noninflammatory states, trauma
Group 2†	Cloudy	Inflammatory arthritis; excludes most patients with osteoarthritis
Group 3	Thick exudate, brownish	Septic arthritis; occasionally seen in gout
Group 4	Hemorrhagic	Trauma, bleeding disorders, tumors, fractures

*From Curran, J. F., et al.: Clin. Orthop. Relat. Res. *173*:28, 1983.
†Inflammatory fluids will clot and should be collected in heparin-containing tubes. All group 2 or 3 fluids should be cultured when the diagnosis is uncertain.

neuron lesions, there may be hyperreflexia or excessive reflex action. To test a reflex properly, the examiner should tap the tendon five or six times to uncover any fading reflex response indicative of developing root signs. To be of clinical significance, findings must show asymmetry between bilateral reflexes unless it is a central lesion. The examiner should not be overly concerned if the reflexes are absent, diminished, or excessive on both sides when tested unless there is a suspected central lesion. This difference is especially true in young people.

At the same time, the examiner should check the cutaneous distribution of the various peripheral nerves and the dermatomes around the joint being examined. One must remember that the dermatomes will vary from person to person, and there is considerable overlap.[3, 5] Although the sensory distribution of peripheral nerves may vary from person to person, they tend to be much more consistent than dermatomes.

The examiner should test for altered sensation by running his or her relaxed hands and fingers over the area to be tested. Following this quick sensory ''scanning'' examination, if the patient feels a difference in sensation between the two sides of the body, the examiner should note where the difference is so that the area can be ''mapped out'' in greater detail. A pinwheel, pin, cotton batting, and/or brush can be used for this purpose.

The examiner should also look for possibilities of referred pain and try to remember which structure could refer pain to the joint being assessed and ensure that these structures are normal and are not, in fact, referring pain to the joint. If a patient complains of low back pain but the lumbar spine is found to be normal, the examiner may want to look at the hip or sacroiliac joints because they may refer pain to the lumbar spine.

Joint Play Movements

All synovial and secondary cartilaginous joints, to some extent, are capable of an active range of motion, termed *voluntary movement*. In addition, there is a small range of movement that can be obtained only passively by the examiner; this movement is called *joint play*, or *accessory movement*. These accessory movements are not under voluntary control; they are necessary, however, for full painless function of the joint and full range of motion of the joint. Joint dysfunction signifies a loss of joint play movement.

The existence of joint play movement is necessary for full pain-free voluntary movement to occur. An essential part of the detailed assessment of any joint includes an examination of its joint play movements. If any joint play movement is found to be absent, this movement must be freed before functional voluntary movement can be fully restored. In most joints, this movement is less than 4 mm in any one direction.

LOOSE PACKED (RESTING) POSITION

To test joint play movement, the examiner places the joint in a resting position, which is the position of a joint in its range of motion where the joint is under the least amount of stress; it is also the position in which the joint capsule has its greatest capacity.[6] The resting position (sometimes called the loose pack position) is one of minimal congruency between the articular surfaces and the joint capsule, with the ligaments being in the position of greatest laxity and passive separation of the joint surfaces being greatest.

Table 1–6. Resting (Loose Packed) Positions of Joints

Joint(s)	Position
Facet (spine)	Midway between flexion and extension
Temporomandibular	Mouth slightly open (freeway space)
Glenohumeral	55° Abduction, 30° horizontal adduction
Acromioclavicular	Arm resting by side in normal physiologic position
Sternoclavicular	Arm resting by side in normal physiologic position
Ulnohumeral (elbow)	70° Flexion, 10° supination
Radiohumeral	Full extension and full supination
Proximal radioulnar	70° Flexion, 35° supination
Distal radioulnar	10° Supination
Radiocarpal (wrist)	Neutral with slight ulnar deviation
Carpometacarpal	Midway between abduction-adduction and flexion-extension
Metacarpophalangeal	Slight flexion
Interphalangeal	Slight flexion
Hip	30° Flexion, 30° abduction and slight lateral rotation
Knee	25° Flexion
Talocrural (ankle)	10° Plantar flexion, midway between maximum inversion and eversion
Subtalar	Midway between extremes of range of movement
Midtarsal	Midway between extremes of range of movement
Tarsometatarsal	Midway between extremes of range of movement
Metatarsophalangeal	Neutral
Interphalangeal	Slight flexion

This position may be the anatomic resting position that is usually considered in the midrange, or it may be just outside the range of pain and spasm. The advantage of the loose packed position is that the joint surface contact areas are reduced and are always changing to decrease friction and erosion in the joints. The position also provides proper joint lubrication and allows the movements of spin, slide, and roll in a joint; thus, this is the ideal position for joint play mobilizations. Examples of resting positions are shown in Table 1–6.

CLOSE PACKED (SYNARTHRODIAL) POSITION

The close packed position should be avoided as much as possible during an assessment. In this position, the two joint surfaces fit together precisely; that is, they are fully congruent. The joint surfaces are tightly compressed; the ligaments and capsule of the joint are maximally tight; and the joint surfaces cannot be separated by distractive forces. Examples of the close packed position of most joints are shown in Table 1–7.

Table 1–7. Close Packed Positions of Joints

Joint(s)	Position
Facet (spine)	Extension
Temporomandibular	Clenched teeth
Glenohumeral	Abduction and lateral rotation
Acromioclavicular	Arm abducted to 30°
Sternoclavicular	Maximum shoulder elevation
Ulnohumeral (elbow)	Extension
Radiohumeral	Elbow flexed 90°, forearm supinated 5°
Proximal radioulnar	5° Supination
Distal radioulnar	5° Supination
Radiocarpal (wrist)	Extension with ulnar deviation
Metacarpophalangeal (fingers)	Full flexion
Metacarpophalangeal (thumb)	Full opposition
Interphalangeal	Full extension
Hip	Full extension and medial rotation*
Knee	Full extension and lateral rotation of tibia
Talocrural (ankle)	Maximum dorsiflexion
Subtalar	Supination
Midtarsal	Supination
Tarsometatarsal	Supination
Metatarsophalangeal	Full extension
Interphalangeal	Full extension

*Some authors include abduction, e.g., Kaltenborn.[6]

Palpation

Initially, palpation for tenderness plays no part in the assessment, since "referred" tenderness is very real and can be misleading. Only when the tissue at fault has been identified is palpation for tenderness used to determine the exact extent of the lesion within that tissue, and only then is palpation done if the tissue lies superficially and within easy reach of the fingers. Tenderness often does enable the examiner to name the affected ligament or the specific section or exact point of the tearing or bruising.

To palpate properly, the examiner must ensure that the area to be palpated is as relaxed as possible. For this to be done, the body part must be supported as much as possible. As the ability to develop palpation develops, the examiner should be able to:

1. Discriminate differences in tissue tension (e.g., effusion, spasm).

2. Distinguish differences in tissue texture.

3. Identify shapes, structures, and tissue type and thus detect abnormalities.

4. Determine tissue thickness and texture and thus determine whether it is pliable, soft, and resilient.

5. Feel variations in temperature.

6. Feel pulses, tremors, and fasciculations.

7. Determine the state of the periarticular tissues.

8. Feel dryness or excessive moisture of the skin.

9. Note any abnormal sensation, e.g., dysesthesia, diminished sensation; hyperesthesia, increased sensation; and anesthesia, absence of sensation.

Palpation of a joint and surrounding area must be carried out in a systematic fashion to ensure that all structures are examined. This procedure involves having a starting point and working from that point to surrounding tissues to ensure their normality or the possibility of pathologic involvement. The examiner must work slowly and carefully, applying light pressure initially and working into a deeper pressure of palpation, "feeling" for pathologic conditions. The uninvolved side should be palpated first so that the patient has some idea of what to expect. Any differences or abnormalities should be noted.

Roentgenograms

The examiner may view the x-ray films.[7, 8] X-rays are part of the electromagnetic spectrum and have the ability to penetrate tissue to varying degrees. The x-ray plates that are developed following exposure to the roentgen rays enable the examiner to see any fractures, dislocations, foreign bodies, or radiopaque substances that may be present. The main function of x-ray examination is to rule out or exclude serious disease, such as infection (osteomyelitis), ankylosing spondylitis, or neoplasm. In soft-tissue injuries, clinical findings should take precedence over x-ray findings. It is desirable to know whether an x-ray has been taken so that, if necessary, the examiner can obtain this information. The examiner should be aware of obvious unusual x-ray findings that distract attention from other tissue that is actually the cause of the pain. Such x-ray abnormalities are significant only if clinical examination bears out their relevance. With experience, the examiner becomes able to detect on x-ray examination many important soft-tissue changes, such as effusion in joints, tendinous calcifications, ectopic bone in muscle, tissue displaced by tumor, and the presence of air or foreign body material in the tissues. Roentgenograms may also be used to give an indication of bone loss. For osteoporosis to be evident on film, approximately 30 to 35 per cent of the bone must be lost.

When viewing bone films, the examiner should note whether the following features vary from normal:

1. Overall size and shape of bone.
2. Local size and shape of bone.
3. Thickness of the cortex.
4. Trabecular pattern of the bone.
5. General density of the whole bone.
6. Local density change.
7. Margins of local lesions.
8. Any break in continuity of the bone.
9. Any periosteal change.
10. Any soft-tissue change.
11. Relationship between bones.
12. Thickness of the cartilage (cartilage space within joints).

The examiner should keep in mind the maturity of the individual when viewing films. Skeletal changes occur with age, and the appearance and fusion of epiphysis, as an example, may be important in interpreting the pathology of the condition seen. Soft-tissue structures can be seen as well as bone, providing there is something to outline them; i.e., the joint capsule may be silhouetted by the pericapsular fat, or a cardiac shadow may be silhouetted by air in the lungs. Anatomic variations and anomalies must all be ruled out before pathology can be ruled in; i.e., accessory navicular, bipartate patella, or os trigonum may all be confused with fractures by the unsuspecting examiner. The fabella is often confused with a loose body in the knee in the anteroposterior projection x-ray film.

The basic principle of roentgen ray use is as

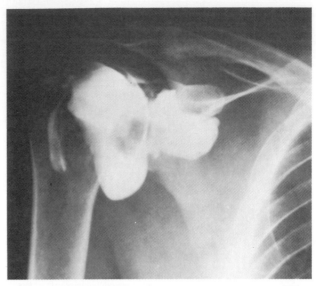

Figure 1–4. Normal arthrogram, shoulder in external rotation. Note the good dependent fold and the outline of the bicipital tendon. (From Neviaser, T. J.: Orthop. Clin. North Am. *11*:209, 1980.)

follows: The greater the density of the tissue, the less penetration by x-rays; thus, the greater the density of the tissue, the whiter it will appear on the film. This fact is illustrated by varying degrees of white, gray, and black on the film. In order of descending degree of density are the following structures: metal, bone, soft tissue, water, fat, and air. This difference gives the six basic densities on the x-ray plate. When viewing the x-rays, the examiner must identify the film, noting the name, age, date, and sex of the individual and must identify the type of projection taken. For example, it should be noted if the view is an anteroposterior, lateral, tunnel, skyline, weight-bearing, or stress type.

In addition to basic x-ray films, there are special

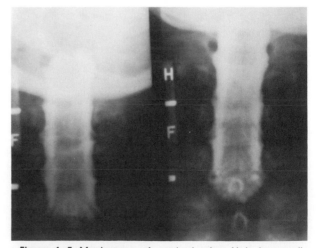

Figure 1–5. Myelogram of cervical spine. Note how radiopaque dye fills root sheaths.

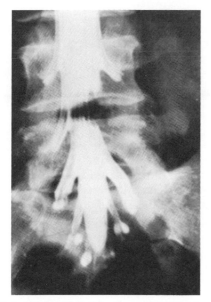

Figure 1–6. Myelogram of lumbar spine showing extrusion of nucleus pulposus of L4-L5. Note how radiopaque dye fills dural recesses. (From Selby, D. K., et al.: Orthop. Clin. North Am. *8*:82, 1977.)

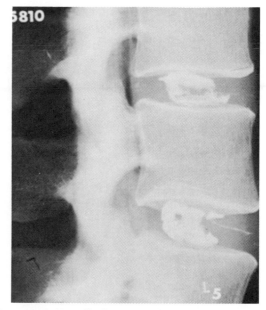

Figure 1–7. Normal discogram shown with barium paste. (From Farfan HF: Mechanical Disorders of the Low Back. Philadelphia, Lea & Febiger, 1973, p. 96.)

techniques which may often be used in orthopedics. For example, *arthrograms* are used to outline structures within a joint (Fig. 1–4), most commonly the knee. There are three types of arthrograms:

1. *Air.* Air is used to outline the joint structures.

2. *Dye or contrast.* A radiopaque dye is used to outline the joint structures.

3. *Double-contrast.* Air and radiopaque dye are used to outline the joint structures.

Another specialized technique is a *myelogram* (Figs. 1–5 and 1–6). A radiopaque dye is placed within the epidural space and is allowed to flow

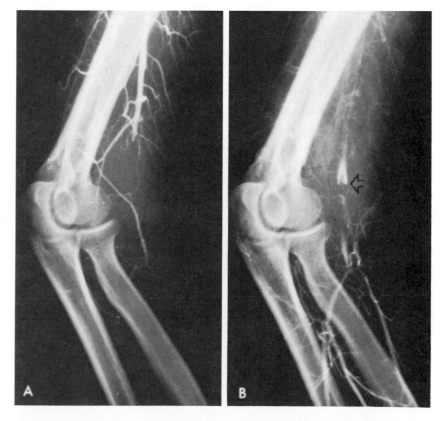

Figure 1–8. Occlusion of brachial artery. (*A*) Arteriogram of a young man with a previously reduced elbow dislocation and an ischemic hand shows an occluded brachial artery. (*B*) A later film shows fresh clot (arrow) in the brachial artery and reconstituted radial and ulnar arteries. Primary repair and thrombectomy treated the ischemic symptoms. (From McLean, G., and D. B. Frieman: Orthop. Clin North Am. *14*:267, 1983.)

to different levels of the spinal cord. This technique is used to detect disc disease, nerve root entrapment, spinal stenosis, and tumors of the spinal cord. Extradural techniques can be used as well. In epidural venography, radiopaque dye is allowed to flow through the epidural veins. This technique can yield supplementary information as to the state of the disc.

Discography involves injecting a radiopaque dye into the disc in order to reproduce signs of disc disease and localize the level of impingement (Fig. 1–7).

With a *venogram* and *arteriogram*, radiopaque dye is injected into specific vessels to outline abnormal conditions (Fig. 1–8). This technique may be used to diagnose arteriosclerosis, to investigate tumors, or to demonstrate blockage after trauma.

Increasing use is being made of *bone scans* (Fig. 1–9). With this technique, chemicals labeled with isotopes, such as technetium pyrophosphate, may be used to localize specific organs that concentrate the particular chemical. The isotope may be localized where there is a high level of activity relative to the rest of a bone. Thus, the bone scan can be used to detect stress fractures and tumors.

Tomograms have also become a common technique. Cuts of film are taken at specific levels of

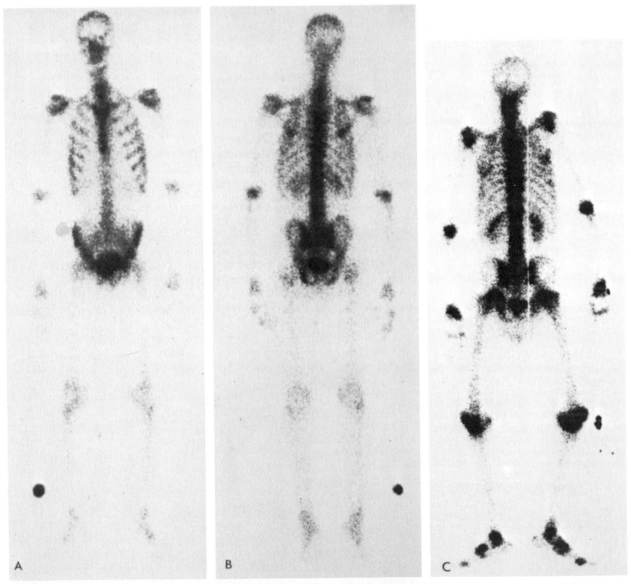

Figure 1–9. Whole body bone scans. (*A*) Normal adult anterior scan. (*B*) Normal adult posterior scan. (*C*) Posterior scan showing joint involvement of rheumatoid arthritis. (From Goldstein, H. A.: Orthop. Clin. North. Am. *14*:244, 250, 1983.)

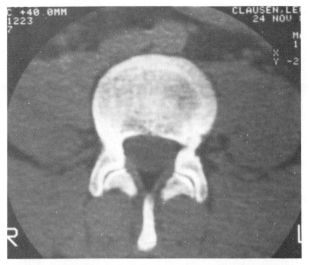

Figure 1–10. Computed tomographic (CT) scan demonstrates the junction of the superior aspect of the left pedicle with the vertebral body. The superior and inferior articular facets, the ligamentum flavum, and the spinous process are shown. (From Chafetz, N., and H. K. Genant: Orthop. Clin. North. Am. *14*:151, 1983.)

the body. This technique can be used to clearly define complicated fractures or to outline structures deep within the body. Plane tomograms or computer isotomograms (CT scans) can be used, particularly for soft tissues (Fig. 1–10).

Roentgenograms may also be used to determine the maturity index of an individual. A special film of the wrist is taken in order to assess skeletal maturity (Fig. 1–11). These films can be compared with established films in a bone atlas compiled by Greulich and Pyle.[9] This technique is often done prior to epiphysiodesis and leg-lengthening procedures.

Conclusion

Having completed all parts of the assessment, the examiner can look at the pertinent objective and subjective facts, note the significant signs and symptoms to determine what is causing the patient's problems, and design a proper treatment regimen based on the findings. If the assessment is not followed through completely, the treatment regime may not be implemented properly and this may lead to unwarranted extended care of the patient and increase health care costs.

Occasionally, patients present with a mixture of signs and symptoms that indicates two or more possible problem areas. Only by adding up the positive findings and subtracting the negative findings can the examiner determine the probable cause of the problem. In many cases, the decision may be an "educated guess," since very few problems are "textbook perfect." Only the examiner's knowledge, clinical experience, and diagnosis followed by trial treatment can conclusively delineate the problem.

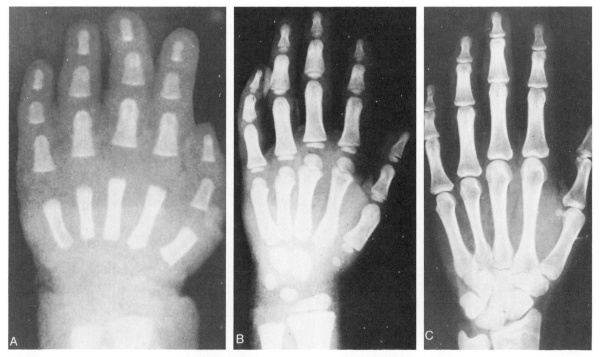

Figure 1–11. X-ray films showing skeletal maturity. (*A*) Male, newborn. (*B*) Male, 5 years old. (*C*) Female, 17 years old.

REFERENCES

CITED REFERENCES

1. Cyriax, J.: Textbook of Orthopedic Medicine, vol. 1: Diagnosis of Soft Tissue Lesions, 8th ed. London, Bailliere Tindall, 1982.
2. Williams, P., and R. Warwick (eds.): Gray's Anatomy, 36th British ed. Philadelphia, W. B. Saunders Co., 1980.
3. Keegan, J. J., and E. D. Garrett: The segmental distribution of the cutaneous nerves in the limbs of man. Anat. Rec. 101:409, 1948.
4. Daniels, L., and C. Worthingham: Muscle Testing: Techniques of Manual Examination. Philadelphia, W. B. Saunders Co., 1980.
5. Hockaday, J. M., and C. W. M. Whitty: Patterns of referred pain in the normal subject. Brain 90:481, 1967.
6. Kaltenborn, F. M.: Mobilization of the Extremity Joints: Examination and Basic Treatment Techniques. Oslo, Olaf Norlis Bokhandel, 1980.
7. Jones, M. D.: Basic Diagnostic Radiology. St. Louis, C. V. Mosby Co., 1969.
8. Miller, W. T.: Introduction to Clinical Radiology. New York, MacMillan, 1982.
9. Greulich, W. W., and S. U. Pyle: Radiographic Atlas of Skeletal Development of the Wrist and Hand. Stanford, Calif., Stanford University Press, 1959.

GENERAL REFERENCES

Bonica, J. J.: The Management of Pain. Philadelphia, Lea & Febiger, 1953.
Cervical Spine Research Society: The Cervical Spine. Philadelphia, J. B. Lippincott Co., 1983.
Chafetz, N., and H. K. Genant: Computed tomography of the lumbar spine. Orthop. Clin. North Am. 14:147, 1983.
Curran, J. F., M. H. Ellman, and N. L. Brown: Rheumatologic aspects of painful conditions affecting the shoulder. Clin. Orthop. Rel. Res. 173:27, 1983.
Farfan, H. F.: Mechanical Disorders of the Low Back. Philadelphia, Lea & Febiger, 1973.
Gartland, J. J.: Fundamentals of Orthopedics. Philadelphia, W. B. Saunders Co., 1979.
Goldstein, H. A.: Bone scintigraphy. Orthop. Clin. North Am. 14:243, 1983.
Grieves, G. P.: Common Vertebral Joint Problems. London, Churchill Livingstone, 1981.
Hammond, M. J.: Clinical examination and the physiotherapist. Aust. J. Physiother. 15:47, 1969.
Hoppenfeld, S.: Physical Examination of the Spine and Extremities. New York, Appleton-Century-Crofts, 1976.
Judge, R. D., G. D. Zuidema, and F. T. Fitzgerald: Clinical Diagnosis: A Physiologic Approach. Boston, Little, Brown & Co., 1982.
MacConnaill, M. A., and J. V. Basmajian: Muscles and Movements: A Basis for Human Kinesiology. Baltimore, Williams and Wilkins Co., 1977.
McLean, G., and D. B. Freiman: Angiography of skeletal disease. Orthop. Clin. North Am. 14:257, 1983.
Neviaser, T. J.: Arthrography of the shoulder. Orthopedic Clin. North Am. 11:205, 1980.
Saunders, H. D.: Evaluation and Treatment of Musculoskeletal Disorders. Minneapolis, H. D. Saunders, 1982.
Selby, D. K., A. J. Meril, K. J. Wagner, and R. R. G. Winans: Water-soluble myelography. Orthop. Clin. North Am. 8:79, 1977.
Squire, L. F., W. M. Colaiace, and N. Strutynsky: Exercises in Diagnostic Radiology, vol. III, Bone. Philadelphia, W. B. Saunders Co., 1972.

2

Cervical Spine

Examination of the cervical spine involves determining whether the injury or pathology occurs in the cervical spine or in a portion of the upper limb. Cyriax called this assessment the *scanning examination*.[1] In the initial assessment of a patient who complains of pain in the neck and/or upper limb, this procedure is always carried out unless the examiner is absolutely sure of where the lesion is localized. If the injury is in the neck, the scanning examination is definitely called for. Once the lesion site has been determined, a more detailed assessment of the affected area is performed if it is outside the cervical spine.

The cervical spine is a complicated area to assess properly, and adequate time must be allowed to ensure that as many causes or problems are examined as possible. Many conditions affecting the cervical spine can manifest in other parts of the body, and the examiner must be aware of this.

Applied Anatomy

The cervical spine consists of several joints. The *atlanto-occipital joints* (C0-C1) are the two uppermost joints. The principal motion at these two joints is flexion-extension (15–20°) or nodding of the head. In addition, side flexion is approximately 10° whereas rotation is negligible. The *atlas* (C1) has no vertebral body as such.

During development, the vertebral body of C1 has evolved into the *odontoid process*, which is part of C2. The *atlanto-occipital joints* are ellipsoid in type and act as a pair or in unison. Along with the atlantoaxial joints, these joints are the most complex articulation of the axial skeleton.

The *atlantoaxial joints* (C1-C2) constitute the most mobile articulation of the spine. Flexion-extension is approximately 10°, and side flexion is approximately 5°. Rotation, which is approximately 50°, is the primary movement of these joints. With rotation, there is a decrease in height of the cervical spine at this level as the vertebrae approximate because of the shape of the facet joints. The odontoid process of C2 acts as a pivot point for the rotation. This middle, or median, joint is classified as a *pivot* (*trochoidal*) type of joint. The lateral atlantoaxial, or facet, joints are classed as *plane* joints. Generally, if a person can talk and chew, there is probably some motion occurring at C1-C2.

It must be remembered that rotation past 50° in the cervical spine may lead to kinking of the contralateral vertebral artery; the ipsilateral vertebral artery may kink at 45° of rotation. This kinking may lead to vertigo, nausea, tinnitus, "drop attacks," and visual disturbances, stroke, or death.

There are 14 *facet*, or *apophyseal*, joints in the cervical spine. The upper four facet joints in the two upper thoracic vertebrae are often included in the examination of the cervical spine. The superior facets of the cervical spine face upward, backward, and medially; the anterior facets face downward, forward, and laterally. This plane facilitates flexion and extension, but it prevents rotation and/or side flexion without both occurring to some degree together. These joints move primarily by gliding and are classified as *synovial*, or *diarthrodial*, type of joints. The capsules are lax to allow for sufficient movement. At the same time, they provide support and a check-rein type of restriction. The greatest flexion-extension of the facet joints occurs between C5 and C6; however, there is almost as much movement between C4-C5 and C6-C7. The neutral or resting position of the cervical spine is slightly extended. The close packed position of the facet joints is complete extension. The facet joints are highly innervated by the recurrent *meningeal* or *sinuvertebral* nerve.

Some anatomists[2-5] refer to the *costal* or *uncovertebral processes* as *uncunate joints* or *joints of von Lushka*. These structures were described by von Lushka in 1858. The uncus gives a "saddle" form to the upper aspect of the cervical vertebra, which is more pronounced posterolaterally. It has the effect of limiting side flexion. Extending from the uncus is a "joint" that appears to form because of a weakness in the annulus fibrosus. The portion of the vertebra above, which "articulates" or conforms to the uncus, is called the *échancrure*, or notch. Notches are found from C3 to T1, but according to most of the authors,[2-5] they are not seen until the ages of 6 to 9 and are fully developed by the age of 18. There is some controversy as to whether they should be classified as real joints because some authors believe they are the result of degeneration of the disc. Degeneration does tend to occur faster in the cervical spine than in any other parts of the spine.

The *intervertebral disc* makes up approximately 25 per cent of the height of the cervical spine. No disc is found between the atlas and the occiput (C0-C1) or between the atlas and the axis (C1-C2). It is the disc rather than the vertebrae that gives the cervical spine its lordotic shape. The *nucleus pulposus* functions as a buffer to axial compression in distributing compressive forces, while the annulus fibrosus acts to withstand tension within the disc. Although it is generally believed that the intervertebral disc has no innervation, research indicates there may be some innervation on the periphery of the annulus fibrosus.[6]

There are seven vertebrae in the cervical spine, with the body of the vertebra supporting the weight of those above it. The facet joints may bear some of the weight of the vertebrae above, but this weight is minimal. However, this slight amount of weight bearing can lead to spondylitic changes in these joints. The outer ring of the vertebral body is made of cortical bone, and the inner part of cancellous bone covered with the cartilaginous end plate. The vertebral arch protects the spinal cord; the spinous processes, the majority of which are bifid in the cervical spine, provide for attachment of muscles. The transverse processes have basically the same function. In the cervical spine, the spinous processes are at the level of the facet joints of the same vertebra. Generally, the spinous process is considered to be absent or at least rudimentary on C1. This is why the first palpable vertebra descending from the external occipital protuberance is the spinous process of C2.

Patient History

In addition to the questions listed under patient history in Chapter 1, the examiner should ask the following:

1. What is the patient's usual activity or pasttime?

2. What are the sites and boundaries of the pain? Have the patient point to the location(s). Symptoms do not go down the arm for a C4 nerve root injury or for nerve roots above that level.

3. Is there any radiation of pain? It is helpful to remember this and correlate it with dermatome findings when doing palpation. Is the pain deep? Superficial? Shooting? Burning? Aching?

4. Is there paresthesia ("pins and needles")? This sensation is present if pressure is applied to the nerve root. It may become evident if pressure is relieved from a nerve trunk.

5. Which activities aggravate the problem? Which activities ease the problem?

6. Is the condition improving? Worsening? Staying the same?

7. What can be learned about the patient's sleeping position? Is there any problem sleeping? How many pillows does the patient use, and what type are they (feather, foam)? What type of mattress does the patient use (hard, soft)?

8. Does the patient have any headaches? If so, where? How frequently do they occur? How intense are they? How long do they last? Acute headaches may be the result of infection, poisoning, or impending cerebral vascular accident (CVA). Throbbing and pulsating headaches tend to be the migraine type. Any aching and pain in the forehead may indicate the possibility of a sinusitis or an occipital or suboccipital lesion. Pain in the temporal area is often due to migraine, temporal arteritis, eye or ear disturbances, temporomandibular joint problems, or tension. Occipital pain may be due to eyestrain, hyperextension injury, or a disc injury. Pain that is worse in the morning may be due to sinusitis, migraine, or

Table 2–1. Chief Functions and Distributions of the Cranial Nerves*

Nerve	Afferent	Efferent
I. Olfactory	Smell: nose	
II. Optic	Sight: eye	
III. Oculomotor		Vol. motor: levator of eyelid, sup., med., and inf. recti, inf. oblique of eyeball
		Autonomic: smooth muscle of eyeball
IV. Trochlear		Vol. motor: sup. oblique of eyeball
V. Trigeminal	Touch, pain: skin of face, mucous membranes of nose, sinuses, mouth, anterior tongue	Vol. motor: muscles of mastication
VI. Abducens		Vol. motor; lat. rectus of eyeball
VII. Facial	Taste: anterior tongue	Vol. motor; facial muscles Autonomic: lacrimal, submandibular and sublingual glands
VIII. Vestibulocochlear	Hearing: ear Balance: ear	
IX. Glossopharyngeal	Touch, pain: posterior tongue, pharynx	Vol. motor: unimportant muscle of pharynx
	Taste: posterior tongue	Autonomic: parotid gland
X. Vagus	Touch, pain: pharynx, larynx, bronchi	Vol. motor: muscles of palate, pharynx, and larynx
	Taste: tongue, epiglottis	Autonomic: thoracic and abdominal viscera
XI. Accessory		Vol. motor: sternocleidomastoid and trapezius
XII. Hypoglossal		Vol. motor: muscles of tongue

*From Hollinshead, W. H., and D. B. Jenkins: Functional Anatomy of the Limbs and Back. Philadelphia, W. B. Saunders Co., 1981, p. 358.

hypertension; pain that is worse in the afternoon is often due to tension or eyestrain. Pain at night may be due to an intracranial disease, whereas pain on bending is often due to sinusitis or migraine.

9. Does a position change alter the headache or pain? If so, which position(s)?

10. Does the patient experience dizziness or faintness? Complete passing out is sometimes called a *drop attack*.

11. Are there any lower limb symptoms? This finding may indicate a severe problem affecting the spinal cord.

12. Does the patient complain of any subjective restrictions when performing movements? If so, which movements are subjectively restricted?

13. Does the patient experience any tingling in the extremities?

14. Are symptoms improving or deteriorating?

15. Is there any difficulty in swallowing (dysphagia), or are there any voice changes? Such a change may be due to neurologic problems, mechanical pressure, or muscle incoordination. One must remember that swallowing becomes more difficult as the neck is extended and that the voice will become weaker as well.

16. What is the patient's age? Spondylosis is often seen in persons 25 years or older and is present in 60 per cent of those older than 45 years

of age and in 85 per cent of those older than 65 years of age. Symptoms of osteoarthritis do not tend to appear until a person is 60 years of age or older.

17. Is pain affected by coughing? Sneezing? Straining? If so, an increase in intrathoracic or intra-abdominal pressure may be causing the problem.

18. Does the patient exhibit or complain of any sympathetic symptoms? There may be injury to the cranial nerves or the sympathetic nervous system, which lies in the soft tissues of the neck anterior and lateral to the cervical vertebrae. The cranial nerves and their functions are shown in Table 2–1. Some of the sympathetic symptoms the examiner may see are "ringing" in the ears, dizziness, blurred vision, photophobia, rhinorrhea, sweating, lacrimation, and hypothemia (loss of strength).

Observation

For a proper observation, the patient must be suitably undressed. A male should wear only shorts, and a female should wear a bra and shorts. In some cases, the bra may have to be removed to determine whether there are any problems such as thoracic outlet syndrome, thoracic symptoms being referred to the cervical spine, or functional restriction of movement of the ribs. The examiner should note the willingness of the patient to move and the pattern of movement demonstrated.

The patient may be seated or standing. The examiner should note the following:

1. Head and neck posture (Fig. 2–1). Is the head in the midline, or is there evidence of torticollis (Fig. 2–2), Klippel-Feil syndrome, or other neck deformity?

2. Shoulder levels. Usually the dominant side will be slightly lower than the nondominant side.

3. Muscle spasm or any asymmetry. Is there any atrophy of the deltoid muscle (circumflex or axillary nerve palsy) or torticollis (spasm, prominence or tightness of the sternocleidomastoid muscle [Fig. 2–2])?

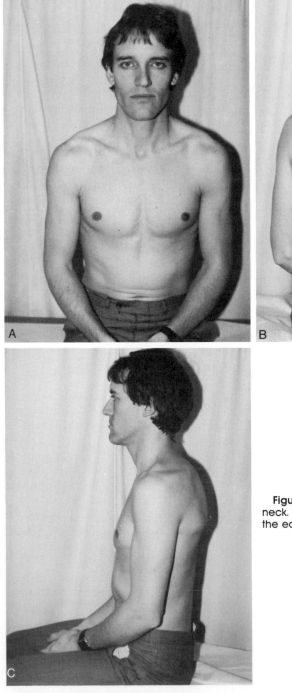
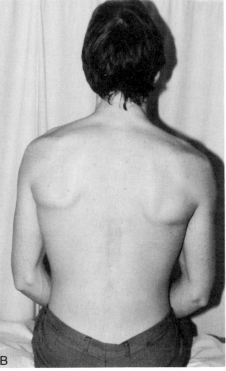

Figure 2–1. Observation views of head and neck. Note lower right shoulder and scapula; the ear is anterior to the shoulder.

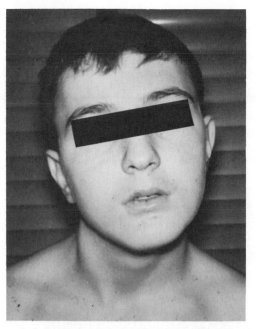

Figure 2–2. Example of torticollis showing prominent sternocleidomastoid muscle on the right. (From Gartland, J. J.: Fundamentals of Orthopaedics. Philadelphia, W. B. Saunders Co., 1979, p. 312.)

4. Facial expression. The examiner should observe the patient's facial expression as the patient moves from position to position, does different movements, and explains the problem. Such observation should give the examiner an idea of how much the patient is subjectively suffering.

5. Bony and soft-tissue contours. If the cervical spine is injured, the head tends to be tilted and rotated away from the pain and the face is tilted upward. If the patient is hysterical, the head tends to be tilted and rotated toward the pain and the head tilted down.

6. Evidence of ischemia in either upper limb.

7. Normal sitting posture. The nose should be in line with the manubrium and xiphoid process of the sternum. From the side, the ear lobe should be in line with the acromion process and the high point on the iliac crest for proper postural alignment. The examiner should remember as well that referred pain from conditions such as spondylosis tends to be in the shoulder and arm rather than the neck. It should also be remembered that the normal curve of the cervical spine is a lordotic type of curvature.

Examination

A complete examination of the cervical spine must be done, not only of the neck but also of the upper limb. Many of the symptoms that occur in the upper limb can be originating from the neck. Unless there is a history of definite trauma to a peripheral joint, a screening examination must be done to rule out problems within the neck.

ACTIVE MOVEMENTS

The first movements that are carried out are the active movements of the cervical spine, with the patient in the sitting position. The examiner is looking for differences in range of movement and the patient's willingness to do the movement. The range of motion taking place in this phase is the summation of all movements of the whole cervical spine, not just at one level. This combined movement allows for greater mobility in the cervical spine while still providing a firm support for the trunk and appendages. The range of motion available in the cervical spine is due to many factors, such as the flexibility of the intervertebral disc, the shape and inclination of the articular processes of the facet joints, and the slight laxity of the ligaments and joint capsules.

The movements should be done in a particular order so that the most painful movements are done last.[1] This is important so that there will be no residual pain carryover from the previous movement. When asking the individual to do the active movements, the examiner must remember to look for limitation of movement and possible reasons for pain, spasm, stiffness, or blocking. As the patient reaches the full range of active movement, passive overpressure may be applied very carefully—but only if the movement appears to be full and pain-free. The overpressure will help to test the end feel of the movement. The examiner must be careful when applying overpressure to rotation.[7] In this position, the vertebral artery is often compressed; this can lead to a decrease in blood supply to the brain. Should this occur, the patient will complain of dizziness or may feel faint. If the patient exhibits these symptoms, the examiner must use extreme care during these movements and during the following treatment.

The examiner can differentiate between movement in the upper and lower cervical spine. During flexion, "nodding" occurs in the upper cervical spine while "flexion" occurs in the lower cervical spine. If this nodding movement does not occur, it indicates restriction of movement in the upper cervical spine; if flexion does not occur, it indicates restriction of motion in the lower cervical spine.

It must be remembered that movement can occur between C1 and C2 alone but not between the other cervical vertebra. That is, if one vertebra moves, the ones adjacent to it are bound to move as well.

The active movements that should be carried out in the cervical spine are as shown in Figure 2–3:

1. Flexion.
2. Extension.
3. Side flexion (left and right).
4. Rotation (left and right).

Flexion. For flexion, or forward bending, the maximum range of motion is 80 to 90° and the extreme of range of motion is normally found when the chin is able to reach the chest with the mouth closed. Up to two finger widths between the chin and chest is considered normal, however. In flexion, the intervertebral disc widens posteriorly and narrows anteriorly. The intervertebral foramen is 20 to 30 per cent larger on flexion than on extension. The vertebra will shift forward in flexion and backward in extension. Also, the mastoid process will move away from the C1 transverse process on flexion and extension.

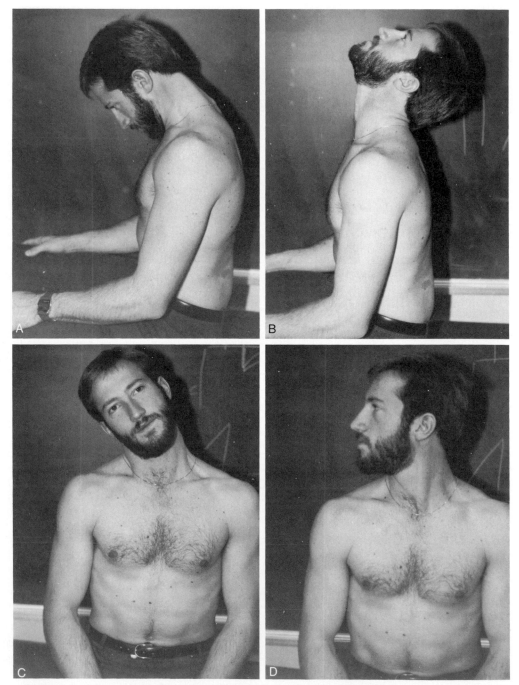

Figure 2–3. Active movements of the cervical spine. (*A*) Flexion. (*B*) Extension. (*C*) Side flexion. (*D*) Rotation.

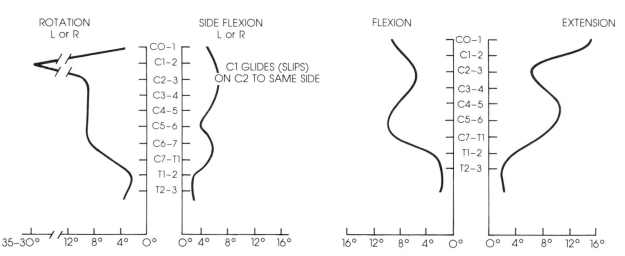

Figure 2–4. Average active range of motion in the cervical spine. Individuals will vary widely, depending on age, body type, and so on. (Adapted from Grieve, G. P.: Common Vertebral Joint Problems. New York, Churchill Livingstone, 1981, pp. 41, 42.)

Extension. Extension, or backward bending, is normally limited to 70°. Because there is no anatomic block to stop movement going past this position, the result may often lead to problems seen during whiplash or cervical strain. Normally, the plane of the nose and forehead should be nearly horizontal. When the head is held in extension, the atlas tilts upward, resulting in posterior compression between the atlas and occiput.

Side Flexion. Side, or lateral, flexion is approximately 20 to 45° to the right and left. Most of the side flexion occurs between the occiput and C1 and between C1 and C2. When the patient does the movement, the examiner should ensure that the ear is taken to the shoulder and not the shoulder to the ear.

Rotation. Normally, rotation is 70 to 90° right and left and the chin does not quite reach the plane of the shoulder. Remember that rotation and side flexion always occur together in the cervical spine. This combined movement may or may not be visible, depending on the movement involved. Rotation and side flexion occur together as a result of the shape of the articular surfaces of the facet joints; this shape is coronally oblique.

Figure 2–4 depicts active range of motion of the cervical spine.

PASSIVE MOVEMENTS

If the patient does not have full range of motion or the examiner has not applied overpressure to determine the end feel of the movement, the patient should be asked to lie down in a supine position. The examiner then passively tests flexion, extension, side flexion and rotation as in the active movements.

These movements are done to determine the end feel of each movement. This may give the examiner an idea of the pathology involved. The normal end feels of the cervical spine motions are tissue stretch for all four movements. As with active movements, the most painful movements are done last. The examiner should also note if a capsular pattern (side flexion and rotation equally limited, extension less limited) is present.

RESISTED ISOMETRIC MOVEMENTS

The same movements that were done actively are done (flexion, extension, side flexion, and rotation) and there should be no movement. It is better for the examiner to say: "Don't let me move you," rather than to tell the patient to "contract the muscle as hard as possible." In this way, the examiner can be sure that the movement is as isometric as possible and that a minimal amount of movement will occur (Fig. 2–5). The examiner should ensure that these movements are done with the cervical spine in the neutral position and that painful movements are done last. Using Table 2–2, the examiner should attempt to determine which muscles are at fault. By looking at the various combinations of muscles that cause the movement, the examiner may be able to decide which muscle is at fault (Fig. 2–6).

PERIPHERAL JOINTS

Once the resisted isometric movements to the cervical spine have been completed, the peripheral joints should be quickly scanned to rule out obvious pathology in the extremities.[1] The following joints are scanned bilaterally.

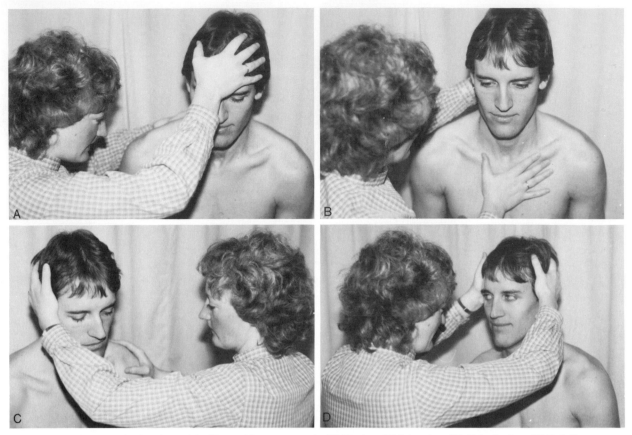

Figure 2–5. Positioning for resisted isometric movements. (*A*) Flexion. (*B*) Extension. (*C*) Side flexion. (*D*) Rotation.

Table 2–2. Muscles of the Cervical Spine: Their Actions and Nerve Supply

Action	Muscles Acting	Nerve Supply
Forward flexion of head	1. Rectus capitis anterior	C1, C2
	2. Rectus capitis lateralis	C1, C2
	3. Longus capitis	C1, C2, C3
	4. Hyoid muscles	Inferior alveolar nerve
		Facial nerve
		Hypoglossal nerve
		Ansa cervicalis
	5. Obliquus capitus superior	C1
	6. Sternocleidomastoid (if head in neutral or flexion)	Accessory
		C2
Extension of head	1. Splenius capitis	C4, C5, C6
	2. Semispinalis capitis	C1–C8
	3. Longissimus capitis	C6–C8
	4. Spinalis capitis	C6–C8
	5. Trapezius	Accessory
		C3, C4
	6. Rectus capitis posterior minor	C1
	7. Rectus capitis posterior major	C1
	8. Obliquus capitis superior	C1
	9. Obliquus capitis inferior	C1
	10. Sternocleidomastoid (if head in some extension)	Accessory
		C2

Table 2–2. Muscles of the Cervical Spine: Their Actions and Nerve Supply *(Continued)*

Action	Muscles Acting	Nerve Supply
Rotation of head (Muscles on one side contract)	1. Trapezius (face moves to opposite side)	Accessory C3, C4
	2. Splenius capitis (face moves to the same side)	C4–C6
	3. Longissimus capitis (face moves to same side)	C6–C8
	4. Semispinalis capitis (face moves to same side)	C1–C8
	5. Obliquus capitis inferior (face moves to same side)	C1
	6. Sternocleidomastoid (face moves to same side)	Accessory C2
Side flexion of head	1. Trapezius	Accessory C3, C4
	2. Splenius capitis	C4-C6
	3. Longissimus capitis	C6-C8
	4. Semispinalis capitis	C1-C8
	5. Obliquus capitis inferior	C1
	6. Rectus capitis lateralis	C1-C2
	7. Longus capitis	C1-C3
Flexion of neck	1. Longus coli	C2-C6
	2. Scalenus anterior	C4-C6
	3. Scalenus medius	C3-C8
	4. Scalenus posterior	C6-C8
Extension of neck	1. Splenius cervicis	C6, C7, C8
	2. Semispinalis cervicis	C1-C6, C7, C8
	3. Longissimus cervicis	C6-C8
	4. Levator scapulae	C3-C4 Dorsal scapular
	5. Iliocostalis cervicis	C6, C7, C8
	6. Spinalis cervicis	C6-C8
	7. Multifidus	C1-C6, C7, C8
	8. Interspinalis cervicis	C1-C8
	9. Trapezius	Accessory C3, C4
	10. Rectus capitus posterior major	C1
	11. Rotatores brevis	C1-C8
	12. Rotatores longi	C1-C8
Side flexion of neck	1. Levator scapulae	C3-C4 Dorsal scapular
	2. Splenius cervicis	C4-C6
	3. Iliocostalis cervicis	C6-C8
	4. Longissimus cervicis	C6-C8
	5. Semispinalis cervicis	C1-C8
	6. Multifidus	C1-C8
	7. Intertransversarii	C1-C8
	8. Scaleni	C3-C8
	9. Sternocleidomastoid	Accessory C2
	10. Obliquus capitis inferior	C1
	11. Rotatores brevi	C1-C8
	12. Rotatores longi	C1-C8
	13. Longus coli	C2-C6
Rotation* of neck (muscles on one side contracting)	1. Levator scapulae (face moves to same side)	C3-C4 Dorsal scapular
	2. Splenius cervicis (face moves to same side)	C4-C6
	3. Iliocostalis cervicis (face moves to same side)	C6-C8
	4. Longissimus cervicis (face moves to same side)	C6, C7, C8
	5. Semispinalis cervicis (face moves to same side)	C1-C8
	6. Multifidus (face moves to opposite side)	C1-C8
	7. Intertransversarii (face moves to same side)	C1-C8
	8. Scaleni (face moves to opposite side)	C3-C8
	9. Sternocleidomastoid (face moves to opposite side)	Accessory C2
	10. Obliquus capitis inferior (face moves to same side)	C1
	11. Rotatores brevis (face moves to same side)	C1-C8
	12. Rotatores longi (face moves to same side)	C1-C8

*Occurs in conjunction with side flexion due to direction of facet joints.

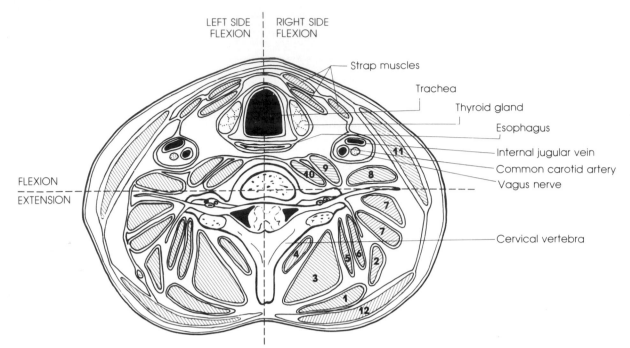

Figure 2–6. Anatomic relations of the lower cervical spine. (*1*) Splenius capitis. (*2*) Splenius cervicis. (*3*) Semispinalis cervicis and capitis. (*4*) Multifidus and rotatores. (*5*) Longissimus capitis. (*6*) Longissimus cervicis. (*7*) Levator scapulae. (*8*) Scalenus posterior. (*9*) Scalenus medius. (*10*) Scalenus anterior. (*11*) Sternocleidomastoid. (*12*) Trapezius.

Temporomandibular Joint. The examiner checks the movement of the joint by placing the index or little finger in the patient's ears (Fig. 2–7). The pulp aspect of the finger is placed forward

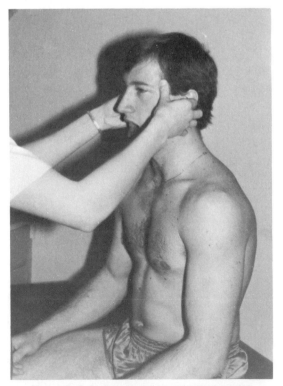

Figure 2–7. Testing temporomandibular joints.

to feel for equality of movement of the condyles of the temporomandibular joints and clicking or grinding and also to make sure that the ear is clear. As the patient opens his mouth, the condyle will move forward. At the same time, the examiner should observe the patient open and close the mouth and should watch for any lateral deviation during the movement.

Shoulder Girdle. The examiner quickly scans this complex of joints by asking the patient to actively elevate the arm through abduction, followed by active elevation through forward flexion. In addition, the examiner quickly tests medial and lateral rotation of each shoulder. Any pattern of restriction should be noted. If the patient is able to reach full abduction without difficulty or pain, the examiner may decide that there is no problem with the shoulder complex.

Elbow Joints. The elbow joints are moved through flexion, extension, supination, and pronation. Any restriction of movement or abnormal sign and symptom should be noted, as it may be indicative of pathology.

Wrist and Hand. The patient actively performs flexion, extension, and radial and ulnar deviation of the wrist. Active movement (flexion, extension, abduction, adduction, and opposition) are done for the fingers and thumb. These actions can be accomplished by having the patient make a fist and then spreading his fingers and thumb wide. Again, any alteration in sign and symptom or restriction of motion should be noted.

MYOTOMES

Having completed the scanning examination of the peripheral joints, the examiner should go on to determine muscle power and possible neurologic weakness by testing the myotomes (Fig. 2–8). Myotomes are tested by the following isometric movements (Table 2–3):

1. Neck flexion, C1–2.
2. Neck side flexion, C3.
3. Shoulder elevation, C4.
4. Shoulder abduction C5.
5. Elbow flexion and/or wrist extension, C6.
6. Elbow extension and/or wrist flexion, C7.
7. Thumb extension and/or ulnar deviation, C8.
8. Abduction and/or adduction of hand intrinsics, T1.

With the patient in a sitting position, the examiner puts the test joint(s) in a neutral position and applies resisted isometric pressure. The contraction should be held for at least 5 seconds so that weakness, if any, can be noted. Where applicable, both sides are tested at the same time to provide a comparison. The examiner must not apply pressure over the joints because this action may mask symptoms or the true problem.

To test neck flexion, the patient's head should be slightly flexed. The examiner applies pressure to the forehead while stabilizing the trunk hand between the scapulae (Fig. 2–8A). 1 neck side flexion, the examiner places one hand above the patient's ear and applies a side flexion force while stabilizing the trunk with the other hand on the opposite shoulder (Fig. 2–8B). Both right and left side flexion must be tested.

The examiner then asks the patient to elevate the shoulders to about one half of full elevation. The examiner applies a downward force on both of the patient's shoulders while the patient attempts to hold them in position.

For testing of shoulder abduction, the examiner asks the patient to abduct the arms to about 75° to 80° with the elbows flexed to 90° and the forearms pronated or in neutral. The examiner applies a downward force on the humerus while the patient attempts to hold the arms in position.

To test elbow flexion and extension, the examiner asks the patient to put his arms by his side, with the elbows flexed to 90° and forearms in neutral. The examiner applies a downward isometric force to the forearms to test the elbow flexors (C6 myotome) and an upward isometric force to test the elbow extensors (C7 myotome).

For testing of wrist movements (flexion, extension, ulnar deviation) the patient's arms are by the side, elbows at 90°, forearms pronated and

Table 2–3. Myotomes of the Upper Limb

Nerve Root	Test Action	Muscles
C1-2	Neck flexion	Rectus lateralis, rectus capitis anterior, longus capitis, longus coli, longus cervicis, sternocleidomastoid
C3	Neck side flexion	Longus capitis, longus cervicis, trapezius, scalenus medius
C4	Shoulder elevations	Diaphragm, trapezius, levator scapulae, scalenus anterior, scalenus medius
C5	Shoulder abduction	Rhomboid major and minor, deltoid, supraspinatus, infraspinatus, teres minor, biceps, scalenus anterior and medius
C6	Elbow flexion and wrist extension	Serratus anterior, latissimus dorsi, subscapularis, teres major, pectoralis major (clavicular head), biceps, coracobrachialis, brachialis, brachioradialis, supinator, extensor carpi radialis longus, scalenus anterior, medius and posterior
C7	Elbow extension and wrist flexion	Serratus anterior, latissimus dorsi, pectoralis major (sternal head), pectoralis minor, triceps, pronator teres, flexor carpi radialis, flexor digitorum superficialis, extensor carpi radialis longus, extensor carpi radialis brevis, extensor digitorum, extensor digiti minimi, scalenus medius and posterior
C8	Thumb extension and ulnar deviation	Pectoralis major (sternal head), pectoralis minor, triceps, flexor digitorum superficialis, flexor digitorum profundus, flexor pollicis longus, pronator quadratus, flexor carpi ulnaris, abductor pollicis longus, extensor pollicis longus, extensor pollicis brevis, extensor indicis, abductor pollicis brevis, flexor pollicis brevis, opponens pollicis, scalenus medius and posterior
T1	Hand intrinsics	Flexor digitorum profundus, intrinsic muscles of the hand (except extensor pollicis brevis), flexor pollicis brevis, opponens pollicis

Muscles listed may be supplied by additional nerve roots; only primary nerve root sources are listed.

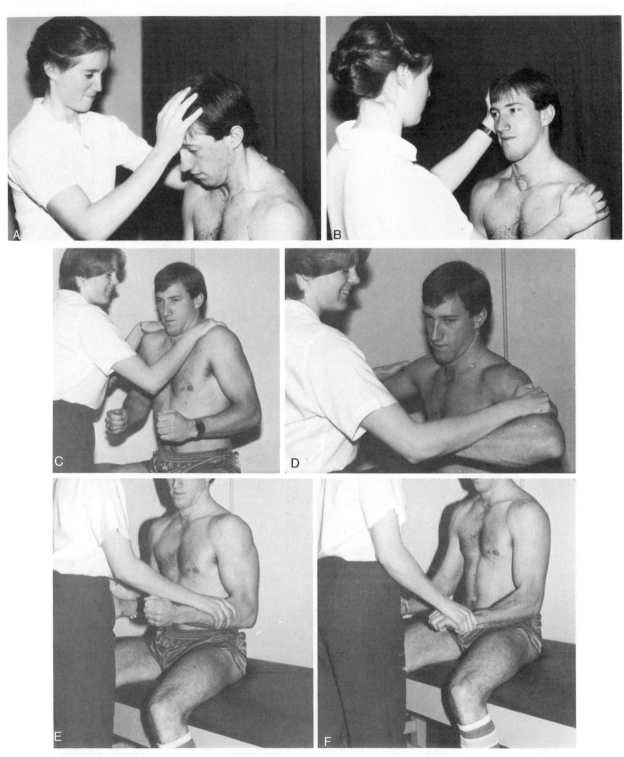

Figure 2–8. Positioning to test myotomes. (*A*) Neck flexion (C1, C2). (*B*) Neck side flexion (C3). (*C*) Shoulder evaluation (C4). (*D*) Shoulder abduction (C5). (*E*) Elbow flexion (C6). (*F*) Wrist extension (C6).

Illustration continued on opposite page

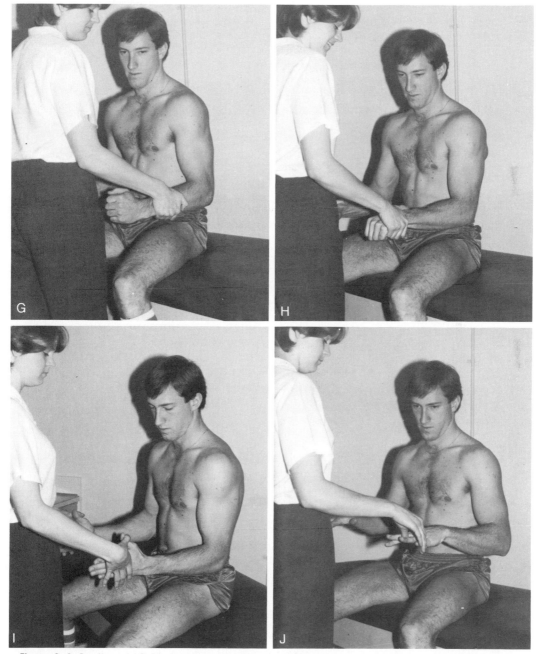

Figure 2–8 *Continued.* (*G*) Elbow extension (C7). (*H*) Wrist flexion (C7). (*I*) Thumb extension (C8). (*J*) Finger abduction (T1).

wrists, hands and fingers in neutral. The examiner applies a downward force to the hands to test wrist extension (C7 myotome), an upward force to test wrist flexion (C6 myotome) and a lateral force (radially deviated) to test ulnar deviation (C8 myotome) while the patient holds the position.

In the test for thumb extension, the patient extends the thumb, but not quite to full range of motion. The examiner applies an isometric force to the thumbs into flexion. For testing of hand intrinsics, the patient squeezes a piece of paper between the fingers while the examiner tries to pull it away; the patient may squeeze the examiner's fingers; or the patient may abduct the fingers slightly with the examiner isometrically adducting them.

SPECIAL TESTS

There are several special tests that may be performed if the examiner feels they are relevant.

Foraminal Compression Test. The patient bends or side flexes the head to one side (Fig. 2–9). The examiner carefully presses straight down on the head. A test result is classified as positive if pain radiates into the arm toward which the head is side flexed during compression and indicates pressure on a nerve root. The distribution of the pain and altered sensation can give some indication as to which nerve root is involved.

Distraction Test. Placing one hand under the patient's chin and the other hand around the occiput, the examiner slowly lifts the patient's head (Fig. 2–10). The test would be classified as positive if the pain is relieved or decreased when the head is lifted or distracted. It is indicative of pressure on nerve roots that has been relieved. This test may be used to check the shoulder as well. By the patient's moving the arms while

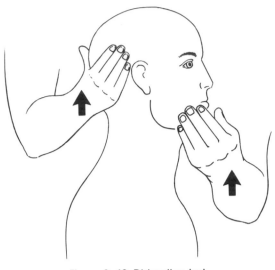

Figure 2–10. Distraction test.

traction is applied, the symptoms are often relieved or lessened in the shoulder. In this case, the test would still be indicative of nerve root pressure in the cervical spine.

Shoulder Depression Test. The examiner side flexes the patient's head while applying a downward pressure on the opposite shoulder (Fig. 2–11). If the pain is increased, it indicates (1) irritation or compression of the nerve roots, (2) foraminal encroachments such as osteophytes in the area, or (3) adhesions around the dural sleeves of the nerve and adjacent joint capsule on the side being stretched.

Vertebral Artery (Cervical Quadrant) Test. With the patient supine, the examiner passively takes the patient's head and neck into extension and side flexion.[8] When this movement is

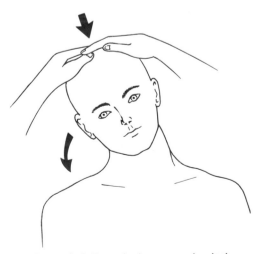

Figure 2–9. Foraminal compression test.

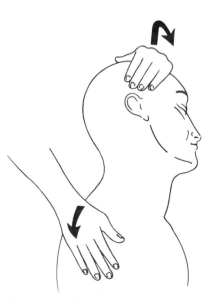

Figure 2–11. Shoulder depression test.

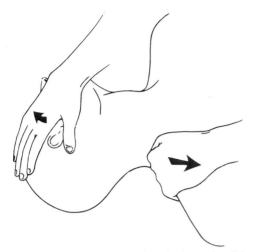

Figure 2–12. Vertebral artery (cervical quadrant) test.

achieved, the examiner rotates the patient's neck to the same side and holds it for about 30 seconds. A positive test will provoke referring symptoms if the side to which the head is taken is affected. This is a test for nerve root compression in the lower cervical spine (Fig. 2–12). To test the upper cervical spine, the examiner "pokes" the patient's chin followed by extension, side flexion, and rotation. This test must be done with care. Dizziness or nystagmus that occurs indicates that the vertebral arteries are being compressed.

Brachial Plexus Tension Test. The patient lies supine, fully elevates the shoulders through abduction, with the elbows extended to the point just short of the onset of pain, and holds this position. The patient externally rotates the shoulders to the point just short of the onset of pain and maintains this position. The forearm is then supinated. While the examiner supports the shoulder and forearm in this position, the patient flexes his elbow. Reproduction of symptoms implies problems of cervical origin, probably the C5 nerve root. In addition, if the cervical spine is then flexed, symptoms will increase.

Lhermitte's Sign. The patient is in the long leg sitting position on the examining table. The examiner passively flexes the patient's head and hips (with legs straight) at the same time. A positive test is indicated by a sharp pain down the spine and into the upper or lower limbs. It is indicative of dural irritation in the spine. The test is similar to a combination of the Brudzinski and double straight leg raise test (described in Chapter 8, Lumbar Spine).

Shoulder Abduction Test. The patient is in sitting or lying position, and the examiner passively or the patient actively elevates the arm through abduction so that the hand or forearm rests on top of the head (Fig. 2–13).[9] A decrease in or relief of symptoms indicates a cervical extradural compression problem such as a herniated disc, epidural vein compression or nerve root compression usually in the C5-C6 area.

Valsalva Test. The examiner asks the patient to take a deep breath and hold it while bearing down, as if moving the bowels. A positive test is indicated by increased pain, which may be due to increased intrathecal pressure. This increased pressure within the spinal cord is usually due to a space-occupying lesion, such as a herniated disc, a tumor, or osteophytes. Test results may be very subjective. The test should be done with care and caution because the patient may become dizzy and pass out while performing the test or shortly afterwards as the procedure can block the blood supply to the brain.

Temperature Test. The examiner alternately applies hot and cold test tubes just behind the patient's ears on each side of the head; each side is done in turn. A positive test is associated with the inducement of vertigo, which indicates inner ear problems in the individual.

Dizziness Test. The examiner actively rotates the patient's head as far as possible to the right and then to the left. The patient's shoulders are then actively rotated as far to the right as possible and to the left as possible while keeping the eyes looking straight ahead. If the patient experiences dizziness in both cases, the problem lies in the vertebral arteries. If the patient experiences dizziness only when the head is rotated, the problem lies within the semicircular canals of the inner ear.

REFLEXES AND CUTANEOUS DISTRIBUTION

The following reflexes should be checked for differences between the two sides, as in Figure 2–14: biceps (C6), the brachioradialis (C6), the

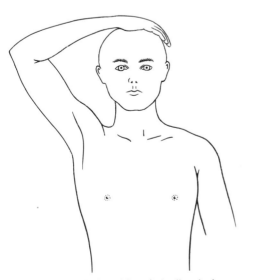

Figure 2–13. Shoulder abduction test.

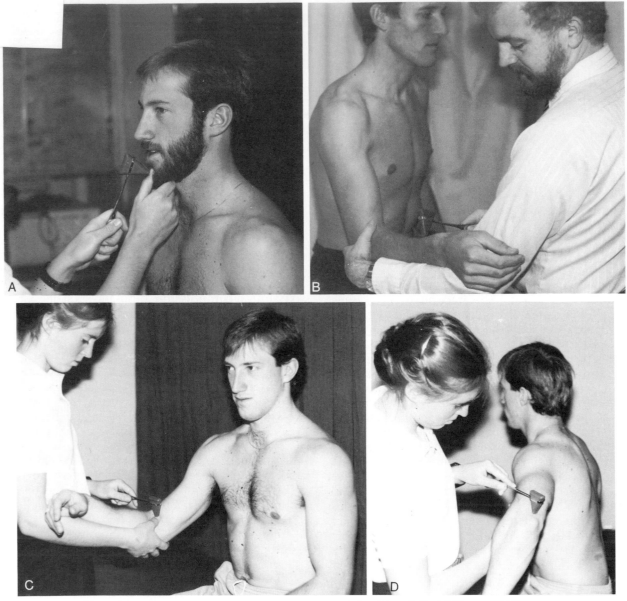

Figure 2–14. Testing of upper limb reflexes. (*A*) Jaw. (*B*) Brachioradialis. (*C*) Biceps. (*D*) Triceps.

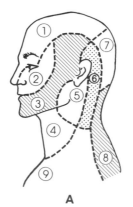

A

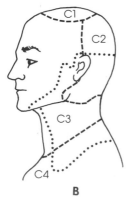

B

Figure 2–15. (*A*) Sensory nerve distribution of the head, neck, and face. (*1*) Ophthalmic nerve. (*2*) Maxillary nerve. (*3*) Mandibular nerve. (*4*) Transverse cutaneous nerve of neck (C2-3). (*5*) Greater auricular nerve (C2-3). (*6*) Lesser auricular nerve (C2). (*7*) Greater occipital nerve (C2-3). (*8*) Cervical dorsal rami (C3-4-5). (*9*) Suprascapular nerve (C5-6). (*B*) Dermatome pattern of the head, neck, and face. C3 is shown in dotted lines because of overlap.

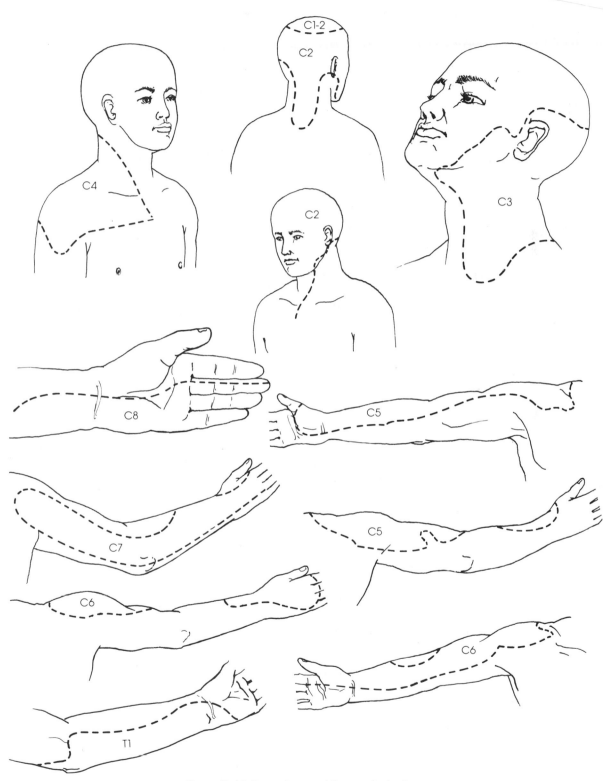

Figure 2–16. Dermatomes of the cervical spine.

triceps (C7-8), and the jaw jerk (cranial nerve V). The reflexes are tested with a reflex hammer. The examiner tests the biceps and jaw jerk reflexes by placing the thumb over the patient's biceps tendon or midpoint of the chin and then tapping the thumbnail with the reflex hammer to elicit the reflex. The brachioradialis and triceps reflexes are tested by tapping of the tendon or muscle directly.

The examiner then checks the *dermatome pattern* of the various nerve roots as well as the distribution of the peripheral nerves (Fig. 2–15 and 2–16). Dermatomes vary from person to person and overlap a great deal, and the accompanying diagrams are estimations only. For example, in the thoracic spine, one dermatome may be completely absent with no loss of sensation. The examiner tests sensation by running relaxed hands over the patient's head (sides and back), down over the shoulders, upper chest and back, and down the arms, being sure to cover all aspects of the arm. If any difference is noted between the sides in this "sensation scan," the examiner may then use a pinwheel, pin, cotton batting and/or brush to map out the exact area of sensory difference.

JOINT PLAY MOVEMENTS

The joint play movements that are carried out in the cervical spine are, for the most part, general movements involving the whole cervical spine and are not limited to one specific joint. The following joint play movements should be performed, and the examiner should note any decreased range of motion, pain, or difference in end feel:

1. Side glide of the cervical spine (general).
2. Anterior glide of the cervical spine (general).
3. Posterior glide of the cervical spine (general).
4. Traction glide of the cervical spine (general).
5. Rotation of the occiput on C1 (specific).
6. Posteroanterior central vertebral pressure (specific).
7. Posteroanterior unilateral vertebral pressure (specific).
8. Transverse vertebral pressure (specific).

Side Glide. The examiner holds the patient's head and moves it from side to side, keeping it in the same plane as the shoulder (Fig. 2–17).[10]

Anterior and Posterior Glide. The examiner holds the patient's head with one hand around the occiput and one hand around the chin, taking care to ensure the patient is not choked.[10] The examiner then draws the head forward for anterior glide (Fig. 2–18) and posteriorly for posterior glide. When doing these movements, the examiner must prevent flexion and extension of the head.

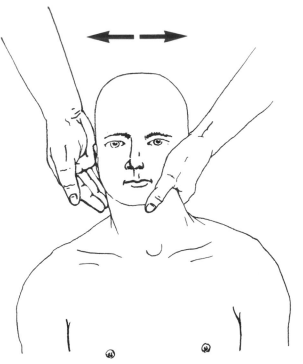

Figure 2–17. Side glide of the cervical spine. Glide to the right is illustrated.

Traction Glide. The examiner places one hand around the patient's chin and the other hand on the occiput.[10] Traction is then applied in a straight longitudinal direction, with the majority of the pull being through the occiput (Fig. 2–19).

Rotation of the Occiput on C1. The examiner holds the patient's head and in this position palpates the transverse processes of C1 (Fig. 2–20). The examiner must first find the mastoid process on each side, then move the fingers inferiorly and anteriorly until a hard bump is palpated. (These bumps are the transverse processes of C1.) Palpation in the area of C1 transverse process is generally painful so care must be taken. If the examiner then rotates the head while palpating the transverse processes, the transverse

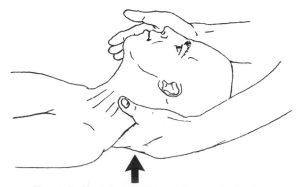

Figure 2–18. Anterior glide of the cervical spine.

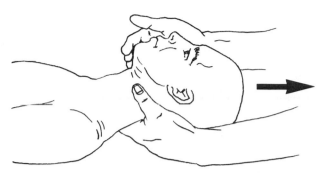

Figure 2–19. Traction glide of the cervical spine.

process on the side to which the head is rotated will normally disappear. If this disappearance does not occur, there is restriction of movement between C0 and C1 on that side.

Vertebral Pressures. For the last three joint play movements (Fig. 2–21), the patient lies prone, the forehead resting in his hands.[8] The examiner palpates the spinous processes of the cervical spine, starting at the C2 spinous process and working downward to the T2 spinous process. The position of the examiner's hands, fingers, and thumbs in performing *posteroanterior central vertebral pressures* are shown in Figure 2–21A. Pressure is then applied through the examiner's thumbs, and the vertebra is pushed forward. The examiner must take care to apply pressure slowly with carefully controlled movements so as to "feel" the movement, which in reality is minimal. This "springing test" may be repeated several times to determine the quality of the movement.

For *posteroanterior unilateral vertebral pressure*, the examiner's fingers move laterally away

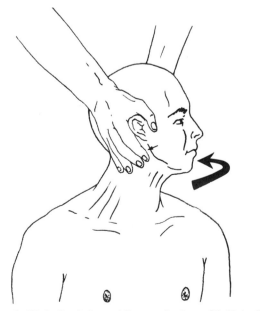

Figure 2–20. Left rotation of the occiput on C1. Note the index finger (small arrow) palpating the right transverse process of C1.

from the tip of the spinous process so that the thumbs rest on the lamina or transverse process of the cervical or thoracic vertebrae (Fig. 2–21B). Anterior "springing" pressure is applied as in the central pressure technique. Both sides should be done and compared.

For *transverse vertebral pressure*, the examiner's thumbs are placed along the side of the spinous process of the cervical or thoracic spine (Fig. 2–21C). The examiner then applies a transverse "springing" pressure to the side of the spinous process, feeling for the quality of movement.

PALPATION

If, after completing the scanning examination of the cervical spine, the examiner decides the problem is in another joint, palpation should be delayed until that joint is completely examined. However, during palpation of the cervical spine, the examiner should note any tenderness, muscle spasm, or other signs and symptoms that may indicate the source of the pathology. As with any palpation, the examiner should note the texture of the skin and surrounding bony and soft tissues on the posterior, lateral, and anterior aspects of the neck. Usually, the patient is palpated while supine so that maximum relaxation of the neck muscles is possible. To palpate the posterior structures, the examiner stands behind the patient and "cups" the patient's head in his hands while palpating with the fingers of both hands. For the lateral and anterior structures, the examiner stands at the patient's side. If the examiner suspects that the problem is in the cervical spine, palpation is done on the following structures (Fig. 2–22).

Posterior Aspect

External Protuberance of the Occiput. The protuberance may be found in posterior midline. The examiner palpates the posterior skull in midline and moves caudally until coming to a point where the fingers "dip" inward. The point just prior to the dip is the external occipital protuberance.

Spinous Processes and Facet Joints of Cervical Vertebrae. The spinous process of C2, C6, and C7 are the most obvious. If the examiner palpates the occiput of the skull and descends in the midline, the C2 spinous process will be palpated as the first bump. The next spinous processes that are most obvious are C6 and C7. The examiner can differentiate between C6 and C7 by passively flexing and extending the neck. With this movement, the C6 spinous process will move in and out while the C7 spinous process remains stationary. The facet joints may be palpated 1.5 to 3 mm

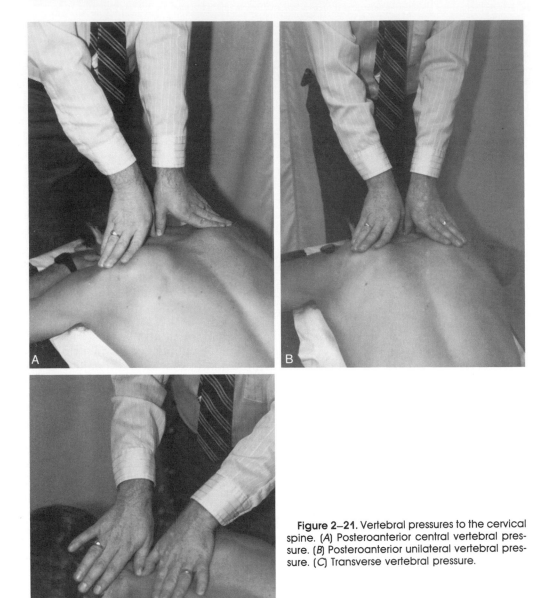

Figure 2–21. Vertebral pressures to the cervical spine. (*A*) Posteroanterior central vertebral pressure. (*B*) Posteroanterior unilateral vertebral pressure. (*C*) Transverse vertebral pressure.

lateral to the spinous process. The muscles in the adjacent area may be palpated for tenderness, swelling, and other signs of pathology. Careful palpation should also include the suboccipital structures.

Mastoid Processes (Below and Behind Ear Lobe). If the examiner palpates the skull following the posterior aspect of the ear, there will be a point on the skull where the finger again "dips" inward. The point just prior to the dip is the mastoid process.

Lateral Aspect

Transverse Processes of Cervical Vertebrae. The C1 transverse process is the easiest to palpate. The examiner first palpates the mastoid processes, then moves inferiorly and slightly anteriorly until a hard bump is felt. If the examiner then applies slight pressure to the bump, the patient will say it feels uncomfortable. These bumps are the transverse processes of C1. The other transverse process may be palpated if the musculature is sufficiently relaxed. Once the C1 transverse process has been located, the examiner moves inferiorly, feeling for similar "bumps." The bumps will not be directly inferior, but will normally follow the lordotic path of the cervical vertebrae. These structures will be situated more interiorly than one may suspect (Fig. 2–22).

Lymph Nodes and Carotid Arteries. The lymph nodes are palpable only if they are swollen. The nodes lie along the line of the sternocleidomastoid muscle. The carotid pulse may be palpated in the midportion of the neck between the sternocleidomastoid muscle and the trachea. The examiner should determine whether the pulse is normal and equal on both sides.

Temporomandibular Joints, Mandible, and Parotid Glands. The temporomandibular joints may be palpated anterior to the external ear. The examiner either may palpate directly over the joint or may place the little or index finger (pulp forward) in the external ear to feel for movement in the joint. The examiner can then move the fingers along the length of the mandible, feeling for any abnormalities. The angle of the mandible is at the level of C2 vertebra. Normally, the parotid gland is not palpable because it lies over the angle of the mandible. If it is swollen, however, it is palpable as a soft, boggy structure.

Anterior Aspect

Hyoid Bone, Thyroid Cartilage, and First Cricoid Ring. The hyoid bone may be palpated as part of the superior part of the trachea above the thyroid cartilage anterior to the C2-C3 vertebrae. The thyroid cartilage lies anterior to the C4-C5 vertebrae. With the neck in a neutral position, the

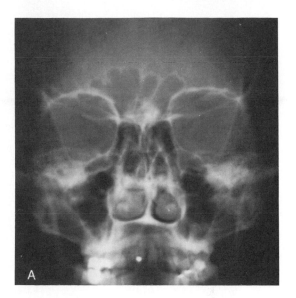

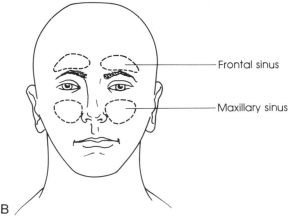

Figure 2–23. Paranasal sinuses. Radiograph (*A*) and illustration (*B*).

thyroid cartilage can be easily moved. In extension, it is tight and crepitations may be felt. Adjacent to the cartilage is the thyroid gland, which the examiner should palpate. If the gland is abnormal, it will be tender and enlarged. The cricoid ring is the first part of the trachea and lies above the site for an emergency tracheostomy. The ring will move when the patient swallows. Rough palpation of the ring may cause the patient to gag. While palpating the hyoid bone, the examiner should ask the patient to swallow. Normally, the bone should move and cause no pain.

Paranasal Sinuses. Returning to the face, the examiner should palpate the paranasal sinuses (frontal and maxillary) for signs of tenderness and swelling (Fig. 2–23).

First Three Ribs. The examiner palpates the manubrium sternum and, moving the fingers laterally, follows the path of the first three ribs posteriorly. The examiner should palpate the ribs individually and with care, since it is difficult to palpate the ribs as they pass under the clavicle.

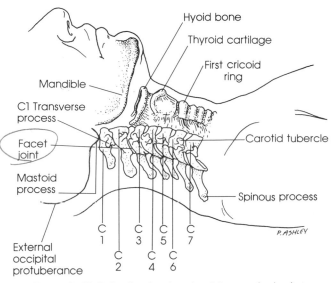

Figure 2–22. Palpation landmarks of the cervical spine.

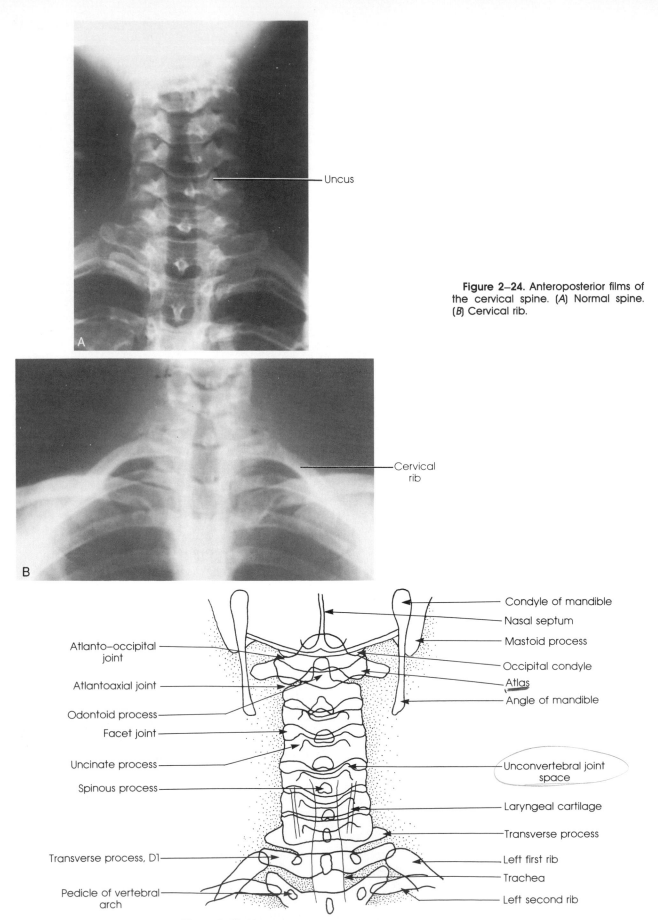

Uncus

A

B

Figure 2–24. Anteroposterior films of the cervical spine. (*A*) Normal spine. (*B*) Cervical rib.

Cervical rib

Condyle of mandible
Nasal septum
Mastoid process
Occipital condyle
Atlas
Angle of mandible

Atlanto–occipital joint
Atlantoaxial joint
Odontoid process
Facet joint
Uncinate process
Spinous process

Unconvertebral joint space

Laryngeal cartilage
Transverse process
Left first rib
Trachea
Left second rib

Transverse process, D1
Pedicle of vertebral arch

Figure 2–25. Diagram of anteroposterior cervical spine film.

As the ribs are palpated, the examiner should feel for rib movement during the patient's breathing action to ensure normal and equal mobility on both sides. A hypomobile rib may refer pain to the shoulder area.

Supraclavicular Fossa. Superior to the clavicle, the examiner can palpate the supraclavicular fossa. Normally, the fossa is a smooth indentation. The examiner should palpate for swelling following trauma (fractured clavicle?), for abnormal soft tissue (swollen glands?), or for abnormal bony tissue (cervical rib?). In addition, the examiner should palpate the sternocleidomastoid muscle along its length for signs of pathology, especially in cases of torticollis.

X-RAY EXAMINATION OF THE CERVICAL SPINE

Anteroposterior View. The examiner should look for or note (Figs. 2–24 and 2–25):

1. The shape of the vertebra.
2. The presence of any lateral wedging.
3. The presence of a cervical rib.

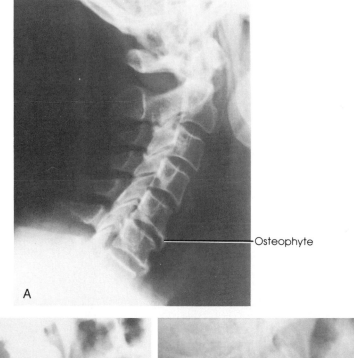

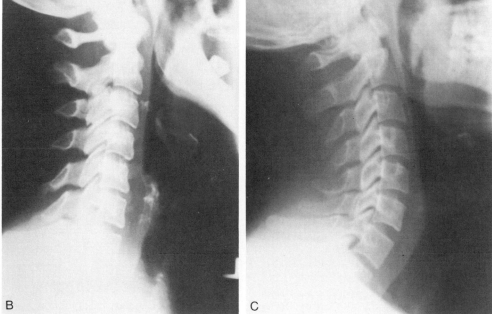

Figure 2–26. Lateral radiograph of the cervical spine. (*A*) Normal curve showing osteophytic lipping. (*B*) Cervical spine in flexion. (*C*) Cervical spine in extension.

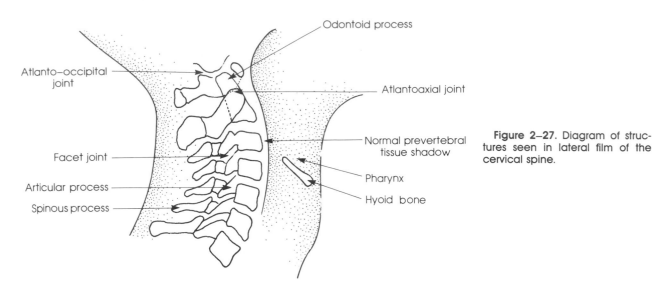

Figure 2–27. Diagram of structures seen in lateral film of the cervical spine.

Lateral View. The examiner should look for or note (Figs. 2–26 and 2–27):

1. Normal or abnormal curvature. The curvature may be highly variable, since 20 per cent of "normals" have a straight or slightly kyphotic curve in neutral.

2. "Kinking" of the cervical spine. Kinking may be indicative of a subluxation or dislocation in the cervical spine.

3. General shape of the vertebra. Is there any fusion, collapse, or wedging? The examiner should count the vertebrae because x-ray films do not always show C7 or T1.

4. Displacement.

5. Disc space. Is it normal? Narrow?

6. Lipping (Fig. 2–26A).

7. Osteophytes.

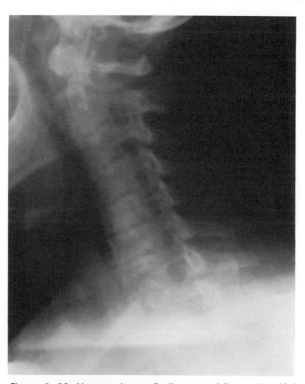

Figure 2–28. Abnormal x-ray findings on oblique view. Note loss of normal curve, narrowing at C4, C5, and C6; osteophytes and lipping of C4, C5, and C6; and encroachment on intervertebral foramen at C4-5, C5-6, and C6-7.

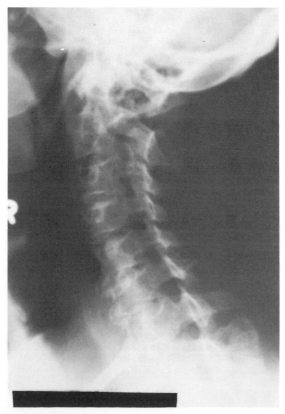

Figure 2–29. Oblique radiograph of the cervical spine showing intervertebral foramen and facet joints. Severe lipping in lower cervical spine and spondylosis are also evident.

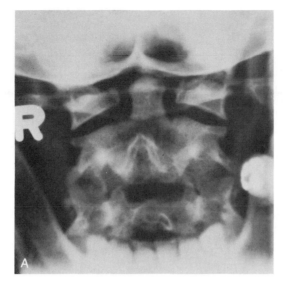

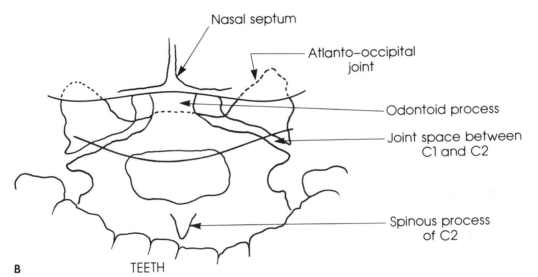

Figure 2–30. Through the mouth radiograph (*A*) and illustration (*B*). Illustration is not identical to radiograph.

Figure 2–31. Diagram of pillar view showing facet joints.

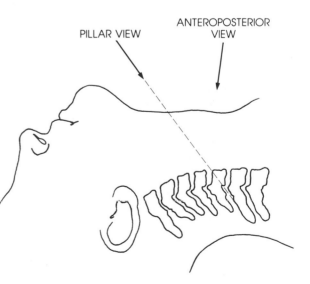

8. Prevertebral soft-tissue width. Measured at the level of the anteroinferior border of the C3 vertebra, this is normally 2.6 to 4.8 mm in width.

9. Subluxation of the facets.

10. Abnormal soft-tissue shadows.

11. Forward shifting of C1 on C2. This finding would indicate instability between C1 and C2. Normally, the joint space between the odontoid process and the anterior arch of the atlas does not exceed 3 mm in the adult.

12. Instability. Instability is present when more than 3.5 mm of horizontal displacement of one vertebra occurs in relation to the adjacent vertebra.

Oblique Films. The examiner should look for or note (Figs. 2–28 and 2–29):

1. Lipping of the joints of von Lushka.

2. Overriding of the facet joints.

3. Facet joints and intervertebral foramen (Fig. 2–29). The oblique view is used primarily to evaluate these structures.

"Through-the-Mouth" View. With this view, the examiner is looking at the relation of the odontoid process to the adjacent bones (Fig. 2–30).

Pillar View. This view is used to evaluate the facet joints and their articular processes (Fig. 2–31).

Précis of the Cervical Spine Assessment

History
Observation
Examination
  Active movements
    Flexion
    Extension
    Side flexion (right and left)
    Rotation (right and left)
  Passive movements (as in active movements)
  Resisted isometric movements (as in active movements)
  Peripheral joint scan
    Temporomandibular joints (open and close mouth)
    Shoulder girdle (elevation through abduction and forward flexion, medial and lateral rotation)
    Elbow (flexion, extension, supination, pronation)
    Wrist (flexion, extension, radial and ulnar deviation)
    Fingers and thumb (flexion, extension, abduction, adduction, circumduction)
  Mytomes
    Neck flexion (C1-C2)
    Neck side flexion (C3)
    Shoulder elevation (C4)
    Shoulder Abduction (C5)
    Elbow flexion (C6) and/or extension (C7)
    Wrist flexion (C7) and/or extension (C6)
    Thumb Extension and/or ulnar deviation (C8)
    Hand intrinsics (T1)
  Special tests
  Reflexes and cutaneous distribution
  Joint play movements
    Slide glide of cervical spine
    Anterior glide of cervical spine
    Posterior glide of cervical spine
    Traction glide of cervical spine
    Rotation of occiput on C1
    Posteroanterior central vertebral pressure
    Posteroanterior unilateral vertebral pressure
    Transverse vertebral pressure
  Palpation
  X-ray viewing

Following any examination, the patient should always be warned of the possibility of exacerbation of symptoms as a result of the assessment.

REFERENCES

CITED REFERENCES

1. Cyriax, J.: Testbook of Orthopaedic Medicine, vol. 1: Diagnosis of Soft Tissue Lesions. London, Bailliere Tindall, 1982.
2. Boreades, A. G., and J. Gershon-Cohen: Luschka joints of the cervical spine. Radiology 66:181, 1956.
3. Hall, M. C.: Luschka's Joint. Springfield, Ill., Charles C Thomas, 1965.
4. Silberstein, C. E.: The evolution of degenerative changes in the cervical spine and an investigation into the "joint of Luschka." Clin. Orthop. Relat. Res. 40:184, 1965.
5. Willis, T. A.: Luschka's joints. Clin. Orthop. Relat. Res. 46:121, 1966.
6. Ferlic, D.: The nerve supply of the cervical intervertebral disc in man. Johns Hopkins Hosp. Bull. 113:347, 1963.
7. Toole, J., and S. H. Tucker: Influence of head position upon cervical circulation. Arch. Neurol. 2:616, 1960.
8. Maitland, G. D.: Vertebral Manipulation. London, Butterworths, 1973.
9. Davidson, R. I., E. J. Dunn, and J. N. Metzmaker: The shoulder abduction test in the diagnosis of radicular pain in cervical extradural compressive monoradiculopathies. Spine 6:441, 1981.
10. Mennell, J. M.: Joint Pain. Boston, Little, Brown & Co., 1964.

GENERAL REFERENCES

Bateman, J. E.: The Shoulder and Neck. Philadelphia, W. B. Saunders Co., 1972.
Bonica, J. J.: The Management of Pain. Philadelphia, Lea & Febiger, 1953.
Cailliet, R.: Neck and Arm Pain. Philadelphia, F. A. Davis Co., 1964.
Cervical Spine Research Society: The Cervical Spine. Philadelphia, J. B. Lippincott, 1983.
Crouch, J. E.: Functional Human Anatomy. Philadelphia, Lea & Febiger, 1973.
Edwards, B. C.: Combined movements in the cervical spine (C2-7): Their value in examination and technique choice. Aust. J. Physiother. 26:165, 1980.
Ferlic, D.: The range of motion of the 'normal' cervical spine. Johns Hopkins Hosp. Bull. 110:59, 1962.
Fielding, J. W.: Normal and selected abnormal motion of the cervical spine from the second cervical vertebra to the

seventh cervical vertebra based on cineroentgenography. J. Bone Joint Surg. 46A:1799, 1964.

Fielding, J. W., G. V. B. Cochran, J. F. Lawsing, and M. Hohl: Tears of the transverse ligament of the atlas—a clinical and biomechanical study. J. Bone Joint Surg. 56A:1683, 1974.

Frykholm, R.: Lower cervical vertebrae and intervertebral discs—surgical anatomy and pathology. Acta Chir. Scand. 101–102:345, 1951–1952.

Grieve, G. P.: Mobilisation of the Spine. New York, Churchill Livingstone, 1979.

Grieve, G. P.: Common Vertebral Joint Problems. New York, Churchill Livingstone, 1981.

Hohl, M.: Normal motions in the upper portion of the cervical spine. J. Bone Joint Surg. 46A:1777, 1964.

Hohl, M., and H. R. Baker: The atlanto-axial joint—roentgenographic and anatomic study of normal and abnormal motion. J. Bone Joint Surg. 46A:1739, 1964.

Hohl, M.: Soft-tissue injuries of the neck. Clin. Orthop. Relat. Res. 109:42, 1975.

Hollinshead, W. H., and D. B. Jenkins: Functional Anatomy of the Limbs and back. Philadelphia, W. B. Saunders Co., 1981.

Hoppenfeld, S.: Physical Examination of the Spine and Extremities. New York, Appleton-Century-Crofts, 1976.

Jackson, R.: The Cervical Syndrome. Springfield, Ill., Charles C Thomas, 1976.

Judge, R. D., G. D. Zuidema, and F. T. Fitzgerald: Clinical Diagnosis—A Physiological Approach. Boston, Little, Brown & Co., 1982.

Kapandji, I. A.: The Physiology of Joints, vol. 3: The Trunk and the Vertebral Column. New York, Churchill Livingstone, 1974.

Liebgott, B.: The Anatomical Basis of Dentistry. Philadelphia, W. B. Saunders Co., 1982.

Lysell, E.: Motion in the cervical spine. Acta Orthop. Scand. (Suppl.) 123:1–61, 1969.

Macnab, I.: Cervical spondylosis. Clin. Orthop. Relat. Res. 109:69, 1975.

Maigne, R.: Orthopaedic Medicine—A New Approach to Vertebral Manipulation. Springfield, Ill., Charles C Thomas, 1972.

Mathews, J. A., and J. Pemberton: Radiologic anatomy of the neck. Physiotherapy 65:77, 1979.

McRae, R.: Clinical Orthopaedic Examination. New York, Churchill Livingstone, 1976.

Panjabi, M. M.: Cervical spine mechanics as a function of transection of components. J. Biomech. 8:327, 1975.

Patterson, R. H.: Cervical ribs and the scalenus muscle syndrome. Ann. Surg. 111:531, 1940.

Pedersen, H. E., C. F. J. Blunck, and E. Gardner: The anatomy of lumbosacral posterior rami and meningeal branches of spinal nerves (sinu-vertebral nerves). J. Bone Joint Surg. 38A:377, 1956.

Penning, L.: Functional pathology of the cervical spine. New York, Excerpta Medica Foundation, 1968.

Rothman, R. H.: The acute cervical disc. Clin. Orthop. Relat. Res. 109:59, 1975.

Rothman, R. H., and F. A. Simeone: The Spine. Philadelphia, W. B. Saunders Co., 1982.

Southwick, W. O. and K. Keggi: The normal cervical spine. J. Bone Joint Surg. 46A:1767, 1964.

Sunderland, S.: Meningeal-neural relations in the intervertebral foramen. J. Neurosurg. 40:756, 1974.

Travell, J. G., and D. G. Simons: Myofacial Pain and Dysfunction—The Trigger Point Manual. Baltimore, Williams and Wilkins, 1983.

Weir, D. C.: Roentgenographic signs of cervical injury. Clin. Orthop. Relat. Res. 109:9, 1975.

Wells, P.: Cervical dysfunction and shoulder problems. Physiotherapy 68:66, 1982.

White, A. A., R. M. Johnson, M. M. Panjabi, and W. O. Southwick: Biomechanical analysis of clinical stability in the cervical spine. Clin. Orthop. Relat. Res. 109:85, 1975.

White, A. A., and M. M. Panjabi: The clinical biomechanics of the occipito-atlantoaxial complex. Orthop. Clin. North Am. 9:867, 1978.

White, A. A., and M. M. Panjabi: Clinical Biomechanics of the Spine. Philadelphia, J. B. Lippincott Co., 1978.

Williams, P., and R. Warwick (eds.): Gray's Anatomy, 36th British ed. Philadelphia, W. B. Saunders Co., 1980.

Wyke, B.: Neurology of the cervical spine joints. Physiotherapy 65:72, 1979.

3

Temporomandibular Joints

The temporomandibular joint is one of the most frequently used joints in the body, but it probably receives the least amount of attention. In any examination of the head and neck, this joint should be included. Without these joints, we would be severely hindered when talking, eating, yawning, kissing, or sucking. Much of the work in this chapter has been developed from the teachings of Rocabado.[1]

Applied Anatomy

The temporomandibular joint is a synovial, condylar, and hinge-type joint with fibrocartilaginous surfaces and an articular disc; this disc completely divides each joint into two cavities (Fig. 3–1). There are two joints, one on either side of the jaw. Both joints must be considered together in any examination. Along with the teeth, these joints are considered to be a "trijoint complex."

Gliding or *sliding* movement occurs in the upper cavity of the joint, whereas rotation or hinge movement occurs in the lower cavity. Rotation occurs from the beginning to the midrange of movement. The upper head of the *lateral pterygoid muscles* draw the disc, or *meniscus*, anteriorly and prepare for condylar rotation during movement. The rotation occurs through the two condylar heads between the articular disc and the condyle. In addition, the disc provides congruent contours and lubrication for the joint. Gliding, which occurs as a second movement, is a translatory movement of the condyle and disc along the slope of the articular eminence. Both the gliding and the rotation are essential for opening and closing of the mouth (Fig. 3–2). The capsule of the temporomandibular joints is thin and loose. In the resting position the mouth is slightly opened so that the teeth are not in contact. In the close packed position, the teeth are tightly clenched and the heads of the condyles are in the posterior aspect of the joint. *Centric occlusion* occurs with maximum contact of the teeth, and it is the position assumed by the jaw when in swallowing.

The temporomandibular joints will actively displace only anteriorly and slightly laterally. When the mouth is opening, the condyles of the joint rest on the articular eminences, and any sudden movement, such as a yawn, may displace one or both condyles forward.

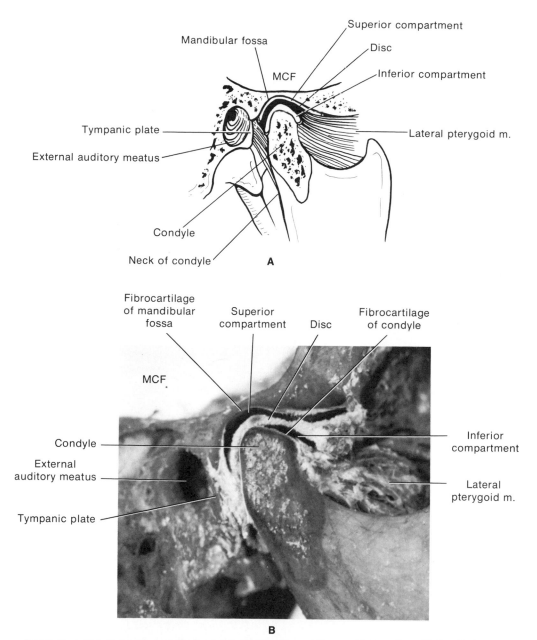

Figure 3–1. The temporomandibular joint. (A) Diagram of the sagittal section. (B) Sagittal section. (From Liebgott, B.: The Anatomical Basis of Dentistry. Philadelphia, W. B. Saunders Co., 1982, p. 292.)

The temporomandibular joints are innervated by branches of the auriculotemporal and masseteric branches of the mandibular nerve.

The *temporomandibular,* or *lateral, ligament* restrains movement of the lower jaw and prevents compression of the tissues behind the condyle. In reality, this collateral ligament is a thickness in the joint capsule.

The *sphenomandibular* and *stylomandibular ligaments* act as restraints to keep the condyle, disc, and temporal bone firmly opposed. The stylomandibular ligament is a specialized band of deep cerebral fascia with thickening of the parotid fascia.

In the human being, there are 20 deciduous, or temporary ("baby") teeth and 32 permanent teeth (Fig. 3–3). There are no premolars. The temporary teeth are shed between the ages of 6 and 13. Missing teeth, abnormal eruption, malocclusion, or dental caries (decay) may lead to problems of the temporomandibular joint. By convention, the teeth are divided into four quadrants—the upper left, the upper right, the lower left, and the lower right quadrant (Fig. 3–4).

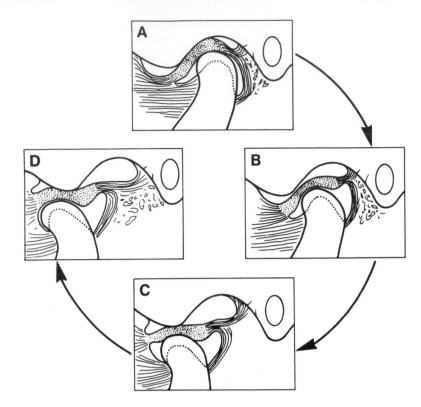

Figure 3–2. Normal temporomandibular joint function during opening movement, as seen by arthrography. The disc is the stippled structure between the condyle below and the temporal bone above. (*A*) Mandible in the closed position. (*B-D*) Progressive stages of opening. The disc slides forward with the condyle as it translates to, and sometimes over, the articular eminence. The superior stratum of the bilaminar zone becomes stretched, the inferior stratum does not. (After D. D. Blaschke, reproduced with permission, from Solberg, W. K., and G. T. Clark: Temporomandibular Joint Problems: Biologic Diagnosis and Treatment. Chicago, Quintessence Publishing, 1980, p. 73.)

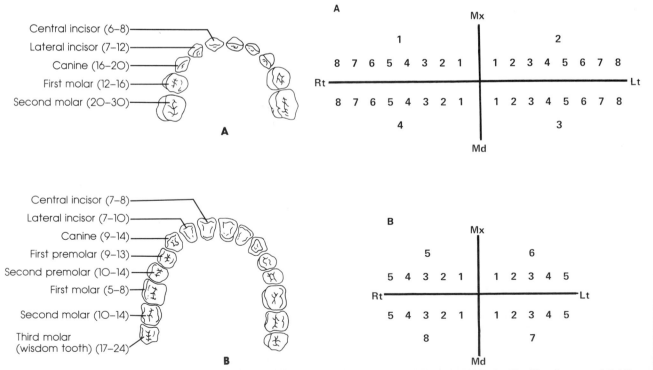

Figure 3–3. Teeth in a child (*A*) and adult (*B*). Numbers indicate age (in months for a child, in years for an adult) when teeth erupt.

Figure 3–4. Numerical symbols for dentition for an adult (*A*) and child (*B*). (From Liebgott, B.: The Anatomical Basis of Dentistry. Philadelphia, W. B. Saunders Co., 1982, p. 331.)

Patient History

In addition to the questions listed under Patient History in Chapter 1, the examiner should ascertain the following information from the patient:

1. Is there pain on opening or closing the mouth?

2. Is there pain on eating?

3. What movements of the jaw cause pain?

4. Do any of these actions cause pain or discomfort? Yawning? Chewing? Swallowing? Speaking? Shouting? If so, where?

5. Does the patient breathe through the nose or the mouth? If the patient is a "mouth breather," the tongue does not sit in the proper position against the palate. In the young, if the tongue does not push against the palate, developmental abnormalities may occur because the tongue provides internal pressure to shape the mouth. The buccinator and orbicularis oris muscle complex provides external pressure to counterbalance the internal pressure of the tongue. Loss of normal neck balance will often result in the individual's becoming a mouth breather and an upper respiratory breather, using the accessory muscles of respiration. Conditions such as adenoids and upper respiratory tract infections may cause the same problems.

6. Does the patient grind the teeth or hold them tightly? *Bruxism* is the forced clenching and grinding of the teeth, especially during sleep. If the front teeth are in contact and the back ones are not, facial and temporomandibular pain may develop as a result of malocclusion.

7. Are any teeth missing? If so, which ones and how many? The presence or absence of teeth and their relationship to one another must be noted on a table similar to the one shown in Figure 3–4. Their presence or absence can have an effect on the temporomandibular joints and their muscles. If some teeth are missing, it may lead to deviation of the teeth to fill in the space, thus altering the vertical dimension. The examiner should watch the patient's jaw movement while the patient is talking.

8. Are any teeth painful or sensitive? This finding may be indicative of dental caries or abscess. Tooth pain may lead to incorrect biting when chewing, putting abnormal stresses on the temporomandibular joints.

9. Are there any ear problems such as hearing loss, ringing in the ears, blocking of the ears, earache, or dizziness? Any symptoms such as these may be due to inner ear, cervical spine, or temporomandibular joint problems.

10. Has the mouth or jaw ever locked? If the jaw has locked in the closed position, the locking is probably due to a disc, with the condyle being posterior to the disc. If locking occurs in the open position, it is probably due to subluxation of the joint (Fig. 3–5).

11. Does the patient smoke a pipe, use a ciga-

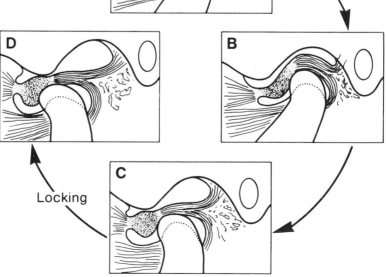

Figure 3–5. Mechanism of blocking mandibular depression at one point caused by marked anterior displacment of the articular disc. (*A*) Rest position. (*B*) As the condyle translates forward, it impinges on the disc but is unable to ride over it. (*C, D*) This blocks full forward translation and thereby full jaw opening. (After D. D. Blaschke, reproduced with permission, from Solberg, W. K., and G. T. Clark: Temporomandibular Joint Problems: Biologic Diagnosis and Treatment. Chicago, Quintessence Publishing, 1980, p. 77.)

Locking

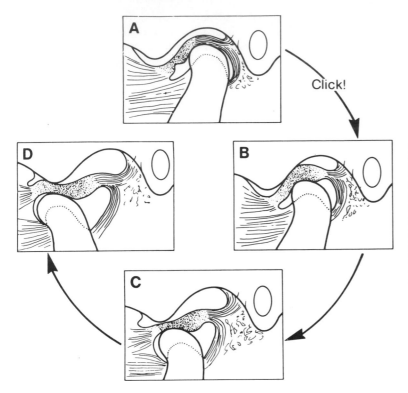

Figure 3–6. Mechanism of early click caused by slight anterior displacement of the articular disc. (*A*) Rest position. (*B*) As the condyle begins to translate forward, it must override a thickness of posterior disc material, causing a click. This seats the condyle in the central, thin part of the disc. (*C, D*) After the click, mandibular opening and translation of the condyle proceed with apparently normal disc mechanics. (After D. D. Blaschke, reproduced with permission from Wolberg, W. K., and G. T. Clark: Temporomandibular Joint Problems: Biologic Diagnosis and Treatment. Chicago, Quintessence Publishing, 1980, p. 75.)

rette holder, chew gum, bite the nails, chew hair, purse or chew lips, continually move the mouth, or have any other nervous habits? All these activities place additional stress on the temporomandibular joints.

12. Does the patient ever feel dizzy or faint?

13. Has the patient complained of any "clicking"? Normally, the condyles of the temporomandibular joint slide out of the concavity and onto the rim of the disc. Clicking may occur when the condyle slides back off the rim into the center (Fig. 3–6). There may be a partial anterior displacement (subluxation) of the disc, which the condyle must override to reach its normal position when the mouth is fully open. This override may cause a click as well. The clicking may be due to uncoordinated muscle action of the lateral pterygoid muscles, a crack or perforation in the disc, osteoarthrosis, or occlusal imbalance. Normally, the upper head of the lateral pterygoid muscle pulls the disc forward. If the disc does not move first, the condyle will click over the disc as the condyles are pulled forward by the lower head of the lateral pterygoid muscle.

14. Has the patient noticed any voice changes? Changes may be due to muscle spasm.

15. Has the patient ever been seen by (a) a dentist? (b) a periodontist (a dentist who specializes in the study of tissues around the teeth and diseases of these tissues)? (c) an orthodontist (a dentist who specializes in correction and prevention of irregularities of the teeth)? (d) an endodontist (a dentist who specializes in the treatment of diseases of the tooth pulp, root canal, and periapical areas)? or (e) an ear, nose, and throat specialist?

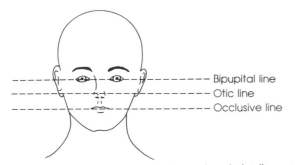

Figure 3–7. Normally, bipupital, otic, and occlusive lines are all parallel.

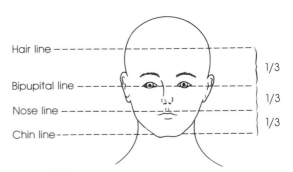

Figure 3–8. Divisions of the face (vertical dimension).

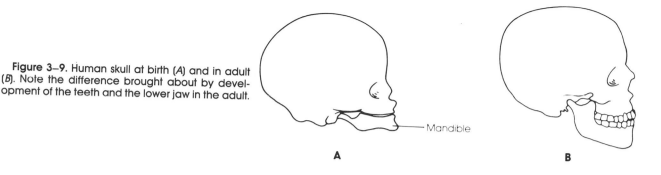

Figure 3–9. Human skull at birth (*A*) and in adult (*B*). Note the difference brought about by development of the teeth and the lower jaw in the adult.

Mandible

A   B

Observation

When assessing a temporomandibular joint, the examiner must also assess the posture of the cervical spine and head. For example, it is necessary that the head be "balanced" on the cervical spine. The bipupital, otic, and occlusive lines should be parallel to each other (Fig. 3–7). The examiner should then determine whether the face is equally divided horizontally between right and left (symmetric). If the head is normally developed vertically, in the adult it may be divided into three parts (Fig. 3–8). In children, elderly persons, or those with massive tooth loss, the lower third is not well developed or it has recessed (Fig. 3–9). The examiner should notice whether there is any paralysis, which could be indicated by *ptosis* (drooping of an eyelid) or by drooping of the mouth on one side (Bell's palsy). The examiner should note whether there is any *malocclusion* that may result in a faulty bite. Malocclusion is a major factor in the development of disc problems of the temporomandibular joint.

The examiner should note whether there is any *crossbite* or *overbite* (Fig. 3–10).

In crossbite the mandibular teeth are unilaterally, bilaterally, or in pairs in buccoversion (they lie anterior to the maxillary teeth). In overbite the anterior maxillary teeth extend below the anterior mandibular teeth when the jaw is in centric occlusion. Any orthodontic appliances or false teeth present should also be noted for fit and possible sore spots. Is there any appearance of crossbite in which the mandible moves to the left or right as the patient's mouth is opened and closed?

The examiner should also notice whether there is normal *vertical dimension*. Vertical dimension is the distance between any two arbitrary points on the face, one of these points being above and the other point being below the mouth, usually in midline. Usually, the upper and lower teeth are used to measure vertical dimension. In the child, the lower third of the face is poorly developed because of lack of teeth. As the teeth grow, the lower third develops into its normal proportion.

The examiner should note whether the patient demonstrates normal bony and soft-tissue contours. If the patient bites down, do the masseter muscles bulge as they normally should? Is the patient able to move the tongue properly? Can the patient move the tongue up to and against the palate? Can the tongue be protruded? Is the patient able to "click" the tongue? All these factors will give the examiner some idea of the mobility of the structures of the mouth and jaw and their neurologic mechanisms. In addition, the examiner should be aware of any poor habits, such as biting the nails or chewing the hair, that may affect the temporomandibular joints.

Figure 3–10. Examples of crossbite and overbite.

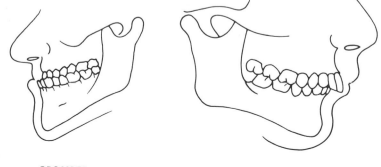

CROSSBITE   OVERBITE

Examination

The examiner must remember that many problems of the temporomandibular joints may be the result of or related to problems in the cervical spine or teeth.

ACTIVE MOVEMENTS

With the patient in the sitting position, the examiner watches the active movements occurring, noting whether they deviate from what would be considered normal range of motion and whether the patient is willing to do the movement.

The patient is first asked to carry out active movements of the neck. The most painful movements, if any, should be done last. These movements include:

1. Flexion.
2. Extension.
3. Side flexion (left and right).
4. Rotation (left and right).

During *flexion* of the neck, the mandible moves up and forward and the posterior structures of the neck become tight. During *extension*, the mandible moves down and back and the anterior structures of the neck become tight. The examiner should note whether the patient can flex and extend the neck while keeping the mouth closed or whether the patient must open the mouth to do these movements. The patient should be asked to place a fist under the chin and then open the mouth. If the mouth opens in this way, movement of the neck into extension is occurring. This test movement would be especially important if the patient subjectively feels that there is a loss of neck extension.

If *side flexion* of the neck occurs to the right, maximum occlusion will occur on the right and vice versa. Side flexion and *rotation* of the neck occur to the same side. Thus, if these movements occur to the right, maximum occlusion will occur to the right.

Having observed the neck movements, the examiner goes on to note the active movements of the temporomandibular joints. These movements include (1) opening and closing of the mouth, (2) protrusion of the mandible, and (3) lateral deviation of the mandible.

Opening and Closing of Mouth

With opening and closing of the mouth, the normal arc of movement of the jaw is smooth and unbroken; that is, both temporomandibular joints are working in unison with no asymmetry or sideways movement. If deviation occurs to the left on opening (Fig. 3–11), the left temporomandibular joint is said to be hypomobile. If, on opening the mouth, the deviation is a "c" type curve, hypomobility is evident toward the side of the deviation; if, on opening the mouth, the deviation is an "s" type curve, the problem is probably muscular imbalance. The chin deviates toward the affected side and is usually the result of spasm of the pterygoid or masseter muscles or an obstruction in the joint. The mandible should open and close in a straight line (Fig. 3–12). The examiner should then determine whether the patient's mouth can functionally be opened. The functional opening is determined by having the patient try to place two or three flexed proximal interphalangeal joints within the mouth opening (Fig. 3–13). This space should be approximately 35 to 40 mm. If the space is less than this, the temporomandibular joint is said to be hypomobile. As the mouth opens, the examiner should palpate the external auditory meatus with the finger (fleshy part anterior). The patient is then

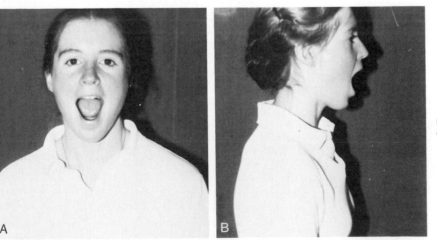

Figure 3–11. Active opening of mouth. (*A*) Anteroposterior view. Note deviation to left. (*B*) Side view.

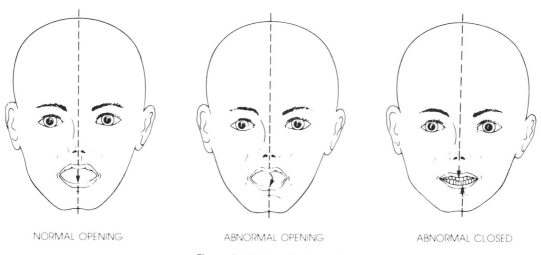

NORMAL OPENING   ABNORMAL OPENING   ABNORMAL CLOSED

Figure 3–12. Mandibular motion.

asked to close the mouth. When the examiner first feels the condyle touch the finger, the temporomandibular joints are in the resting position. This resting position of the temporomandibular joints is called the *freeway space*. Normally, the space between the front teeth at this point is 2 to 4 mm. If this space is greater than 4 mm, the temporomandibular joints are said to be hypermobile.

If rotation does not occur at the temporomandibular joint, the mouth will not open. There may be gliding at the temporomandibular joint, but rotation has not occurred.

Protrusion of the Mandible

The examiner asks the patient to protrude or jut the lower jaw out past the upper teeth. The

patient should be able to do this without difficulty.

The patient should then purse the lips in an attempt to whistle. If the patient is unable to do this or to wink or close an eye on one side, the symptoms may be indicative of Bell's palsy (paralysis of the facial nerve).

Lateral Deviation of the Mandible

Next, the examiner should measure the mandible from the posterior aspect of the temporomandibular joint to the notch of the chin (Fig. 3–14). Both sides are measured and compared for equality. Any difference indicates a developmental problem or structural change so that the patient might not be able to get balancing in the midline. When charting any changes, the examiner should note opening deviation as well as the functional opening and any lateral deviation (Fig. 3–15). The opening and lateral deviation of the mandible can be measured with a millimeter ruler. When using the ruler, the examiner should pick a midline point from which to measure. This same ruler can be used to measure protrusion. Any lateral deviation from the normal opening position or abnormal protrusion to one side indicates that the lateral pterygoid, masseter, or temporalis muscle, the disc, or the lateral ligament on the opposite side is affected.

PASSIVE MOVEMENTS

Very seldom are passive movements carried out for the temporomandibular joints except when the examiner is attempting to determine the end feel of the joints. The normal end feel of these

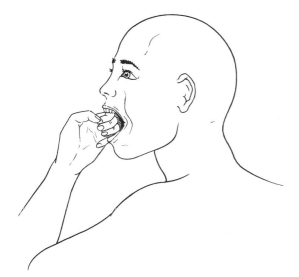

Figure 3–13. Functional opening "knuckle" test.

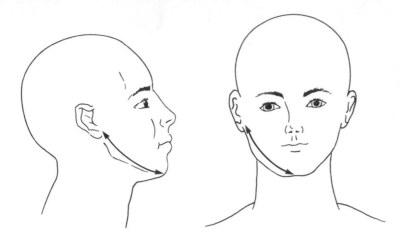

Figure 3–14. Measuring the mandible.

joints is tissue stretch on opening and teeth contact ("bone to bone") on closing.

RESISTED ISOMETRIC MOVEMENTS

Resisted isometric movements of the temporomandibular joints are relatively difficult to test.

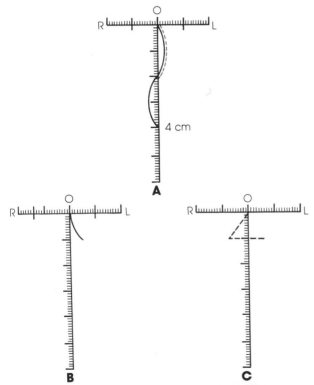

Figure 3–15. Charting temporomandibular motion. (A) Deviation R & L on opening; maximum opening: 4 cm; lateral deviation equal (1 cm each direction); protrusion on functional opening (dashed lines). (B) Capsule-ligamentous pattern; opening limited to 1 cm; lateral deviation greater to R than L; deviation to L on opening. (C) Protrusion is 1 cm; lateral deviation to R on protrusion (indicates weak lateral pterygoid on opposite side).

The jaw should be in the resting position. The examiner applies firm but gentle resistance to the joints by asking the patient to hold the position; the patient is not to let the examiner move it. The movements tested are shown in Figure 3–16 and Table 3–1:

1. Opening of the mouth (depression).
2. Closing of the mouth (elevation or occlusion).
3. Lateral deviation of the jaw.

SPECIAL TESTS

The *Chvostek test* is used to determine whether there is pathology involving the seventh cranial (facial) nerve (Fig. 3–17). The examiner taps the parotid gland overlying the masseter muscle. If the facial muscles twitch, the result is positive.

The examiner can listen to (auscultate) the temporomandibular joints during movement (Fig. 3–18). The movements "listened to" include opening and closing of the mouth, lateral deviation of the mandible to the right and left, and mandibular protrusion and occlusion. Normally, only on occlusion would a sound be heard. This is a single, solid sound, not a "slipping" sound. A slipping sound could occur when the teeth are not "hitting" simultaneously. When the examiner is listening, each movement should be done four or five times to ensure a correct diagnosis.

REFLEXES AND CUTANEOUS DISTRIBUTION

The reflex of the temporomandibular joint is called the jaw reflex (Fig. 3–19). The examiner's thumb is placed on the chin of the patient with the patient's mouth relaxed and open in the resting position. The examiner then taps the thumb nail with a neurologic hammer. If the reflex occurs, it will close the mouth and is an indication of the test of cranial nerve V.

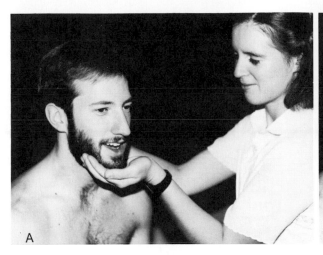
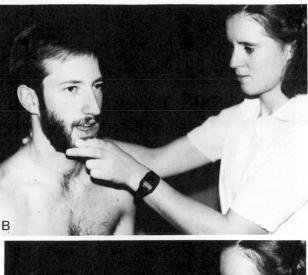

Figure 3–16. Resisted isometric movements for the muscles controlling the temporomandibular joint. (*A*) Opening of the mouth (depression). (*B*) Closing of the mouth (elevation or occlusion). (*C*) Lateral deviation of the jaw.

Table 3–1. Muscles of the Temporomandibular Joint: Their Action and Nerve Supply

Action	Muscles Acting	Nerve Supply
Opening of mouth (depression of mandible)	1. Lateral (external) pterygoid 2. Mylohyoid* 3. Geniohyoid* 4. Digastric*	Mandibular Inferior alveolar Hypoglossal Inferior alveolar Facial
Closing of mouth (elevation of mandible or occlusion)	1. Masseter 2. Temporalis 3. Medial (internal) pterygoid	Mandibular Mandibular Mandibular
Protrusion of mandible	1. Lateral (external) pterygoid 2. Medial (internal) pterygoid 3. Masseter* 4. Mylohyoid* 5. Geniohyoid* 6. Digastric* 7. Stylohyoid* 8. Temporalis (anterior fibers)*	Mandibular Mandibular Mandibular Inferior alveolar Hypoglossal Inferior alveolar Facial Facial Mandibular
Retraction of mandible	1. Temporalis (posterior fibers) 2. Masseter* 3. Digastric* 4. Stylohyoid* 5. Mylohyoid* 6. Geniohyoid*	Mandibular Mandibular Inferior alveolar Facial Inferior alveolar Inferior alveolar Hypoglossal
Lateral deviation of mandible	1. Lateral (external) pterygoid (ipsilateral muscle) 2. Medial (internal) pterygoid (contralateral muscle) 3. Temporalis* 4. Masseter*	Mandibular Mandibular Mandibular Mandibular

*Act only when assistance is required.

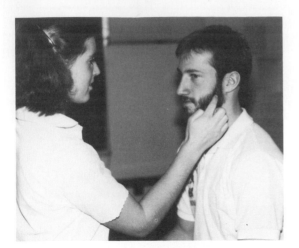

Figure 3–17. Chvostek test.

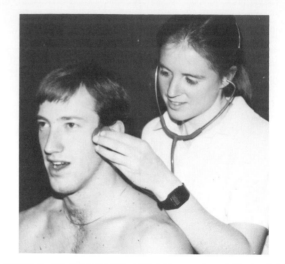

Figure 3–18. Auscultation of the temporomandibular joint.

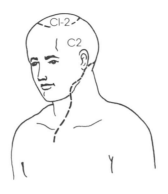

Figure 3–19. Testing of the jaw reflex.

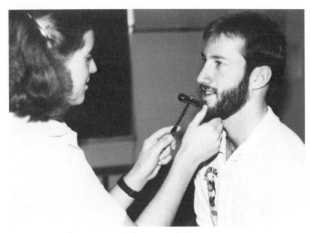

Figure 3–20. Dermatomes of the head.

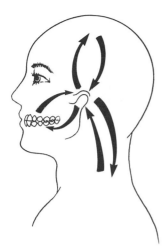

Figure 3–21. Referred pain patterns to and from the temporomandibular joint from and to the teeth, head, or neck.

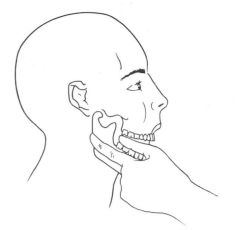

Figure 3–22. Joint play of the temporomandibular joint.

The examiner must be aware of the dermatomal patterns for the head and neck (Fig. 3–20) as well as peripheral nerve distribution (Fig. 2–15A). The examiner must remember that pain may be referred to or from the temporomandibular joint from or to the teeth, neck, or head (Fig. 3–21).

JOINT PLAY MOVEMENTS

The joint play movements of the temporomandibular joints are then determined (Fig. 3–22). Wearing rubber gloves, the examiner places both thumbs on the lower teeth inside the mouth and both index fingers on the mandible outside the mouth. The mandible is then pushed open at the temporomandibular joint, and the examiner can feel the tissue stretch of the joint.

PALPATION

To palpate the temporomandibular joint, the examiner places the finger (padded part anteriorly) in the external auditory canal and asks the patient to actively open and close the mouth. As this is being done, the examiner determines whether both sides are moving simultaneously and whether the movement is smooth. If the patient feels pain on closing, the posterior capsule is usually involved. The freeway space may be palpated in a similar fashion; the examiner's fingers feel the condyle during closing.

The examiner then places the index fingers over the mandibular condyles and feels for elicited pain or tenderness on opening and closing of the mouth. The examiner may also palpate the pterygoid, the temporalis, and the masseter muscles and any other soft tissues for tenderness or indi-

cations of pathology. This procedure is followed by palpation of the following structures:

Mandible. The examiner palpates the mandible along its whole length, feeling for any differences between the left and right sides. As the examiner moves along the superior aspect of the angle of the mandible, the fingers will pass over the parotid gland. Normally, the gland is not palpable, but with pathology (e.g., mumps) the site will feel "boggy" rather than hard and bony, which is normal.

Teeth. The examiner should note the position, absence, or tenderness of the teeth. The examiner wears a rubber glove and palpates inside the mouth. At the same time, the interior cheek region and gums may be palpated for pathology.

Hyoid Bone (Anterior to C2–3 Vertebra). While palpating the hyoid bone (see Figure 2–23), the examiner asks the patient to swallow. Normally, the bone should move and cause no pain. The hyoid bone is part of the superior trachea.

Thyroid Cartilage (Anterior to C4–5 Vertebra). When the neck is in the neutral position, the thyroid cartilage can be easily moved; while in extension, it is tight and the examiner may feel crepitations. The thyroid gland, which is adjacent to the cartilage, may be palpated at the same time. If abnormal or inflamed, it will be tender and enlarged.

Mastoid Processes. The examiner should palpate the skull following the posterior aspect of the ear. The examiner will come to a point on the skull where the finger "dips" inward (see Figure 2–23). The point just prior to the dip is the mastoid process.

Cervical Spine. Beginning on the posterior aspect at the occiput, the examiner should systematically palpate the posterior structures of the neck (spinous processes, facet joints, and muscles of the suboccipital region) working from the head toward the shoulders. On the lateral aspect, the

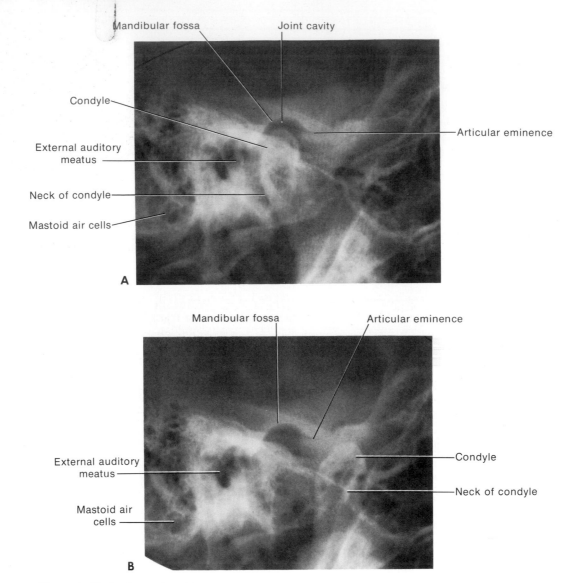

Figure 3–23. Radiographs of the right temporomandibular joint. (*A*) Mouth closed. (*B*) Mouth open. (From Liebgott, B.: The Anatomical Basis of Dentistry. Philadelphia, W. B. Saunders Co., 1982, p. 295. Courtesy of Dr. Fireman.)

transverse processes of the vertebrae, the lymph nodes (palpable only if swollen), and the muscles should be palpated. Anteriorly, the sternocleidomastoid muscles should be palpated for tenderness. A more detailed description of the palpation of these structures is given in Chapter 2.

X-RAY EXAMINATION OF THE TEMPOROMANDIBULAR JOINTS

Anteroposterior View. The examiner should look for condylar shape and normal contours.

Lateral View. The examiner should look for (1) a condylar shape and contours, (2) position of condylar heads in the opened and closed positions (Fig. 3–23), (3) amount of condylar move-

ment (closed versus open), and (4) relation of temporomandibular joint to other bony structures of the skull and cervical spine (Fig. 3–24).

Précis of the Temporomandibular Joint Assessment

History
Observation
Examination
   Active movements
      Neck flexion
      Neck extension
      Neck side flexion (left and right)

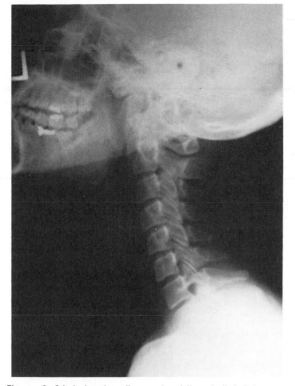

Figure 3–24. Lateral radiograph of the skull, left temporomandibular joint, and cervical spine.

Neck rotation (left and right)
Extend neck by opening mouth
Assess functional opening
Assess freeway space
Open mouth
Close mouth
Measure mandibular length
Measure protrusion of mandible
Measure lateral deviation of mandible (left and right)
Passive movements (as in Active movements, if necessary)
Resisted isometric movements
  Open mouth
  Close mouth
  Lateral deviation of jaw
Special tests
Reflexes and cutaneous distribution
Joint play movements
Palpation
X-ray viewing

Following any examination the patient should always be warned of the possibility of exacerbation of symptoms resulting from the assessment.

REFERENCES

CITED REFERENCE

1. Rocabado, M.: Course notes, Course on temporomandibular joints. Edmonton, Canada, 1979.

GENERAL REFERENCES

Anthony, C. P. and N. J. Kotthoff: Textbook of Anatomy and Physiology. St. Louis, C. V. Mosby Co., 1971.

Crouch, J. E.: Functional Human Anatomy. Philadelphia, Lea & Febiger, 1973.

Dawson, P. E.: Evaluation, Diagnosis, and Treatment of Occlusal Problems. St. Louis, C. V. Mosby Co., 1984.

Eversaul, G. A.: Dental Kinesiology. Las Vegas, G. A. Eversaul, 1977.

Fain, W. D. and J. M. McKinney: The TMJ examination form. J. Craniomandibular Pract. 3:139, 1985.

Gelb, H.: Clinical Management of Head, Neck and TMJ Pain and Dysfunction. Philadelphia, W. B. Saunders Co., 1977.

Gelb, H.: An orthopaedic approach to occlusal imbalance and temporomandibular joint dysfunction. Dent. Clin. North Am. 23:181, 1979.

Gelb, H., and J. Tarte: A two-year clinical dental evaluation of 200 cases of chronic headache: The craniocervical-mandibular syndrome. J. Am. Dent. Assoc. 91:1230, 1975.

Helland, M. M.: Anatomy and function of the temporomandibular joint. J. Orthop. Sports Physical Ther. 1:145–152, 1980.

Hollinshead, W. H., and D. B. Jenkins: Functional Anatomy of the Limbs and Back. Philadelphia, W. B. Saunders Co., 1981.

Hoppenfeld, S.: Physical Examination of the Spine and Extremities. New York, Appleton-Century-Crofts, 1976.

Liebgott, B.: The Anatomical Basis of Dentistry. Philadelphia, W. B. Saunders Co., 1982.

Maitland, G. D.: The Peripheral Joints: Examination and Recording Guide. Adelaide, Australia, Virgo Press, 1973.

Silver, C. M., S. D. Simon, and A. A. Savastano: Meniscus injuries of the temporomandibular joint. J. Bone Joint Surg. 38A:541, 1956.

Thilander, B.: Innervation of the temporomandibular joint capsule in man. Transactions of the Royal Schools of Dentistry No. 7, 1961.

Travell, J.: Temporomandibular joint pain referred muscles of the head & neck. J. Prosthet. Dent. 10:745, 1960.

Travell, J. G., and D. G. Simons: Myofacial Pain and Dysfunction: The Trigger Point Manual. Baltimore, Williams & Wilkins, 1983.

Williams, P., and R. Warwick (eds.): Gray's Anatomy, 36th British ed. Philadelphia, W. B. Saunders Co., 1980.

4

The Shoulder

The prerequisite to any treatment of a patient with pain in the shoulder region is a precise and comprehensive picture of the signs and symptoms as they present at the examination and how they behaved until that time. This knowledge ensures that the techniques used will be suited to the condition and that the degree of success will be estimated against this understood background. Shoulder pain can be due to intrinsic disease of the shoulder joints or pathology in the periarticular structures, or it may originate from the spine, chest, or visceral structures. The shoulder complex is difficult to assess because of its many structures (most of which are located in a small area); its many movements; and the many lesions that can occur either inside or outside the joints. Influences such as referred pain plus the possibility of more than one lesion at one time, as well as the difficulty in deciding what weight to give to each response, make the examination even more difficult to understand. Assessment of the shoulder region often necessitates an evaluation of the cervical spine to rule out referred symptoms, and the examiner must always be prepared to include the cervical spine in any shoulder assessment.

Applied Anatomy

The *glenohumeral joint* is a multiaxial ball-and-socket synovial joint that depends on muscles rather than bones or ligaments for its support and integrity. The *labrum*, which is a ring of fibrocartilage, surrounds and slightly deepens the glenoid cavity of the scapula. Only part of the humeral head is in contact with the glenoid at

any one time. This joint has three axes and three degrees of freedom. The resting position of the glenohumeral joint is 55° of abduction and 30° of horizontal adduction. The close packed position of the joint is full abduction and external rotation. When relaxed, the humerus sits in the upper part of the glenoid cavity; with contraction of the rotator cuff muscles, it is pulled down into the lower, wider part of the glenoid cavity. If this "dropping down" does not occur, full abduction is impossible. The capsular pattern of the glenohumeral joint is lateral rotation most limited, followed by abduction and medial rotation. Branches of the posterior cord and the suprascapular, axillary, and lateral pectoral nerves innervate the joint.

The *acromioclavicular joint* is a plane synovial joint that augments the range of motion in the humerus. The bones making up this joint are the acromion process of the scapula and the lateral end of the clavicle. The joint has two degrees of freedom. The capsule, which is fibrous, surrounds the joint. An articular disc may be found within the joint. Rarely does it separate the acromion and clavicular articular surfaces. This joint depends on ligaments (primarily the acromioclavicular and coracoclavicular) for its strength. In the resting position of the joint, the arm rests by the side in the normal standing position. In the close packed position of the acromioclavicular joint, the arm is abducted to 90°. The indication of a capsular pattern in the joint is pain at the extreme range of motion. This joint is innervated by branches of the suprascapular and lateral pectoral nerve.

The *sternoclavicular joint*, along with the acromioclavicular joint, enables the humerus to move through a full 180° of abduction. It is a saddle-shaped synovial joint with two degrees of freedom and is made up of the medial end of the clavicle, the manubrium sternum, and the cartilage of the first rib. There is a substantial disc between the two bony joint surfaces, and the capsule is thicker anteriorly than posteriorly. The disc separates the articular surfaces of the clavicle and sternum and adds significant strength to the joint because of attachments, thus preventing medial displacement of the clavicle. Like the acromioclavicular joint, it depends on ligaments for its strength. The movements possible at this joint and the acromioclavicular joint are elevation, depression, protrusion, retraction, and rotation. The close packed position of the sternoclavicular joint is full or maximum rotation of the clavicle, which occurs when the upper arm is in full elevation. The resting position and capsular pattern are the same as with the acromioclavicular joint. The joint is innervated by branches of the anterior supraclavicular nerve and the nerve to the subclavius muscle.

Although the *scapulothoracic "joint"* is not a true joint, it does function as an integral part of the shoulder complex and must be considered in any assessment. Some texts call this structure *scapulocostal joint*. This joint consists of the body of the scapula and the muscles covering the posterior chest wall. Because it is not a true joint, it does not have a capsular pattern or a close packed position. The resting position of this joint would be the same as for the acromioclavicular joint.

Patient History

In addition to the general history questions which were presented in Chapter 1, there are a number of questions to be asked that apply to the shoulder.

1. What is the patient unable to do functionally?

2. What is the extent and behavior of the patient's pain? For example, deep, boring, toothache-like pain in the neck and/or shoulder region may be indicative of *thoracic outlet syndrome* (Fig. 4–1). Strains of the rotator cuff usually cause dull toothache, as in pain that is worse at night,

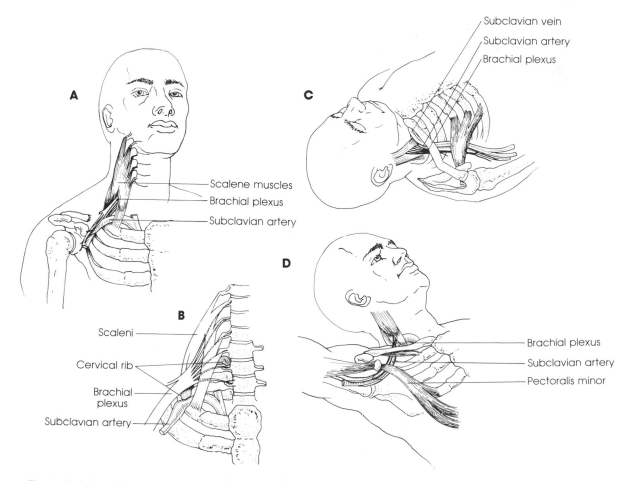

Figure 4–1. Location and causes of thoracic outlet syndrome. (*A*) Scalenus anterior syndrome. (*B*) Cervical rib syndrome. (*C*) Costoclavicular space syndrome. (*D*) Hyperabduction syndrome.

whereas acute calcific tendinitis usually causes a "red-hot," burning type of pain.

3. Are there any movements that cause the patient pain or problems? If so, which ones? The examiner must always keep in mind that cervical spine movements may also cause pain in the shoulder. Persons who have had recurrent dislocations of the shoulder may find that any movement involving lateral rotation will bother them because this movement is involved in anterior dislocations of the shoulder. Acromioclavicular pain is especially evident above 90° abduction.

4. What is the patient's age? Many problems of the shoulder can be age-related. For example, rotator cuff degeneration usually occurs when the patients are in their 40s and 50s. Calcium deposits may occur between the ages of 20 and 40. Chondrosarcomas may be seen in those over the age of 30 years, whereas *frozen shoulder* is seen in individuals between the ages of 45 and 60 if it is due to causes other than trauma.

5. Are there any activities that cause or increase the pain? For example, bicipital tendinitis is often seen in skiers and may be the result of holding on to a ski tow; in cross-country skiing it may be the result of poling (using the pole for propulsion).

6. Do any positions relieve the pain? Patients with nerve root pain may find that elevation of the arm over the head gives relief of symptoms.

7. Is there any indication of muscle spasm, deformity, bruising, wasting, paresthesia, or numbness?

8. If there was an injury, what exactly was the mechanism of injury? Did the patient fall on an outstretched hand, which could potentially indicate a fracture or dislocation of the glenohumeral joint? Did the patient fall on or receive a blow to the tip of the shoulder? This finding may indicate an acromioclavicular dislocation or subluxation.

9. Does the patient support the upper limb or hesitate to move it? This action could mean that one of the joints of the shoulder complex is unstable or that there is an acute problem in the shoulder.

10. How long has the problem bothered the patient? For example, idiopathic frozen shoulder will go through three stages of 3 to 5 months each.[1] The condition becomes progressively worse over a 3- to 5-month period, stays the same for a 3- to 5-month period, and then progressively improves over a 3- to 5-month period.

11. Does the patient complain of the limb feeling weak and heavy after activity? Does the limb tire easily? Are there any *venous* symptoms, such as swelling or stiffness, which may extend all the way to the fingers? Are there any *arterial* symptoms, which may be indicated by coolness or

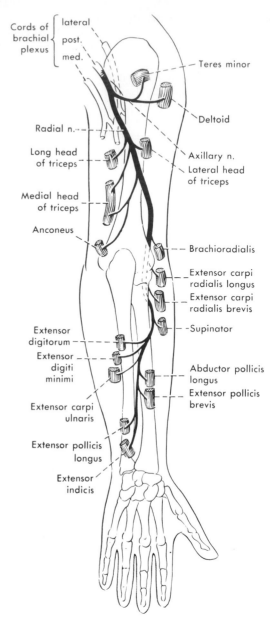

Figure 4–2. Motor distribution of the radial and axillary nerves. (From Hollinshead, W. H., and D. B. Jenkins: Functional Anatomy of the Limbs and Back, 5th ed. Philadelphia, W. B. Saunders Co., 1981, p. 132.)

pallor in the upper limb? These complaints may be the result of pressure on an artery or vein or both. An example is thoracic outlet syndrome (Fig. 4–1), in which pressure may be applied to the vascular and/or neurologic structures as they enter the upper limb in three locations: at the scalene triangle, at the costoclavicular space, and under pectoralis minor and the coracoid process.[2, 3]

12. Is there any indication of nerve injury? The examiner should evaluate the nerves and the muscles supplied by the nerves to determine this.

Any history of weakness, numbness, or paresthesia may indicate nerve injury. For example, the suprascapular nerve may be injured as it passes through the suprascapular notch under the transverse scapular ligament, leading to atrophy and paralysis of the supraspinatus and infraspinatus muscles. The examiner should listen to the history carefully, since this condition could mimic a third-degree (rupture) strain of the supraspinatus tendon. Another potential nerve injury is one to the circumflex (axillary) nerve (Fig. 4–2) following dislocation of the glenohumeral joint. In this case, the deltoid muscle and the teres minor muscle will be atrophied and weak or paralyzed. The radial nerve (Fig. 4–2) is sometimes injured as it winds around the posterior aspect of the shaft of the humerus. The injury is frequently seen when the humeral shaft is fractured. If the nerve is damaged in this location, the extensors of the elbow, wrist, and fingers will be affected as well as an altered sensation in the radial nerve sensory distribution.

13. Which hand is dominant? Often the dominant shoulder will be lower than the nondominant shoulder and the range of motion may not be the same for both. Usually the dominant shoulder will show greater muscularity.

Observation

The patient must be suitably undressed so that the examiner can observe the normal bony and soft-tissue contours of both shoulders and determine whether they are normal and symmetric. When observing the shoulder, the examiner looks at the entire upper limb because the hand may show some vasomotor changes that may be the result of problems in the shoulder. These changes may include shiny skin, loss of hair, swelling, and muscle atrophy.

ANTERIOR VIEW

When looking at the patient from the anterior view (Fig. 4–3), the examiner should begin by ensuring that the head and neck are in the midline of the body, followed by observation of the shoulders. The examiner should look for the possibility of a *step deformity* (Fig. 4–4) over the shoulder area. Such a deformity may be due to an acromioclavicular dislocation, with the distal end of the clavicle lying superior to the acromion process. If the deformity appears when traction is applied to the arm, it may be due to multidirectional instability, leading to inferior subluxation of the glenohumeral joint. This sign is referred to as a *sulcus sign* because of the appearance of a sulcus below the acromion process. Flattening of the normally round deltoid muscle may indicate an anterior dislocation of the glenohumeral joint or paralysis of the deltoid muscle (Fig. 4–5). The examiner should note any abnormal bumps or alignment in the bones that may indicate past injury such as a fracture of the clavicle.

As mentioned earlier, in most individuals the dominant side will be lower than the nondominant side. This difference may be due to the extra use of the dominant side, resulting in the ligaments, joint capsules, and muscles becoming stretched, allowing the arm to "sag" slightly. Individuals such as tennis players[4] and others

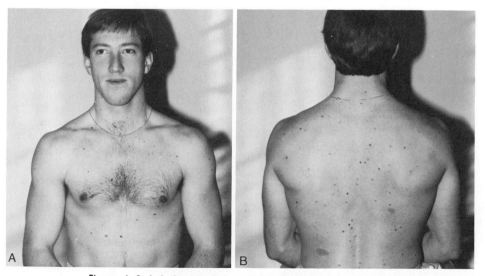

Figure 4–3. Anterior (A) and posterior (B) views of the shoulder.

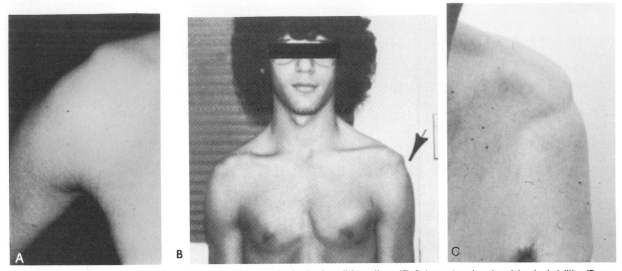

Figure 4–4. (*A*) Step deformity resulting from acromioclavicular dislocation. (*B*) Sulcus sign for shoulder instability. (From Warren, R. F.: Clin. Sports Med. 2:339, 1983.) (*C*) Subluxation of glenohumeral joint following stroke (paralysis of deltoid muscle).

who stretch their upper limbs will show even greater differences along with gross hypertrophy of the muscles on the dominant side (Fig. 4–6).

The examiner notes whether the patient is able to assume the normal functional position for the shoulder, which is forward flexion to 45° and abduction to 60°, with the arm in neutral or no rotation. The examiner should be aware that if the patient's arm is then medially rotated to bring the hand into midline, the biceps tendon is forced against the lesser tuberosity of the medial wall of the bicipital (intertubercular) groove (Fig. 4–7). If this position is maintained for long periods of time, there may be increased wear of the biceps tendon, which may lead to bicipital tendonitis. The bicipital groove may vary in width and depth, possibly leading to problems if the shoulder is overused. Especially wide or deep grooves lead to the greatest problems. The wide grooves tend to allow the tendon too much lateral movement, leading to inflammation; the deep grooves tend to be too narrow, compressing the tendon.[5]

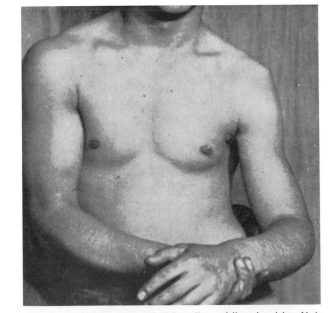

Figure 4–5. Subcoracoid dislocation of the shoulder. Note the prominent acromion, the arm held away from the side, the flat deltoid. (From McLaughlin. Trauma, p. 246.)

POSTERIOR VIEW

When viewing the patient from behind (Fig. 4–3), the examiner again notes bony and soft-tissue contours. The spines of the scapulae, which begin medially at the level of the third (T3) thoracic vertebra, should be at the same angle. The scapula itself should extend from the T2 spinous process to the T7 spinous process of the thoracic vertebrae. The inferior angle of the scapulae should be equidistant from the spine. The examiner should note the possible presence of (1) "winging" of the scapula, a condition in which the medial border moves away from the posterior chest wall (see Fig. 4–14) or (2) *Sprengel's deformity*, which is a congenitally high or undescended scapula (Fig. 4–8).[6, 7] With this deformity, the scapular muscles are poorly developed or replaced by a fibrous band. The condition may be unilateral or bilateral, and the range of the shoulder abduction is decreased, although functional disability may be slight. Usually the scapula is smaller than normal and is medially rotated.

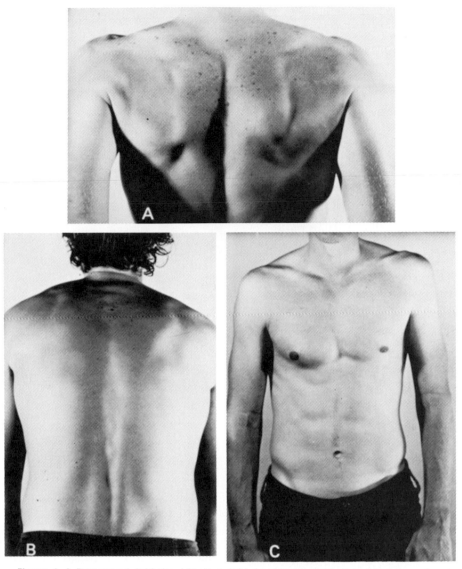

Figure 4–6. Depressed right shoulder in a right dominant individual, in this case, a tennis player. (*A*) Hypertrophy of playing shoulder muscles. (*B*) With muscles relaxed, the distance between spinous processes and medial border of scapula is widened on the right. (*C*) Depressed shoulder. (From Priest, J. D., and D. A. Nagel: Am. J. Sports Med. *4*:33, 1976.)

Figure 4–7. Different shapes of the bicipital groove. (Modified from Hitchcock, H. H., and C. O. Bechtol: J. Bone Joint Surg. *30A*:267, 1948.

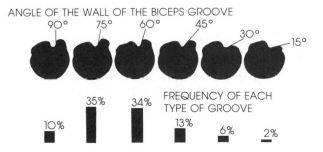

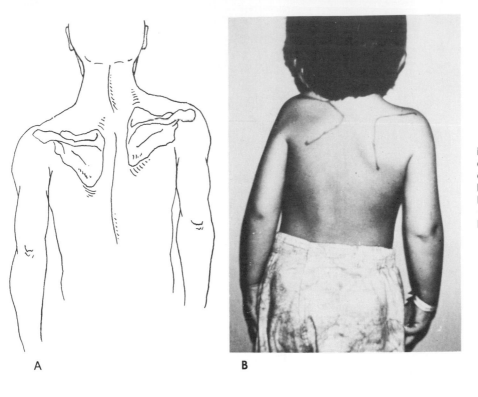

Figure 4–8. Sprengel's deformity. (*A*) Note the elevated shoulder on the right. (*B*) Deformity is on the left. (From Gartland, J. J.: Fundamentals of Orthopaedics. Philadelphia, W. B. Saunders Co., 1979, p. 73. Photo courtesy of Dr. Roshen Irani.)

A   B

Examination

Because assessment of the shoulder may include an assessment of the cervical spine, the examination may be an extensive one. If there is any doubt in the examiner's mind as to the location of the lesion, a cervical spine assessment should be performed.

As with any assessment, the examiner is comparing one side of the body with the other. This comparison is necessary because of the individual differences between normal people.

ACTIVE MOVEMENTS

The first movements to be examined are the active movements. These movements are usually done in such a way that the painful movements are performed last. The movements that should be carried out actively in the shoulder region include:

1. Elevation through abduction (170–180°).
2. Elevation through forward flexion (160–180°).
3. Lateral rotation (80–90°).
4. Medial rotation (60–100°).
5. Extension (50–60°).
6. Adduction (50–75°).
7. Horizontal adduction/abduction (cross flexion/cross extension) (130°).
8. Circumduction (200°).

Active elevation through abduction is normally 170 to 180°. The extreme of the range of motion is found when the arm is abducted and lies against the head on the same side (Fig. 4–9). Active elevation through forward flexion is normally 160 to 180° and is the extreme of the range of motion in the same position as active elevation through abduction. Active lateral rotation is normally 80 to 90°. Care must be taken when applying overpressure because this movement potentially could lead to anterior dislocation of the glenohumeral joint, especially in those with recurrent dislocation problems. Active medial rotation is normally 60 to 100°.

Active extension is normally 50 to 60°. The examiner must ensure that the movement is in the shoulder and not in the spine, since some patients may flex the spine forward, giving the appearance of increased shoulder extension. Adduction is normally 50 to 75° if the arm is brought in front of the body. Horizontal flexion is normally 130°. To accomplish this movement, the patient first abducts the arm to 90° and then moves the arm across the front of the body. Horizontal extension is approximately 45°. After abducting the arm to 90°, the patient moves the straight arm in a backward direction. Circumduc-

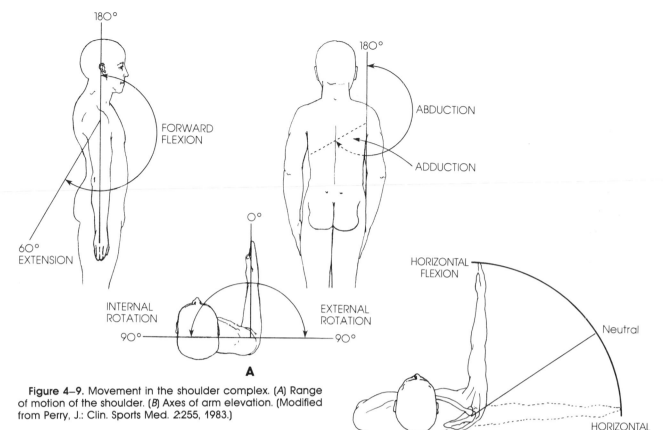

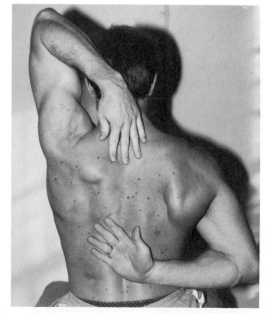

Figure 4–9. Movement in the shoulder complex. (*A*) Range of motion of the shoulder. (*B*) Axes of arm elevation. (Modified from Perry, J.: Clin. Sports Med. 2:255, 1983.)

tion is normally about 200° and involves taking the arm in a circle on the vertical plane.

When examining these movements, the examiner may ask the patient to do the movements in combination. For example, *Apley's scratch test* combines medial rotation with adduction and lateral rotation with abduction (Fig. 4–10). By doing the examination this way, many examiners feel they are decreasing the time taken to do the assessment. As well, by doing the combined movements, the examiner is given some idea of the functional capacity of the patient. For example, in order for one to comb the hair, for a woman to do a back zipper, or for a man to reach his wallet in his back pocket, abduction combined with lateral rotation and adduction combined with medial rotation are needed. When using this method, however, the examiner must take care to notice which movements are restricted and which ones are not, because several movements are performed at the same time. Often, the dominant shoulder will show greater restriction than the nondominant shoulder even in "normal" individuals.

As the patient elevates the upper extremity by abducting the shoulder, the examiner should note whether a painful arc is present (Fig. 4–11).[8] A painful arc may be due to subacromial bursitis, calcium deposits, or a tendinitis of the rotator cuff muscles. The pain is the result of pinching

inflamed or tender structures under the acromion process and the coracoacromial ligament. Initially, the structures are not pinched under the acromion process, so that the patient is able to

Figure 4–10. Apley scratch test. The left arm is in lateral rotation and abduction, and the right arm is in medial rotation and adduction.

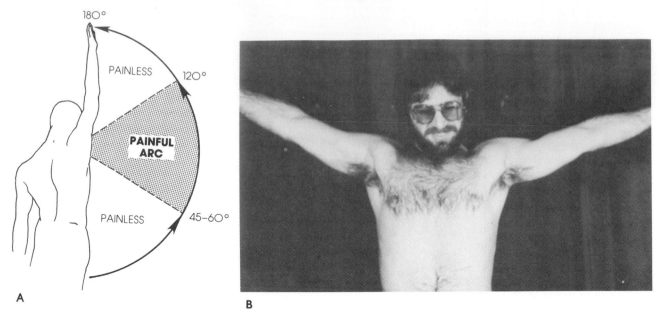

Figure 4–11. Painful arc in the shoulder. (*A*) In the case of acromioclavicular joint problems only, the range 120–180° would elicit pain. (*B*) This athlete demonstrates a painful arc, in this case maximal at approximately 115° of adduction in the coronal plane. This is indicative of impingement. (From Hawkins, R. J., and P. E. Hobeika: Clin. Sports Med. *2*:391, 1983.)

abduct 45 to 60° with little difficulty. As the patient abducts further (60 to 120°), the structures become pinched and the patient is often unable to abduct fully because of pain. If full abduction is possible, however, the pain will diminish after approximately 120° as the pinched soft tissues have passed under the acromion process and are no longer being pinched. Often the pain is greater going up (against gravity) than coming down and there is more pain on active abduction than passive abduction. If the movement is very painful, the individual often elevates the arm through forward flexion in an attempt to decrease the pain. If the examiner finds the pain is greater as

the patient reaches full elevation, this finding would lead the examiner to consider the possibility of an acromioclavicular joint problem. Table 4–1 presents the signs and symptoms of three types of painful arc in the shoulder, with the superior type being the most common. The examiner may find that the arc of pain may also be present during elevation through forward flexion, although the pain is usually less severe on this movement. The interconnection of the subacromial, subcoracoid, and subscapularis bursae with each other and with the glenohumeral joint capsule will often give a broad area of signs and symptoms.

Table 4–1. Classification of Glenohumeral Painful Arcs*

	Anterior	Posterior	Superior
Night pain	Yes	Yes	Maybe
Age	50+	50+	40+
Sex ratio	F > M	F > M	M > F
Aggravated by	Lateral rotation and abduction	Medial rotation and abduction	Abduction
Tenderness	Lesser tuberosity	Posterior aspect of greater tuberosity	Greater tuberosity
Acromioclavicular joint involvement	No	No	Often
Calcification (if present)	Supraspinatus, infraspinatus, and/or subscapularis	Supraspinatus and/or infraspinatus	Supraspinatus and/or subscapularis
Third-degree strain biceps brachii (long-head)	No	No	Occasional
Prognosis	Good	Very good	Poor (without surgery)

*From Kessel, L., and M. Watson: J. Bone Joint Surg. *59B*:166, 1977.[8]

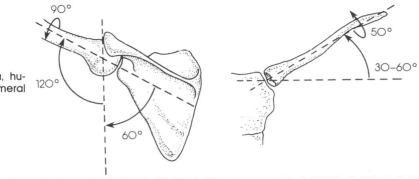

Figure 4–12. Movement of the scapula, humerus, and clavicle during scapulohumeral rhythm.

When examining the movement of elevation through abduction, the examiner must take the time to observe the *scapulohumeral rhythm* (Fig. 4–12) anteriorly and posteriorly.[9, 10] That is, during 180° of abduction, there is a 2:1 ratio of movement of the humerus to the scapula, with 120° of movement occurring at the glenohumeral joint and 60° occurring at the scapulothoracic joint. During this total movement, there are three phases:

1. In the first phase of 30° of movement, the outer end of the clavicle elevates 12 to 15° while the scapula is said to be "setting." This setting phase means that the scapula may rotate in, rotate out, or not move at all. The angle between the scapular spine and the clavicle will also increase 10°, but there will be no rotation of the clavicle.

2. During the next 60° of elevation (second phase), the clavicle will elevate 30 to 36° and there will be a 2:1 ratio of scapulohumeral movement. There is still no rotation of the clavicle at this stage.

3. During the final 90° of motion (third phase), there continues to be a 2:1 ratio of scapulohu-

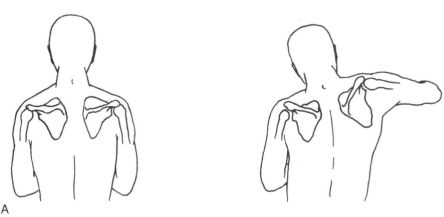

A

Figure 4–13. Reverse scapulohumeral rhythm (notice shoulder hiking). The cause is frozen shoulder (*A*) and tear of rotator cuff (*B*). (B is from Beetham, W. P., et al.: Physical Examination of the Joints. Philadelphia, W. B. Saunders Co., 1965, p. 41.)

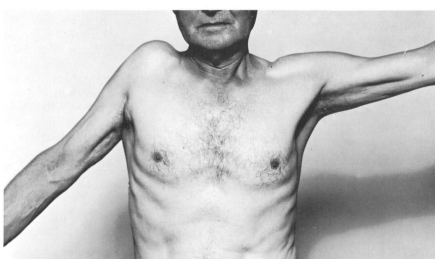

B

meral movement and the angle between the scapular spine and the clavicle increases a further 10°. It is in this stage that the clavicle will rotate posteriorly 30 to 60°. At the same time, the clavicle will rotate upward 50° on a long axis. Also during this final stage, the humerus laterally rotates 90° so that the greater tuberosity of the humerus avoids the acromion process.

If the clavicle does not rotate and elevate, elevation through abduction at the glenohumeral joint is limited to 120°. If the glenohumeral joint does not move, elevation through abduction is limited to 60°, which occurs totally in the scapulothoracic joint. If there is no lateral rotation of the humerus during abduction, the total movement available is 120°, 60° of which occurs at the glenohumeral joint and 60° of which occurs at the scapulothoracic articulation. The normal end of range of motion is reached when there is contact of a surgical neck of humerus against the acromion process. *Reverse scapulohumeral rhythm* (Fig. 4–13) means that the scapula moves more than the humerus. This is seen in conditions such as frozen shoulder; the patient appears to "hitch" the whole shoulder complex rather than produce a smooth coordinated abduction movement.

It must be remembered that the biceps tendon does not move in the bicipital groove during movement but that the humerus moves over the fixed tendon. From adduction to full elevation of abduction, a given point in the groove moves along the tendon at least 4 cm. If the examiner wanted to keep excursion of the biceps tendon to a minimum, the arm should be elevated with the humerus in medial rotation. Elevation of the arm with the humerus laterally rotated causes maximum excursion of the biceps tendon.

As the patient does the various movements, the examiner watches to see whether the various components of the shoulder complex move in normal sequence and whether the patient exhibits any apprehension when doing the movement. Any apprehension suggests the possibility of instability. The examiner should also watch for winging of the scapula, which is indicative of injury to the serratus anterior muscle or the long thoracic nerve. If the scapula appears to wing, the examiner asks the patient to forward flex the shoulder to 90°. The examiner then pushes the straight arm toward the patient's body while the patient resists. If there is weakness of the serratus anterior muscle or its nerve, this movement will cause the scapula to wing, which means the medial border of the scapula will move away from the chest wall and protrude posteriorly. Winging of the scapula may also be tested by having the patient standing and leaning against the wall. The patient is then asked to do a "push-

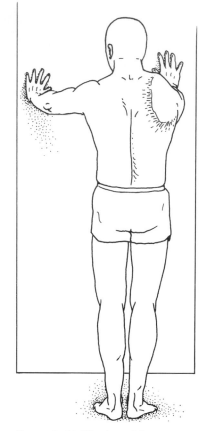

Figure 4–14. Winging of the scapula.

up" away from the wall while the examiner watches for possible winging of the scapula (Fig. 4–14).

Injury to other nerves in the shoulder region must not be overlooked. As previously mentioned, damage to the suprascapular nerve will affect the supraspinatus and infraspinatus muscles, whereas injury to the musculocutaneous nerve will lead to paralysis of the coracobrachialis, biceps, and brachialis muscles. These changes will affect elbow flexion and supination and forward flexion of the shoulder. There will also be a loss of the biceps reflex. Injury to the circumflex (axillary) nerve will lead to paralysis of the deltoid and teres minor muscles, thus affecting abduction and lateral rotation of the shoulder. There will also be a sensory loss over the deltoid insertion area. Damage to the radial nerve will affect all the extensor muscles of the upper limb. In the shoulder, the triceps muscles may be paralyzed so that the patient will be unable to actively extend the elbow against gravity.

PASSIVE MOVEMENTS

If, during the active movements, the range of motion is not full and the examiner is unable to

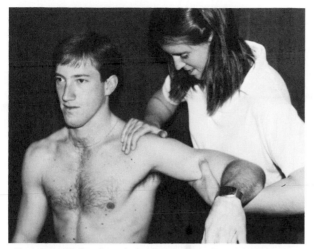

Figure 4–15. Passive abduction of the glenohumeral joint.

test the end feel, all passive movements of the shoulder should be performed to determine the end feel and passive range of motion. These movements include:

1. Elevation through forward flexion of the arm.
2. Elevation through abduction of the arm.
3. Elevation through abduction of the glenohumeral joint only (Fig. 4–15).
4. Lateral rotation of the arm.
5. Medial rotation of the arm.
6. Extension of the arm.
7. Adduction of the arm.
8. Horizontal adduction/abduction of the arm.
9. Quadrant test.

Particular attention is paid to the passive medial and lateral rotation if the examiner suspects a problem with the glenohumeral joint capsule. The examiner must remember that *subcoracoid*

bursitis may limit full lateral rotation while *subacromial bursitis* may limit full abduction because of compression or pinching of these structures. Even if overpressure on active movement has been applied, it is still necessary for the examiner to perform elevation through abduction of the glenohumeral joint only and the Quadrant test. The examiner should find these end feels on passive movements of the shoulder:

1. Elevation through forward flexion: tissue stretch.
2. Elevation through abduction: bone to bone or tissue stretch.
3. Lateral rotation: tissue stretch.
4. Medial rotation: tissue stretch.
5. Extension: tissue stretch.
6. Adduction: tissue approximation or tissue stretch.
7. Horizontal adduction: tissue stretch.
8. Horizontal abduction: tissue approximation.
9. Elevation through abduction of glenohumeral joint: bone to bone or tissue stretch.

To test the *quadrant position*,[11] the examiner stabilizes the scapula and clavicle by placing the forearm under the patient's scapula of the arm to be tested and the hand extends over the shoulder to hold the trapezius muscle to prevent shoulder shrugging (Fig. 4–16). To test the position, the upper limb is elevated to rest alongside the patient's head with the shoulder externally rotated. The patient's shoulder is then adducted. As adduction occurs on the coronal plane, a point (quadrant position) will be reached where the arm will move forward slightly from the coronal plane. At approximately 60° of adduction (from the arm beside the head), this position of maximum forward movement will occur even if a backward pressure is applied. As the shoulder is

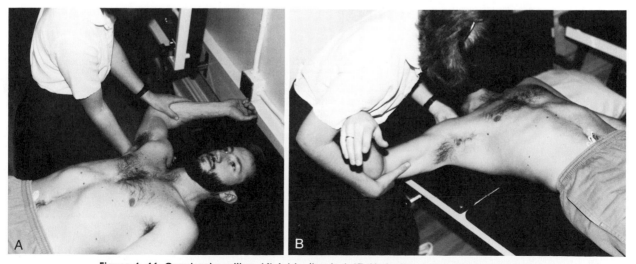

Figure 4–16. Quadrant position. (*A*) Adduction test. (*B*) Abduction test (locked quadrant).

further adducted, it will fall back to the same coronal plane as previously. The quadrant position indicates the position at which the arm has medially rotated during its descent to the patient's side. When doing the movement, the examiner not only should feel the movement but also should determine the quality of the movement.

Similarly, the quadrant position may be found by abducting the medially rotated shoulder while maintaining extension. In this case, the quadrant position is reached (approximately 120° abduction) when the shoulder will no longer abduct because it is prevented from laterally rotating. This position is referred to as the *locked quadrant position*. If the arm is allowed to move forward, lateral rotation will occur and full abduction can be achieved. In addition to these movements, passive elevation through abduction of the glenohumeral joint with the clavicle and scapula fixed is also performed by the examiner to determine the amount of abduction in the glenohumeral joint alone. Normally this movement should be 120°.

The *capsular pattern* of the shoulder is lateral rotation showing the greatest restriction, followed by abduction and medial rotation. Each of these movements has a capsular end feel. Other movements may be limited, but not in the same order and not with as much restriction. Finding of limitation, but not in the order described, is indicative of a *noncapsular pattern*.

RESISTED ISOMETRIC MOVEMENTS

Having completed the active and passive movements, which are done in standing, sitting or lying supine (in the case of Quadrant test), the patient lies supine to do the resisted isometric movements (Fig. 4–17). During the active movements, the examiner should have noted which movements caused discomfort or pain so that this

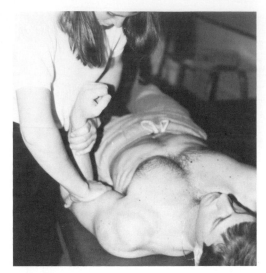

Figure 4–17. Positioning of the patient for resisted isometric movements.

information can be correlated with those of resisted isometric movements. By carefully noting which movements cause pain when doing the tests isometrically, the examiner should be able to determine which muscle or muscles are at fault (Table 4–2). For example, if the patient experiences pain primarily on medial rotation, but also on abduction and adduction, a suspected problem would be in the subscapularis muscle, since the other muscles involved in these actions are involved in actions that were found to be pain-free. To do the resisted isometric tests, the examiner positions the patient's arm at the side with the elbow flexed to 90°. The movements tested isometrically are:

1. Forward flexion of the shoulder.
2. Extension of the shoulder.
3. Adduction of the shoulder.
4. Abduction of the shoulder.
5. Medial rotation of the shoulder.
6. Lateral rotation of the shoulder.

Table 4–2. Muscles About the Shoulder: Their Actions and Nerve Supply (Including Nerve Root Deviation)

Action	Muscles Performing Action	Nerve Supply	Nerve Root Deviation
Forward flexion	1. Deltoid (anterior fibers)	Circumflex (axillary)	C5, C6 (posterior cord)
	2. Pectoralis major (clavicular fibers)	Lateral pectoral	C5, C6 (lateral cord)
	3. Coracobrachialis	Musculocutaneous	C5, C6, C7 (lateral cord)
	4. Biceps (when strong contraction required)	Musculocutaneous	C5, C6, C7 (lateral cord)
Extension	1. Deltoid (posterior fibers)	Circumflex (axillary)	C5, C6 (posterior cord)
	2. Teres major	Subscapular	C5, C6 (posterior cord)
	3. Teres minor	Circumflex (axillary)	C5, C6 (posterior cord)
	4. Latissimus dorsi	Thoracodorsal	C6, C7, C8 (posterior cord)
	5. Pectoralis major (sternocostal fibers)	Lateral pectoral	C5, C6 (lateral cord)
		Medial pectoral	C8, T1 (medial cord)
	6. Triceps (long head)	Radial	C5, C6, C7, C8, T1 (posterior cord)

Table continued on following page

Table 4–2. Muscles About the Shoulder: Their Actions and Nerve Supply
(Including Nerve Root Deviation) *(Continued)*

Action	Muscles Performing Action	Nerve Supply	Nerve Root Deviation
Horizontal adduction	1. Pectoralis major 2. Deltoid (anterior fibers)	Lateral pectoral Circumflex (axillary)	C5, C6 (lateral cord) C5, C6 (posterior cord)
Horizontal abduction	1. Deltoid (posterior fibers) 2. Teres major 3. Teres minor 4. Infraspinatus	Circumflex (axillary) Subscapular Circumflex (axillary) Suprascapular	C5, C6 (posterior cord) C5, C6 (posterior cord) C5, C6 (brachial plexus trunk) C5, C6 (brachial plexus trunk)
Abduction	1. Deltoid 2. Supraspinatus 3. Infraspinatus 4. Subscapularis 5. Teres minor 6. Long head of biceps (if arm externally rotated first, trick movement)	Circumflex (axillary) Suprascapular Suprascapular Subscapular Circumflex (axillary) Musculocutaneous	C5, C6 (posterior cord) C5, C6 (brachial plexus trunk) C5, C6 (brachial plexus trunk) C5, C6 (posterior cord) C5, C6 (posterior cord) C5, C6, C7 (lateral cord)
Adduction	1. Pectoralis major 2. Latissimus dorsi 3. Teres major 4. Subscapularis	Lateral pectoral Thoracodorsal Subscapular Subscapular	C5, C6 (lateral cord) C6, C7, C8 (posterior cord) C5, C6 (posterior cord) C5, C6 (posterior cord)
Medial rotation	1. Pectoralis major 2. Deltoid (anterior fibers) 3. Latissimus dorsi 4. Teres major 5. Subscapularis (when arm is by side)	Lateral pectoral Circumflex (axillary) Thoracodorsal Subscapular Subscapular	C5, C6 (lateral cord) C5, C6 (posterior cord) C6, C7, C8 (posterior cord) C5, C6 (posterior cord) C5, C6 (posterior cord)
Lateral rotation	1. Infraspinatus 2. Deltoid (posterior fibers) 3. Teres minor	Suprascapular Circumflex (axillary) Circumflex (axillary)	C5, C6 (brachial plexus trunk) C5, C6 (posterior cord) C5, C6 (posterior cord)
Elevation of scapula	1. Trapezius (upper fibers) 2. Levator scapulae 3. Rhomboid major 4. Rhomboid minor	Accessory C3, C4 nerve roots C3, C4 nerve roots Dorsal scapular Dorsal scapular Dorsal scapular	Cranial nerve XI C3, C4 C5 (C4), C5 (C4), C5
Depression of scapula	1. Serratus anterior 2. Pectoralis major 3. Pectoralis minor 4. Latissimus dorsi 5. Trapezius (lower fibers)	Long thoracic Lateral pectoral Medial pectoral Thoracodorsal Accessory C3, C4 nerve roots	C5, C6, (C7) C5, C6 (lateral cord) C8, T1 (medial cord) C6, C7, C8 (posterior cord) Cranial nerve XI C3, C4
Protraction (forward movement) of scapula	1. Serratus anterior 2. Pectoralis major 3. Pectoralis minor 4. Latissimus dorsi	Long thoracic Lateral pectoral Medial pectoral Thoracodorsal	C5, C6 (C7) C5, C6 (lateral cord) C8, T1 (medial cord) C6, C7, C8 (posterior cord)
Retraction (backward movement) of scapula	1. Trapezius 2. Rhomboid major 3. Rhomboid minor	Accessory Dorsal scapular Dorsal scapular	Cranial nerve XI (C4) C5 (C4) C5
Lateral (upward) rotation of inferior angle of scapula	1. Trapezius (upper and lower fibers) 2. Serratus anterior	Accessory C3, C4 nerve roots Long thoracic	Cranial nerve XI C3, C4 C5, C6, (C7)
Medial (downward) rotation of inferior angle of scapula	1. Levator scapulae 2. Rhomboid major 3. Rhomboid minor 4. Pectoralis minor	C3, C4 nerve roots Dorsal scapular Dorsal scapular Dorsal scapular Medial pectoral	C3, C4 C5 (C4), C5 (C4), C5 C8, T1 (medial cord)
Flexion of elbow	1. Brachialis 2. Biceps brachii 3. Brachioradialis 4. Pronator teres 5. Flexor carpi ulnaris	Musculocutaneous Musculocutaneous Radial Median Ulnar	C5, C6, (C7) C5, C6 C5, C6, (C7) C6, C7 C7, C8
Extension of elbow	1. Triceps 2. Anconeus	Radial Radial	C6, C7, C8 C7, C8, (T1)

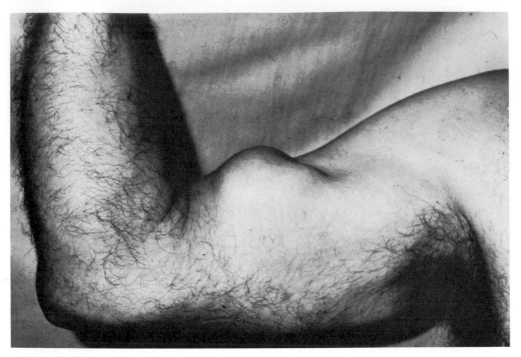

Figure 4–18. Rupture of the long head of the biceps brachii caused by the patient's awkward catch of partner in gymnastics. Bunching of muscle is attended by complete loss of function of the long head. (From O'Donoghue, D. H.: Treatment of Injuries to Athletes, 4th ed. Philadelphia, W. B. Saunders Co., 1984, p. 53.)

7. Flexion of the elbow.
8. Extension of the elbow.

Resisted isometric elbow flexion and extension must be performed because some of the muscles act over the elbow as well as the shoulder. The examiner should watch for the possibility of a third-degree strain (rupture) of the long head of biceps tendon when testing isometric elbow flexion (Fig. 4–18).

SPECIAL TESTS

Only those special tests believed by the examiner to have relevance should be done.

Yergason's Test. With the patient's elbow flexed to 90° and stabilized against the thorax with the forearm pronated, the examiner resists supination while the patient laterally rotates the arm against resistance (Fig. 4–19).[12] A positive

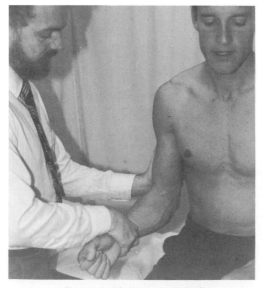

Figure 4–19. Yergason's test.

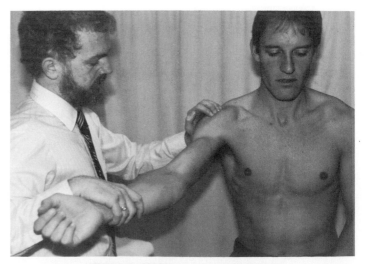

Figure 4–20. Biceps test (Speed's test).

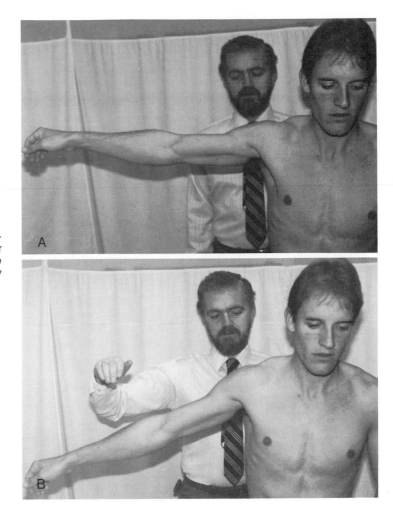

Figure 4–21. Drop-arm test. (*A*) The patient abducts the arm to 90°. (*B*) The patient tries to lower the arm slowly and is unable to do so; instead, the arm drops to his side. Examiner's hand is simply illustrating the start position.

result elicits tenderness in the bicipital groove, or the tendon may pop out of the groove and is indicative of bicipital tendinitis. This test is not a particularly effective one, since the tendon does not move in the bicipital groove during the test and biceps tendon pain tends to occur on motion rather than on tension.

Speed's Test (Biceps Test). The examiner resists shoulder forward flexion by the patient while the patient's forearm is supinated and the elbow is completely extended (Fig. 4–20). A positive test elicits increased tenderness in the bicipital groove and is indicative of bicipital tendinitis. Speed's test is more effective than Yergason's test because the bone moves over the tendon during the test.

Drop-Arm Test. The examiner abducts the patient's shoulder to 90° and then asks the patient to slowly lower it to the side in the same arc of movement (Fig. 4–21). A positive test is indicated if the patient is unable to return the arm to the side slowly or has severe pain when attempting to do so. A positive result indicates a tear in the rotator cuff complex.

Ludington's Test. The patient clasps both hands on top of the head, allowing the interlocking fingers to support the weight of upper limbs (Fig. 4–22). This action allows maximum relaxation of the biceps tendon in its resting position. The patient then alternately contracts and relaxes the biceps muscles. While the patient does the contractions and relaxations, the examiner palpates the biceps tendons, which will be felt on the

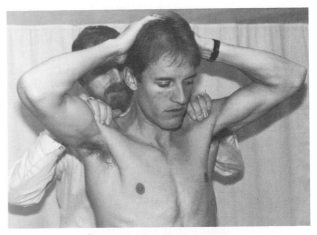

Figure 4–22. Ludington's test.

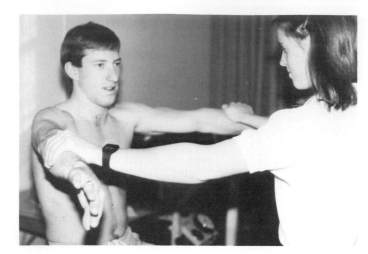

Figure 4-23. Supraspinatus test.

uninvolved side but not on the affected side if
the test result is positive. A positive result indicates a rupture of the long head of biceps tendon.

Supraspinatus Test. The patient's shoulder is
abducted to 90° with neutral (no) rotation and
resistance to abduction is given by the examiner
(Fig. 4–23). The shoulder is then medially rotated
and angled forward 30° so that the patient's
thumbs point toward the floor. Resistance to abduction is again given while the examiner looks
for weakness or pain, reflecting a positive test
result. A positive test result indicates a tear of the
supraspinatus tendon or muscle.

Impingement Sign. The patient's arm is forcibly
abducted through forward flexion by the examiner
causing a "jamming" of the greater tuberosity
against the anteroinferior acromial surface.[13] The
patient's face will show pain, reflecting a positive
test result (Fig. 4–24). The test is indicative of an
overuse injury to the supraspinatus and sometimes to the biceps tendon.

Transverse Humeral Ligament Test. The patient's shoulder is abducted and medially rotated
by the examiner. The examiner's fingers are then
placed along the bicipital groove and the patient's
shoulder is laterally rotated. If the examiner feels
the tendon snap in and out of the groove as the
lateral rotation occurs, this is an indication of a
positive test result. A positive result is indicative
of a torn transverse humeral ligament.

**Apprehension Test for Anterior Shoulder Dis-
location.** The examiner abducts and laterally rotates the patient's shoulder slowly (Fig. 4–25). A
positive test is indicated by a look or feeling of
apprehension or alarm on the patient's face, and
the patient will resist further motion. The patient
may also state that this is what it felt like when
the shoulder was previously dislocated. It is imperative that this test be done slowly. If the test
is done too quickly, there is always the chance
that the humerus will dislocate.

Posterior Apprehension Test. The examiner

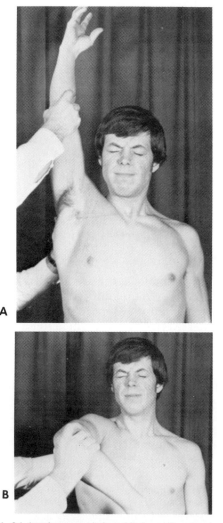

Figure 4-24. Impingement sign. (*A*) A positive impingement
sign is present if pain and its resulting facial expression are
produced when the arm is forcibly flexed forward by the
examiner, jamming the greater tuberosity against the anteroinferior surface of the acromium. (*B*) An alternative method
of demonstrating the impingement sign is by forcibly internally
rotating the proximal humerus when the arm is forward flexed
to 90°. (From Hawkins, R. J., and J. C. Kennedy: Am. J. Sports
Med. *8*:391, 1980.

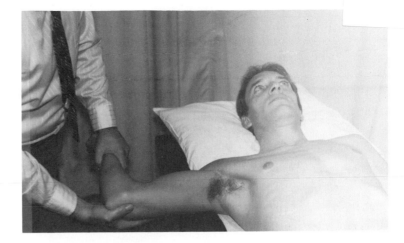

Figure 4–25. Anterior apprehension test.

forward flexes and medially rotates the patient's shoulder (Fig. 4–26). The examiner then applies a posterior force on the patient's elbow. A positive result is indicated by a look or feeling of apprehension or alarm on the patient's face, and the patient will resist further motion. The test is indicative of a posterior dislocation of the humerus.

Allen Maneuver. The examiner flexes the patient's elbow to 90° while the shoulder is extended horizontally and laterally rotated (Fig. 4–27). The patient then rotates the head away from the test side. The examiner palpates the radial pulse, which will become absent (disappear) when the head is rotated away from the test side. This indicates a positive test result for *thoracic outlet syndrome*. It must be remembered that when doing any thoracic outlet test that the examiner must find the pulse before positioning the patient and that even in a "normal" individual, the pulse may be diminished.

Adson Maneuver. This is probably the most common means of testing for thoracic outlet syndrome. The patient's head is rotated to face the tested shoulder (Fig. 4–28). The patient then extends the head while the examiner laterally rotates and extends the patient's shoulder. The examiner locates the radial pulse, and the patient is instructed to take a deep breath and hold it. A disappearance of the pulse is indicative of a positive test.

Halstead Maneuver. The examiner finds the radial pulse and applies a downward traction on the tested extremity while the patient's neck is hyperextended and the head rotated to the opposite side (Fig. 4–29). Absence or disappearance of a pulse indicates a positive test for thoracic outlet syndrome.

Costoclavicular Syndrome Test. The examiner palpates the radial pulse while then drawing the patient's shoulder down and back (Fig. 4–30). A positive test is indicated by an absence of the pulse and possibly thoracic outlet syndrome. This test is particularly effective in patients who complain of symptoms while wearing a backpack or heavy coat.

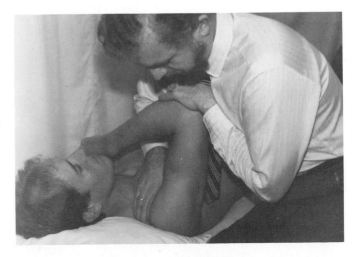

Figure 4–26. Posterior apprehension test.

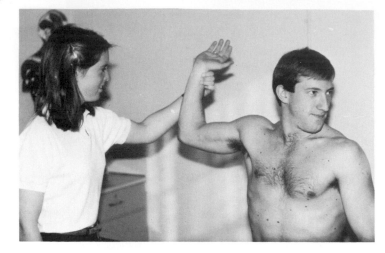

Figure 4–27. Allen maneuver.

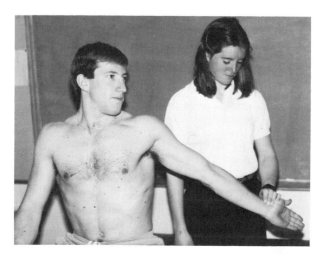

Figure 4–28. Adson maneuver.

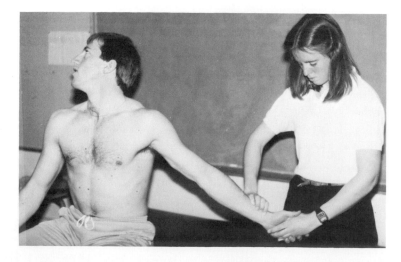

Figure 4–29. Halstead maneuver.

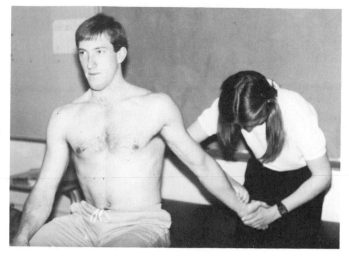

Figure 4–30. Costoclavicular syndrome test.

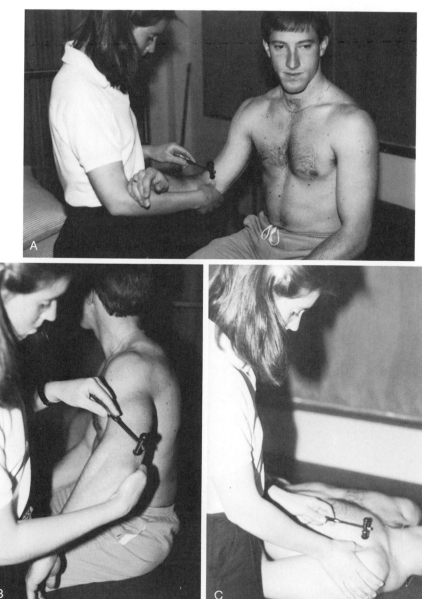

Figure 4–31. Positioning to test the reflexes about the shoulder. (*A*) Biceps. (*B*) Triceps. (*C*) Pectoralis major.

REFLEXES AND CUTANEOUS DISTRIBUTION

The reflexes that are often assessed in the shoulder region include the pectoralis major (C6–C7), the biceps (C5–C6), and the triceps (C7) (Fig. 4–31). The examiner must also be aware of the dermatomal patterns of the nerve roots (Fig. 4–32) as well as the cutaneous distribution of the peripheral nerves (Fig. 4–33). The examiner should remember that dermatomes will vary from person to person; thus, the accompanying diagrams are estimations only. A test for altered sensation is performed by running the relaxed hands and fingers over the neck, shoulder, and anterior and posterior chest area. Any difference in sensation should be noted. These differences can be mapped out more exactly using a pinwheel, pin, cotton batting, and/or brush.

True shoulder pain rarely extends below the

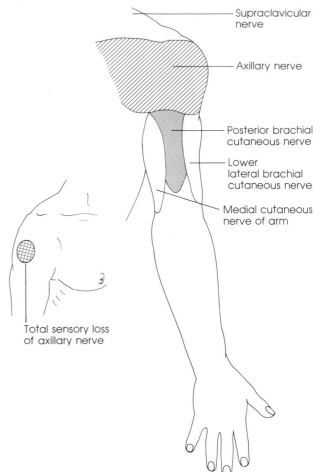

Figure 4–33. Cutaneous distribution of peripheral nerves about the shoulder.

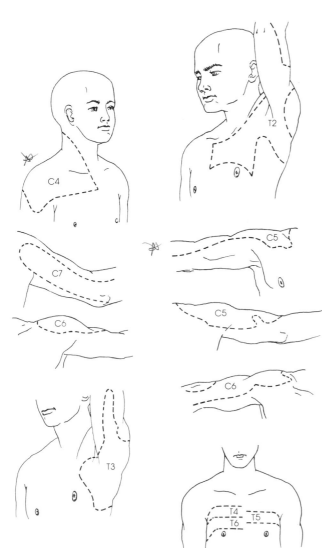

Figure 4–32. Dermatomal pattern of the shoulder. Dermatomes on one side only are illustrated.

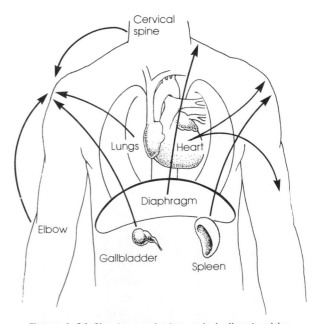

Figure 4–34. Structures referring pain to the shoulder.

elbow. Pain in the acromioclavicular and sterno-clavicular joints tends to be localized to the affected joint and usually does not spread or radiate. Pain can be referred to the shoulder from many structures,[14] including the cervical spine, elbow, lungs, heart, diaphragm, gallbladder, and spleen (Fig. 4–34).

JOINT PLAY MOVEMENTS

Joint play movements[11, 15] are usually performed with the patient lying supine. The examiner compares the amount of available movement on the affected side with the movement on the unaffected side.

The joint play movements performed at the shoulder are shown in Figure 4–35 and include the following:

1. Backward glide of the humerus.
2. Forward glide of the humerus.
3. Lateral distraction of the humerus.
4. Caudal glide of the humerus (long arm traction).
5. Backward glide of the humerus in abduction.
6. Lateral distraction of the humerus in abduction.
7. Anteroposterior and cephalocaudal movement of the clavicle at the acromioclavicular joint.
8. Anteroposterior and cephalocaudal movement of the clavicle at the sternoclavicular joint.
9. General movement of the scapula to determine mobility.

To perform the backward joint play movement of the humerus, the examiner grasps the patient's upper limb, placing one hand around the humerus as high up in the axilla as possible. The other hand is placed around the humerus above and near the elbow (Fig. 4–35A). The examiner then applies a backward force, keeping the patient's arm parallel to the body so that no rotation or torsion occurs at the glenohumeral joint.

Forward joint play movement of the humerus is carried out in a similar fashion, with the examiner's hands, as shown in Figure 4–35B. The examiner applies an anterior force, keeping the patient's arm parallel to the body so that no rotation or torsion occurs at the glenohumeral joint.

To apply a lateral distraction joint play movement to the humerus, the examiner places his or her hands, as shown in Figure 4–35C. Then a lateral distraction force is applied to the glenohumeral joint, with the patient's arm kept parallel to the body so that no rotation or torsion occurs at the glenohumeral joint.

Caudal glide joint play movement is performed with the patient in the same supine position. The examiner grasps above the patient's wrist with one hand and palpates below the distal spine of the scapula posteriorly and below the icle anteriorly over the glenohumera with the other hand (Fig. 4–35E). The exam then applies a traction force to the shoulder while palpating to see whether the head of the humerus drops down (moves distally) in the glenoid cavity as it normally should. If the patient complains of pain in the elbow, the test may be done with the hands positioned as in Figure 4–35D.

The examiner then abducts the patient's arm to 90°, grasping above the patient's wrist with one hand while stabilizing the thorax with the other hand. The examiner then applies a "long arm" traction force to determine joint play in this position.

With the patient's arm abducted to 90°, the examiner then grasps the humerus with both hands as close to the thorax as possible and applies a backward force, keeping the patient's arm parallel to the body. This movement is a backward joint play movement of the humerus in abduction (Fig. 4–35F).

To assess the acromioclavicular and sternoclavicular joints, the examiner gently grasps the clavicle as close to the joint to be tested as possible and moves it in and out and up and down while palpating the joint with the other hand. A comparison of the amount of movement available is made between the two sides (Fig. 4–35G and H).

For a determination of mobility of the scapula, the patient lies on one side to fixate the thorax with the arm relaxed by the side. The uppermost scapula is tested in this position. The examiner faces the patient, placing the lower hand (farthest from the head) under the patient's arm so that the patient's arm rests on the examiner's forearm. The hand of the examiner's same arm holds the upper (cranial) dorsal surface of the patient's scapula. By holding the scapula in this way, the examiner is able to move it medially, laterally, caudally, cranially, and away from the thorax (Fig. 4–35I).

PALPATION

When palpating the shoulder complex, the examiner should note any muscle spasm, tenderness, abnormal "bumps," or other signs and symptoms that may indicate the source of pathology. The examiner should perform palpation in a systematic manner, beginning with the anterior structures and working around to the posterior structures. Findings on the injured side should be compared with those on the unaffected, or "uninjured," side. Any differences between the two sides should be noted, since they may give an indication of the cause of the patient's problems.

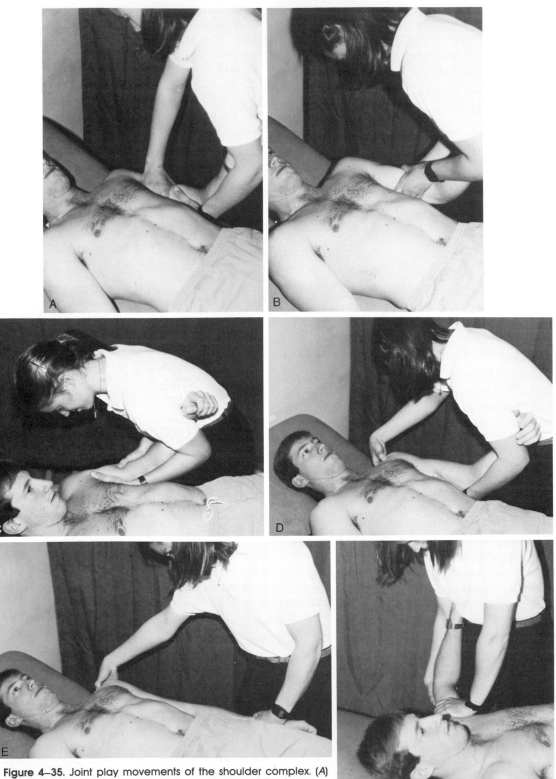

Figure 4–35. Joint play movements of the shoulder complex. (*A*) Backward glide of the humerus. (*B*) Forward glide of the humerus. (*C*) Lateral distraction of the humerus. (*D*) Long arm traction. (*E*) Long arm traction applied below elbow. (*F*) Backward glide of the humerus in abduction.

Illustration continued on opposite page.

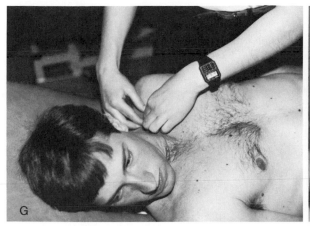

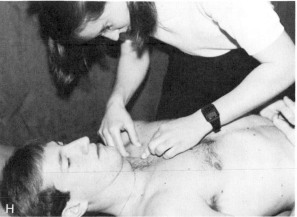

Figure 4–35 *Continued.* (*G*) Joint play of the acromioclavicular joint. (*H*) Joint play of the sternoclavicular joint. (*I*) General movement of the scapula to determine mobility.

Anterior Structures

The anterior structures of the shoulder may be palpated with the patient supine lying, or sitting (Fig. 4–36A).

Clavicle. The clavicle should be palpated along its full length for tenderness or abnormal bumps, such as a callus formation following a fracture, and to ensure that it is in its resting position relative to the uninjured side. That is, it may be rotated anteriorly or posteriorly more than the unaffected side or one end may be higher than that of the uninjured side, indicating a possible subluxation or dislocation at the sternoclavicular or acromioclavicular joint.

Sternoclavicular Joint. The sternoclavicular joint should be palpated for normal positioning relative to the sternum and first rib. Palpation should also include supporting ligaments and sternocleidomastoid muscle. Adjacent to the joint, the suprasternal notch may be palpated. From the notch, the examiner moves the fingers laterally and posteriorly to palpate the first rib. The examiner should apply slight caudal pressure to the first rib on both sides and note any difference. Spasm of the scalene muscles or pathology in the area may result in elevation of the first rib on the affected side.

Acromioclavicular Joint. Like the sternoclavicular joint, the acromioclavicular joint should be palpated for normal positioning and tenderness. Likewise, supporting ligaments (acromioclavicular and coracoclavicular) and the trapezius, subclavius, and deltoid (anterior, middle, and posterior fibers) muscles should be palpated for tenderness and spasm.

Coracoid Process. The coracoid process may be palpated approximately 2.5 cm below the junction of the lateral one third and medial two thirds of the clavicle. The short head of the biceps and coracobrachialis muscles originate from, and pectoralis minor inserts into, this process.

Sternum. In the midline of the chest, the examiner should palpate the three portions of the sternum (manubrium, body, and xiphoid process), noting any abnormality or tenderness.

Ribs and Costal Cartilage. Adjacent to the sternum, the examiner should palpate the sternocostal and costochondral articulations, noting any swelling, tenderness, or other abnormality. These "articulations" are sometimes sprained or subluxed or a costochondritis (Tietze's syndrome) may be evident. The examiner should palpate the ribs as they extend around the chest wall, looking for any potential pathology.

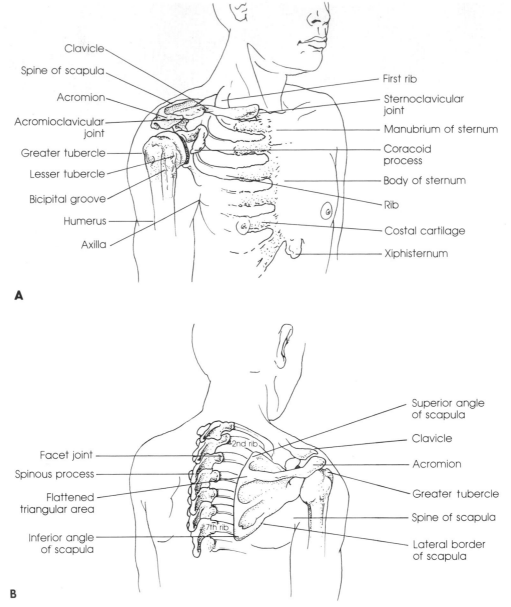

Figure 4–36. Landmarks of the shoulder region. (*A*) Anterior view. (*B*) Posterior view.

Humerus and Rotator Cuff Muscles. Moving laterally from the chest and caudally from the acromion process, the examiner should palpate the humerus and its surrounding structures for potential pathology. The examiner first palpates the lateral tip of the acromion process and then moves inferiorly to the greater tuberosity of the humerus. The examiner should then laterally rotate the humerus. During palpation, the long head of the biceps in the bicipital groove will slip under the fingers, followed by the lesser tuberosity of the humerus (Fig. 4–37). As with all palpation, the testing should be done gently and carefully to prevent causing the patient undue pain. By alternately laterally and medially rotating the humerus, the smooth progression over the three structures will normally be noted. It will also be noted that the lesser tuberosity is at the level of the coracoid process. If the examiner then palpates along the lesser tuberosity and the lip of the bicipital groove, the fingers will rest on the tendon of subscapularis muscle. Moving laterally over the bicipital groove to its other lip, the examiner may then palpate the insertion of pectoralis major muscle. The patient is then asked to further medially rotate the humerus so that the forearm rests behind the back, and the examiner palpates just inferior to the anterior aspect of the acromion process for the supraspinatus tendon. Any tenderness of the tendon should be noted. The examiner then passively abducts the patient's shoulder to 80 to 90° and palpates the notch

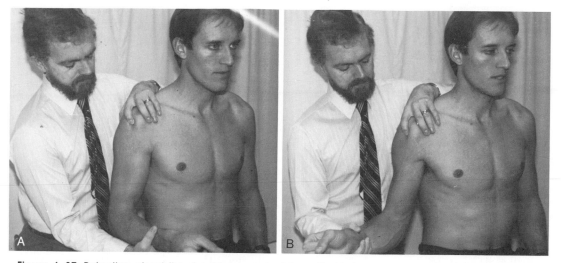

Figure 4–37. Palpation about the shoulder—greater tuberosity (A), bicipital groove, and lesser tuberosity (B).

formed by the acromion-spine of the scapula and the clavicle. In the notch, the examiner will be palpating the musculotendinous junction of the supraspinatus muscle.

Axilla. With the shoulder slightly abducted (20 to 30°), the examiner may palpate the structures of the axilla–latissimus dorsi muscle (posterior wall), pectoralis major muscle (anterior wall), serratus anterior muscle (medial wall), lymph nodes (palpable only if swollen), and the brachial artery. The patient is then asked to lie prone "on the elbows" with the shoulders slightly laterally rotated and the elbow slightly adducted in relation to the shoulder. The examiner then palpates just inferior to the most lateral aspect of the scapula for the insertion of the infraspinatus muscle. Just distal to this insertion, the examiner may be able to palpate the insertion of teres minor.

Posterior Structures

To complete the palpation, the patient may be either sitting or lying prone with the upper limb by the trunk (Fig. 4–36B).

Spine of Scapula. From the acromion process the examiner moves along the spine of the scapula, noting any tenderness or abnormality.

Scapula. The examiner follows the spine of the scapula to the medial border of the scapula and then the outline of the scapula, which normally extends from the spinous process of T2 to the spinous process of T7. The examiner then moves around the inferior angle of the scapula and along the lateral border of the scapula. After the borders of the scapula have been palpated, the posterior surface (supraspinatus and infraspinatus muscles) may be palpated for tenderness, atrophy, or spasm.

Spinous Processes of Lower Cervical and Tho-

racic **Spine**. In the midline, the examiner may palpate the cervical and thoracic spinous processes for any abnormality. This is followed by palpation of the trapezius muscle.

Triceps Tendon. Inferior to the posterior aspect of the acromion process, the examiner may palpate the tendon of the long head of triceps as it originates from the infraglenoid tubercle.

X-RAY EXAMINATION OF THE SHOULDER COMPLEX

Anteroposterior View. With this view (Fig. 4–38), the examiner should note:

1. The relation of the humerus to the glenoid cavity.

2. The relation of the clavicle to the acromion process.

3. Whether the epiphyseal plate of the humeral head is present, and if so, whether it is normal.

4. Whether there are any calcifications in any

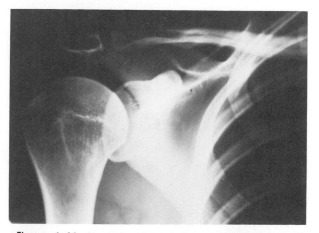

Figure 4–38. Normal anteroposterior radiograph of the shoulder.

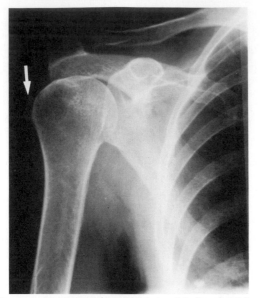

Figure 4–39. Calcium deposit (arrow) in the shoulder.

of the tendons (Fig. 4–39), especially those of the supraspinatus or infraspinatus muscles.

A stress anteroposterior radiograph may be used to "gap" the injured acromioclavicular joint to see whether there has been a third-degree sprain or to show an inferior laxity at the glenohumeral joint (Fig. 4–40). Medial rotation of the humerus with this view may show a defect on the lateral aspect of the humeral head from recurrent dislocations. This defect is called a Hill-Sach lesion. The examiner should look at the *acromiohumeral interval* (the distance between the acromion process and the humerus) and see whether it is normal.[17] The normal interval is 7 to 14 mm (Fig. 4–41). If this distance decreases, it is potentially an indication of rotator cuff tears.

Axial Lateral View. For this view to be obtained, the patient must be able to abduct the shoulder. The examiner should note:

1. The relation of the glenoid cavity, humerus, scapula, and clavicle.

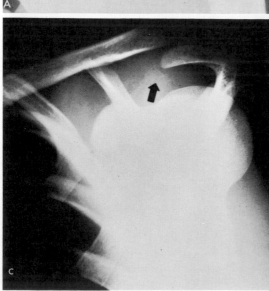

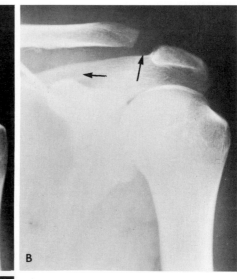

Figure 4–40. Stress radiograph for third-degree acromioclavicular sprain. (*A*) With the patient supine, no dislocation is noted. (*B*) Standing with 4 pounds suspended from the wrist. Note particularly the widening at the acromioclavicular joint and also the difference in distance between the clavicle and coracoid. (*C*) Lateral view of the acromioclavicular joint in showing the complete separation. (From O'Donoghue, D. H.: Treatment of Injuries to Athletes, 4th ed. Philadelphia, W. B. Saunders Co., 1984, p. 142.)

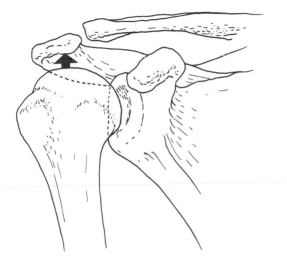

Figure 4–41. Acromiohumeral interval.

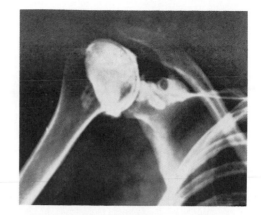

Figure 4–43. Typical arthrographic picture in adhesive capsulitis. Note the absence of dependent axillary fold and poor filling of the biceps. (From Neviaser, J. S.: J. Bone Joint Surg. *44A*:1328, 1962.)

2. The acromioclavicular joint. This view is the best for observing this joint.

3. Any calcification in the subscapularis, infraspinatus, and teres minor muscles.

Arthrogram. An arthrogram of the shoulder is useful for delineating many of the soft tissues and recesses around the glenohumeral joint (Fig. 4–42).[18–20] For example, normally the glenohumeral joint will hold approximately 16 to 20 ml of solution. With adhesive capsulitis (idiopathic frozen shoulder), the amount the joint will hold may decrease to 5 to 10 ml. The arthrogram will show a decrease in the capacity of the joint and obliteration of the axillary fold. Also, there is an almost complete lack of filling of the subscapular bursa with adhesive capsulitis (Fig. 4–43). Tearing of any structures such as the supraspinatus tendon may result in extravasation of the radiopaque dye.

Angiogram. In the case of thoracic outlet syndromes and other arterial impingement type syndromes, angiograms are sometimes used to demonstrate blockage of the subclavian artery during certain moves (Fig. 4–44).

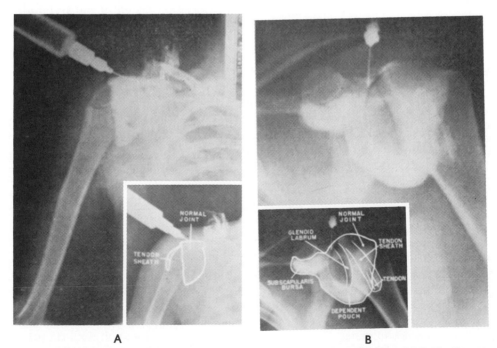

A   **B**

Figure 4–42. Normal arthrograms of the shoulder in a child (*A*) and an adult (*B*). (From Kerwin, G. A., et al.: J. Bone Joint Surg. *39A*:1270, 1957.)

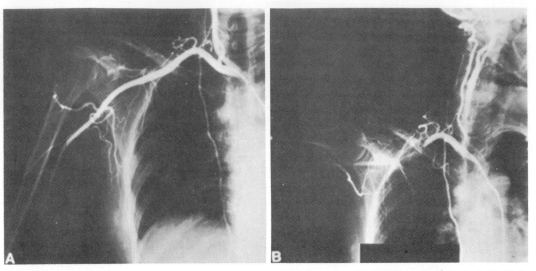

Figure 4–44. Angiograms of the subclavian artery with the arm at rest (A) and abducted (B). Note complete obstruction of the subclavian artery (B). (From Brown, C.: Clin. Orthop. Relat. Res. *173*:55, 1983.)

Précis of the Shoulder Complex Assessment

History
Observation
Examination
  Active movements
    Elevation through forward flexion of the arm
    Elevation through abduction of the arm
    Medial rotation of the arm
    Lateral rotation of the arm
    Adduction of the arm
    Horizontal adduction/abduction of the arm
    Circumduction of the arm
  Passive movements
    Elevation through abduction of the arm
    Elevation through forward flexion of the arm
    Elevation through abduction at the glenohumeral joint only
    Lateral rotation of the arm
    Medial rotation of the arm
    Extension of the arm
    Adduction of the arm
    Horizontal adduction/abduction of the arm
  Resisted isometric movements
    Forward flexion of the shoulder
    Extension of the shoulder
    Abduction of the shoulder
    Adduction of the shoulder
    Medial rotation of the shoulder
    Lateral rotation of the shoulder
    Flexion of the elbow
    Extension of the elbow
  Special tests
  Reflexes and cutaneous distribution
  Joint play movements
    Backward glide of the humerus
    Forward glide of the humerus
    Lateral distraction of the humerus
    Long arm traction
    Backward glide of the humerus in abduction
    Lateral distraction of the humerus in abduction
    Anteroposterior and cephalocaudal movement of the clavicle at the acromioclavicular joint
    Anteroposterior and cephalocaudal movement of the clavicle at the sternoclavicular joint
    General movement of the scapula to determine mobility
  Palpation
  X-ray viewing

Following any examination, the patient should always be warned of the possibility of exacerbation of symptoms resulting from the assessment.

REFERENCES

CITED REFERENCES

1. Cyriax, J.: Textbook of Orthopaedic Medicine, vol. I: Diagnosis of Soft Tissue Lesions. London, Bailliere Tindall, 1982.
2. Nichols, H.M.: Anatomic structures of the thoracic outlet syndrome. Clin. Orthop. Relat. Res. *51*:17, 1967.
3. Riddell, D.H. Thoracic outlet syndrome: Thoracic and vascular aspects. Clin. Orthop. Relat. Res. *51*:53, 1967.
4. Priest, J.D., and D.A. Nagel: Tennis shoulder. Am. J. Sports Med. *4*:28, 1976.
5. Hitchcock, H.H., and C.O. Bechtol: Painful shoulder: Observation on the role of the tendon of the long head of the biceps brachii in its causation. J. Bone Joint Surg. *30A*:263, 1948.
6. Carson, W.C., W.W. Lovell, and T.E. Whitesides: Congenital elevation of the scapula. J. Bone Joint Surg. *63A*:1199, 1981.
7. Cavendish, M.E.: Congenital elevation of the scapula. J. Bone Joint Surg. *54B*:395, 1972.
8. Kessel, L., and M. Watson: The painful arc syndrome. J. Bone Joint Surg. *59B*:166, 1977.

9. Reid, D.C.: The shoulder girdle: Its function as a unit in abduction. Physiotherapy 55:57, 1969.
10. Saha, S.K.: Mechanics of shoulder movements and a plea for the recognition of "zero position" of glenohumeral joint. Clin. Orthop. Relat. Res. 173:3, 1983.
11. Maitland, G.D.: Peripheral Manipulation. London, Butterworths, 1977.
12. Yergason, R.M.: Supination sign. J. Bone Joint Surg. 13:160, 1931.
13. Hawkins, R.J., and J.C. Kennedy: Impingement syndrome in athletics. Am. J. Sports Med. 8:151, 1980.
14. Brown, C.: Compressive, invasive referred pain to the shoulder. Clin. Orthop. Rel. Res. 173:55, 1983.
15. Kaltenborn, E.M.: Mobilization of the Extremity Joints. Oslo, Olaf Norlis Bokhandle, 1980.
16. McRae, R.: Clinical Orthopedic Examination. London, Churchill Livingstone, 1976.
17. Weiner, D.S., and I. Macnab: Superior migration of the humeral head. J. Bone Joint Surg. 52B:524, 1970.
18. Kernwein, G.A., B. Rosenberg, and W.R. Sneed.: Arthrographic studies of the shoulder joint. J. Bone Joint Surg. 39A:1267, 1957.
19. Neviaser, J.S.: Arthrography of the shoulder joint: Study of the findings of adhesive capulitis of the shoulder. J. Bone Joint Surg. 44A:1321, 1962.
20. Reeves, B: Arthrography of the shoulder. J. Bone Joint Surg. 48B:424, 1966.

GENERAL REFERENCES

Adams, J.C.: Outline of Orthopaedics. London, E & S Livingstone, 1968.
American Orthopaedic Association: Manual of Orthopaedic Surgery. Chicago, 1972.
Bateman, J.E.: The Shoulder and Neck, 2nd ed. Philadelphia, W.B. Saunders Co., 1978.
Bateman, J.E.: Neurologic painful conditions affecting the shoulder. Clin. Orthop. Relat. Res. 173:44, 1983.
Beetham, W.P., H.F. Polley, C.H. Slocum, and W.F. Weaver: Physical Examination of the Joints. Philadelphia, W.B. Saunders Co., 1965.
Cailliet, R.: Shoulder Pain. Philadelphia, F.A. Davis Co., 1966.
Dempster, W.T.: Mechanisms of shoulder movement. Arch. Phys. Med. Rehabil. 436:49, 1965.
First Aid. St. John's Ambulance. Ottawa, The Runge Press Ltd., 1963.
Foster, C.R.: Multidirectional instability of the shoulder in the athlete. Clin. Sports Med. 2:355, 1983.
Gartland, J.J.: Fundamentals of Orthopaedics. Philadelphia, W.B. Saunders Co., 1979.
Hawkins, R.J., and P.E. Hobeika: Impingement syndrome in the athletic shoulder. Clin. Sports Med. 2:391, 1983.
Hollinshead, W.H., and D.B. Jenkins: Functional Anatomy of the Limb and Back. Philadelphia, W.B. Saunders Co., 1981.
Hoppenfeld, S.: Physical Examination of the Spine and Extremities. New York, Appleton-Century-Crofts, 1976.
Jobe, F.W.: Painful athletic injuries of the shoulder. Clin. Orthop. Relat. Res. 173:117, 1983.
Judge, R.D., G.D. Zuidema, and F.T. Fitzgerald: Clinical Diagnosis: A Physiological Approach. Boston, Little, Brown & Co., 1982.
Kapandji, I.A.: The Physiology of the Joints, vol. I: Upper Limb. New York, Churchill Livingstone, 1970.
Lippman, R.K.: Frozen shoulder; periarthritis; bicipital tenosynovitis. Arch. Surg. 47:283, 1943.
Ludington, N.A.: Rupture of the long head of biceps flexor cubiti muscle. Ann. Surg. 27:358, 1923.
Naffzinger, H.C. and W.T. Grant: Neuritis of the brachial plexus mechanical in origin: The scalenus syndrome. Clin. Orthop. Relat. Res. 51:7, 1967.
Neer, C.S.: Impingement lesions. Clin. Orthop. Relat. Res. 173:70, 1983.
Neviaser, J.S.: Adhesive capsulitis and the stiff and painful shoulder. Orthop. Clin. North Am. 11:327, 1980.
Neviaser, R.J.: Anatomic considerations and examination of the shoulder. Orthop. Clin. North Am. 11:187, 1980.
Neviaser, R.J.: Lesions of the biceps and tendinitis of the shoulder. Orthop. Clin. North Am. 11:343, 1980.
Neviaser, R.J.: Painful conditions affecting the shoulder. Clin. Orthop. Relat. Res. 173:63, 1983.
Neviaser, R.J.: Tears of the rotator cuff. Orthop. Clin. North Am. 11:295, 1980.
O'Donoghue, D.H.: Treatment of Injuries to Athletes, 4th ed. Philadelphia, W.B. Saunders Co., 1984.
Overton, L.M.: The causes of pain in the upper extremities: A differential diagnosis study. Clin. Orthop. Relat. Res. 51:27, 1967.
Perry, J.: Anatomy and biomechanics of the shoulder in throwing, swimming, gymnastics, and tennis. Clin. Sports Med. 2:247, 1983.
Post, M., R. Silver, and M. Singh: Rotator cuff tear: Diagnosis and treatment. Clin. Orthop. and Relat. Res. 173:78, 1983.
Rathburn, J.B., and I. Macnab: The microvascular pattern of the rotator cuff. J. Bone Joint Surg. 52B:540, 1970.
Reid, D.C.: Functional Anatomy and Joint Mobilization. Edmonton, University of Alberta Press, 1970.
Sarrafian, S.K.: Gross and functional anatomy of the shoulder. Clin. Orthop. Relat. Res. 173:44, 1983.
Tank, R., and J. Halbach: Physical therapy evaluation of the shoulder complex in athletes. J. Orthop. Sports Phys. Ther. 3:108, 1982.
Wiles, P., and R. Sweetnam: Essentials of Orthopaedics. London, J.A. Churchill Ltd., 1965.
Yocum, L.A.: Assessing the shoulder: History, physical examination, differential diagnosis, and special tests used. Clin. Sports Med. 2:281, 1983.

5

Elbow Joints

The elbow's primary role in the upper limb complex is to help position the hand in the appropriate location to perform its function. Once the shoulder has positioned the hand in a gross fashion, the elbow allows for adjustments in height and length of the limb to position the hand correctly. In addition, the forearm rotates, partly at the elbow, to place the hand in the most effective position to perform its function.

Applied Anatomy

The elbow consists of a complex set of joints that require careful assessment for proper treatment. The treatment must be geared to the pathology of the condition, since the joint responds poorly to trauma, harsh treatment, or incorrect treatment (see Figure 5–23).

Because they are closely related, the joints of the elbow complex make up a compound synovial joint, with injury to any one part affecting the other components as well. The elbow articulations are made up of the *ulnohumeral joint* and the *radiohumeral joint*. In addition, the complexity of the elbow articulations is further increased by the *superior radioulnar joint*, which has continuity with the elbow articulations. These three joints make up the *cubital articulations*. The capsule and joint cavity are continuous for all three joints. The combination of these joints allows two degrees of freedom at the elbow. The *trochlear joint* allows one degree of freedom (flexion-extension) while the radiohumeral and superior radioulnar joints allow the other degree of freedom (rotation).

The *ulnohumeral*, or *trochlear joint*, is found between the trochlea of the humerus and the trochlear notch of the ulna, and it is classified as a *uniaxial hinge joint*. The bones of this joint are shaped so that the axis of movement is not horizontal but passes downward and medially, going through an arc of movement. This position leads to the carrying angle at the elbow[1] (Fig. 5–1). The resting position of this joint is with the elbow flexed to 70° and the forearm supinated 10°. The neutral position (0°) is midway between supination and pronation in the "thumb-up" position (Fig. 5–2). The capsular pattern is flexion more limited than extension, and the close packed position is extension with the forearm in supination. On full extension, the medial part of the olecranon process is not in contact with the trochlea; on full flexion, the lateral part of the olecranon process is not in contact with the trochlea. This change allows the side-to-side joint play movement necessary for supination and pronation. A small amount of rotation occurs at this joint. In early flexion, 5° of medial rotation occurs; in late flexion, 5° of lateral rotation occurs.

The *radiohumeral joint* is a uniaxial hinge joint between the capitulum of the humerus and the head of the radius. The resting position is with the elbow flexed to 70° and the forearm supinated to 10°. The close packed position of the joint is with the elbow flexed to 90° and the forearm supinated 5°. As with the trochlear joint, the capsular pattern is flexion more limited than extension.

The ulnohumeral and radiohumeral joints are supported medially by the *ulnar collateral ligament*, a fan-shaped structure, and laterally by the *radial collateral ligament*, a cord-like structure.

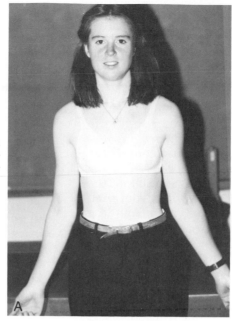
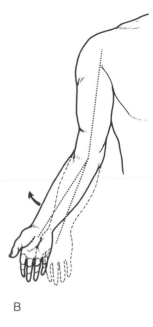

Figure 5–1. (A) Carrying angle of the elbow. (B) Excessive valgus carrying angle. (From American Orthopaedic Association: Manual of Orthopaedic Surgery. Chicago, 1972, p. 138.)

The ulnar collateral ligament has two parts, which along with the flexor carpi ulnaris muscle form the *cubital tunnel* through which passes the *ulnar nerve* (see Figure 5–18). Any injury or blow to the area, or injury that increases the carrying angle, will put an abnormal stress on the nerve as it passes through the tunnel. This can lead to problems such as *tardy ulnar palsy*, a condition that can occur many years after the original injury.

The *superior radioulnar joint* is a uniaxial pivot joint. The head of the radius is held in proper relation to the ulna and humerus by the *annular ligament*, which makes up four fifths of the joint. The resting position of this joint is supination of

35° and elbow flexion of 70°. The close packed position is supination of 5°. The capsular pattern of this joint is equal limitation of supination and pronation.

The three elbow articulations are innervated by branches from the musculocutaneous, median, ulnar, and radial nerves.

The *middle radioulnar articulation* is not a true joint, but is made up of the radius and ulna and the *interosseous membrane* between the two bones. The interosseous membrane is tense only midway between supination and pronation (neutral position). Although this "joint" is not part of the elbow joint complex, it is affected by injury to the elbow joints; conversely, injury to this area can affect the mechanics of the elbow articulations. The interosseous membrane prevents proximal displacement of the radius on the ulna. The displacement is most likely to occur with pushing movements. The *oblique cord* connects the radius and ulna, running from the lateral side of the *ulnar tuberosity* to the radius slightly below the *radial tuberosity*. Its fibers run at right angles to those of the interosseous membrane. The cord assists in preventing displacement of the radius on the ulna, especially those movements involving pulling.

Patient History

In addition to the general history questions presented in Chapter 1, the following information should be ascertained:

1. What is the patient's usual activity or pastime?

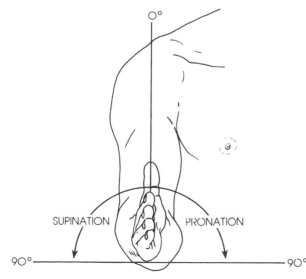

Figure 5–2. "Thumb-up" or neutral (zero) position between supination and pronation.

2. What are the details of the present pain and other symptoms? What are the sites and boundaries of the pain? The pain may be radiating and could ache or be worse at night. Aching pain over the lateral epicondyle that radiates may be indicative of a "tennis elbow" problem.

3. How old is the patient? What is the patient's occupation? Tennis elbow (lateral epicondylitis) problems usually occur in persons 35 years of age or older and in those who use a great deal of wrist flexion and extension in their occupations. If the patient is a child who complains of pain in the elbow and lacks supination on examination, the examiner could potentially suspect a dislocation of the head of the radius. This type of injury is often seen in young children. A parent may give the child a sharp "come-along" tug on the arm, leading to a dislocation of the head of the radius.

4. Does the patient complain of any abnormal nerve distribution pain? The examiner should note whether there is any tingling or numbness and, if so, where it is for reference when checking dermatomes and peripheral nerve distribution later in the examination.

5. Are any movements impaired? Which movements does the patient feel are restricted? If flexion or extension is limited, two joints may be involved—the ulnohumeral and radiohumeral. If supination or pronation is problematic, any one of five joints could be involved—the radiohumeral, superior radioulnar, middle radioulnar, inferior radioulnar, or ulnomeniscocarpal.

6. Does the patient have any history of previous injury or trauma? This question is especially important in regard to the elbow because the ulnar nerve may be affected by tardy ulnar palsy.

Observation

The patient must be suitably undressed so that both arms are exposed to allow comparison of both sides.

The examiner first places the patient's arms in the anatomic position to determine whether there is a normal carrying angle[1] (see Figure 5–1). In the adult this would be a slight valgus deviation between the humerus and the ulna and is best viewed with the forearm supinated and elbow extended. In males the normal carrying angle is 5 to 10°; in females it is 10 to 15°. If the carrying angle is greater than 15°, it is called *cubitus valgus*; if it is less than 5 to 10°, it is called *cubitus varus*.

If swelling exists, all three joints of the elbow complex would be affected because they have a common capsule. With swelling, the joint would be held in its resting position with the elbow held in approximately 70° of flexion. It is in the resting

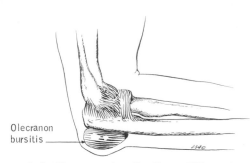

Figure 5–3. Olecranon bursitis. (From O'Donoghue, D. H.: Treatment of Injuries to Athletes. Philadelphia, W. B. Saunders Co., 1976, p. 275.)

position that the joint has maximum volume. Moreover, there may be localized swelling in the case of olecranon bursitis ("student's elbow") (Fig. 5–3).

The examiner should look for normal bony and soft-tissue contours anteriorly and posteriorly. Often athletes, such as pitchers and other throwers, will show a much larger arm on their throwing side.

The examiner should note whether the patient can assume the normal position of function of the elbow (Fig. 5–4). A normal functional position is 90° of flexion, with the forearm midway between supination and pronation.[2] In this position, the olecranon process of the ulna and the medial and lateral epicondyle of the humerus will normally form an isosceles triangle (Fig. 5–5). When the arm is fully extended, the three points normally form a straight line.[3] The forearm may also be considered in a functional position when slightly pronated, as in writing. From this position, forward flexion of the shoulder enables the person to bring food to the mouth; supination of the forearm decreases the amount of shoulder flexion necessary to accomplish this.

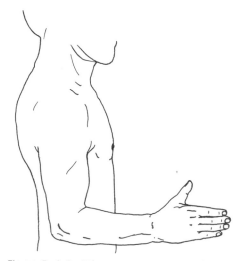

Figure 5–4. Position of function of the elbow.

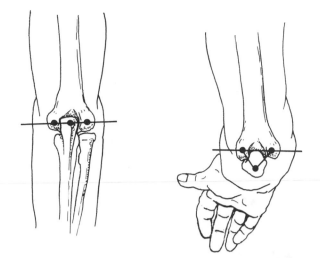

Figure 5–5. Relation of the medial and lateral epicondyles and the olecranon at the elbow in extension and flexion.

Examination

ACTIVE MOVEMENTS

Examination is performed with the patient in the sitting position. As always, active movements are done first, and it is important to remember that the most painful movements are done last. The active movements include:

1. Flexion of the elbow (140–150°).
2. Extension of the elbow (0–10°).
3. Supination of the forearm (90°).
4. Pronation of the forearm (80–90°).

Active elbow *flexion* is 140 to 150°, and the end feel is usually tissue approximation. In thin individuals, the end feel may be bone to bone as a result of the coronoid process hitting against the coronoid fossa.

Active elbow *extension* is 0°, although up to a 10° hyperextension may be exhibited, especially in women. This hyperextension is considered normal if it is equal on both sides and if there is no history of trauma. The end feel of active elbow extension is bone to bone.

Active *supination* should be 90°, and the end feel should be tissue stretch (Fig. 5–6).

For active *pronation*, the range of motion is approximately the same (80 to 90°), and the end feel is tissue stretch. It should be noted, however, that for both supination and pronation only 75° or thereabouts occurs in the forearm articulations. The remaining 15° is the result of wrist action.

PASSIVE MOVEMENTS

If the range of motion is full on active movements, overpressure may be gently applied to test the end feel in each direction. If the movement is not full, passive movements should be carried out to test the end feel, including:

1. Flexion of the elbow.
2. Extension of the elbow.
3. Supination of the forearm.
4. Pronation of the forearm.

In addition to the end feel tests during passive movements, the examiner should note whether a capsular pattern is present. The capsular pattern for the elbow complex as a whole is more limitation of flexion than extension.

RESISTED ISOMETRIC MOVEMENTS

For proper testing of the muscles of the elbow complex, the movement must be resisted and isometric. The patient is seated, and the following movements are tested (Fig. 5–7 and Table 5–1):

1. Elbow flexion.
2. Elbow extension.
3. Supination.
4. Pronation.
5. Wrist flexion.
6. Wrist extension.

It is necessary to carry out wrist extension and

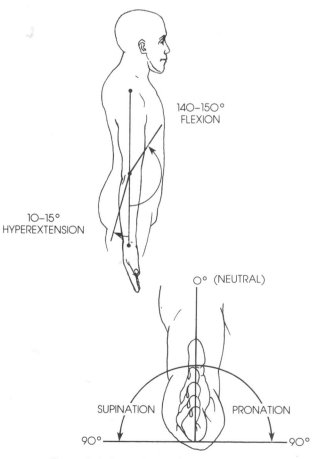

140–150° FLEXION

10–15° HYPEREXTENSION

0° (NEUTRAL)

SUPINATION   PRONATION

90°   90°

Figure 5–6. Range of motion at the elbow.

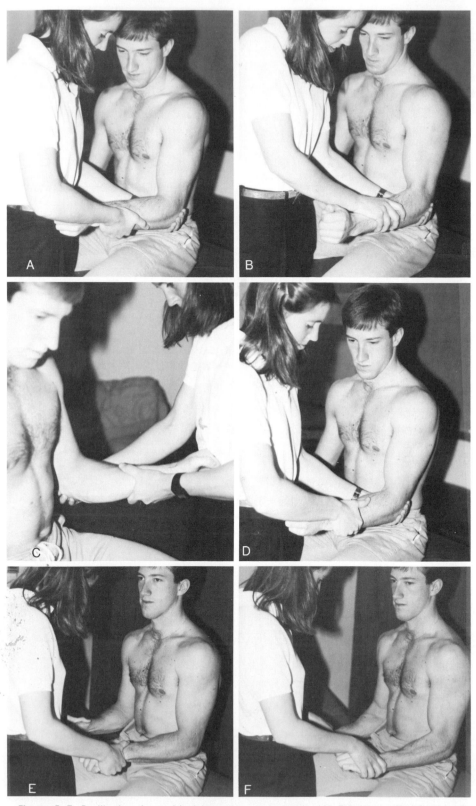

Figure 5–7. Positioning for resisted isometric movements. (*A*) Extension. (*B*) Flexion. (*C*) Pronation. (*D*) Supination. (*E*) Wrist flexion. (*F*) Wrist extension.

Table 5–1. Muscles about the Elbow: Their Actions and Nerve Supply, Including Root Derivations

Action	Muscles Involved	Nerve Supply	Nerve Root Deviation
Flexion of elbow	1. Brachialis	Musculocutaneous	C5, C6 (C7)
	2. Biceps brachii	Musculocutaneous	C5, C6
	3. Brachioradialis	Radial	C5, C6, (C7)
	4. Pronator teres	Median	C6, C7
	5. Flexor carpi ulnaris	Ulnar	C7, C8
Extension of elbow	1. Triceps	Radial	C6, C7, C8
	2. Anconeus	Radial	C7, C8, (T1)
Supination of forearm	1. Supinator	Posterior interosseous (radial)	C5, C6
	2. Biceps brachii	Musculocutaneous	C5, C6
Pronation of forearm	1. Pronator quadratus	Anterior interosseous (median)	C8, T1
	2. Pronator teres	Median	C6, C7
	3. Flexor carpi radialis	Median	C6, C7
Flexion of wrist	1. Flexor carpi radialis	Median	C6, C7
	2. Flexor carpi ulnaris	Ulnar	C7, C8
Extension of wrist	1. Extensor carpi radialis longus	Radial	C6, C7
	2. Extensor carpi radialis brevis	Posterior interosseous (radial)	C7, C8
	3. Extensor carpi ulnaris	Posterior interosseous (radial)	C7, C8

flexion because there are a large number of muscles that act over the wrist as well as the elbow.

SPECIAL TESTS

Only those special tests that the examiner feels have relevance should be tested.

Ligamentous Instability Test. The patient's arm is stabilized with one of the examiner's hands at the elbow and the other hand placed above the patient's wrist. With the patient's elbow slightly flexed (20 to 30°) and stabilized with the examiner's hand, an adduction or varus force is applied at the distal forearm by the examiner to test the lateral collateral ligament (Fig. 5–8). The examiner applies the force several times with increasing pressure while noting any alteration in pain or the range of motion. An abduction or valgus force at the distal forearm is then applied in a similar fashion to test the medial collateral ligament. The examiner should note any laxity, decreased mobility, or altered pain that may be present compared with the uninvolved elbow.

Tinel's Sign (at the Elbow). The area of the ulnar nerve in the groove (between the olecranon process and medial epicondyle) is tapped. A positive sign is indicated by a tingling sensation in the ulnar distribution of the forearm and hand distal to the point of compression (Fig. 5–9). The test gives an indication of the rate of regeneration of the sensory fibers of a nerve. The most distal point at which the abnormal sensation is felt represents the limit of nerve regeneration.

Pinch Grip Test. The patient is asked to pinch the tips of the index finger and thumb together.

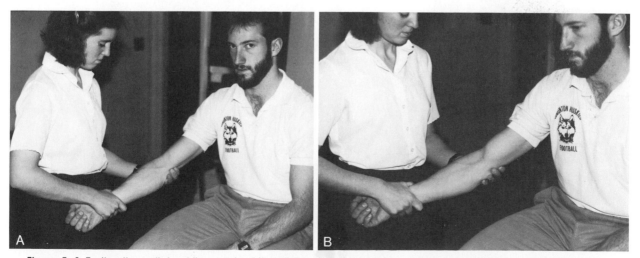

Figure 5–8. Testing the collateral ligaments of the elbow. (*A*) Lateral collateral ligament. (*B*) Medial collateral ligament.

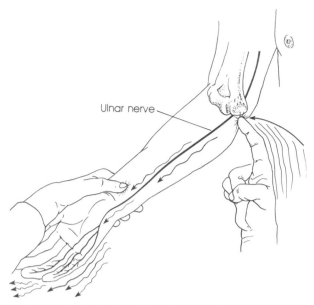

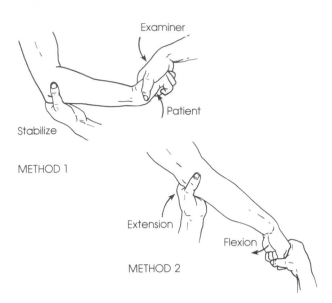

Figure 5–9. Tinel's sign at the elbow for the ulnar nerve.

Figure 5–10. Tests for tennis elbow.

Normally there should be a tip-to-tip pinch. If, however, on attempting this test, the patient is unable to pinch tip to tip and instead has an abnormal pulp-to-pulp pinch of the index finger and thumb, it is indicative of a positive sign for pathology to the anterior interosseous nerve, a branch of the median nerve. This may indicate an entrapment of the anterior interosseous nerve as it passes between the two heads of pronator teres muscle (see Figure 5–16).[4]

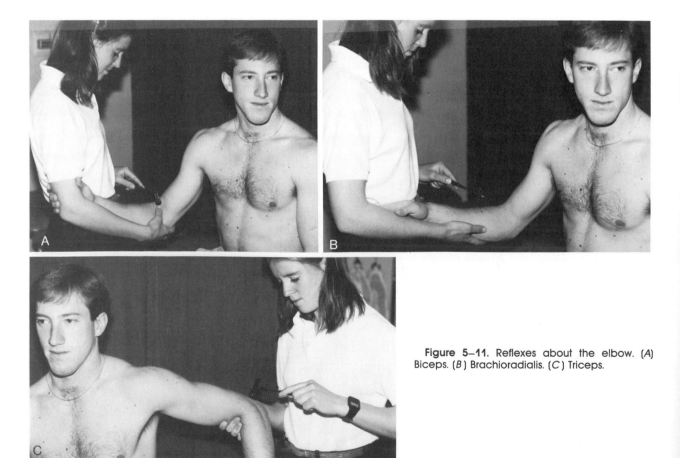

Figure 5–11. Reflexes about the elbow. (A) Biceps. (B) Brachioradialis. (C) Triceps.

Tennis Elbow Test (Method One). The elbow is stabilized by the examiner's thumb, which rests on the patient's lateral epicondyle (Fig. 5–10). The patient is then asked to make a fist, pronate the forearm, and radially deviate and extend the wrist while the examiner resists the motion. A positive sign is indicated by a sudden severe pain in the area of the lateral epicondyle of the humerus. The epicondyle may be palpated to indicate the origin of the pain. This test is sometimes called *Cozen's test.*

Tennis Elbow Test (Method Two). While palpating the lateral epicondyle, the examiner pronates the patient's forearm, flexes the wrist fully, and extends the elbow (Fig. 5–10). A positive test is indicated by pain over the lateral epicondyle of the humerus. The examiner may palpate the epicondyle at the same time.

Medial Epicondylitis (Golfer's Elbow) Test. While the examiner palpates the patient's medial epicondyle, the patient's forearm is supinated and the elbow and wrist are extended by the examiner. A positive sign is indicated by pain over the medial epicondyle of the humerus.

Elbow Flexion Test. The patient is asked to completely flex the elbow and to hold it in the flexed position for 5 minutes. A positive test is indicated by tingling or paresthesia in the ulnar nerve distribution of the forearm and hand. The test helps to determine whether a cubital tunnel syndrome is present.

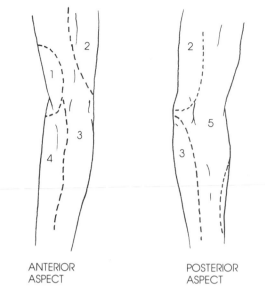

Figure 5–13. Sensory nerve distribution about the elbow. (*1*) Lower lateral cutaneous nerve of forearm (radial). (*2*) Medial cutaneous nerve of arm. (*3*) Medial cutaneous nerve of forearm. (*4*) Lateral cutaneous nerve of forearm (musculocutaneous nerve). (*5*) Posterior cutaneous nerve of forearm (radial nerve).

REFLEXES AND CUTANEOUS DISTRIBUTION

The reflexes about the elbow that are often checked include the biceps (C5), brachioradialis (C6), and triceps (C7) (Fig. 5–11). The examiner should also check the dermatomes around the elbow and the cutaneous distribution of the various nerves, noting any difference (Figs. 5–12 and 5–13). Pain may be referred to the elbow from the neck (often mimicking tennis elbow), the shoulder, or the wrist (Fig. 5–14).

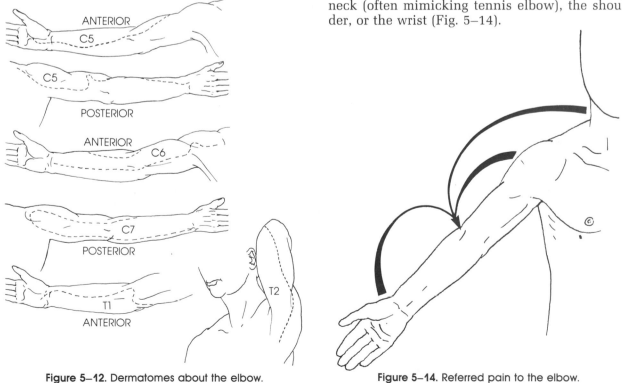

Figure 5–12. Dermatomes about the elbow.

Figure 5–14. Referred pain to the elbow.

r Interosseous Nerve

Neurologically, the examiner must be aware of potential injury or pinching of the various nerves about the elbow. The anterior interosseous nerve, which is a branch of the median nerve, is sometimes pinched or entrapped as it passes between the two heads of pronator teres muscle leading to functional impairment of flexor pollicis longus, the lateral half of flexor digitorum profundus, and pronator quadratus muscles. The condition is called *anterior interosseous nerve syndrome* (Fig. 5–15),[4] characterized by a pinch deformity (Fig. 5–16). The deformity results from the paralysis of the flexors of the index finger and thumb. This leads to extension of the distal interphalangeal joint of the index finger and the interphalangeal joint of the thumb. The resulting pinch is pulp to pulp rather than tip to tip. If the median nerve is damaged or pinched just prior to the anterior interosseous branch being given off, it may be called *pronator syndrome*; in this case, the flexor carpi radialis, palmaris longus, and flexor digitorum muscles are affected in addition to those affected by the anterior interosseous nerve syndrome. In both cases, the sensory distribution of the median nerve will be affected.

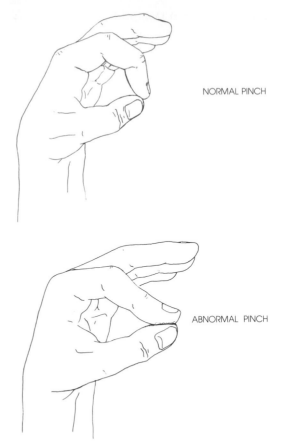

NORMAL PINCH

ABNORMAL PINCH

Figure 5–16. Normal versus abnormal pinch seen in anterior interosseous nerve syndrome.

Median Nerve

The median nerve may also be pinched or compressed above the elbow as it passes under the *ligament of Struthers*, an anomalous structure found in about 1 per cent of the population (Fig. 5–17).[5] The ligament runs from an abnormal spur on the shaft of the humerus to the medial epicon-

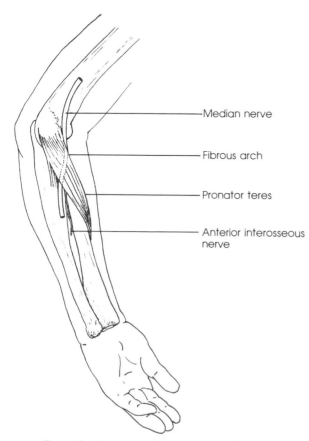

Median nerve

Fibrous arch

Pronator teres

Anterior interosseous nerve

Figure 5–15. Anterior interosseous syndrome.

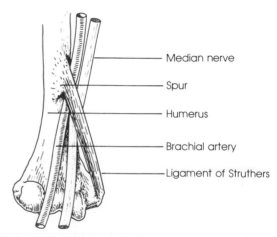

Median nerve

Spur

Humerus

Brachial artery

Ligament of Struthers

Figure 5–17. Compression of the median nerve by ligament of Struthers.

dyle of the humerus. Since the brachial artery sometimes accompanies the nerve through this tunnel, it may also be compressed, resulting in possible vascular as well as neurologic symptoms. In this case, the neurologic involvement would include the pronator teres muscle as well as those muscles affected by the pronator syndrome. The condition may also be called the *humerus supracondylar process syndrome*.

Ulnar Nerve

In the elbow region, the ulnar nerve is most likely to be injured, compressed, or stretched in the cubital tunnel (Fig. 5–18).[5] This tunnel, which is relatively long, can cause trapping of the nerve as the nerve passes through it or as the nerve passes between the two heads of the flexor carpi ulnaris muscle. When the elbow is flexed, greater stretch is placed on the nerve. Thus, symptoms are more likely to occur when the elbow is flexed. It is usually in the cubital tunnel area that the ulnar nerve is affected, leading to tardy ulnar palsy.

Radial Nerve

The major branch of the radial nerve in the forearm is the *posterior interosseous nerve*, which is given off in front of the lateral epicondyle of the humerus.[5, 6] This branch may be compressed as it passes between the two heads of supinator in the *arcade* or *canal of Frohse*, a fibrous arch in the supinator muscle occurring in 30 per cent of the population (Fig. 5–19). Compression leads to functional involvement of the forearm extensor muscles. There is no sensory deficit. This condi-

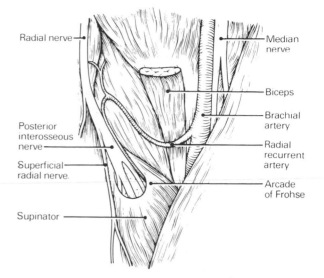

Figure 5–19. Canal or arcade of Frohse. (From Wadsworth, T. G.: The Elbow. New York, Churchill Livingstone, 1982.)

tion, called *radial tunnel syndrome*, may mimic tennis elbow.

JOINT PLAY MOVEMENTS

When examining the joint play movements (Fig. 5–20), the examiner must compare the injured side with the good side. The following joint play movements should be performed on the elbow:

1. Radial deviation of the ulna and radius on the humerus.
2. Ulnar deviation of the ulna and radius on the humerus.
3. Distraction of the olecranon process on the humerus in 90° of flexion.
4. Anteroposterior glide of the radius on the humerus.

The first two movements are performed in a fashion similar to those in the collateral ligament tests. The examiner stabilizes the patient's elbow by holding the patient's humerus firmly and places the other hand above the patient's wrist, abducting and adducting the patient's forearm. The patient's elbow is straight (extended) during the movement, and the end feel should be bone to bone.

To distract the olecranon process, the examiner flexes the patient's elbow to 90°. Wrapping both hands around the patient's forearm close to the elbow, the examiner then applies a distractive force at the elbow, ensuring that no torque is applied.

To test anteroposterior glide of the radius on the humerus, the examiner stabilizes the patient's forearm. The patient's arm is held between the examiner's body and arm. The examiner places the thumb of the other hand over the anterior

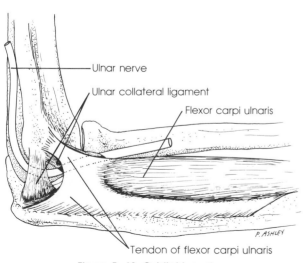

Figure 5–18. Cubital tunnel.

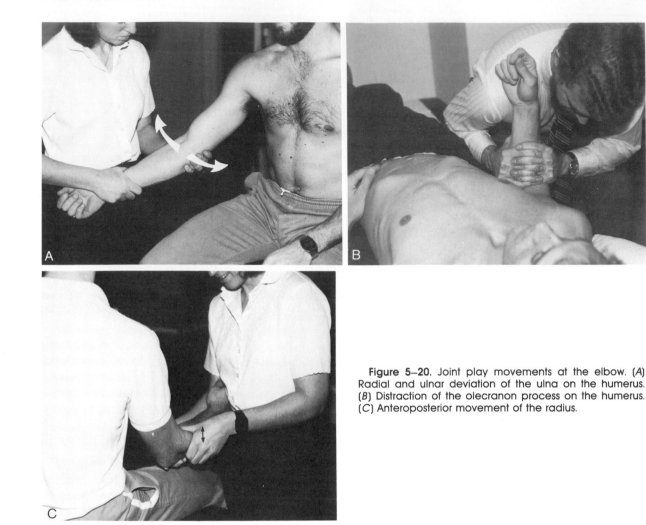

Figure 5–20. Joint play movements at the elbow. (*A*) Radial and ulnar deviation of the ulna on the humerus. (*B*) Distraction of the olecranon process on the humerus. (*C*) Anteroposterior movement of the radius.

radial head while the index finger is over the posterior radial head. The examiner then pushes the radial head posteriorly with the thumb and anteriorly with the index finger. This movement must be performed with care because it can be very painful to the patient.

PALPATION

With the patient's arm relaxed, the examiner begins palpation on the anterior aspect, moves to the medial aspect and then the lateral aspect, followed finally by the posterior aspect. The patient may sit or lie supine, whichever is more comfortable. The examiner is looking for any tenderness, abnormality, change in temperature or in texture of the tissues, or abnormal "bumps."

As with all palpation, the injured side must be compared with the "normal," or uninjured side.

Anterior Aspect

The following structures are palpated.
Cubital Fossa. The fossa is bound by the pronator teres muscle medially, the brachioradialis muscle laterally, and an imaginary line joining the two epicondyles superiorly. Within the fossa, the biceps tendon and brachial artery may be palpated. After crossing the elbow joint, the brachial artery divides into two branches, the radial artery and the ulnar artery. The examiner must be aware of the brachial artery because it has the potential of being injured in severe trauma (e.g., fracture or dislocation). Trauma to this area may

lead to compartment syndromes such as *Volk-mann's ischemic contracture*. The median and musculocutaneous nerves are also found in the fossa, but they are not palpable. Pressure on the median nerve may cause symptoms in its cutaneous distribution.

Coronoid Process and Head of Radius. Within the cubital fossa, if the examiner palpates carefully so as not to hurt the patient, the coronoid process of the ulna and the head of the radius may be palpated. Palpation of the radial head will be facilitated by supinating and pronating the forearm. The examiner may palpate the head of the radius from the posterior aspect at the same time by placing the fingers over the head on the posterior aspect and thumb over it on the anterior aspect. In addition to the muscles previously mentioned, the biceps and brachialis muscles may be palpated for potential abnormality.

Medial Aspect

Moving to the medial aspect of the elbow, the examiner palpates the following structures.

Medial Epicondyle. Originating from the medial epicondyle are the *wrist flexor–forearm pronator* groups of muscles. The muscle bellies and their insertion into the bone should both be palpated. Tenderness over the epicondyle where the muscles insert is sometimes called *golfer's elbow* or *tennis elbow* of the medial epicondyle.

Medial (Ulnar) Collateral Ligament. This fan-shaped ligament may be palpated as it extends from the medial epicondyle to the medial margin of the coronoid process anteriorly and olecranon process posteriorly.

Ulnar Nerve. If the examiner moves posteriorly behind the medial epicondyle, the fingers will rest over the ulnar nerve in the cubital tunnel (proximal part). Usually the nerve is not directly palpable, but pressure on the nerve will often cause abnormal sensations in its cutaneous distribution. It is this nerve that is struck when "one hits the funny bone."

Lateral Aspect

The following structures are palpated.

Lateral Epicondyle. The wrist extensor muscles originate from the lateral epicondyle, and their muscle bellies, as well as their insertion into the epicondyle, should be palpated. It is at this point of insertion of the common extensor tendon that lateral tennis elbow originates. When palpating, the examiner should remember that the extensor carpi radialis longus muscle inserts above the epicondyle along a short ridge extending from the epicondyle to the humeral shaft. At the same time the examiner palpates the brachioradialis and supinator muscles on the lateral aspect of the elbow.

Lateral (Radial) Collateral Ligament. This cord-like ligament may be palpated as it extends from the lateral epicondyle of the humerus to the annular ligament and lateral surface of the ulna.

Annular Ligament. Distal to the lateral epicondyle, the annular ligament and head of the radius may be palpated if not previously done. The palpation is facilitated by supination and pronation of the forearm.

Posterior Aspect

Finally, the following structures should be palpated, as in Figure 5–21.

Olecranon Process and Olecranon Bursa. The olecranon process is best palpated with the elbow flexed to 90°. If the examiner then grasps the skin overlying the process, the olecranon bursa may be palpated. The examiner should note any synovial thickening or the presence of any *rice bodies*, which are small seeds of fragmented fibrous tissue that can act as further irritants to the bursa should it be affected.

Triceps Muscle. The triceps muscle, inserting into the olecranon process, should be palpated both at its insertion and along its length for any signs of abnormality.

X-RAY EXAMINATION OF THE ELBOW COMPLEX

Anteroposterior View. The examiner should note the relations of the epicondyles, trochlea, capitulum, radial head, radial tuberosity, coronoid process, and olecranon process (Fig. 5–22). Any loose bodies, calcification, myositis ossificans, joint space narrowing, or osteophytes should be identified. If the examiner is looking at a young child, the epiphysial plate should be noted to see if it is normal for each bone.

Lateral View. The examiner should note the relations of the epicondyles, trochlea, capitulum, radial head, radial tuberosity, coronoid process, and olecranon process. As with the anteroposterior view, any loose bodies, calcifications of the joint (Fig. 5–23), myositis ossificans, dislocations (Fig. 5–24), joint space narrowing, or osteophytes should be noted.

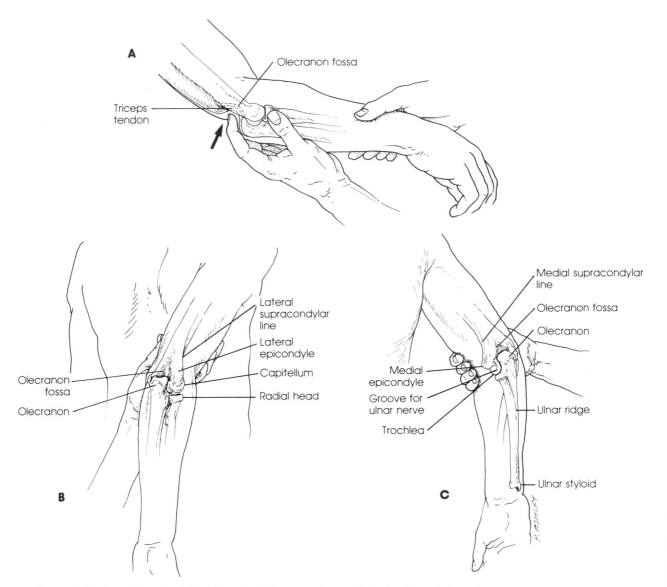

Figure 5–21. Palpation about the elbow. (*A*) Olecranon fossa. (*B*) Posterolateral view of the elbow. (*C*) Posteromedial view of the elbow.

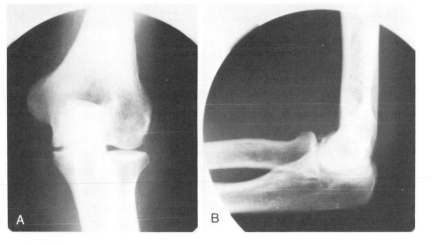

Figure 5–22. Anteroposterior (*A*) and lateral (*B*) radiographs of the elbow.

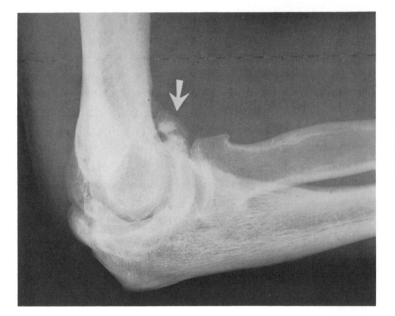

Figure 5–23. Excessive ossification following dislocation of elbow treated by early active use. (From O'Donoghue, D. H.: Treatment of Injuries to Athletes, 4th ed. Philadelphia, W. B. Saunders Co., 1984, p. 232.)

Figure 5–24. Lateral film of a dislocated elbow, showing the lower end of the humerus resting on the ulna in front of the coronoid. Note fragmentation of the coronoid. (From O'Donoghue, D. H.: Treatment of Injuries to Athletes, 4th ed. Philadelphia, W. B. Saunders Co., 1984, p. 227.)

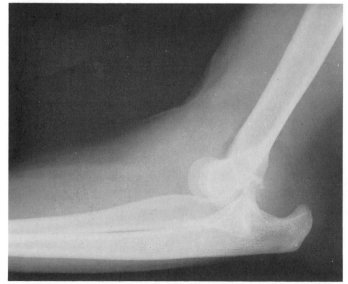

Précis of the Elbow Assessment

History
Observation
Examination
  Active movements
    Elbow flexion
    Elbow extension
    Supination
    Pronation
  Passive movements (as in Active movements, if
    necessary)
  Resisted isometric movements
    Elbow flexion
    Elbow extension
    Supination
    Pronation
    Wrist flexion
    Wrist extension
  Special tests
  Reflexes and cutaneous distribution
  Joint play movements
    Radial deviation of ulna and radius on hume-
      rus
    Ulnar deviation of ulna and radius on humerus
    Distraction of olecranon process on humerus in
      90° of flexion
    Anteroposterior glide of radius on humerus
  Palpation
  X-ray viewing

Following any examination, the patient should
always be warned of the possibility of exacerbation of symptoms as a result of the assessment.

REFERENCES

CITED REFERENCES

1. Beals, R. K.: The normal carrying angle of the elbow: Clin. Orthop. Relat. Res. *119*:194, 1976.

2. Kapandji, A. I.: The Physiology of the Joints, vol. I: Upper Limb. New York: Churchill Livingstone, 1970.
3. American Orthopaedic Association: Manual of Orthopaedic Surgery. Chicago, 1972.
4. Wiens, E., and S. Lane: The anterior interosseous nerve syndrome. Can. J. Surg. *21*:354, 1978.
5. Spinner, M., and P. S. Spencer: Nerve compression lesions of the upper extremity: A clinical and experimental review. Clin. Orthop. Relat. Res. *104*:46, 1974.
6. Wadsworth, T. G.: The Elbow. New York, Churchill Livingstone, 1982.

GENERAL REFERENCES

Chusid, J. G., and J. J. McDonald: Correlative Neuroanatomy and Functional Neurology. Los Altos, Lange Medical Publications, 1961.
Conwell, H. E.: Injuries to the elbow. Clin. Symp., *22*:35, 1970.
Cyriax, J.: Textbook of Orthopaedic Medicine, vol. I: Diagnosis of Soft Tissue Lesions. London, Bailliere Tindall, 1982.
Hollinshead, W. H., and D. B. Jenkins.: Functional Anatomy of the Limbs and Back. Philadelphia, W. B. Saunders Co., 1981.
Hoppenfeld, S.: Physical Examination of the Spine and Extremities. New York, Appleton-Century-Crofts, 1976.
Ishizuki, M.: Functional anatomy of the elbow joint and three-dimensional quantitative motion analysis of the elbow joint. J. Jpn. Orthop. Assoc. 53:989, 1979.
Judge, R. D., G. D. Zuidema, and F.T. Fitzgerald: Clinical Diagnosis: A Physiological Approach. Boston, Little, Brown and Co., 1982.
Kaltenborn, F. M.: Mobilization of the Extremity Joints. Oslo, Olaf Norlis Bolchandel, 1980.
London, J. T.: Kinematics of the elbow. J. Bone Joint Surg. 63A:529, 1981.
Maitland, G. D.: The Peripheral Joints: Examination and Recording Guide. Adelaide, Australia, Virgo Press, 1973.
O'Donoghue, D. H.: Treatment of Injuries to Athletes. Philadelphia, W. B. Saunders Co., 1976, 1984.
Roles, N. C., and R. H. Maudsley: Radial tunnel syndrome: Resistant tennis elbow as a nerve entrapment. J. Bone Joint Surg. 54B:499, 1972.
Williams, P. L., and R. Warwick (eds.): Gray's Anatomy. Philadelphia, W. B. Saunders Co., 1980.

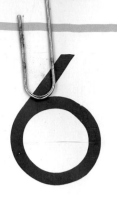

Forearm, Wrist, and Hand

The hand and wrist are the most active and intricate parts of the upper extremity. Because of this, they are vulnerable to injury and do not respond well to serious injury. Their mobility is enhanced by a wide range of movement at the shoulder and complementary movement at the elbow. In addition, the ten bones, the 17 articulations, and the 19 intrinsic and 20 extrinsic muscles of the wrist and hand provide a tremendous variability of movement. As well as being an expressive organ of communication, the hand acts as both a motor and sensory organ, providing information such as temperature, thickness, texture, depth, and shape as well as the motion of an object. It is this sensual acuity that enables the examiner to accurately examine and palpate during an assessment.

The assessment of the hand should be done with two objectives in mind. First, the injury or lesion should be assessed as accurately as possible to ensure proper treatment. Second, the examiner should evaluate the remaining function to determine whether the patient will have any incapacity in everyday life.

Although the joints of the forearm, wrist, and hand are discussed separately, it must be remembered that these joints do not act in isolation but as functional groups. Thus, the position of one joint will influence the position and action of another joint. For example, if the wrist is flexed, the interphalangeal joints will not fully flex, primarily because of passive insufficiency of the finger extensions.

Applied Anatomy

The *distal radioulnar joint* is a uniaxial pivot joint that has one degree of freedom. Although the radius moves over the ulna, the ulna does not remain stationary. It moves back and laterally during pronation and forward and medially during supination. The resting position of the joint is 10° of supination, and the close packed position is 5° of supination. The capsular pattern of the distal radioulnar joint is equal limitation of supination and pronation.

The *radiocarpal (wrist) joint* is a biaxial ellipsoid joint. The radius articulates with the scaphoid and lunate. The lunate and triquetrum also articulate with the cartilaginous disc (triangular-shaped) and not the ulna. The disc extends from the ulnar side of the distal radius and attaches to the ulna at the base of the ulnar styloid process. The disc adds stability to the wrist. It creates a close relationship between the ulna and carpal bones and binds the distal ends of the radius and ulna together. With the disc in place, the radius bears 60 per cent of the load and the ulna 40 per cent. If the disc is removed, the radius transmits 95 per cent of the axial load and the ulna 5 per cent.[1] Thus, the cartilaginous disc acts as a cushion for the wrist joint. The disc can be damaged by forced extension and pronation. The distal end of the radius is concave and the proximal row of carpals is convex, but the curvatures are not equal. The joint has two degrees of freedom, and the resting position is neutral with slight ulnar deviation. The close packed position is extension, and the capsular pattern is equal limitation in all directions.

The *intercarpal joints* are considered to be the joints between the individual bones of the proximal row of carpal bones (scaphoid, lunate, and triquetrum) and the joints between the individual bones of the distal row of carpal bones (trapezium, trapezoid, capitate, and hamate). They are bound together by small intercarpal ligaments (dorsal, palmar, and interosseous) that allow only a slight amount of gliding movement between the bones. The close packed position is extension, and the resting position is neutral or slight flexion. The *pisotriquetral joint* is considered separately because the pisiform sits on the triquetrum and does not take a direct part in the other intercarpal movements.

The *midcarpal joints* form a compound articulation between the proximal and distal rows of carpal bones with the exception of the pisiform bone. On the medial side, the scaphoid, lunate, and triquetrum articulate with the capitate and hamate, forming a compound *sellar joint*. On the lateral aspect, the scaphoid articulates with the trapezoid and trapezium, forming another compound sellar joint. As with the intercarpal joints, these articulations are bound together by dorsal and palmar ligaments; however, there are no interosseous ligaments between the proximal and distal row of bones. Therefore, greater movement exists at the midcarpal joints than at the intercarpal joints. The close packed position of these joints is extension with ulnar deviation, and the resting position is neutral or slight flexion with ulnar deviation.

At the thumb, the *carpometacarpal (CMC) joint* is a saddle-shaped (sellar) joint that has three degrees of freedom, whereas the second to fifth carpometacarpal joints are plane joints.[2] The capsular pattern of the carpometacarpal joint of the thumb is abduction most limited followed by extension. The resting position is midway between abduction and adduction and midway between flexion and extension. The close packed position of the carpometacarpal joint of the thumb is full opposition. For the second to fifth carpometacarpal joints, the capsular pattern of restriction is equal limitation in all directions. The bones of these joints are held together by dorsal and palmar ligaments. In addition, the thumb articulation has a strong lateral ligament extending from the lateral side of the trapezium to the radial side of the base of the first metacarpal, and the medial four articulations have an interosseous ligament similar to that found in the carpal articulations.

The carpometacarpal articulations of the fingers allow only gliding movement. The carpometacar-pal articulation of the thumb is unique in that it allows flexion, extension, abduction, adduction, rotation and circumduction. It is able to do this because of the shape of this articulation, which, as previously mentioned, is saddle-shaped. Because of the many movements possible at this joint, the thumb is able to adopt any position relative to the palmar aspect of the hand.[2]

The plane *intermetacarpal joints* have only a small amount of gliding movement between them and do not include the thumb articulation. They are bound together by palmar, dorsal, and interosseous ligaments.

The *metacarpophalangeal (MCP) joints* are condyloid joints. The second and third metacarpophalangeal joints tend to be immobile and are the primary stabilizing factor of the hand while the fourth and fifth joints are more mobile. The collateral ligaments of these joints are tight on flexion and relaxed on extension. These articulations are also bound by palmar ligaments and deep transverse metacarpal ligaments. Each joint has two degrees of freedom. The first metacarpophalangeal joint has three degrees of freedom, thus facilitating the movement of the carpometacarpal joint of the thumb.[2] The close packed position of the first metacarpophalangeal joint is maximum opposition, and the close packed position for the second to fifth metacarpophalangeal joints is maximum flexion.[3] The resting position of the metacarpophalangeal joints is slight flexion, whereas the capsular pattern is more limitation of flexion than extension.

The *interphalangeal (IP) joints* are uniaxial hinge joints with each joint having one degree of freedom. The close packed position of the *proximal interphalangeal (PIP) joints* and *distal interphalangeal (DIP) joints* is full extension; the resting position is slight flexion. The capsular pattern of these joints is flexion more limited than extension. The bones of these joints are bound together by a fibrous capsule and by the palmar and collateral ligaments. During flexion, there is some rotation in these joints so that the pulp of the fingers faces more fully the pulp of the thumb (see Fig. 6–23).

Patient History

In addition to the general history questions presented in Chapter 1, the following information should be ascertained:

1. What is the patient's usual activity or pastime?

2. What is the patient's occupation?

3. What are the sites and boundaries of pain and any abnormal sensation that are present?

4. Are the symptoms improving, getting worse, or staying the same?

extensor tendons (which are flat or ovoid). Within the hand, there is a surgical "no man's land" (Fig. 6–1), which is a region between the distal palmar crease and the midportion of the middle phalanx of the fingers. Damage to the flexor tendons in this area requiring surgical repair usually leads to the formation of adhesive bands that restrict gliding. The tendons may become ischemic in this area as well, being replaced by scar tissue. Because of this, the prognosis following surgery in this area is poor.

9. What is the mechanism of injury? For example, a fall on the outstretched hand may lead to a lunate dislocation, or extension of the fingers may cause dislocation of the fingers. A rotational force applied to the wrist or near it may lead to a *Galleazzi fracture*, a fracture of the radius and dislocation of the distal end of the ulna.

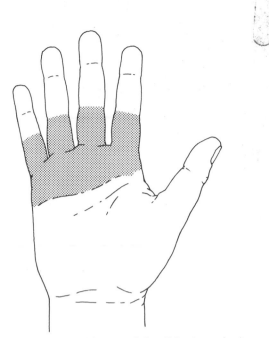

Figure 6–1. Surgical "no-man's land" (palmar view).

5. When did the injury or onset occur, and how long has the patient been incapacitated? These two questions are not necessarily the same; for instance, a burn may occur at a certain time, but incapacity may not occur until hypertrophic scarring appears.

6. What things is the patient functionally unable to do?

7. Has the person ever injured the forearm, wrist, or hand before?

8. Which part of the forearm, wrist, or hand is injured? If the flexor tendons (which are round, have synovial sheaths and have a longer excursion than the extensor tendons) are injured, they respond much more slowly to treatment than do

Observation

While observing the patient and viewing the hands from both the anterior and posterior aspects, the examiner should note the patient's willingness and ability to use the hand.

The bone and soft tissue contours of the forearm, wrist, and hand should be normal and any deviation noted. The posture of the hand at rest will often demonstrate common deformities. The examiner should note any muscle wasting on the thenar eminence (median nerve), first dorsal interosseous muscle (C7 nerve root), or hypothenar eminence (ulnar nerve) that may be indicative of nerve or nerve root injury.

Any localized swellings (such as a ganglion) that are usually seen on the dorsum of the hand should be recorded (Fig. 6–2). In the wrist and

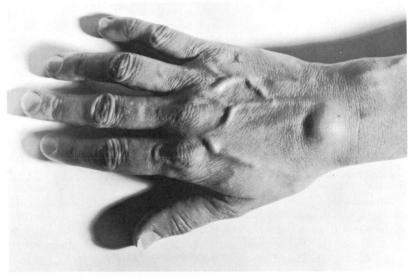

Figure 6–2. Ganglion or small cystic swelling on the dorsum of the right hand just distal to the wrist joint. (From Polley, H. F., and G. G. Hunder: Rheumatologic Interviewing and Physical Examination of the Joints. Philadelphia, W. B. Saunders Co., 1978, p. 96.)

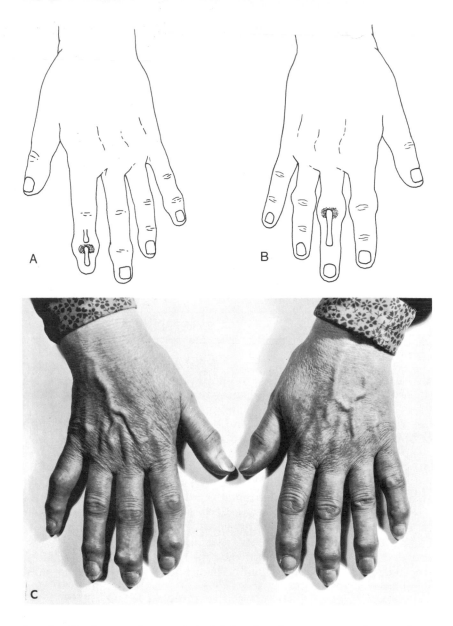

Figure 6-3. Heberden's and Bouchard's nodes. (*A*) Heberden's nodes. (*B*) Bouchard's nodes. (*C*) Degenerative joint disease (osteoarthritis) of both hands. Osteoarthritic enlargement of the distal interphalangeal joints (Heberden's nodes) and the proximal interphalangeal joints (Bouchard's nodes) is present. The metacarpophalangeal joints are not affected. (*C* is from Polley, H. F., and G. G. Hunder: Rheumatologic Interviewing and Physical Examination of the Joints. Philadelphia, W. B. Saunders Co., 1978, p. 120.)

hand, effusion and synovial thickening is most evident on the dorsal and radial aspect. Swelling of the metacarpophalangeal and interphalangeal joints is most obvious on the dorsal aspect.

Because the dominant hand tends to be larger than the nondominant hand, the examiner should remember that if the patient has an area on the fingers that lacks sensation, this area will be avoided when lifting or identifying objects and instead will use another finger with normal sensitivity.

Any vasomotor changes should be recorded. These changes may be indicative of a peripheral vascular disease, diabetes mellitus, Raynaud's disease, or reflex neurovascular syndromes such as shoulder-hand syndrome or Sudeck's atrophy. The vasomotor changes seen could include loss of hair on the hand, brittle fingernails, increase or decrease in sweating of the palm, shiny skin,

radiographic evidence of osteoporosis, or any difference in temperature between the two limbs.

The examiner should note any hypertrophy of one or more fingers. Hypertrophy of the bone may be seen in Paget's disease, neurofibromatosis, or arteriovenous fistula.

The presence of Heberden's or Bouchard's nodes (Fig. 6-3) should be recorded. Heberden's nodes appear on the dorsal surface of the distal interphalangeal joints and are associated with osteoarthritis. Bouchard's nodes are on the dorsal surface of the proximal interphalangeal joints. They are often associated with gastrectasis and rheumatoid arthritis.

Any ulcerations may indicate neurologic or circulatory problems. Any alteration in color of the limb with changes in position may indicate a circulatory problem.

The examiner should note any rotational or

angulated deformities of the fingers, which may be indicative of previous fracture. The fingers, when extended, generally are slightly rotated toward the thumb.

Scars, if present, may indicate recent surgery or past injury. A scar may result in decreased mobility in a joint if the formation of scar tissue is sufficient.

The examiner should take time to observe the fingernails. "Spoon-shaped" nails are often the result of fungal infection, "clubbed" nails may be due to hypertrophy of the underlying soft tissue or to respiratory or cardiac problems (see Figures 6–13 and 6–15). Table 6–1 gives an indication of other pathologic processes that may affect the fingernails.

Table 6–1. Glossary of Nail Pathology*

Condition	Description	Occurrence
Beau's lines	Transverse lines or ridges marking repeated disturbances of nail growth	Systemic diseases, toxic or nutritional deficiency states of many types, trauma (from manicuring)
Defluvium unguium (onychomadesis)	Complete loss of nails	Certain systemic diseases such as scarlet fever, syphilis, leprosy, alopecia areata, and exfoliative dermatitis
Diffusion of lunula unguis	"Spreading" of lunula	Dystrophies of the extremities
Eggshell nails	Nail plate thin, semitransparent bluish-white, with a tendency to curve upward at the distal edge	Syphilis
Fragilitas unguium	Friable or brittle nails	Dietary deficiency, local trauma
Hapalonychia	Nails very soft, split easily	Following contact with strong alkalis; endocrine disturbances, malnutrition, syphilis, chronic arthritis
Hippocratic nails	"Watch-glass nails" associated with "drumstick fingers"	Chronic respiratory and circulatory diseases, especially pulmonary tuberculosis; hepatic cirrhosis
Koilonychia	"Spoon nails"; nails are concave on the outer surface	In dysendocrinisms (acromegaly), trauma, dermatoses, syphilis, nutritional deficiencies, hypothyroidism
Leukonychia	White spots or striations or rarely the whole nail may turn white (congenital type)	Local trauma, hepatic cirrhosis, nutritional deficiencies and many systemic diseases
Mees' lines	Transverse white bands	Hodgkin's granuloma, arsenical and thallium toxicity, high fevers, local nutritional derangement
Moniliasis of nails	Infections (usually paronychial) caused by yeast forms (Candida albicans)	Frequently in food-handlers, dentists, dishwashers, gardeners
Onychatrophia	Atrophy or failure of development of nails	Trauma, infection, dysendocrinism, gonadal aplasia, and many systemic disorders
Onychauxis	Nail plate is greatly thickened	Mild persistent trauma, systemic diseases such as peripheral stasis, peripheral neuritis, syphilis, leprosy, hemiplegia, or at times may be congenital
Onychia	Inflammation of the nail matrix causing deformity of the nail plate	Trauma, infection, many systemic diseases
Onychodystrophy	Any deformity of the nail plate, nail bed, or nail matrix	Many diseases; trauma; or may be caused by chemical agents (poisoning, allergy)
Onychogryposis	"Claw nails"—extreme degree of hypertrophy, sometimes with horny projections arising from the nail surface	May be congenital or related to many chronic systemic diseases (see onychauxis above)
Onycholysis	Loosening of the nail plate beginning at the distal or free edge	Trauma, injury by chemical agents, many systemic diseases
Onychomadesis	Shedding of all the nails (defluvium unguium)	Dermatoses such as exfoliative dermatitis, alopecia areata, psoriasis, eczema, nail infection, severe systemic diseases, arsenical poisoning
Onychophagia	Nail biting	Neurosis
Onychorrhexis	Longitudinal ridging and splitting of the nails	Dermatoses, nail infections, many systemic diseases, senility, injury by chemical agents, and hyperthyroidism
Onychoschizia	Lamination and scaling away of nails in thin layers	Dermatoses, syphilis, injury by chemical agents
Onychotillomania	Alteration of the nail structures caused by persistent neurotic picking of the nails	Neurosis
Pachyonychia	Extreme thickening of all the nails. The nails are more solid and more regular than in onychogryposis	Usually congenital and associated with hyperkeratosis of the palms and soles
Pterygium unguis	Thinning of the nail fold and spreading of the cuticle over the nail plate	Associated with vasospastic conditions such as Raynaud's phenomenon and occasionally with hypothyroidism

*From Berry, T. J.: The Hand As a Mirror of Systemic Disease. Philadelphia, F. A. Davis Co., 1963.

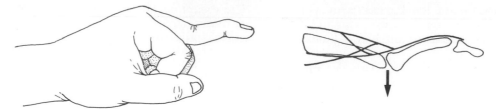

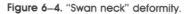

Figure 6–4. "Swan neck" deformity.

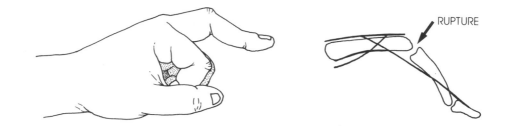

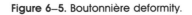

Figure 6–5. Boutonnière deformity.

RUPTURE

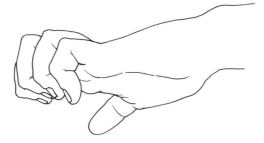

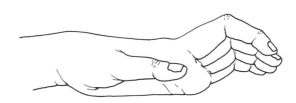

Figure 6–6. "Claw" fingers.

Figure 6–7. "Ape hand" deformity.

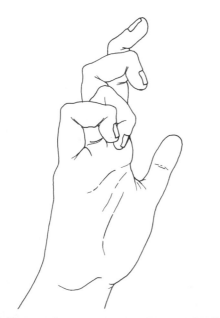

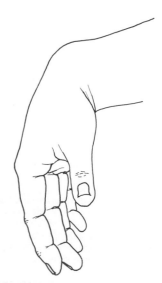

Figure 6–8. "Bishop's hand" or "benediction hand" deformity.

Figure 6–9. Drop-wrist deformity.

COMMON HAND AND FINGER DEFORMITIES

Deformities of the hand and fingers that may be seen include the following:

Swan Neck Deformity. This deformity usually involves only the fingers. There is flexion of the metacarpophalangeal and distal interphalangeal joints. In addition to this, there is extension of the proximal interphalangeal joint. The condition is a result of contracture of the intrinsic muscles and is often seen in rheumatoid arthritis or following trauma (Fig. 6–4).

Boutonnière Deformity. Extension of the metacarpophalangeal and distal interphalangeal joints and flexion of the proximal interphalangeal joint are seen. The deformity is the result of a rupture of the central tendinous slip of the extensor hood and is most common following trauma or in rheumatoid arthritis (Fig. 6–5).

Claw Fingers. This deformity results from the loss of intrinsic muscle action and the overaction of the extrinsic extensor muscles on the proximal phalanx of the fingers. The metacarpophalangeal joints are hyperextended, and the proximal and distal interphalangeal joints are flexed. The deformity is most commonly due to a combined median and ulnar nerve palsy (Fig. 6–6).

"Trigger Finger." Also known as digital tenovaginitis stenosans, this deformity is the result of a thickening of the flexor tendon sheath, which causes sticking of the tendon when the patient attempts to flex the finger. A low-grade inflammation of the proximal fold of the flexor tendon leads to swelling and constriction (stenosis) in the digital flexor tendon. When the patient attempts to flex the finger, the tendon sticks, and the finger "lets go," often with a snap. As the condition worsens, the finger will flex but eventually will not let go, and it will have to be

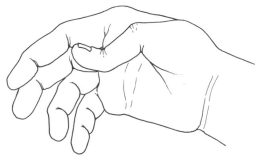

Figure 6–10. "Z" deformity of the thumb.

passively extended. The condition is more likely to occur in middle-aged women, whereas "trigger thumb" is more common in young children. The condition usually occurs in the third or fourth finger. It is most commonly associated with rheumatoid arthritis and tends to be worse in the morning.

"Ape Hand" Deformity. There is wasting of the thenar eminence of the hand as a result of a median nerve palsy and the thumb falls back in line with the fingers due to the pull of the extensor muscles. The patient is also unable to oppose or flex the thumb (Fig. 6–7).

Bishop's or Benediction Hand Deformity. There is wasting of the hypothenar muscles of the hand, the interossei muscles, and the two medial lumbrical muscles because of ulnar nerve palsy (Fig. 6–8).

Drop-Wrist Deformity. The extensor muscles of the wrist are paralyzed as a result of a radial nerve palsy, and the wrist and fingers cannot be extended (Fig. 6–9).

"Z" Deformity of the Thumb. The thumb is flexed at the metacarpophalangeal joint and extended at the interphalangeal joint (Fig. 6–10).

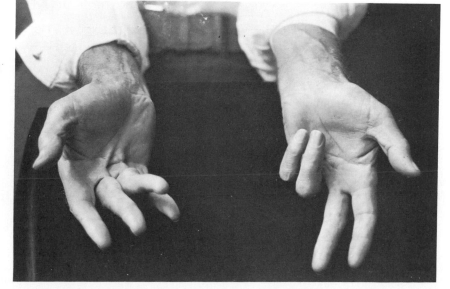

Figure 6–11. Dupuytren's contracture in both hands showing flexion contractures of the fourth and fifth digits of the left hand and less severe contractures in the third, fourth, and fifth digits of the right hand. Note the puckering of palmar skin and presence of bands extending from the concavity of the palm to the proximal interphalangeal joints of the third and fourth digits of the right hand. (From Polley, H. F., and G. G. Hunder: Rheumatological Interviewing and Physical Examination of the Joints. Philadelphia, W. B. Saunders Co., 1978, p. 98.)

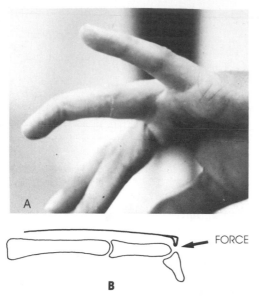

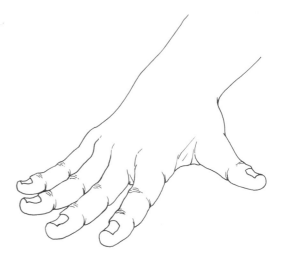

Figure 6–13. "Spoon" nails.

Figure 6–12. Mallet finger. (*A*) Patient actively attempting to extend finger. (*B*) Mechanism of injury. Tendon is ruptured or avulsed from bone.

The deformity may be due to heredity, or it may be associated with rheumatoid arthritis.

Dupuytren's Contracture. This condition is the result of contracture of the palmar fascia. There is a fixed flexion deformity of the metacarpophalangeal and proximal interphalangeal joints (Fig. 6–11). Dupuytren's contracture is usually seen in the ring or little finger, and the skin is often adherent to the fascia. It affects men more often than women and is usually seen in the 50- to 70-year-old age group.

Mallet Finger. A mallet finger deformity is the result of a rupture or avulsion of the extensor tendon where it inserts into the distal phalanx of the finger. The rupture or avulsion results in the distal phalanx resting in a flexed position (Fig. 6–12).

OTHER PHYSICAL FINDINGS

The hand is the terminal part of the upper limb. Many pathologic conditions manifest themselves in this structure and may lead the examiner to suspect pathologic conditions elsewhere in the body. Some of these conditions may include:

1. Generalized or continued body exposure to radiation produces brittle nails, longitudinal nail ridges, skin keratosis (thickening), and ulceration.

2. The Plummer-Vinson syndrome produces spoon-shaped nails (Fig. 6–13). This condition is a dysphasia with atrophy in the mouth, pharynx, and upper esophagus.

3. Psoriasis may cause scaling, deformity, and fragmentation and detachment of the nails.

4. Hyperthyroidism produces nail atrophy and ridging with warm, moist hands.

5. Vasospastic conditions produce a thin nail fold and *pterygium* (abnormal extension) of the cuticle.

6. Avitaminosis and chronic alcoholism produce transverse, or "Beau's," lines in the nails (Fig. 6–14).

7. Many arterial diseases produce a lack of linear growth with thick, dark nails.

8. Lues (syphilis) produces a hypertrophic overgrowth of the nail plate. The nails break and crumple easily.

9. Chronic respiratory disorders produce clubbing of the nails (Fig. 6–15).

10. Subacute bacterial endocarditis may produce "Osler's nodes," which are small, tender nodes in the finger pads.

11. Congenital heart disease may produce cyanosis and nail clubbing.

12. Neurocirculatory aesthesia (loss of strength and energy) produces cold, damp hands.

13. Parkinson's disease produces a typical hand tremor known as "pill roller hand" (Fig. 6–16).

14. Causalgic states produce a painful, swollen, hot hand.

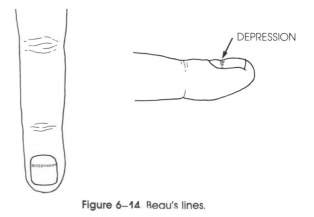

Figure 6–14. Beau's lines.

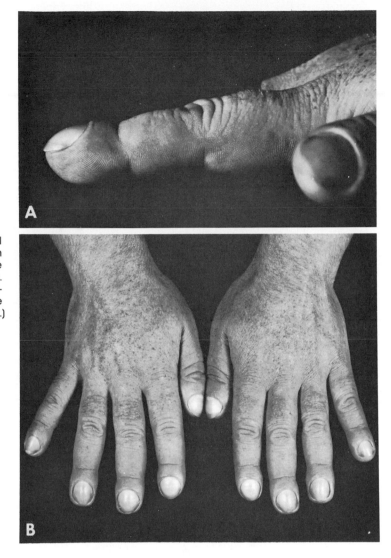

Figure 6–15. Clubbing of distal interphalangeal joints and rounding of the nails in a patient with hypertrophic osteoarthropathy. (*A*) Close-up, side view of index finger. (*B*) Dorsal aspect of both hands. (From Polley, H. F., and G. G. Hunder: Rheumatological Interviewing and Physical Examination of the Joints. Philadelphia, W. B. Saunders Co., 1978, p. 122.)

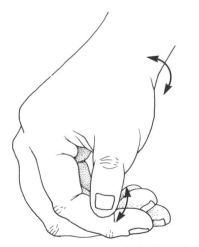

Figure 6–16. "Pill rolling" hand seen in Parkinson's disease.

15. *"Opera glove" anesthesia* is seen in hysteria, leprosy, and diabetes. It is a condition in which there is numbness from the elbow to the fingers (Fig. 6–17).

16. *Raynaud's disease* produces a cold, mottled, painful hand. It is an idiopathic vascular disorder characterized by intermittent attacks of pallor and cyanosis of the extremities brought on by cold or emotion.

17. Rheumatoid arthritis produces a warm, wet hand as well as joint swelling, dislocations, or subluxations and ulnar deviation of the wrist.

18. The deformed hand of Volkmann's ischemic contracture is one that is very typical for a compartment syndrome following a fracture or dislocation of the elbow (Fig. 6–18).

Table 6–2 gives further examples of physical findings of the hand.

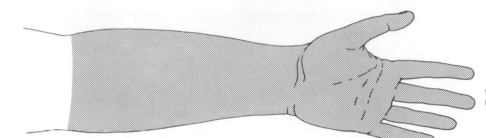

Figure 6–17. "Opera glove" anesthesia showing area of abnormal sensation.

Table 6–2. Outline of Physical Findings of the Hand*

I. Variations in size and shape of hand
  A. Large, blunt fingers (spade hand)
    1. Acromegaly
    2. Hurler's disease (gargoylism)
  B. Gross irregularity of shape and size
    1. Paget's disease of bone
    2. Maffucci's syndrome
    3. Neurofibromatosis
  C. Spider fingers, slender palm (arachnodactyly)
    1. Hypopituitarism
    2. Eunuchism
    3. Ehlers-Danlos syndrome, pseudoxanthoma elasticum
    4. Tuberculosis
    5. Asthenic habitus
    6. Osteogenesis imperfecta
  D. Sausage-shaped phalanges
    1. Rickets (beading of joints)
    2. Granulomatous dactylitis (tuberculosis, syphilis)
  E. Spindliform joints (fingers)
    1. Early rheumatoid arthritis
    2. Systemic lupus erythematosus
    3. Psoriasis
    4. Rubella
    5. Boeck's sarcoidosis
    6. Osteoarthritis
  F. Cone-shaped fingers
    1. Pituitary obesity
    2. Fröhlich's dystrophy
  G. Unilateral enlargement of hand
    1. Arteriovenous aneurysm
    2. Maffucci's syndrome
  H. Square dry hands
    1. Cretinism
    2. Myxedema
  I. Single, widened, flattened distal phalanx
    1. Sarcoidosis
  J. Shortened fourth and fifth metacarpals (bradymetacarpalism)
    1. Pseudohypoparathyroidism
    2. Pseudo-pseudohypoparathyroidism
  K. Shortened, incurved fifth finger (symptom of Du Bois)
    1. Mongolism
    2. "Behavioral problem"
    3. Gargoylism (broad, short, thick-skinned hand)
  L. Malposition and abduction, fifth finger
    1. Turner's syndrome (gonadal dysgenesis, webbed neck, etc.)
  M. Syndactylism
    1. Congenital malformations of the heart, great vessels
    2. Multiple congenital deformities
    3. Laurence-Moon-Biedl syndrome
    4. In normal individuals as an inherited trait
  N. Clubbed fingers
    1. Subacute bacterial endocarditis
    2. Pulmonary causes
      a. Tuberculosis
      b. Pulmonary arteriovenous fistula
      c. Pulmonic abscess
      d. Pulmonic cysts
      e. Bullous emphysema
      f. Pulmonary hypertrophic osteoarthropathy
      g. Bronchogenic carcinoma
    3. Alveolocapillary block
      a. Interstitial pulmonary fibrosis
      b. Sarcoidosis
      c. Beryllium poisoning
      d. Sclerodermatous lung
      e. Asbestosis
      f. Miliary tuberculosis
      g. Alveolar cell carcinoma
    4. Cardiovascular causes
      a. Patent ductus arteriosus
      b. Tetralogy of Fallot
      c. Taussig-Bing complex
      d. Pulmonic stenosis
      e. Ventricular septal defect
    5. Diarrheal states
      a. Ulcerative colitis
      b. Tuberculous enteritis
      c. Sprue
      d. Amebic dysentery
      e. Bacillary dysentery
      f. Parasitic infestation (G-I tract)
    6. Hepatic cirrhosis
    7. Myxedema
    8. Polycythemia
    9. Chronic urinary tract infections (upper and lower)
      a. Chronic nephritis
    10. Hyperparathyroidism (telescopy of distal phalanx)
    11. Pachydermoperiostosis (syndrome of Touraine, Solente and Golé)
  O. Joint disturbances
    1. Arthritides
      a. Osteoarthritis
      b. Rheumatoid arthritis
      c. Systemic lupus erythematosus
      d. Gout
      e. Psoriasis
      f. Sarcoidosis
      g. Endocrinopathy (acromegaly)
      h. Rheumatic fever
      i. Reiter's syndrome
      j. Dermatomyositis
    2. Anaphylactic reaction—serum sickness
    3. Scleroderma
II. Edema of the Hand
  A. Cardiac disease (congestive heart failure)
  B. Hepatic disease
  C. Renal disease
    1. Nephritis
    2. Nephrosis
  D. Hemiplegic hand
  E. Syringomyelia
  F. Superior vena caval syndrome
    1. Superior thoracic outlet tumor
    2. Mediastinal tumor or inflammation
    3. Pulmonary apex tumor
    4. Aneurysm

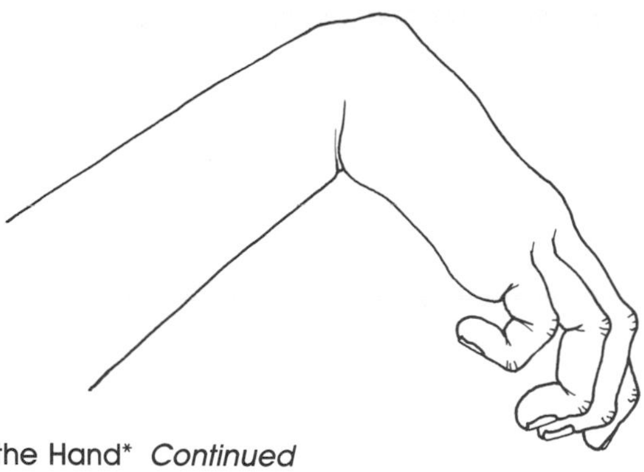

Figure 6–18. Deformity seen with Volkmann's ischemic contracture. Note clawed fingers.

Table 6–2. Outline of Physical Findings of the Hand* *Continued*

G. Generalized anasarca, hypoproteinemia
H. Postoperative lymphedema (radical breast amputation)
I. Ischemic paralysis (cold, blue, swollen, numb)
J. Lymphatic obstruction
    1. Lymphomatous masses in axilla
K. Axillary mass
    1. Metastatic tumor, abscess, leukemia, Hodgkin's disease
L. Aneurysm of ascending or transverse aorta, or of axillary artery
M. Pressure on innominate or subclavian vessels
N. Raynaud's disease
O. Myositis
P. Cervical rib
Q. Trichiniasis
R. Scalenus anticus syndrome
III. Neuromuscular effects
  A. Atrophy
    1. Painless
      a. Amyotrophic lateral sclerosis
      b. Charcot-Marie-Tooth peroneal atrophy
      c. Syringomyelia (loss of heat, cold and pain sensation)
      d. Neural leprosy
    2. Painful
      a. Peripheral nerve disease
        1. Radial nerve (wrist drop)
          a. Lead poisoning, alcoholism, polyneuritis, trauma
          b. Diphtheria, polyarteritis, neurosyphilis, anterior poliomyelitis
        2. Ulnar nerve (benediction palsy)
          a. Polyneuritis, trauma
        3. Median nerve (claw hand)
          a. Carpal tunnel syndrome
            1. Rheumatoid arthritis
            2. Tenosynovitis at wrist
            3. Amyloidosis
            4. Gout
            5. Plasmacytoma
            6. Anaphylactic reaction
            7. Menopause syndrome
            8. Myxedema
  B. Extrinsic pressure on the nerve (cervical, axillary, supraclavicular or brachial)
    1. Pancoast tumor (pulmonary apex)
    2. Aneurysms of subclavian arteries, axillary vessels, or thoracic aorta
    3. Costoclavicular syndrome
    4. Superior thoracic outlet syndrome
    5. Cervical rib
    6. Degenerative arthritis of cervical spine
    7. Herniation of cervical intervertebral disk
  C. Shoulder-hand syndrome
    1. Myocardial infarction
    2. Pancoast tumor
    3. Brain tumor

    4. Intrathoracic neoplasms
    5. Discogenetic disease
    6. Cervical spondylosis
    7. Febrile panniculitis
    8. Senility
    9. Vascular occlusion
    10. Hemiplegia
    11. Osteoarthritis
    12. Herpes zoster
  D. Ischemic contractures (sensory loss in fingers)
    1. Tight plaster cast applications
  E. Polyarteritis nodosa
  F. Polyneuritis
    1. Carcinoma of lung
    2. Hodgkin's disease
    3. Pregnancy
    4. Gastric carcinoma
    5. Reticuloses
    6. Diabetes mellitus
    7. Chemical neuritis
      a. Antimony, benzene, bismuth, carbon tetrachloride, heavy metals, alcohol, arsenic, lead, gold, emetine
    8. Ischemic neuropathy
    9. Vitamin B deficiency
    10. Atheromata
    11. Arteriosclerosis
    12. Embolic
  G. Carpodigital (carpopedal spasm) tetany
    1. Hypoparathyroidism
    2. Hyperventilation
    3. Uremia
    4. Nephritis
    5. Nephrosis
    6. Rickets
    7. Sprue
    8. Malabsorption syndrome
    9. Pregnancy
    10. Lactation
    11. Osteomalacia
    12. Protracted vomiting
    13. Pyloric obstruction
    14. Alkali poisoning
    15. Chemical toxicity
      a. Morphine, lead, alcohol
  H. Tremor
    1. Parkinsonism
    2. Familial disorder
    3. Hypoglycemia
    4. Hyperthyroidism
    5. Wilson's disease (hepatolenticular degeneration)
    6. Anxiety
    7. Ataxia
    8. Athetosis
    9. Alcoholism, narcotic addiction
    10. Multiple sclerosis
    11. Chorea (Sydenham's, Huntington's)

*From Judge, R. D., et al.: Clinical Diagnosis: A Physiological Approach. Boston, Little, Brown and Co., 1982.

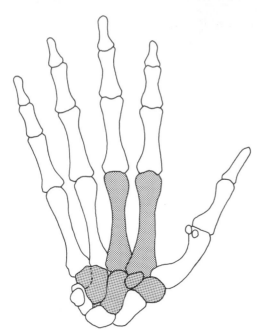

Figure 6–19. Palmar view of hand showing stable segment (stippled areas).

Examination

It is important for the examiner to remember that adduction of the hand (ulnar deviation) is greater than abduction (radial deviation) because of shortness of the ulnar styloid process. Supination of the forearm is stronger than pronation, whereas abduction has a greater range of motion in supination than pronation. Adduction and abduction range of motion is minimal when the wrist is fully extended or flexed. Flexion and extension at the fingers are maximal when the wrist is in neutral (not abducted or adducted); flexion and extension of the wrist are minimal when the wrist is in pronation.

The wrist and hand have a fixed and mobile segment. The fixed segment consists of the distal row of carpal bones (trapezium, trapezoid, capitate, and hamate), and the second and third metacarpals. This is the stabilizing segment of the wrist and hand (Fig. 6–19), and movement between these bones is less than between the bones of the mobile segments. This arrangement allows stability without rigidity and enables the hand to move more discretely and with suppleness. The mobile segment is made up of the five phalanges and the first, fourth, and fifth metacarpal bones.

The functional position of the wrist is extension to 20 to 35° with ulnar deviation of 10 to 15°.[2] This position, sometimes called the *position of rest*, minimizes the restraining action of the long extensor tendons and allows complete flexion of the fingers (Fig. 6–20). In this position, the pulp of the index finger and thumb come into contact to facilitate thumb-finger action. The *position of*

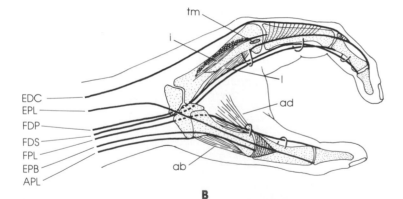

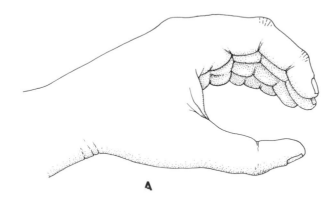

Figure 6–20. Position of function of the hand.
(*A*) Normal view.

(*B*) The hand is in the position of function. Notice in particular that a very small amount of motion in the thumb and fingers is useful motion in that it can be utilized in pinch and grasp. Notice the close relationship of the tendons to bone. The flexor tendons are held close to bone by a pulley-like thickening of the flexor sheath as represented schematically. With the hand in this position, intrinsic and extrinsic musculature is in balance and all muscles are acting within their physiologic resting length.

EDC, Extensor digitorum communis
EPL, Extensor pollicis longus
FDP, Flexor digitorum profundus
FDS, Flexor digitorum sublimis
FPL, Flexor pollicis longus
EPB, Extensor pollicis brevis
APL, Abductor pollicis longus
i, Interossei
tm, Transverse metacarpal ligament
l, Lumbrical
ad, Adductor pollicis brevis
ab, Abductor pollicis brevis

(*B* is from O'Donoghue, D. H.: Treatment of Injuries to Athletes. Philadelphia, W. B. Saunders Co., 1984, p. 287.)

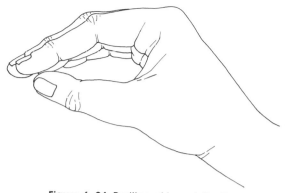

Figure 6–21. Position of immobilization.

wrist immobilization (Fig. 6–21) is extension more than the position of rest, with the metacarpophalangeal joints flexed more as well and the interphalangeal joint extended. In this way, the joints are immobilized so that the potential for contracture is kept to a minimum.

During extension, most of the movement occurs in the radiocarpal joint (approximately 50°) and less occurs in the midcarpal joint (approximately 35°). The motion of extension is accompanied by slight radial deviation and pronation of the forearm. During flexion, most of the movement occurs in the midcarpal joint (approximately 50°) and less occurs in the radiocarpal joint (approximately 35°). This movement is accompanied by slight ulnar deviation and supination of the forearm. Radial deviation occurs primarily between the proximal and distal rows of carpal bones (0 to 20°), with the proximal row moving toward the ulna and the distal row moving radially. Ulnar deviation occurs primarily at the radiocarpal joint (0 to 37°).[2]

ACTIVE MOVEMENTS

Physiologic (Anatomic) Movement

Examination is accomplished with the patient in the sitting position. As always, the most painful movements are done last. In determination of the movements of the hand, the middle finger is considered to be midline (Fig. 6–22). Wrist flexion will decrease as the fingers are flexed, and movements of flexion and extension are limited, usually by the antagonistic muscles and ligaments. The patient should actively perform the following movements:

1. Pronation of the forearm (85 to 90°).
2. Supination of the forearm (85 to 90°).
3. Wrist abduction (radial deviation) (15°).
4. Wrist adduction (ulnar deviation) (30 to 45°).
5. Wrist flexion (80 to 90°).
6. Wrist extension (70 to 90°).
7. Finger flexion (MCP: 85 to 90°; PIP: 100 to 115°; DIP: 80 to 90°).
8. Finger extension (MCP: 30 to 45°; PIP: 0°; DIP: 20°).
9. Finger abduction (20 to 30°).
10. Finger adduction (0°).
11. Thumb flexion (CMC: 45 to 50°; MCP: 50 to 55°; IP: 85 to 90°).
12. Thumb extension (MCP: 0°; IP: 0 to 5°).
13. Thumb abduction (60 to 70°).
14. Thumb adduction (30°).
15. Opposition of little finger and thumb (tip to tip).

Active *pronation* and *supination* are approximately 85 to 90°, although there is variability between individuals and it is more important to compare the movement with the normal side. Approximately 75° of supination and pronation occurs in the forearm articulations. The remaining 15° is the result of wrist action. The normal end feel of both movements is tissue stretch, although in skinny individuals, the end feel of pronation may be bone to bone.

Radial and *ulnar deviations* of the wrist are 15° and 30 to 45°, respectively. The normal end feel of these movements is bone to bone. Wrist flexion is 80 to 90°; wrist extension is 70 to 90°. The end feel of both movements is tissue stretch.

Flexion of the fingers occurs at the metacarpophalangeal joints (85 to 90°), the proximal interphalangeal joints (100 to 115°), and the distal interphalangeal joints (80 to 90°). Extension occurs at the metacarpophalangeal joints (30 to 45°), the proximal interphalangeal joints (0°), and the distal interphalangeal joints (20°). The end feel of finger flexion and extension is tissue stretch. Fin-

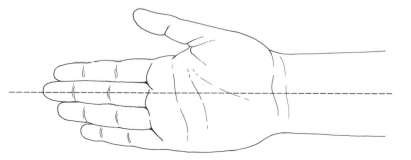

Figure 6–22. Axis or reference position of the hand.

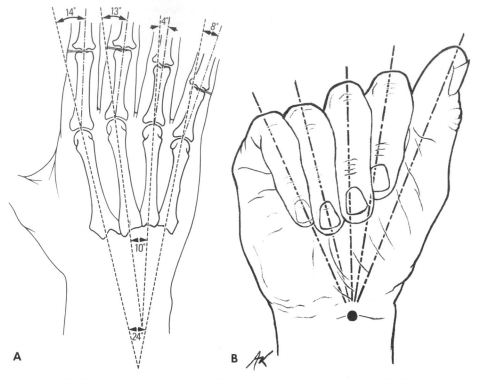

Figure 6–23. Alignment of the fingers. (*A*) Normal physiological alignment. (*B*) Oblique flexion of the last four digits. Only the index ray flexes toward the median axis. Thus, when the last four digits are flexed, separately at the metacarpophalangeal and the proximal interphalangeal joints, their axes converge toward the scaphoid tubercle. (From Tubiana, R.: The Hand. Philadelphia, W. B. Saunders Co., 1981, p. 197 and p. 22.)

ger abduction occurs at the metacarpophalangeal joints (20 to 30°). The end feel is tissue stretch. Finger adduction occurs at the same joint (0°).

The digits are medially deviated slightly in relation to the metacarpal bones (Fig. 6–23). As well, the metacarpals are at an angle to each other. These positions increase the dexterity of the hand and oblique flexion of the medial four digits, but contribute to deformities seen in conditions such as rheumatoid arthritis.

Thumb flexion occurs at the carpometacarpal joint (45 to 50°), the metacarpophalangeal joint (50 to 55°), and the interphalangeal joint (80 to 90°). It is associated with medial rotation of the thumb as a result of the shape of the carpometacarpal joint. Extension of the thumb occurs at the interphalangeal joint (0 to 5°). It is associated with lateral rotation. Flexion and extension takes place in a plane parallel to the palm of the hand. Thumb abduction is 60 to 70°; thumb adduction is 30°. These movements occur in a plane at right angles to the flexion-extension plane.[2]

The examiner must be aware that active movements may be affected because of neurologic as well as contractile problems. For example, the median nerve is sometimes compressed as it passes through the carpal tunnel (Fig. 6–24), affecting its motor and sensory distribution in the hand and fingers. The condition is referred to as *carpal tunnel syndrome*. The nerve may be compressed following trauma (e.g., Colles fracture, lunate dislocation) or by tenosynovitis of the flexor tendons, a ganglion, or collagen disease. Up to 20 per cent of pregnant women may expe-

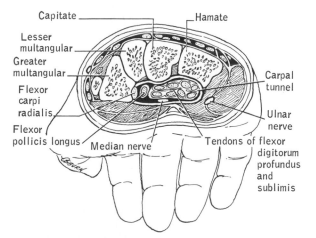

Figure 6–24. Cross section of the wrist showing the carpal tunnel. (From O'Donoghue, D. H.: Treatment of Injuries to Athletes, 4th ed. Philadelphia, W. B. Saunders Co., 1984, p. 258.)

rience some median nerve symptoms caused by fluid retention.

Functional Movement (Grip)

Having completed testing of the anatomic or physiologic active movements, the examiner then assesses the patient's functional active movements. Various grips are attempted, and gross grip strength is often measured by a dynamometer or sphygmomanometer. The average readings for males are 46 kg and 300⁺ mm respectively; average values for females are 23 kg and about 300 mm, respectively.[4]

Grip, regardless of type, consists of four stages:[2, 5]

1. Opening of the hand, which requires the simultaneous action of the intrinsic muscles of the hand and the long extensor muscles.

2. Closing of the fingers to grasp the object and adapt to the object's shape.

3. Regulation of the force exerted in holding the object. The force exerted by an individual will vary depending on the weight, surface characteristics, fragility, and utilization of the object.

4. Release, in which the hand opens to let go of the object.

The thumb, although not always used in gripping, adds another important dimension when it is used. It gives both stability and helps control the direction in which the object will move. Both of these factors are necessary for precision movements. The thumb also increases the power of a grip by acting as a buttress, resisting the pressure of an object held between it and the fingers.

The nerve supply distribution and the functions of the digits also present interesting patterns. Flexion and sensation of the ulnar digits is controlled by the ulnar nerve and is more related to *power* grip. Flexion and sensation of the radial digits is controlled by the median nerve and is more related to *precision grip*. The muscles of the thumb, often used in both types of grip, are supplied by both nerves. In all cases of gripping, opening of the hand or release depends on the radial nerve.

Power Grip. A power grip requires firm control

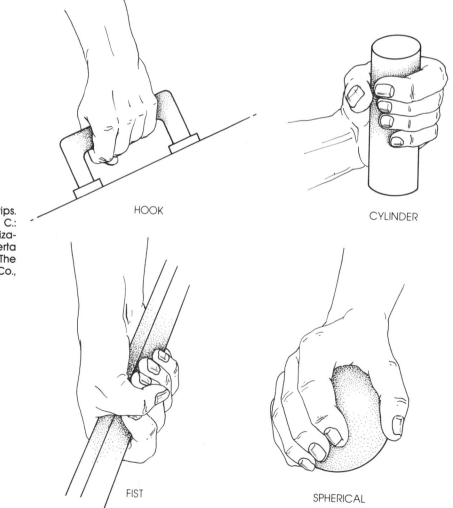

Figure 6–25. Types of power grips. Based on concepts from Reid, D. C.: Functional Anatomy and Joint Mobilization. Edmonton, University of Alberta Bookstore, 1970; and Tubiana, R.: The Hand. Philadelphia, W. B. Saunders Co., 1981.)

HOOK

CYLINDER

FIST

SPHERICAL

and gives greater flexor asymmetry to the hand (Fig. 6–25).[2, 5, 6] With this grip, the digits maintain the object against the palm. The combined effect of joint position brings the hand into line with the forearm. For a power grip to be formed, the fingers are flexed, the wrist is in ulnar deviation, and the wrist is extended. Examples of power grips are the *hook grasp*, in which all or the second and third fingers are used as a hook and may involve the interphalangeal joints only or the interphalangeal and metacarpophalangeal joints (the thumb is not involved); and the *cylinder grasp*, or palmar prehension, in which the thumb is used and the entire hand wraps around an object. With the *fist grasp*, or digital palmar prehension, the hand moves around a narrow object. Another type of power grip is the *spherical grasp*, or palmar prehension, in which there is more opposition and the hand moves around the sphere.

Precision or Prehension Grip. The precision grip is an activity limited mainly to the metacarpophalangeal joints (Fig. 6–26).[2, 5, 6] The palm may or may not be involved, but there is pulp-to-pulp contact between the thumb and fingers and the thumb opposes the fingers. An example is *digital prehension*, in which palmar pinch or *subterminal opposition* is achieved. With this grip, there is pulp-to-pulp pinch and opposition is necessary. An example is holding a pencil. This grip is sometimes called a *precision grip with power*. Another example is lateral prehension or subterminolateral opposition. The thumb and lateral side of the index finger come into contact, and it may be called a "side," "lateral," or "key" pinch. No opposition is needed. An example of this movement is holding keys or a card. Another prehension grip is *tip-to-tip prehension*, or *terminal opposition*. With this positioning, the tip of the thumb is brought into opposition with the tip of another finger. The strength of the pinch may be tested using a pinch meter. The pulp-to-pulp pinch ranges from 2 to 5 gm for males depending on the finger, and from 2 to 4 gm for females. For the side or key pinch, the value is 7 to 8 gm for males and 4 to 5 gm for females.[4]

Functional coordinated movements may be tested by asking the patient to do simple activities, such as fastening a button, tying a shoelace, or tracing a diagram.

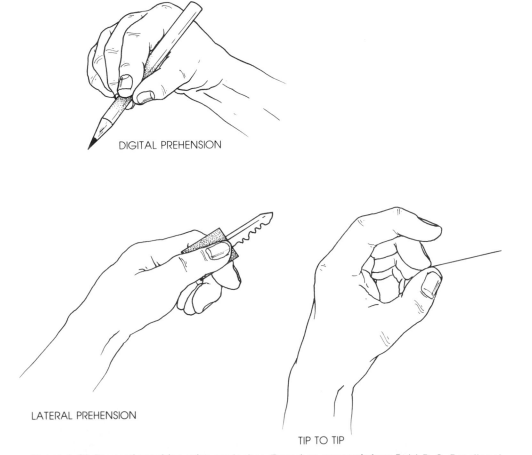

DIGITAL PREHENSION

LATERAL PREHENSION

TIP TO TIP

Figure 6–26. Types of precision grips or pinches. (Based on concepts from Reid, D. C.: Functional Anatomy and Joint Mobilization. Edmonton, University of Alberta Bookstore, 1970; and Tubiana, R.: The Hand. Philadelphia, W. B. Saunders Co., 1981.)

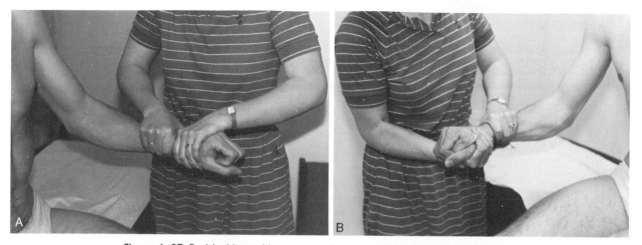

Figure 6–27. Resisted isometric movements of the wrist. (*A*) Flexion. (*B*) Extension.

PASSIVE MOVEMENTS

If, when watching the patient perform the active movements, the examiner feels the range of motion is full, overpressure could be gently applied to test the end feel of the joint in each direction. If the movement is not full, passive movements must be performed by the examiner to test the end feel. At the same time, the examiner must watch for the presence of a capsular pattern. The passive movements are the same as the active movements, and the examiner must remember to test each individual joint.

The capsular pattern of the distal radioulnar joint is full range of motion with pain at the extremes of supination and pronation. At the wrist, the capsular pattern is equal limitation of flexion and extension. At the metacarpophalan-geal and interphalangeal joints, the capsular pattern is flexion more limited than extension. At the trapeziometacarpal joint of the thumb, the capsular pattern is abduction more limited than extension.

RESISTED ISOMETRIC MOVEMENTS

As with the active movements, the resisted isometric movements are done in the sitting position. The movements must be isometric and performed in the neutral position (Figs. 6–27 and 6–28):

1. Pronation of the forearm (see Figure 5–7).
2. Supination of the forearm (see Figure 5–7).
3. Wrist abduction (radial deviation).
4. Wrist adduction (ulnar deviation).

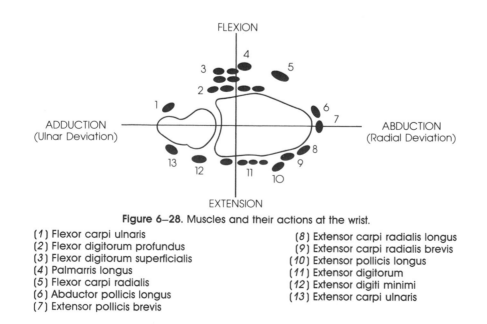

Figure 6–28. Muscles and their actions at the wrist.

(*1*) Flexor carpi ulnaris
(*2*) Flexor digitorum profundus
(*3*) Flexor digitorum superficialis
(*4*) Palmaris longus
(*5*) Flexor carpi radialis
(*6*) Abductor pollicis longus
(*7*) Extensor pollicis brevis

(*8*) Extensor carpi radialis longus
(*9*) Extensor carpi radialis brevis
(*10*) Extensor pollicis longus
(*11*) Extensor digitorum
(*12*) Extensor digiti minimi
(*13*) Extensor carpi ulnaris

Table 6–3. Muscles of the Forearm, Wrist, and Hand: Their Actions and Innervation, Including Nerve Root Derivations

Action	Muscles Involved	Innervation	Nerve Root Deviation
Supination of forearm	1. Supinator	Posterior interosseous (radial)	C5, C6
	2. Biceps brachii	Musculocutaneous	C5, C6
Pronation of forearm	1. Pronator quadratus	Anterior interosseous (median)	C8, T1
	2. Pronator teres	Median	C6, C7
	3. Flexor carpi radialis	Median	C6, C7
Extension of wrist	1. Extensor carpi radialis longus	Radial	C6, C7
	2. Extensor carpi radialis brevis	Posterior interosseous (radial)	C7, C8
	3. Extensor carpi ulnaris	Posterior interosseous (radial)	C7, C8
Flexion of wrist	1. Flexor carpi radialis	Median	C6, C7
	2. Flexor carpi ulnaris	Ulnar	C7, C8
Ulnar deviation of wrist	1. Flexor carpi ulnaris	Ulnar	C7, C8
	2. Extensor carpi ulnaris	Posterior interosseous (radial)	C7, C8
Radial deviation of wrist	1. Flexor carpi radialis	Median	C6, C7
	2. Extensor carpi radialis longus	Radial	C6, C7
	3. Abductor pollicis longus	Posterior interosseous (radial)	C7, C8
	4. Extensor pollicis brevis	Posterior interosseous (radial)	C7, C8
Extension of fingers	1. Extensor digitorum communis	Posterior interosseous (radial)	C7, C8
	2. Extensor indices (second finger)	Posterior interosseous (radial)	C7, C8
	3. Extensor digiti minimi (little finger)	Posterior interosseous (radial)	C7, C8
Flexion of fingers	1. Flexor digitorum profundus	Anterior interosseous (median)	C8, T1
	2. Flexor digitorum superficialis	Median	C7, C8, T1
	3. Lumbricals	1st and 2nd: Median; 3rd and 4th: Ulnar (deep terminal branch)	C8, T1 C8, T1
	4. Interossei	Ulnar (deep terminal branch)	C8, T1
	5. Flexor digiti minimi (little finger)	Ulnar (deep terminal branch)	C8, T1
Abduction of fingers (with fingers extended)	1. Dorsal interossei	Ulnar (deep terminal branch)	C8, T1
	2. Abductor digiti minimi (little finger)	Ulnar (deep terminal branch)	C8, T1
Adduction of fingers (with fingers extended)	Palmar interossei	Ulnar (deep terminal branch)	C8, T1
Extension of thumb	1. Extensor pollicis longus	Posterior interosseous (radial)	C7, C8
	2. Extensor pollicis brevis	Posterior interosseous (radial)	C7, C8
	3. Abductor pollicis longus	Posterior interosseous (radial)	C7, C8
Flexion of thumb	1. Flexor pollicis brevis	Superficial head: median (lateral terminal branch)	C8, T1
		Deep head: ulnar	C8, T1
	2. Flexor pollicis longus	Anterior interosseous (median)	C8, T1
	3. Opponens pollicis	Median (lateral terminal branch)	C8, T1
Abduction of thumb	1. Abductor pollicis longus	Posterior interosseous (radial)	C7, C8
	2. Abductor pollicis brevis	Median (lateral terminal branch)	C8, T1
Adduction of thumb	Adductor pollicis	Ulnar (deep terminal branch)	C8, T1
Opposition of thumb and little finger	1. Opponens pollicis	Median (lateral terminal branch)	C8, T1
	2. Flexor pollicis brevis	Superficial head: median (lateral terminal branch)	C8, T1
	3. Abductor pollicis brevis	Median (lateral terminal branch)	C8, T1
	4. Opponens digiti minimi	Ulnar (deep terminal branch)	C8, T1

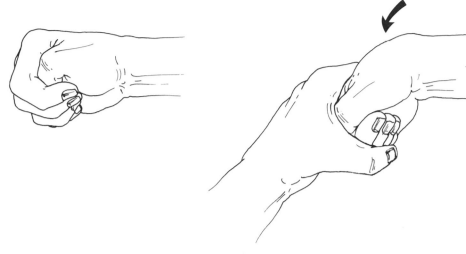

Figure 6–29. Finkelstein test.

5. Wrist flexion.
6. Wrist extension.
7. Finger flexion.
8. Finger extension.
9. Finger abduction.
10. Finger adduction.
11. Thumb flexion.
12. Thumb extension,
13. Thumb abduction.
14. Thumb adduction.
15. Opposition of the little finger and thumb.

SPECIAL TESTS

Only those special tests that the examiner feels have relevance should be performed.

Finkelstein Test. The Finkelstein test[7] is used for determining the presence of de Quervain's or Hoffman's disease, a tenosynovitis in the thumb. The patient makes a fist with the thumb inside the fingers (Fig. 6–29). The examiner stabilizes the forearm and ulnarly deviates the wrist. A positive test is indicated by pain over the abductor pollicis longus and extensor pollicis brevis tendons at the wrist and is indicative of a tenosynovitis in these two tendons. Because the test may cause some discomfort in normal individu-

als, the examiner should compare the pain caused on the affected side relative to the normal side.

Tinel's Sign (at the Wrist). The examiner taps over the carpal tunnel at the wrist (Fig. 6–30). A positive test causes tingling into the thumb, index finger (forefinger), and the middle and lateral half of the ring finger (median nerve distribution). Tinel's sign at the wrist is indicative of a carpal tunnel syndrome. The tingling or paresthesia must be felt distal to the point of pressure for a positive test. The test gives an indication of the rate of regeneration of the sensory fibers of the median nerve. The most distal point at which the abnormal sensation is felt represents the limit of nerve regeneration.

Phalen's (Wrist Flexion) Test. The examiner flexes the patient's wrists maximally and holds this position for 1 minute by pushing both the patient's wrists together (Fig. 6–31). A positive test is indicated by tingling into the thumb, the index finger, and the middle and lateral half of the ring finger. It is indicative of carpal tunnel syndrome caused by pressure on the median nerve.[9]

Bunnel-Littler Test. The metacarpophalangeal joint is held slightly extended while the examiner moves the proximal interphalangeal joint into flexion, if possible (Fig. 6–32).[10] If the test is

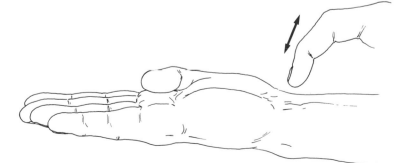

Figure 6–30. Tinel's sign at the wrist.

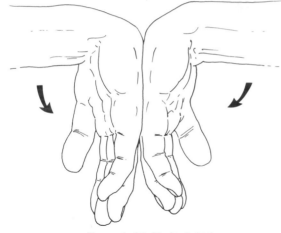

Figure 6–31. Phalen's test.

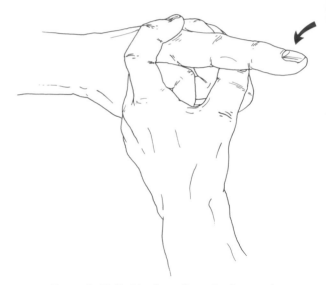

Figure 6–33. Test for the retinacular ligaments.

positive, which is indicated by the proximal interphalangeal joint not being able to be flexed, it means there is a tight intrinsic muscle or contracture of the joint capsule. If the metacarpophalangeal joints are slightly flexed, the proximal interphalangeal joint will fully flex if the intrinsic muscles are tight. It will not flex fully if the capsule is tight. The patient remains passive during the test and does no active movements.

Test for Tight Retinacular Ligaments. The proximal interphalangeal joint is held in a neutral position while the distal interphalangeal joint is flexed by the examiner (Fig. 6–33). If the distal interphalangeal joint does not flex, the retinacular (collateral) ligaments or capsule are tight. If the proximal interphalangeal joint is flexed and the distal interphalangeal joint flexes easily, the retinacular ligaments are tight and the capsule is normal. As with the previous test, the patient remains passive during the test and does no active movements.

Allen Test. The patient is asked to open and close the hand several times as quickly as possible and then squeeze the hand tightly (Fig. 6–34).[9] The examiner's thumb and index finger are placed

over the radial and ulnar arteries. The patient then opens the hand while pressure is maintained over the arteries. One artery is tested by releasing the pressure over that artery to see if the hand flushes. Then the other artery is tested in a similar fashion. Both hands should be tested for comparison. It is a test to determine the patency of the radial and ulnar arteries and to determine which artery provides the major blood supply to the hand.

Froment's Sign. The patient attempts to grasp a piece of paper between the thumb and index finger (Fig. 6–35).[9] When the examiner attempts to pull the paper away, the terminal phalanx of the thumb will flex because of paralysis of the adductor pollicis muscle, indicating a positive test. The test is indicative of an ulnar nerve paralysis.

Wrinkle (Shrivel) Test. The patient's fingers are placed in water for approximately 5 minutes. The examiner then removes the patient's fingers from the water and observes whether the skin over the pulp is wrinkled. Normal fingers will show wrinkling, whereas denervated ones will not. The test is valid only in the first few months following injury.[11]

Weber's Two-Point Discrimination Test. The examiner uses a paper clip to apply pressure on two adjacent points simultaneously in an attempt to find the minimal distance at which the patient can distinguish the two stimuli.[5] This distance is called the *threshold for discrimination*. Coverage values are shown in Figure 6–36. The patient must concentrate on feeling the points and must not be able to see the area being tested. The patient's hand should be immobile on a hard surface. For accurate results, the examiner must ensure that the two points touch the skin simultaneously.

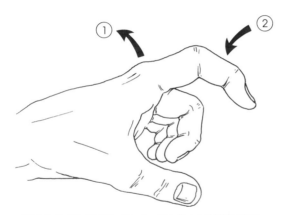

Figure 6–32. Positioning for the Bunnel-Littler test.

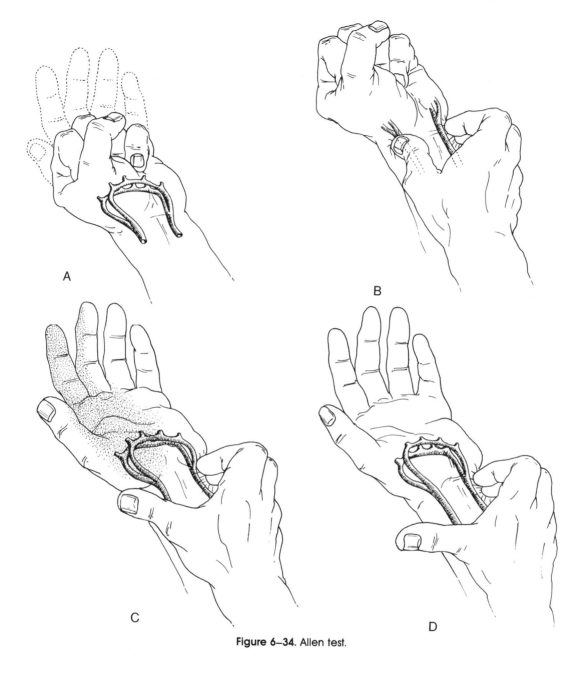

Figure 6–34. Allen test.

Figure 6–35. Froment's sign.

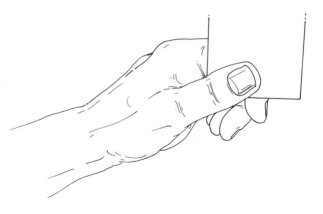

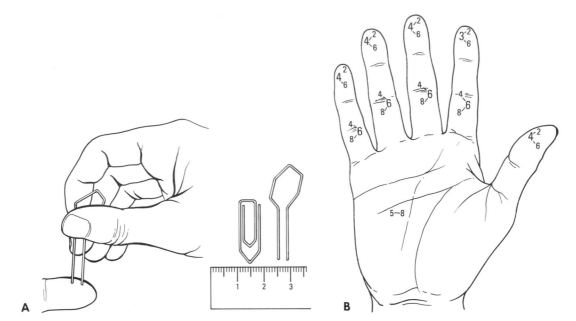

Figure 6–36. Two-point discrimination. (*A*) Technique of performing the two-point discrimination test of Weber. (After Moberg.) (*B*) Values of discriminations in the Weber test in millimeters in the different zones of the palm. The largest figure indicates the average values, the two others the minimum and maximum values. (After Moberg.) (Reprinted form Tubiana, R.: The Hand. Philadelphia, W. B. Saunders Co., 1981, pp. 645 and 646.)

Dellon's Moving Two-Point Discrimination Test. This test is used to predict functional recovery and measures the quickly adapting fibers/receptor system.[5] The examiner moves two blunt points from proximal to distal along the long axis of the limb or digit. One or two points are randomly used as the examiner moves distally. At the same time, the distance between the two points is decreased until the two points can no longer be distinguished.

REFLEXES AND CUTANEOUS DISTRIBUTION

The examiner must be aware of the sensory distribution of the ulnar, median, and radial nerves in the hand (Fig. 6–37). Several sensation tests may be carried out in the hand, such as two-point discrimination and *stereognosis* (the ability to differentiate size and shape of objects). Figure 6–36 shows the normal values for two-point discrimination at different locations in the hand. If

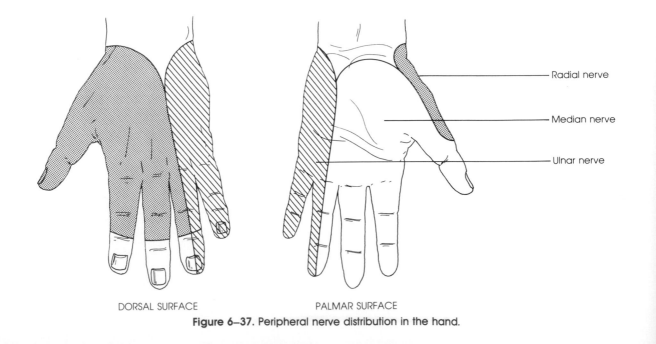

DORSAL SURFACE   PALMAR SURFACE

Figure 6–37. Peripheral nerve distribution in the hand.

from the cervical or upper thoracic spine, shoulder, and elbow. Seldom is wrist or hand pain referred up the limb (Fig. 6–38).

Neurologically, the examiner must be aware of potential injury of the various nerves about the wrist and hand.

The *median nerve* gives off a sensory branch above the wrist before it passes through the carpal tunnel. This sensory branch supplies the skin of the palm (Fig. 6–39). It is important to remember that carpal tunnel syndrome will not affect the median sensory distribution in the palm but will result in altered sensation in the fingers.

The *ulnar nerve* is sometimes compressed as it passes through the pisohamate, or *Guyon's canal* (Fig. 6–40). The nerve may be compressed from trauma, use of crutches, or chronic pressure, for example, as seen in people who cycle long distances, leaning on the handlebars or who extensively use pneumatic jackhammers. The ulnar nerve gives off two sensory branches above the wrist. These branches supply the palmar and dorsal aspects of the hand, as illustrated in Figure 6–37, and do not pass through Guyon's canal. Thus, if the ulnar nerve is compressed in the canal, only the fingers will show an altered sensation.

The examiner can attempt a differential diagnosis of paresthesia in the hand if altered sensation is present. A comparison with a normal dermatome chart should be made, and the examiner should remember that there is a fair amount of variability within the dermatomes (Fig. 6–41). In addition, there are areas of the hand where sensation is more important (Fig. 6–42). Abnormal sensation may mean the following:

    1. Numbness in the thumb only may be due

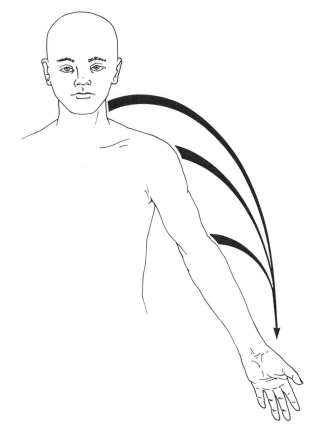

Figure 6–38. Symptoms can be referred to the wrist and hand from the elbow, shoulder, and cervical spine.

the values are three or four times greater than the normal values, sufficient cutaneous sensibility for control and learning is absent and visual control becomes necessary. It must be remembered that pain may be referred to the wrist and the hand

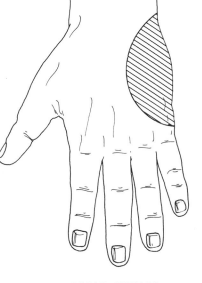
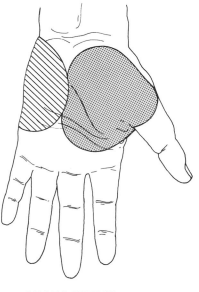

Figure 6–39. Sensory distribution of branches of the ulnar and median nerves given off above the wrist. Diagonal lines = Ulnar nerve; shaded area = median nerve.

DORSAL SURFACE   PALMAR SURFACE

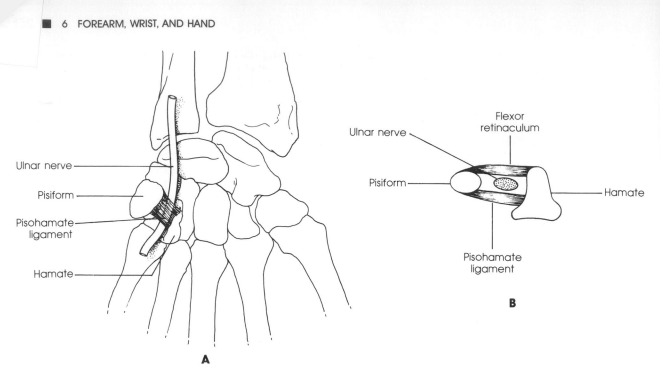

Figure 6–40. Guyon's canal. (*A*) Palmar view. (*B*) Section view showing position of nerve relative to pisohamate ligament and flexor retinaculum.

to pressure on the digital nerve on the outer aspect of the thumb.

2. Pins and needles in the thumb may be due to a contusion of the thenar branch of the median nerve.

3. Paresthesia in the thumb and index finger may be due to a C5 disc lesion or C6 nerve root palsy.

4. Paresthesia in the thumb, index finger, and middle finger may be due to a C5 disc lesion, a C6 nerve root palsy, or a thoracic outlet syndrome.

5. Paresthesia of the thumb, index finger, and

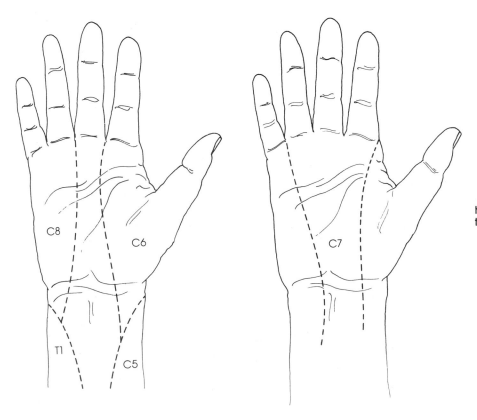

Figure 6–41. Dermatomes of the hand. Note overlap at dermatomes. Both views are palmar.

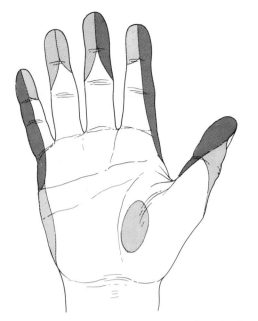

Figure 6–42. Importance of hand sensation. Dark areas indicate where sensation is most important; gray, where sensation is a little less important; white, where sensation is least important. (From Tubiana, R.: The Hand. Philadelphia, W. B. Saunders Co., 1981, p. 74.)

the middle and half of the ring finger on the palmar aspect may be due to an injury to the median nerve, possibly through the carpal tunnel; on the dorsal aspect, it could be due to injury to the radial nerve.

6. Numbness of the thumb and middle finger may be due to a tumor of the humerus.

7. Paresthesia on all five digits in one or both hands may be due to a thoracic outlet syndrome. If it is in both hands, it may be due to a central cervical disc protrusion. The level of protrusion would be indicated by the distribution of the paresthesia.

8. Paresthesia of the index and middle fingers may be due to a trigger finger or "stick" palsy, if it is on the palmar aspect, or a C6 disc lesion or C7 nerve root palsy. On the dorsal aspect of the hand, it may be due to a carpal exostosis or subluxation. Stick palsy is the result of an inordinant amount of pressure from a cane on the ulnar nerve as it passes through the palm.

9. Paresthesia of the index, middle, and ring fingers may be due to a C6 disc lesion, a C7 nerve root injury, or a carpal tunnel syndrome.

10. Paresthesia of all four fingers may be due to a C6 disc lesion or injury to the C7 nerve root.

11. Paresthesia of the middle finger only may be due to a C6 disc lesion or a C7 nerve root lesion.

12. Paresthesia of the middle and ring fingers may be due to a C6 disc lesion, a C7 nerve lesion, or stick palsy.

13. Paresthesia of the middle, ring, and little fingers may be due to a C7 disc lesion or a C8 nerve root palsy. The same would be true if there were paralysis of the ring and little fingers. This paresthesia may also be the result of a thoracic outlet syndrome.

14. Paresthesia on the ulnar side of the ring finger and all of the little finger may be due to pressure of the ulnar nerve at the elbow or in the palm.

JOINT PLAY MOVEMENTS

When assessing joint play movements, the examiner should remember that if the patient complains of inability or pain on wrist flexion, the lesion is probably in the midcarpal joints. If the patient complains of inability or pain on wrist extension, the lesion is probably in the radiocarpal joints because it is in these joints that most of the movement occurs during these actions. If the patient complains of pain or inability on supination and pronation, the lesion is, in all probability, in the ulnameniscocarpal joint or inferior radioulnar joint.

These joint play movements are carried out on the *wrist* (Fig. 6–43):

1. Long axis extension (traction or distraction).
2. Anteroposterior glide.
3. Side glide.
4. Side tilt.

The joint play movement of the *intermetacarpal joints* is anteroposterior glide.

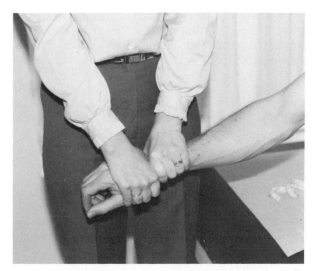

Figure 6–43. Positioning for joint play movements of the wrist.

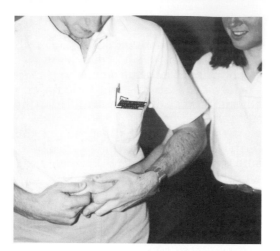

Figure 6–44. Positioning for joint play movements of the fingers.

These joint play movements are carried out on *fingers* (Fig. 6–44):

1. Long axis extension (traction or distraction).
2. Anteroposterior glide.
3. Rotation.
4. Side glide.

The amount of movement obtained by the joint play should be compared with the normal side and should be considered significant only if there is a difference between the two sides.

Wrist

For the wrist, long axis extension is performed by the examiner stabilizing the radius and ulna with one hand (the patient's arm may be flexed to 90° and stabilization applied at the elbow if there is no pathology at the elbow) and placing the other hand just distal to the wrist. The examiner then applies a longitudinal traction movement with the distal hand.

Anteroposterior glide is applied at the wrist in two positions. The examiner first places the stabilizing hand around the distal end of the radius and ulna just proximal to the radiocarpal joint, then places the other hand around the proximal row of carpal bones. If the hands are positioned properly, they should touch each other (Fig. 6–43). The examiner applies an anteroposterior gliding movement of the proximal row of carpal bones on the radius and ulna. Then the stabilizing hand is moved so that it is around the proximal row of carpal bones. The examiner places the mobilizing hand around the distal row of carpal bones. An anteroposterior gliding movement is applied to the distal row of carpal bones on the proximal row.

Side glide is performed in a similar fashion, except that a side-to-side movement is performed instead of an anteroposterior movement. To perform side tilting of the carpals on the radius and ulna, the examiner stabilizes the radius and ulna by placing the stabilizing hand around the distal radius and ulna just proximal to the radiocarpal joint and the mobilizing hand around the patient's hand and radially or ulnarly deviates the hand on the radius and ulna. These joint play movements are general ones involving all carpal bones. To check the joint play movements of the individual carpal bones, *Kaltenborn's technique* should be used.[3]

Intermetacarpal Joints

To accomplish anteroposterior glide at the intermetacarpal joints, the examiner stabilizes one metacarpal bone and moves the adjacent metacarpal anteriorly and posteriorly in relation to the fixed bone. The process is repeated for each joint.

Fingers

The joint play movements for the fingers are the same for the metacarpophalangeal, proximal interphalangeal, and distal interphalangeal joints. The hand position of the examiner just moves further distally.

To perform long axis extension, the examiner stabilizes the proximal segment or bone using one hand while placing the second hand around the distal segment or bone of the particular joint to be tested. With the mobilizing hand, the examiner applies a longitudinal traction to the joint.

Anteroposterior glide is accomplished by stabilizing the proximal bone with one hand. The mobilizing hand is placed around the distal segment of the joint, and the examiner applies an anterior and/or posterior movement to the distal segment, being sure to maintain the joint surfaces parallel to one another. A minimal amount of traction may be applied to bring about slight separation of the joint surfaces.

Rotation of the joints of the fingers is accomplished by stabilizing the proximal segment with one hand. With the other hand, the examiner applies slight traction to the joint to distract the joint surfaces and then rotates the distal segment on the proximal segment.

To perform side glide joint play to the joints of the fingers, the proximal segment is stabilized with one hand, while the examiner applies slight traction to the joint with the mobilizing hand to distract the joint surfaces and then moves the distal segment sideways, keeping the joint surfaces parallel to one another.

Carpal Bones

Kaltenborn suggests ten tests to determine the mobility of each of the carpal bones. The movement between each of the bones is determined in a sequential manner, and both sides are to be tested for comparison.

1. Fixate the capitate and move the trapezoid.
2. Fixate the capitate and move the scaphoid.
3. Fixate the capitate and move the lunate.
4. Fixate the capitate and move the hamate.
5. Fixate the scaphoid and move the trapezoid and trapezium.
6. Fixate the radius and move the scaphoid.
7. Fixate the radius and move the lunate.
8. Fixate the ulna and move the triquetrum.
9. Fixate the triquetrum and move the hamate.
10. Fixate the triquetrum and move the pisiform.

PALPATION

To palpate the forearm, wrist, and hand, the examiner starts proximally and works distally first on the dorsal surface and then on the anterior surface (Fig. 6–45). The muscles of the forearm are first palpated for any signs of tenderness or pathology.

Dorsal Surface

On the dorsal aspect, the examiner begins on the thumb side of the hand and palpates the following structures: (1) the "snuff box"; (2) the carpal bones; and (3) the metacarpal bones and phalanges.

Anatomic "Snuff Box." The snuff box is located between the tendons of extensor pollicis longus

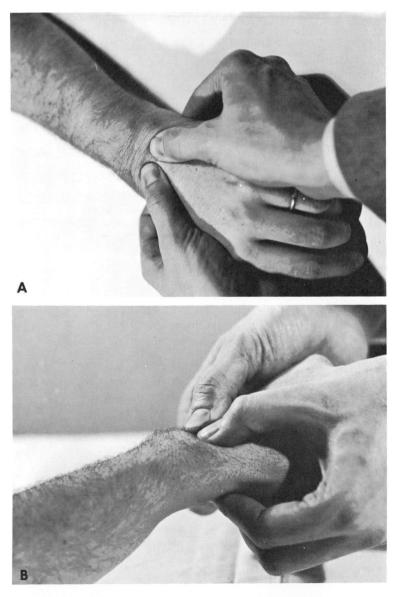

Figure 6–45. Palpation of the left wrist by using both hands. (*A*) Top view. (*B*) Side view. The wrist is being palpated firmly (note blanched nails of examiner's thumbs) by both thumbs and second (index) fingers. The other fingers serve to support and position the patient's hand as partially shown in *B*. (From Polley, H. F., and G. G. Hunder: Rheumatological Interviewing and Physical Examination of the Joints. Philadelphia, W. B. Saunders Co., 1978, p. 101.)

and extensor pollicis brevis and can best be seen by having the patient actively extend the thumb. The scaphoid bone may be palpated inside the snuff box. Tenderness of the scaphoid bone is often treated as a fracture until proven otherwise because of the possibility of avascular necrosis of the bone. Palpating proximally, one finds the radial styloid on the lateral aspect (in the anatomic position) of the wrist. Moving medially over the radius, the examiner will come to the radial (Lister's) tubercle. The extensor pollicis longus tendon moves around the tubercle to enter the thumb, which gives it a different angle of pull from extensor pollicis brevis. The ulnar styloid is palpated on the medial aspect (in the anatomic position) of the wrist. The examiner will note that the radial styloid extends further distally than the ulnar styloid. Palpating over the dorsum of the wrist, crossing the radius and ulna, one should attempt to palpate the six extensor tendon tunnels moving lateral to medial:

1. Tunnel one—abductor pollicis longus and extensor pollicis brevis.

2. Tunnel two—extensor carpi radialis longus and brevis.

3. Tunnel three—extensor pollicis longus.

4. Tunnel four—extensor digitorum and extensor indices.

5. Tunnel five—extensor digiti minimi.

6. Tunnel six—extensor carpi ulnaris.

Carpal Bones. In the anatomic snuff box, the examiner can begin palpating the proximal row of carpal bones, starting with the scaphoid bone. When palpating the carpal bones, the examiner usually palpates them on the anterior and dorsal surface at the same time. The proximal row of carpal bones from lateral to medial (in the anatomic position) are the:

1. Scaphoid.

2. Lunate.

3. Triquetrum (just below the ulnar styloid).

4. Pisiform.

On the anterior aspect, the examiner should take care to ensure proper positioning of the lunate bone. If it dislocates or subluxes, it tends to move in an anterior direction into the carpal tunnel, which may lead to carpal tunnel syndrome symptoms. The pisiform is often easier to palpate if the patient's wrist is flexed. The examiner may then palpate the pisiform where the flexor carpi ulnaris tendon inserts into it.

Returning to the anatomic snuff box and moving distally the examiner palpates the trapezium bone. As this is done, the radial pulse is often palpated in the anatomic snuff box. The distal row of carpal bones from lateral to medial (in the anatomic position) are palpated individually:

1. Trapezium.

2. Trapezoid.

3. Capitate (distal to lunate).

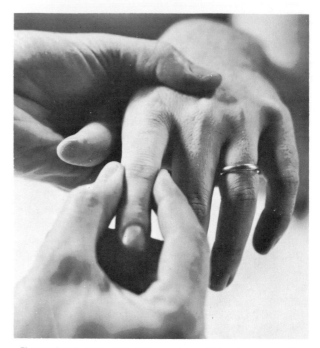

Figure 6–46. Palpation of the proximal interphalangeal joint of the left second finger. The examiner's left hand is supporting the patient's hand while the examiner's right thumb and forefinger are used to palpate simultaneously and alternately the medial and lateral aspects of the joint. The other proximal interphalangeal joints are examined similarly. (From Polley, H. F., and G. G. Hunder: Rheumatological Interviewing and Physical Examination of the Joints. Philadelphia, W. B. Saunders Co., 1978, p. 132.)

4. Hamate (distal to triquetrum; the hook of the hamate on anterior surface is the easiest part to palpate).

Metacarpal Bones and Phalanges. The examiner returns to the trapezium bone and moves further distally to palpate the trapezium, first metacarpal joint, and the metacarpal bone. Moving medially, the examiner palpates each metacarpal bone on the anterior and dorsal surfaces in turn. A similar procedure is carried out for the metacarpophalangeal and interphalangeal joints and the phalanges. These structures are also palpated on their medial and lateral aspects for tenderness, swelling, altered temperature, or other signs of pathology (Fig. 6–46).

To test distal blood flow, the examiner compresses the nail bed and notes the time taken for color to return to the nail. Comparison with the normal side will give some indication of restricted flow.

Anterior Surface

The examiner then moves to the anterior surface to complete the palpation.

Pulses. Proximally, the radial and ulnar pulses are first palpated. The radial pulse on the anterolateral aspect of the wrist on top of the radius is easiest to palpate and is the one most frequently used when "taking a patient's pulse." It runs between the tendons of flexor carpi radialis and abductor pollicis longus. The ulnar pulse may be palpated lateral to the tendon of flexor carpi ulnaris. It is more difficult to palpate because it runs deeper and lies under the pisiform and the palmar fascia.

Tendons. Moving across the anterior aspect, the examiner may be able to palpate the long flexor tendons in a lateral to medial direction:

1. Flexor carpi radialis.
2. Flexor pollicis longus.
3. Flexor digitorum superficialis.
4. Flexor digitorum profundus.
5. Palmaris longus.
6. Flexor carpi ulnaris (inserts into pisiform).

The palmaris longus (if present) lies over the tendons of the flexor digitorum superficialis, which lie over the tendons of the flexor digitorum profundus.

Palmar Fascia and Intrinsic Muscles. The examiner should then move distally to palpate the palmar fascia and intrinsic muscles of the thenar and hypothenar eminence for indications of pathology.

Skin Flexion Creases. From an anatomic point of view, the examiner should note the various skin flexion creases of the wrist, hand and fingers (Fig. 6–47). The flexion creases indicate lines of adherence between the skin and fascia with no intervening adipose tissue. The following creases should be noted:

1. The proximal skin crease of the wrist indicates the upper limit of the synovial sheaths of the flexor tendons.

2. The middle skin crease of the wrist indicates the wrist (radiocarpal) joint.

3. The distal skin crease of the wrist indicates the upper margin of the flexor retinaculum.

4. The radial longitudinal skin crease of the palm encircles the thenar eminence. (Palm readers refer to this line as the "life line.")

5. The proximal transverse line of the palm runs across the shafts of the metacarpal bones, indicating the superficial palmar arterial arch (Fig. 6–48). (Palm readers refer to this line as the "head line.")

6. The distal transverse line of the palm lies over the heads of the second to fourth metacarpals. (Palm readers refer to this line as the "love line.")

7. The proximal skin crease of the fingers is 2 cm distal to the metacarpophalangeal joints.

8. The middle skin crease of the fingers is made up of two lines and lies over the proximal interphalangeal joints.

9. The distal skin crease of the fingers lies over the distal interphalangeal joints.

10. On the flexor and extensor aspect, the skin creases over the proximal and distal interphalangeal joints lie proximal to the joint. On the extensor aspect, the metacarpophalangeal creases lie

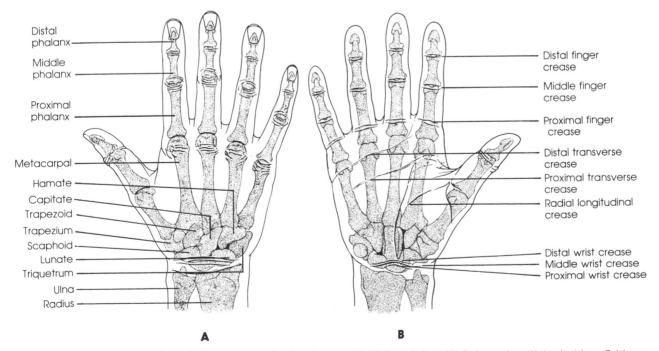

Distal phalanx
Middle phalanx
Proximal phalanx
Metacarpal
Hamate
Capitate
Trapezoid
Trapezium
Scaphoid
Lunate
Triquetrum
Ulna
Radius

Distal finger crease
Middle finger crease
Proximal finger crease
Distal transverse crease
Proximal transverse crease
Radial longitudinal crease
Distal wrist crease
Middle wrist crease
Proximal wrist crease

A   B

Figure 6–47. Bony landmarks and skin creases of the hand and wrist. (*A*) Dorsal view. (*B*) Palmar view. (Adapted from Tubiana, R.: The Hand. Philadelphia, W. B. Saunders Co., 1981, p. 619.)

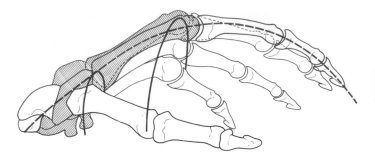

Figure 6–48. Longitudinal and transverse arches of the hand (lateral view). Shaded areas show the fixed part of the skeleton. (From Tubiana, R.: The Hand. Philadelphia, W. B. Saunders Co., 1981, p. 25.)

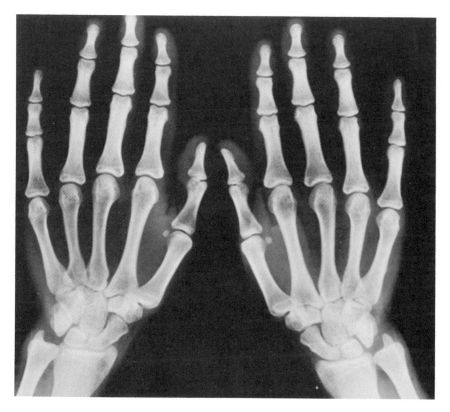

Figure 6–49. Radiograph showing the skeleton of both hands. The thumb metacarpal is the shortest and the index metacarpal by far the longest. The first and second phalanges of the middle and ring finger are longer than those of the index. Note the interlocking design of the carpometacarpal articulations and the saddle shape in opposing planes of the articular surfaces of the trapezium and the base of the first metacarpal. (From Tubiana, R.: The Hand. Philadelphia, W. B. Saunders Co., 1981, p. 21.)

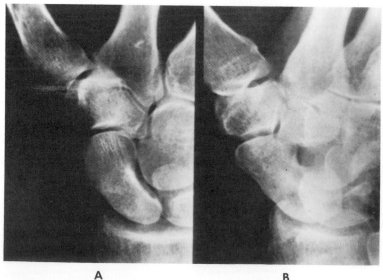

Figure 6–50. Radiograph of the normal scaphoid. (*A*) Posteroanterior view. (*B*) Lateral view. (From Tubiana, R.: The Hand. Philadelphia, W. B. Saunders Co., 1981, p. 659.)

A   B

proximal to the joint; on the flexor aspect, they lie distal to the joint.

Arches. In addition, the examiner should ensure the viability of the arches of the hand (Fig. 6–48). The carpal transverse arch is the result of the shape of the carpal bones, which in part forms the carpal tunnel. The flexor retinaculum forms the roof for the tunnel. The metacarpal transverse arch is formed by the metacarpal bones, and its shape can have great variability because of the mobility of these bones. This arch is most evident when the palm is cupped. The longitudinal arch is made of the carpal bones, metacarpal bones, and phalanges. The keystone of this arch is the metacarpophalangeal joints, which provide stability and support for the arch.

Weakness or atrophy of the intrinsic muscles of the hand will lead to a loss of these arches. The deformity is most obvious with paralysis of the median and ulnar nerves, resulting in an "ape hand" deformity.

RADIOGRAPHIC STUDIES OF THE FOREARM, WRIST, AND HAND

Anteroposterior View. The examiner should note the shape and position of the bones (Fig. 6–49), watching for (1) any evidence of fractures or displacement, (2) any decrease in the joint spaces, and (3) any change in bone density, which may be due to avascular necrosis. If it is due to avascular necrosis, there will be rarefaction and increased density of the bone and possibly sclerosis of the bone. Avascular necrosis is often seen in the scaphoid bone (Figs. 6–50 and 6–51A) following a fracture or in the lunate in Kienböck's disease (Fig. 6–51B).[12]

The anteroposterior view of the wrist and hand is used to determine the skeletal age of an individual.[13] The left hand and wrist are used for study because they are thought to be less influenced by environmental factors. The method used in this technique is based on the fact that after an *ossification center* appears (Fig. 6–52), it changes its shape and size in a systematic manner as the ossification gradually spreads throughout the cartilaginous parts of the skeleton. The wrist and hand are studied because several bones are available for overall comparison. The patient's hand is compared with standard plates[14] until one plate is found that best approximates that of the patient. There is one standard for males and another for females. In two thirds of the population, skeletal age is no more than a year above or below chron-

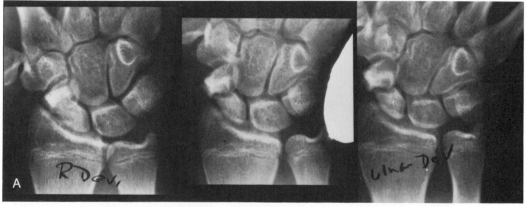

RADIAL DEVIATION NEUTRAL ULNAR DEVIATION

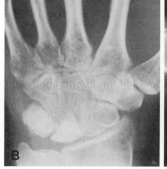
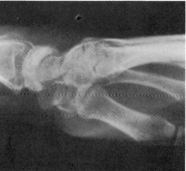

Figure 6–51. Avascular necrosis of the carpal bones. (*A*) Scaphoid fracture in three positions. (From Cooney, W. P., et al.: Clin. Orthop. Relat. Res. *149*:92, 1980.) (*B*) Lunate fracture and sclerosis in Kienböck's disease. (From Beckenbaugh, R. D., et al.: Clin. Orthop. Relat. Res. *149*:99, 1980.)

ANTEROPOSTERIOR VIEW LATERAL VIEW

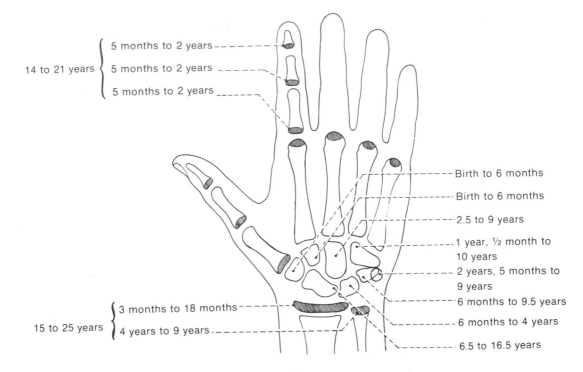

14 to 21 years {
5 months to 2 years ------
5 months to 2 years ------
5 months to 2 years ------

Birth to 6 months
Birth to 6 months
2.5 to 9 years
1 year, ½ month to 10 years
2 years, 5 months to 9 years
6 months to 9.5 years
6 months to 4 years
6.5 to 16.5 years

15 to 25 years {
3 months to 18 months ------
4 years to 9 years ------

A

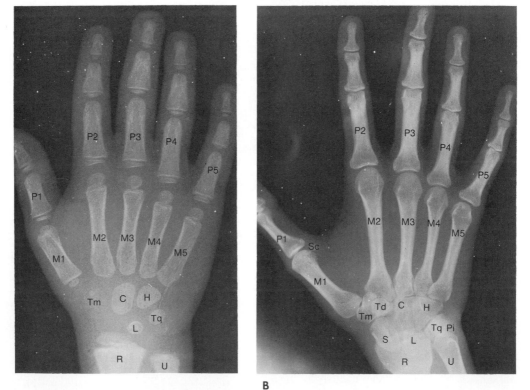

B

Figure 6–52. Ossification centers of the hand.

(*A*) Date of appearance and date of fusion are included. (From Tubiana, R.: The Hand. Philadelphia, W. B. Saunders Co., 1981, p. 11.)

(*B*) Radiographs of the hand and wrist. *Left*: Child, 4- to 5-year-old boy or 3- to 4-year-old girl. *Right*: Adult. C = Capitate; H = hamate; L = lunate; M = metacarpal; P = phalanges; Pi = pisiform; R = radius; S = scaphoid; Td = trapezoid; Tm = trapezium; Tq = triquetrum; U = ulna. (From Liebgott, B.: The Anatomical Basis of Dentistry. Philadelphia, W. B. Saunders Co., 1982, p. 454.)

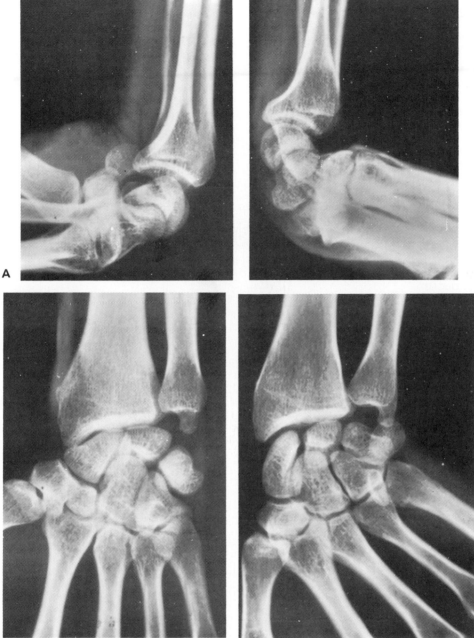

Figure 6–53. (*A*) Radiographs of wrist flexion and extension (lateral views). (*B*) Posteroanterior views of wrist in radial and ulnar deviation. Note the change in the form of the lunate, indicating a slipping toward the front in the radial slant and toward the rear in the ulnar. (From Tubiana, R.: The Hand. Philadelphia, W. B. Saunders Co., 1981, p. 655.)

ologic age. Acceleration or retardation of 3 years or more is considered abnormal. At birth, none of the carpal bones is visible (see Figure 1–11). This method may be used up to age 20, when the bones of the hand and wrist have fused.

Lateral View. The examiner should note the shape and position of bones for any evidence of fractures and/or displacement (Fig. 6–53).

Axial View. The axial view is especially useful if the examiner suspects a problem with the carpal bones (Fig. 6–54).

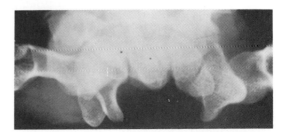

Figure 6–54. Radiograph of the carpal tunnel (axial view). (From Tubiana, R.: The Hand. Philadelphia, W. B. Saunders Co., 1981, p. 662.)

Précis of the Forearm, Wrist, and Hand Assessment

History
Observation
Examination
  Active movements
    Pronation of the forearm
    Supination of the forearm
    Wrist flexion
    Wrist extension
    Radial deviation of wrist
    Ulnar deviation of wrist
    Finger flexion (at MCP, PIP, and DIP joints)
    Finger extension (at MCP, PIP, and DIP joints)
    Finger abduction
    Finger adduction
    Thumb flexion
    Thumb extension
    Thumb abduction
    Thumb adduction
    Opposition of the thumb and little finger
    Functional grip tests
    Pinch tests
    Coordination tests
  Passive movements (as in Active movements, except functional grip, pinch tests and coordination tests if necessary)
  Resisted isometric movements (as in Active movements, in the neutral position)
  Special tests
  Reflexes and cutaneous distribution
  Joint play movements
    Long axis extension at the wrist and fingers (MCP, PIP, and DIP joints)
    Anteroposterior glide at the wrist and fingers (MCP, PIP, and DIP joints)
    Side glide at the wrist and fingers (MCP, PIP, and DIP joints)
    Side tilt at the wrist
    Anteroposterior glide at the intermetacarpal joints
    Rotation at the MCP, PIP, and DIP joints
    Carpal bone mobility
  Palpation
  X-ray viewing

Following any examination, the patient should always be warned of the possibility of exacerbation of symptoms as a result of the assessment.

REFERENCES

CITED REFERENCES

1. Palmer, A.K., and F.W. Werner: The triangular fibrocartilage complex of the wrist: Anatomy and function. J. Hand Surg. 6:152, 1981.
2. Kapandji, I.A.: The Physiology of Joints, vol. I: Upper Limb. New York, Churchill Livingstone, 1970.
3. Kaltenborn, F.M.: Mobilization of the Extremity Joints. Oslo, Olaf Norlis Bokhandel, 1980.
4. Wadsworth, C.T.: Wrist and hand examination and interpretation. J. Orthop. Sports Phys. Ther. 5:108, 1983.
5. Tubiana, R.: The Hand. Philadelphia, W.B. Saunders Co., 1981.
6. Reid, D.C.: Functional Anatomy and Joint Mobilization. Edmonton, University of Alberta Press, 1970.
7. Finkelstein, H.: Stenosing tendovaginitis at the radial styloid process. J. Bone Joint Surg. 12:509, 1930.
8. Moldaver, J.: Tinel's sign—its characteristics and significance. J. Bone Joint Surg. 60A:412, 1978.
9. American Society for Surgery of the Hand: The Hand—Examination and Diagnosis. Aurora, Col., 1978.
10. Hoppenfeld, S.: Physical Examination of the Spine and Extremities. New York, Appleton-Century-Crofts, 1976.
11. O'Riain, S.: Shrivel test: A new and simple test of nerve function in the hand. Br. Med. J. 3:615, 1973.
12. Beckenbaugh, R.D., T.C. Shives, J.H. Dobyns, and R.L. Linschied: Kienbock's disease: The natural history of Kienbock's disease and consideration of lunate fractures. Clin. Orthop. Relat. Res. 149:98, 1980.
13. Hansman, C.F., and M.M. Mresh: Appearance and fusion of ossification centers in the human skeleton. Am. J. Roentgenol. 88:476, 1962.

GENERAL REFERENCES

American Orthopaedic Association: Manual of Orthopaedic Surgery. Chicago, 1972.
Backhouse, K.M.: Functional anatomy of the hand. Physiotherapy 54:114, 1968.
Beetham, W.P., H.F. Polley, C.H. Slocumb, and W.F. Weaver: Physical Examination of the Joints. Philadelphia, W.B. Saunders Co., 1965.
Cailliet, R.: Hand Pain and Impairment. Philadelphia, F.A. Davis Co., 1971.
Coleman, H.M.: Injuries of the articular disc at the wrist. Bone Joint Surg. 42B:522, 1960.
Cooney, W.P., J.H. Dobyns, and R.L. Linschied: Fractures of the scaphoid: A rational approach to management. Clin. Orthop. Relat. Res. 149:90, 1980.
Cooney, W.P., M.J. Lucca, E.Y.S. Chao, and R.L. Linscheid: Kinesiology of the thumb trapeziometacarpal joint. J. Bone Joint Surg. 63A:1371, 1981.
Cyriax, J.: Textbook of Orthopaedic Medicine, vol. I: Diagnosis of Soft Tissue Lesions. London, Bailliere Tindall, 1982.
Gilula, L.A., and P.M. Weeks: Post-traumatic ligamentous instabilities of the wrist. Diagn. Radiol. 129:641, 1978.
Greulich, W.W., and S.U. Pyle: Radiographic Atlas of Skeletal Development of the Wrist and Hand. Stanford, Calif., Stanford University Press, 1959.
Hollinshead, W.H., and D.B. Jenkins.: Functional Anatomy of the Limbs and Back. Philadelphia, W.B. Saunders Co., 1981.
Jacobs, P.: Atlas of Hand Radiographs. Baltimore, University Park Press, 1973.
Johnson, R.P.: The acutely injured wrist and its residuals. Clin. Orthop. Relat. Res. 140:33, 1980.
Judge, R.D., G.D. Zuidema, and F.T. Fitzgerald: Clinical Diagnosis: A Physiological Approach. Boston, Little, Brown and Co., 1982.
Kauer, J.M.G.: Functional anatomy of the wrist. Clin. Orthop. Relat. Res. 149:9, 1980.
Kendall, E.P., and B.K. McCreary: Muscles: Testing and Function. Baltimore, Williams and Wilkins, 1983.
Liebgott, B.: The Anatomical Basis of Dentistry. Philadelphia, W.B. Saunders Co., 1982.
Maitland, G.D.: The Peripheral Joints: Examination and Recording Guide. Adelaide, Australia, Virgo Press, 1973.
McMurtry, R.Y., Y. Youm, A.E. Flatt, and T.E. Gillespie: Kinematics of the wrist. II: Clinical applications. J. Bone Joint Surg. 60A:955, 1978.

McRae, R.: Clinical Orthopaedic Examination. New York, Churchill-Livingstone, 1976.

Mennell, J.M.: Joint Pain. Boston, Little, Brown and Co., 1964.

Mennell, J.M.: Manipulation of the joints of the wrist. Physiotherapy 57:247, 1971.

Nicholas, J.S.: The swollen hand. Physiotherapy 63:285, 1977.

O'Donoghue, D.H.: Treatment of Injuries to Athletes, 4th ed. Philadelphia, W.B. Saunders Co., 1984.

Samman, P.D.: The Nails in Disease. London, Wm. Heinemann Medical Books Ltd., 1965.

Todd, T.W.: Atlas of Skeletal Maturation. St. Louis, C.V. Mosby Co., 1937.

Tucker, W.E.: Manipulative techniques employed in the treatment of injury and osteoarthritis of the fingers and hands. Physiotherapy 57:257, 1971.

Volz, R.G., and J. Benjamin: Biomechanics of the wrist. Clin. Orthop. Relat. Res. 149:112, 1980.

Williams, P., and R. Warwick: Gray's Anatomy, 36th British ed. Philadelphia, W.B. Saunders Co., 1980.

Wynn Parry, C.B.: Rehabilitation of the Hand. London, Butterworths, 1981.

Youm, Y., R.Y. McMurtry, A.E. Flatt, and T.E. Gillespie: Kinematics of the wrist: I. An experimental study of radioulnar deviation and flexion-extension. J. Bone Joint Surg. 60A:423, 1978.

7

Thoracic (Dorsal) Spine

Assessment of the thoracic spine involves examination of the part of the spine that is most rigid because of the associated rib cage. The rib cage in turn provides protection for the heart and lungs. Normally the thoracic spine, being one of the primary curves, exhibits a mild *kyphosis* (posterior curvature); the *cervical* and *lumbar spines* being secondary curves, exhibit a mild *lordosis* (anterior curvature). When the examiner assesses the thoracic spine, it is essential that the cervical and lumbar spine be evaluated at the same time (Fig. 7–1).

Applied Anatomy

The *costovertebral joints* are synovial plane joints located between the ribs and the vertebral body. There are 24 of these joints, and they are divided into two parts. Ribs 1, 10, 11, and 12 articulate with a single vertebra. The other articulations have an intra-articular ligament that divides the joint into two parts so that each rib (ribs 2 through 9) articulates with two adjacent vertebrae and the intervening intervertebral disc.

The *costotransverse joints* are synovial joints found between the ribs and the transverse processes of the vertebra of the same level for ribs 1 through 10. Because ribs 11 and 12 do not articulate with the transverse processes, this joint does not exist for these two levels.

The *costochondral joints* lie between the ribs and the costal cartilage. The *sternocostal joints* are found between the costal cartilage and the sternum. Joints 2 through 6 are synovial, whereas the first costal cartilage is united with the sternum by a synchondrosis. Where a rib articulates with an adjacent rib or costal cartilage, a synovial interchondral joint (ribs 5 through 9) exists.

The superior facet of the T1 vertebra is similar to a facet of the cervical spine. Because of this, T1 is classified as a *transitional vertebra*. The T1 superior facet faces up and back; the inferior facet faces down and forward. The T2 to T11 superior facets face up and back and slightly laterally; the inferior facets face down, forward, and slightly medially (Fig. 7–2). This shape enables slight rotation in the thoracic spine. Thoracic vertebrae 11 and 12 are classified as transitional and the facets of these vertebrae become positioned in a way similar to that of the lumbar facets. The superior facets of these two vertebrae face up, back, and more medially; the inferior facets face forward and slightly laterally. The close packed position of the facet joints in the thoracic spine is extension.

Within the thoracic spine, there are 12 vertebrae, which diminish in size from T1 to T3 and then increase progressively in size to T12. These vertebrae are distinctive in having facets on the body and transverse processes for articulation with the ribs. The spinous processes of these vertebrae face obliquely downward. T7 has the

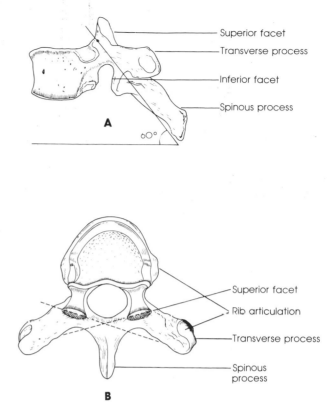

Figure 7–2. T7 Thoracic vertebra. (*A*) Side view. (*B*) Superior view.

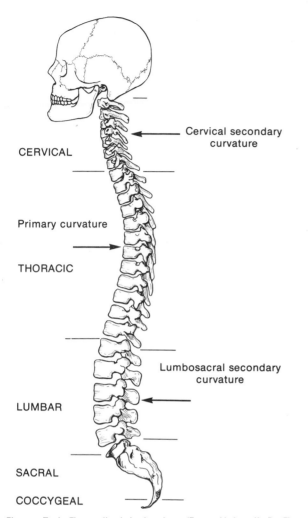

Figure 7–1. The articulated spine. (From Liebgott, B.: The Anatomical Basis of Dentistry. Philadelphia, W. B. Saunders Co., 1982, p. 47.)

greatest spinous process angulation, whereas the upper three thoracic vertebrae have spinous processes that project directly posteriorly. In other words, the spinous processes of these vertebrae are on the same plane as the transverse processes of the same vertebra (Fig. 7–3).

T4, T5, and T6 vertebrae have spinous processes that project downward slightly. In this case, the tips of the spinous processes are on a plane halfway between their own transverse processes and the transverse processes of the vertebrae below. For T7, T8, and T9 vertebrae, the spinous processes project downward, with the tip of the spinous processes being on a plane of the transverse processes of the vertebrae below. For the T10 spinous process, the arrangement is similar to that of the T9 spinous process; i.e., the spinous process is level with the transverse process of the vertebra below. For T11, the arrangement is similar to that of T6; i.e., the spinous process is halfway between the two transverse processes of the vertebra. T12 is similar to T3; i.e., the level

of the transverse process is level with the process of the same vertebra. The location of the spinous processes becomes important if the examiner wishes to perform posteroanterior central vertebral pressures. For example, if the examiner pushes on the spinous process of T8, the body of T9 will also move. In fact, the vertebral body of T8 will likely arc, whereas T9 will move in an anterior direction. T7 is sometimes classified as a transitional vertebra because it is the point at which the lower limb axial rotation alternates with the upper limb axial rotation (Fig. 7–4).

The ribs, which help to stiffen the thoracic spine, articulate with the demifacets on vertebrae T2 to T9. For T1 and T10 vertebrae, there is a whole facet for ribs 1 and 10, respectively. The

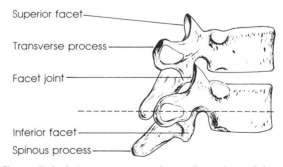

Figure 7–3. Spinous process of one thoracic vertebra at level of body of vertebra below (T7–T9).

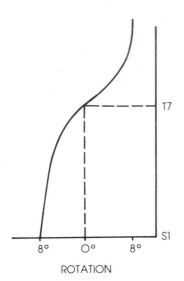

Figure 7–4. Axial rotation of the spine going from left to right on heel strike.

ROTATION

first rib articulates with T1 only; the second rib articulates with T1 and T2; and the third rib articulates with T2 and T3, and so on. Ribs 1 through 7 articulate with the sternum directly and are classified as *true ribs.* Ribs 8, 9, and 10 join with the costocartilage of the rib above and are classified as *false ribs.* Ribs 11 and 12 are classified as *floating ribs* because they do not attach to the sternum or costal cartilages at their distal end.

Ribs 11 and 12 articulate only with the bodies of T11 and T12 vertebrae and not with the transverse processes of the vertebrae or with the costocartilage of the rib above. The ribs are held by ligaments to the body of the vertebra and to the transverse processes of the same vertebrae. Some of these ligaments also bind the ribs to the vertebra above.

At the top of the rib cage, the ribs are relatively horizontal. As the rib cage descends, they run more and more obliquely downward. By the 12th rib, the ribs are more vertical than horizontal. With inspiration, the ribs are pulled up and forward, and this increases the anteroposterior diameter of the ribs. The first six ribs increase the anteroposterior dimension of the chest mainly by rotating around their long axes. Rotation downward of the rib neck is associated with depression, while rotation upward of the same portion is

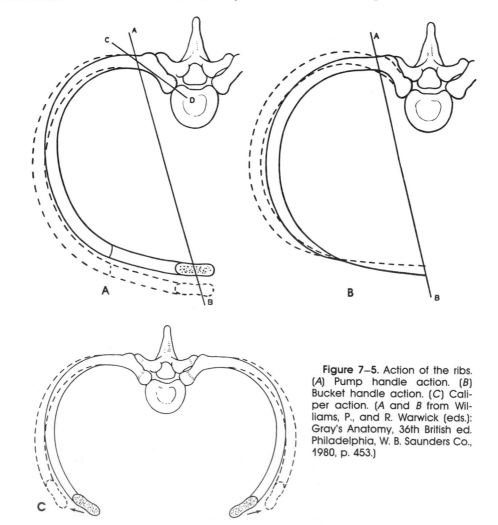

Figure 7–5. Action of the ribs. (*A*) Pump handle action. (*B*) Bucket handle action. (*C*) Caliper action. (*A* and *B* from Williams, P., and R. Warwick (eds.): Gray's Anatomy, 36th British ed. Philadelphia, W. B. Saunders Co., 1980, p. 453.)

associated with elevation. These movements are known as a "pump handle" action and are accompanied by elevation of the manubrium sternum upward and forward (Fig. 7–5).[1–3]

Ribs 7 through 10 mainly increase lateral, or transverse, dimension. To accomplish this, the ribs move upward, backward, and medially to increase the infrasternal angle or downward, forward, and laterally to decrease the angle. These movements are known as a "bucket handle" action. This action is also performed by ribs 2 through 6 but to a much lesser degree (Fig. 7–5).

The lower ribs (ribs 8 through 12) move laterally in what is known as a "caliper" action which increases lateral diameter[2] (Fig. 7–5).

The ribs are quite elastic in children, but they become increasingly brittle with age. In the anterior half of the chest, the ribs are subcutaneous, in the posterior half, they are covered by muscles.

Patient History

A thorough and complete history should include past and present problems. By listening carefully, the examiner is often able to identify the patient's problem and can then go on to use the observation and examination to confirm or refute the impressions established from the history. Information concerning the present pain, its site, nature, and behavior are all important. If any part of the history implicates the cervical or lumbar spine, the examiner must include these areas in the assessment as well.

In addition to the general questions asked in Chapter 1, the following information should be ascertained:

1. What are the details of the present pain and other symptoms? What are the sites and boundaries of the pain? Have the patient point to the location(s). Is there any radiation of pain? The examiner should remember that many of the abdominal structures such as the stomach, liver, and pancreas may refer pain to the thoracic region. Is the pain deep, superficial, shooting, burning, or aching? Does the pain occur on inspiration, expiration, or both?

2. Is there any paresthesia?

3. Which activities aggravate the problem?

4. Which activities ease the problem?

5. Is the condition improving, becoming worse, or staying the same?

6. What is the patient's age and occupation? For example, conditions such as Scheuermann's disease occur in young teenagers between the ages of 13 and 16,

7. Does the patient have any problems with

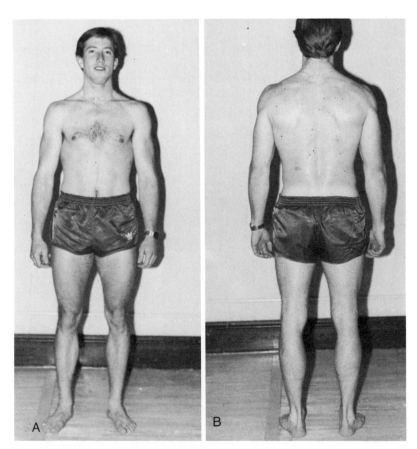

Figure 7–6. Normal posture. (A) Front view. (B) Posterior view.

digestion? Pain may be referred to the thoracic spine or ribs from pathologic conditions in the thorax or abdomen.

8. Does the patient have any difficulty in breathing? If a breathing problem exists, it may be due to some structural deformity (e.g., scoliosis) or thorax pathology.

9. Are the patient's symptoms referred to the legs or arms or head and neck? If so, it is imperative that the examiner assess these areas as well. For example, because shoulder movements may be restricted with thoracic spine problems, the examiner must always be aware that problems in one part of the body may affect other parts of the body.

10. Are the symptoms improving or worsening?

11. Is pain affected by coughing? Sneezing? Straining?

12. Does any particular posture bother the patient?

Observation

The patient must be suitably undressed so that the body is exposed as much as possible. In the case of a female, the bra is often removed to provide a better view of the spine and rib cage. The patient is usually observed first standing and then sitting.

As with any observation, the examiner should note the following:

Any alteration in the overall spinal posture may lead to problems in the thoracic spine. It is important to observe the total body posture from the head to the toes and to look for any deviation from normal (Fig. 7–6).

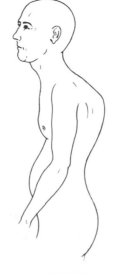

Figure 7–7. Congenital thoracic kyphosis. (From Moe, J. H., et al.: Scoliosis and other spinal deformities. Philadelphia, W. B. Saunders Co., 1978, p. 152.)

Kyphosis. Kyphosis is a condition that is most prevalent in the thoracic spine (Fig. 7–7). The examiner must ensure that a kyphosis is actually present, remembering that a slight kyphosis or posterior curvature is normal and is found in

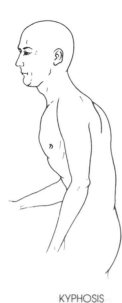

KYPHOSIS

GIBBUS

DOWAGER'S HUMP

Figure 7–8. Kyphotic deformity.

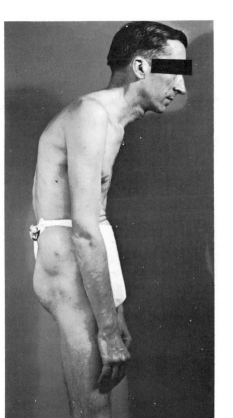

Figure 7–9. Lateral view of patient with ankylosing (rheumatoid) spondylitis showing forward protrusion of head, flattening of anterior chest wall, thoracic kyphosis, protrusion of abdomen, and flattening of lumbar lordosis. This patient also has slight flexion of the hips on the pelvis. (From Polley, H. F., and G. G. Hunder: Rheumatologic Interviewing and Physical Examination of the Joints. Philadelphia, W. B. Saunders, 1978, p. 161.)

every individual. In addition, some individuals have "flat" scapulae, which will give the appearance of an excessive kyphosis. The examiner must ensure that it is actually the spine that has the

excessive curvature. Types of kyphotic deformities are shown in Figure 7–8:[4]

1. *Round back*, or decreased pelvic inclination (20°) with a thoracolumbar or thoracic kyphosis (see Fig. 7–9).

2. *Hump back*, often a localized, sharp, posterior angulation called *gibbus*.

3. *Flat back*, decreased pelvic inclination (20°) with a mobile spine.

4. *Dowager's hump* resulting from postmenopausal osteoporosis.

Scoliosis. This is a deformity in which there is one or more lateral curvatures of the lumbar or thoracic spine. (In the cervical spine, the condition is called *torticollis*.) The curvature may occur in the thoracic spine alone, in the thoracolumbar area, or in the lumbar spine alone (Fig. 7–10). Scoliosis may be nonstructural or structural. Poor posture, hysteria, nerve root irritation, inflammation in the spine area, a leg length discrepancy, or hip contracture can cause nonstructural scoliosis. Structural changes may be genetic, idiopathic, or due to some congenital problem such as a wedge vertebra, hemivertebra, or failure of vertebral segmentation. In other words, there is a structural change in the bone and normal flexibility of the spine is lost.[5]

A number of curve patterns may be present in the scoliosis (Fig. 7–11).[5] The curve patterns are designated according to the level of the apex of the curve (Table 7–1). A *right thoracic curve* has a convexity towards the right, and the apex of the curve is in the thoracic spine. With a *cervical scoliosis* or torticollis, the apex is between C1 and C6. For a *cervicothoracic curve* the apex is at C7 or T1. For a *thoracic curve*, the apex is between T2 and T11. The *thoracolumbar curve* has its apex at T12 or L1. The *lumbar curve* has an apex between L2 and L4, and a *lumbosacral scoliosis* has an apex at L5 or S1. The involvement

Figure 7–10. Idiopathic scoliosis. (A) Postural deformity caused by idiopathic thoracolumbar scoliosis. (B) Asymmetry of posterior thorax accentuated with patient flexed. Note "hump" on the right and "hollow" on the left. (From Gartland, J. J.: Fundamentals of Orthopedics. Philadelphia, W. B. Saunders Co., 1979, p. 341.)

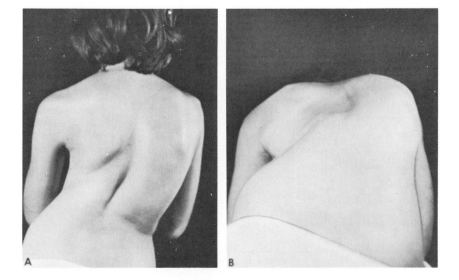

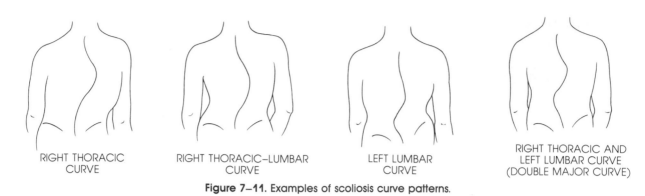

RIGHT THORACIC
CURVE

RIGHT THORACIC–LUMBAR
CURVE

LEFT LUMBAR
CURVE

RIGHT THORACIC AND
LEFT LUMBAR CURVE
(DOUBLE MAJOR CURVE)

Figure 7–11. Examples of scoliosis curve patterns.

of the thoracic spine results in a very poor cosmetic appearance or defect as a result of deformation of the ribs along with the spine.

With a structural scoliosis, the vertebral bodies rotate to the convexity of the curve and become distorted.[6] This rotation, if the thoracic spine is involved, causes the ribs on the convex side of the curve to push posteriorly, causing a rib "hump" and narrowing the thoracic cage on the convex side. As the vertebral body rotates to the convex side of the curve, the spinous process deviates towards the concave side. The ribs on the concave side move anteriorly, causing a "hollow" and a widening of the thoracic cage on the concave side (Fig. 7–12). Lateral deviation may be more evident if the examiner uses a plumb bob (plummet) from the C7 spinous process or external occipital protuberance (Fig. 7–13).

Table 7–1. Curve Patterns and Prognosis in Idiopathic Scoliosis*

	Curve Pattern				
	Primary Lumbar	Thoracolumbar	Combined Thoracic and Lumbar	Primary Thoracic	Cervicothoracic
Incidence (%)	23.6	16	37	22.1	1.3
Average age curve noted (yr.)	13.25	14	12.3	11.1	15
Average age curve stabilized (yr.)	14.5	16	15.5	16.1	16
Extent of curve	D11–L3 (five vertebrae)	D6 or D7–L1 or 1, 2 (six to eight vertebrae)	Dorsal, D6–D10 (five segments) Lumbar, D11–L4 (five segments)	D6–D11 (six segments)	C7 or D1–D4 or D5 (four to six vertebrae)
Apex of curve	L1 or L2	D11 or D2	Dorsal, D7 or D8 Lumbar, L2	D8 or D9 (rotation extreme, convexity usually to right)	D3
Average angular value at maturity (degrees)					
Standing	36.8	42.7	Dorsal, 51.9; lumbar, 41.4	81.4	34.6
Supine	29.1	35	Dorsal, 41.4; lumbar, 37.7	73.8	32.2
Prognosis	Most benign and least deforming of all idiopathic curves	Not severely deforming Intermediate between dorsal and lumbar curves	Good Body usually well aligned, curves even if severe tend to compensate each other High percentage of very severe scoliosis if onset before age of 10 yr.	Worst Progresses more rapidly, becomes more severe and produces greater clinical deformity than any other pattern Five years of active growth during which could increase	Deformity unsightly Poorly disguised because of high shoulder, elevated scapula, and deformed thoracic cage

*Adapted from Ponseti, I. V., and B. Friedman: J. Bone Joint Surg. *32-A*:381, 1950.

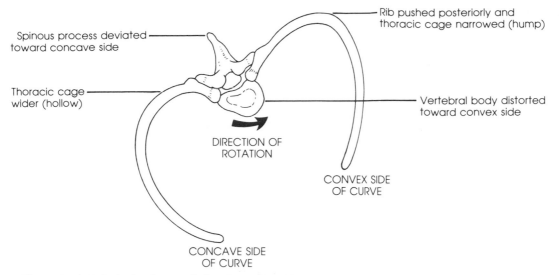

Rib pushed posteriorly and thoracic cage narrowed (hump)

Spinous process deviated toward concave side

Thoracic cage wider (hollow)

Vertebral body distorted toward convex side

DIRECTION OF ROTATION

CONVEX SIDE OF CURVE

CONCAVE SIDE OF CURVE

Figure 7–12. Pathologic changes in the ribs and vertebra with idiopathic scoliosis in the thoracic spine.

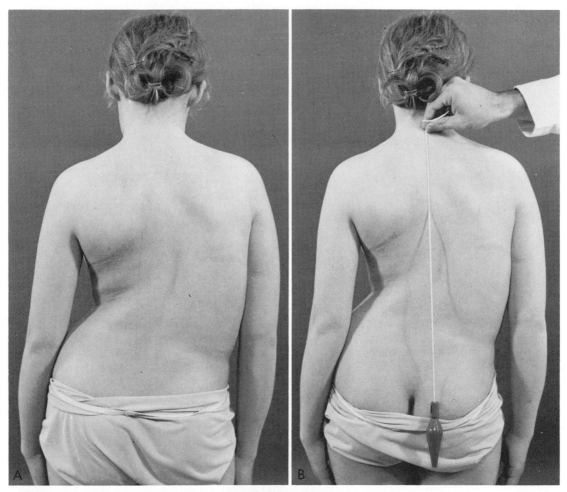

Figure 7–13. Right thoracic idiopathic scoliosis (posterior view).

(*A*) The left shoulder is lower and the right scapula more prominent. Note the decreased distance between the right arm and the thorax, with the shift of the thorax to the right. The left iliac crest appears higher, but this is due to the shift of the thorax with fullness on the right and elimination of the waistline. The "high" hip is thus only apparent, not real.

(*B*) Plumbline dropped from the prominent vertebra of C7 (vertebra prominens) measures the decompensation of the thorax over the pelvis. The distance from the vertical plumbline to the gluteal cleft is measured in centimeters and is recorded noting the direction of deviation. When there is a cervical or cervicothoracic curve, the plumb should fall from the occipital protuberance (inion).

(From Moe, J. H., et al.: Scoliosis and Other Spinal Deformities. Philadelphia, W. B. Saunders Co., 1978, p. 14.)

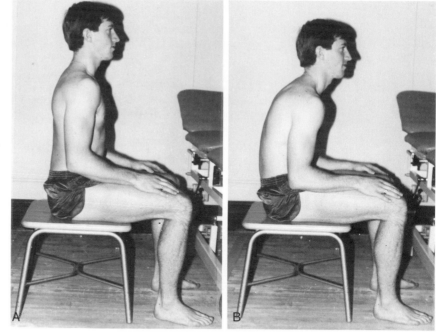

Figure 7–14. Sitting posture. (*A*) Normal position. (*B*) Sag sitting.

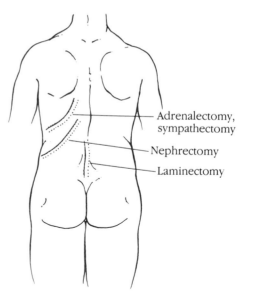

Cholecystectomy — Laparotomy

Appendectomy — Colon or sigmoid resection

Hernia

Adrenalectomy, sympathectomy

Nephrectomy

Laminectomy

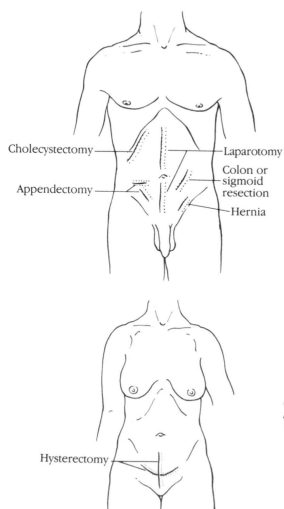

Hysterectomy

Figure 7–15. Common surgical scars of the abdomen and thorax. (From Judge, R. D., et al.: Clinical Diagnosis: A Physiologic Approach. Boston, Little, Brown & Co., 1982, p. 295.)

The examiner should note whether the ribs are symmetric and whether the rib contours are normal and equal on both sides. In idiopathic scoliosis, the rib contours are not normal and there is asymmetry of the ribs. Muscle spasm due to injury may also be evident. The bony and soft-tissue contours should be observed for equality on both sides, or any noticeable difference.

The examiner should note whether the patient sits up properly with the normal spinal curves present and the tip of the ear, tip of the acromion process, and high point of the iliac crest in a straight line as they should be, or does the patient sit in a slumped position (i.e., sag sitting, as in Figure 7–14)?

The skin should be observed for any abnormality or scars. If there are scars, what are they from? (See Figure 7–15.)

Breathing. Does the patient breathe diaphragmatically or apically? Children tend to breath abdominally, whereas women tend to do upper thoracic breathing. Men tend to be upper and lower thoracic breathers. In the aged, the breathing tends to be in the lower thoracic and abdominal regions. The examiner should note the quality of the respiratory movements, at the same time noting the rate, rhythm, and effort needed to inhale and exhale. As well, the presence of any coughing or noisy breathing should be noted. Because the chest wall movement that occurs during breathing displaces the pleural surfaces,

thorax muscles, nerves, and ribs, pain is accentuated by breathing and coughing if any one of these structures is injured.

Chest Deformities. Are there any chest deformities? (See Figure 7–16.)

1. *Pigeon chest* (pectus carinatum). The sternum projects forward and downward like the heel of a boot, increasing the anteroposterior dimension of the chest. This deformity impairs the effectiveness of breathing by restricting ventilation volume.

2. *Funnel chest* (pectus excavatum). This deformity is the result of the sternum being pushed posteriorly by an overgrowth of the ribs.[7] The anteroposterior dimension of the chest is decreased, and the heart may be displaced. On inspiration, this deformity causes a depression of the sternum that affects respiration and may result in kyphosis.

3. *Barrel chest.* The sternum projects forward and upward so that the anteroposterior diameter is increased. It is seen in conditions such as emphysema.

Examination

When carrying out an examination of the thorax and thoracic spine, the examiner must remember

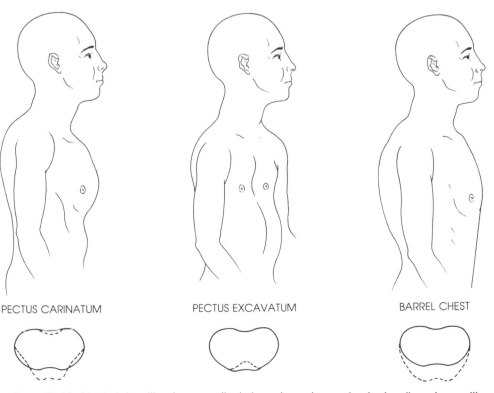

PECTUS CARINATUM   PECTUS EXCAVATUM   BARREL CHEST

Figure 7–16. Chest deformities. Lower vertical views show change in chest wall contours with deformity.

that although the assessment is primarily of the thoracic spine, if the history, observation, or examination indicates symptoms into or from the neck, the upper limb, or the lumbar spine and lower limb, these structures must be examined as well. Thus, the examination of the thoracic spine may be an extensive one. Unless there is a history of specific trauma or injury to the thoracic spine, the examiner must be prepared to assess more

than that area alone. If a problem is suspected above the thoracic spine, the scanning examination of the cervical spine and upper limb (as described in Chapter 2) should be performed. If a problem is suspected below the thoracic spine, the scanning examination of the lumbar spine and lower limb (as described in Chapter 8) should be done. Only examination of the thoracic spine is described here.

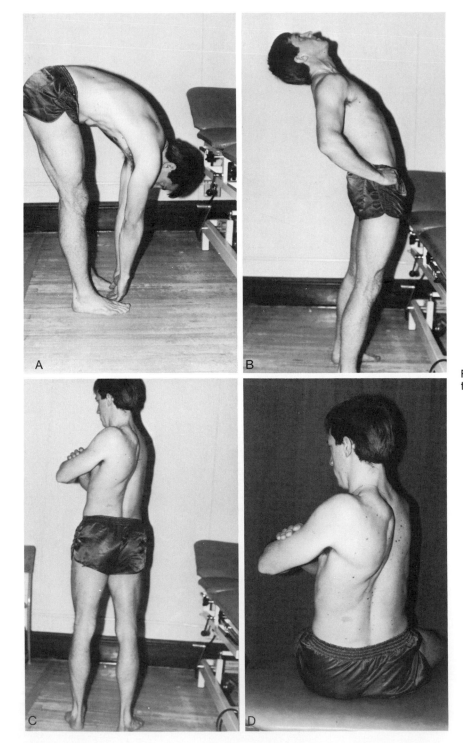

Figure 7–17. Active movement. (*A*) Forward flexion. (*B*) Extension. (*C*) Rotation (standing). (*D*) Rotation (sitting).

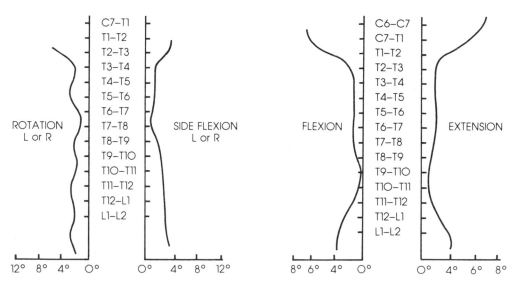

Figure 7–18. Average range of motion in the thoracic spine. (Adapted from Grieve, G. P.: Common Vertebral Joint Problems. New York, Churchill Livingstone, 1981, pp. 41, 42.)

ACTIVE MOVEMENTS

The active movements of the thoracic spine are usually done with the patient standing. It must be remembered that movement will be limited by the rib cage and the long spinous processes of the thoracic spine. When assessing the thoracic spine, the examiner should be sure to note whether the movement occurs in the spine or in the hips. It must be remembered that an individual can touch the toes with a completely rigid spine if there is sufficient range of motion in the hip joints. Likewise tight hamstrings may alter the results. The movements may be done with the patient sitting, in which case the effect of hip movement will be eliminated or decreased. As with any examination, the most painful movements are done last.

These active movements should be carried out in the thoracic spine, as shown in Figure 7–17:

1. Forward flexion (20 to 45°).
2. Extension (25 to 45°).
3. Side flexion (left and right) (20 to 40°).
4. Rotation (left and right) (35 to 50°).
5. Costovertebral expansion (3 to 7.5 cm).
6. Rib motion.

Forward Flexion

For flexion (forward bending), the normal range of motion in the thoracic spine is 20 to 45° (Fig. 7–18). Because the range of motion at each vertebra is difficult to measure, the examiner can use a tape measure to derive an indication of overall movement (Fig. 7–19). These methods are indirect ones. If one wishes to measure the range of motion at each vertebral segment, a series of radiographs would be necessary. The examiner first measures the length of the spine from the C7 spinous process to the T12 spinous process with the patient in the normal standing posture. The patient is then asked to bend forward, and the spine is again measured. A 2.7-cm difference in tape measure length is considered normal.

If the examiner wishes, the spine may be measured from C7 spinous process to S1 with the patient in normal standing position. The patient is then asked to bend forward, and the spine is again measured. A 10-cm difference in tape measure length is considered normal. In this case, the examiner is measuring movement in the lumbar as well as thoracic spine; thus most movement, approximately 7.5 cm, occurs between T12 and S1.

A third method of measuring spinal flexion is to ask the patient to bend forward and try to touch the toes while keeping the knees straight. The examiner then measures from the finger tips to the floor and records the distance. The examiner must keep in mind that with this method, the movement could potentially occur totally in the hip.

The examiner can decide which method to use. It is of primary importance, however, to note on the patient's chart how the measuring was done and which reference points were used.

While the patient is flexed forward the examiner can observe the spine from the "skyline" view (Fig. 7–20). With nonstructural scoliosis, the scoliotic curve will disappear on forward flexion; with structural scoliosis, it will remain. With the skyline view, the examiner is looking for a hump on one side (convex side of curve) and a hollow (concave side of curve) on the other. This "hump and hollow" sequence is due to vertebral rotation, which pushes the ribs and

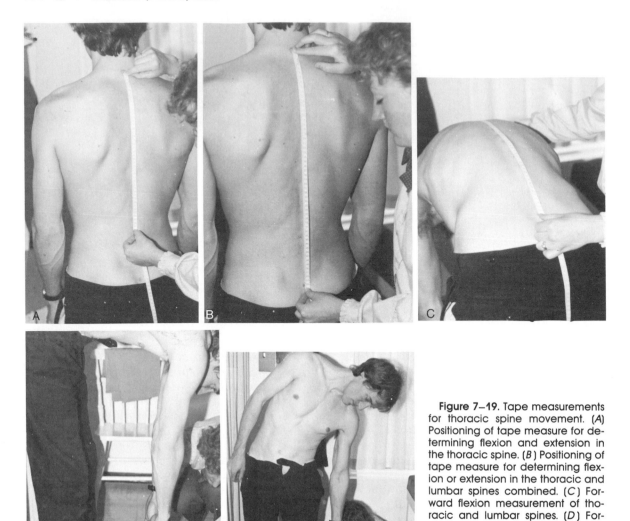

Figure 7–19. Tape measurements for thoracic spine movement. (*A*) Positioning of tape measure for determining flexion and extension in the thoracic spine. (*B*) Positioning of tape measure for determining flexion or extension in the thoracic and lumbar spines combined. (*C*) Forward flexion measurement of thoracic and lumbar spines. (*D*) Forward flexion measurement of thoracic and lumbar spines and hips (fingertips to floor). (*E*) Side flexion tape measurement (fingertips to floor).

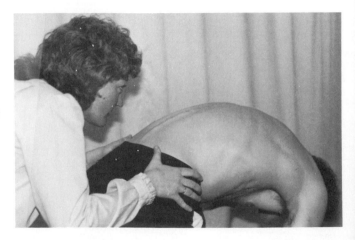

Figure 7–20. Examiner performing "skyline" view of spine for assessment of scoliosis.

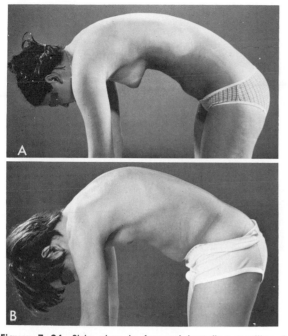

Figure 7-21. Side view in forward bending position for assessment of kyphosis. (*A*) Normal thoracic roundness is demonstrated with a gentle curve to the whole spine. (*B*) An area of increased bending is seen in the thoracic spine, indicating structural changes—Scheuermann's disease, in this example. (From Moe, J. H., et al.: Scoliosis and Other Spinal Deformities. Philadelphia, W. B. Saunders Co., 1978, p. 18.)

muscles out on one side and the paravertebral valley on the opposite side. The vertebral rotation is most evident in the flexed position.

When the patient flexes forward, the thoracic spine should curve forward in a smooth, even manner (Fig. 7-21). The examiner should look for any apparent tightness or sharp angulations such as a gibbus when the movement is performed. If the patient has an excessive kyphosis to begin with, very little forward flexion movement will occur in the thoracic spine.

Extension

Extension (backward bending) in the thoracic spine is normally 25 to 45°. As this movement occurs over 12 vertebrae, the movement between the individual vertebrae is difficult to detect visually. As with flexion, the examiner can use a tape measure and obtain the distance between the same two points (the C7 and T12 spinous processes). Again, a 2.5-cm difference in tape measure length between standing and extension is considered normal. McKenzie advocates having the patient place the hands in the small of the back to add stability while performing the backward movement.[8]

As the patient extends, the thoracic curve should curve backward or at least straighten in a smooth, even manner. The examiner should look for any apparent tightness or angulation when the movement is performed. If the patient shows excessive kyphosis (Fig. 7-22), the kyphotic curvature will remain on extension whether the movement is tested while standing or lying prone.

Side Flexion

Side (lateral) flexion is approximately 20 to 40° to the right and left. The patient is asked to run the hand down the side of the leg as far as possible without bending forward or backward. The examiner can then "eyeball" the angle of side flexion or use a tape measure to determine the length from the finger tips to the floor and compare with the other side. (See Figure 7-19E). Normally, the distances should be equal. In either case, one must remember that movement in the lumbar spine as well as the thoracic spine is being measured. As the patient bends sideways, the spine should curve sideways in a smooth, even manner. The examiner should look for any tightness or abnormal angulation, which may indicate hypomobility or hypermobility at a specific segment when the movement is performed.

Rotation

Rotation in the thoracic spine is approximately 35 to 50°. The patient is asked to cross the arms in front or to place the hands on opposite shoulders and then asked to rotate to the right and left while the examiner eyeballs the amount of rotation, comparing both ways. Again, the examiner must remember that movement in the lumbar spine as well as the thoracic spine is occurring.

Costovertebral Expansion

Costovertebral joint movement is usually determined by measuring chest expansion (Fig. 7-23). The examiner places the tape measure around the chest at the level of the fourth intercostal space. The patient is asked to exhale as much as possible, and the examiner takes a measurement. The patient is then asked to inhale as much as possible and to hold it while the second measurement is taken. The normal difference between inspiration and expiration is 3 to 7.5 cm.

A second method of measuring chest expansion is to measure at three different levels. If this method is used, the examiner must take care to ensure that the levels of measurement are noted for consistency. The levels are (1) under the axillae for apical expansion, (2) at the nipple line or xiphysternal junction for midthoracic expansion, and (3) at the T10 rib level for lower thoracic

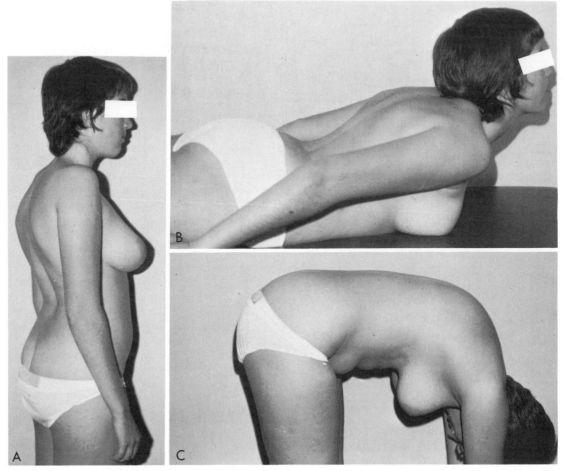

Figure 7–22. Kyphosis and lordosis. (*A*) On physical examination, a definite increase in thoracic kyphosis and lumbar lordosis is visualized. (*B*) Thoracic kyphosis does not fully correct on thoracic extension. (*C*) Lumbar lordosis, on the other hand, usually corrects on forward bending; in this case, some lordosis remains. (From Moe, J. H., et al.: Scoliosis and Other Spinal Deformities. Philadelphia, W. B. Saunders Co., 1978, p. 339.)

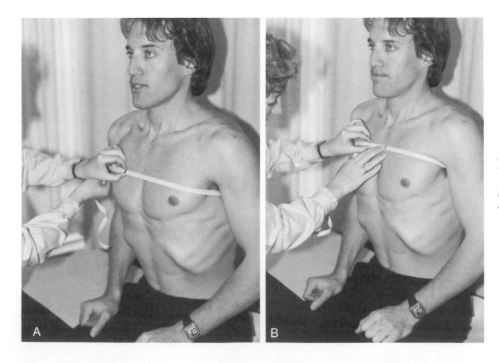

Figure 7–23. Measuring chest expansion. (*A*) Fourth lateral intercostal space. (*B*) Axilla.

Illustration continued on opposite page

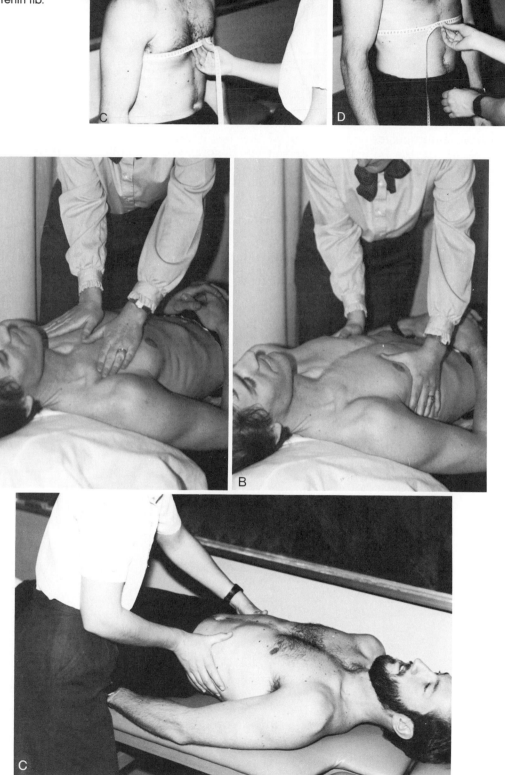

Figure 7–23 *Continued.* (*C*) Nipple line. (*D*) Tenth rib.

Figure 7–24. Feeling rib movement. (*A*) Upper ribs. (*B*) Middle ribs. (*C*) Lower ribs.

expansion. As previously, the measurements are taken at expiration and inspiration.

Following measurement of chest expansion, it is worthwhile for patient to take a deep breath and to cough so that the examiner can determine whether this action causes or alters any pain. If it does, the examiner may suspect a respiratory-related problem.

Rib Motion

The patient is then asked to lie supine. The examiner's hands are placed in a relaxed fashion over the upper chest. In this position, the examiner is feeling anteroposterior movement of the ribs (Fig. 7–24). As the patient inhales and exhales, the examiner should compare both sides for rib movement and see whether the movement is equal on both sides. Any restriction or difference in motion should be noted. If a rib stops moving relative to the other ribs on inhalation, it is classified as a *depressed rib*. If a rib stops moving relative to the other ribs on exhalation, it is classified as an *elevated rib*. It must be remembered that restriction of one rib affects the adjacent ribs. If a depressed rib is implicated, it is usually the uppermost restricted rib that causes the greatest problem. If an elevated rib is present, it is usually the lowest restricted rib that causes

the greatest problem.[3, 9] The examiner then moves the hands down the chest, testing the movement in the middle and lower ribs in a suitable fashion.

To test lateral movement, the examiner's hands are placed around the sides of the rib cage at approximately 45° to the vertical axis of the patient's body. The examiner begins at the level of the axilla and works down the lateral aspect of the ribs, feeling the movement of the ribs during inspiration and expiration and noting any restriction.

PASSIVE MOVEMENTS

Because passive movements in the thoracic spine are difficult to do in a gross fashion, the movement between each vertebra may be performed. The examiner can passively test:

1. Forward flexion.
2. Extension.
3. Side flexion (left and right).
4. Rotation (left and right).

With the patient sitting, the examiner places one hand on the patient's forehead or on top of the head (Fig. 7–25). With the other hand, the examiner palpates over and between the spinous processes of the lower cervical and upper thoracic (C5 to T3) spine and feels for movement between the spinous processes while flexing and extending

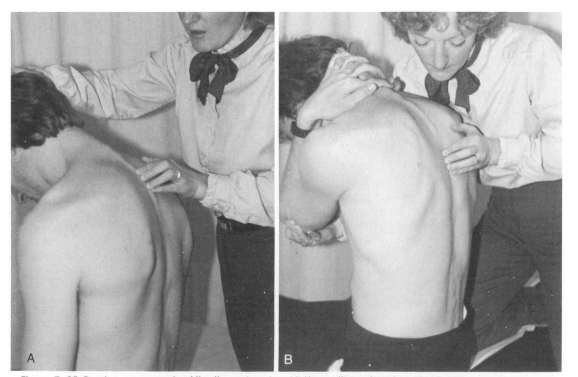

Figure 7–25. Passive movements of the thoracic spine. (*A*) Upper thoracic spine. (*B*) Middle and lower thoracic spine.

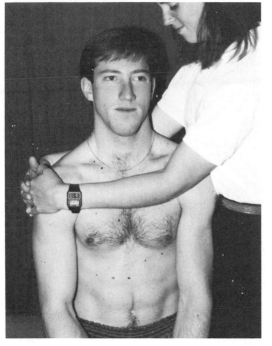

Figure 7–26. Positioning for resisted isometric movements.

the patient's head. Rotation and side flexion may be tested by rotating and side flexing the patient's head. To test the movement properly, the examiner places the middle finger over the spinous process and the index and ring finger on either side of it between the spinous processes of the vertebra being tested and the two adjacent vertebrae. The examiner should feel the movement occurring, assess its quality, and note whether the movement is hypomobile or hypermobile relative to the adjacent vertebra. The hypomobility or hypermobility may be indicative of pathology.[9]

To test the movement of the vertebrae between T3 and T11, the patient sits with the fingers clasped behind the neck and the elbows together in front. The examiner places one hand and arm around the patient's elbows while palpating over and between the spinous processes, as previously described. The examiner then flexes and extends the spine by lifting and lowering the patient's elbows. Rotation and side flexion of the trunk may be performed in a similar fashion to test these movements as well. As before, the examiner should note how much movement is occurring and its quality.[9]

RESISTED ISOMETRIC MOVEMENTS

Resisted isometric movements are performed with the patient in the sitting position. The examiner places one leg behind the patient's but-

tocks and the upper limb around the patient's chest and back (Fig. 7–26). The patient is then asked to carry out the following movements:

1. Forward flexion.
2. Extension
3. Side flexion (left and right).
4. Rotation (left and right).

Since the movement must be isometric, the examiner should say, "Don't let me move you," rather than ask the patient to do the specific movement. The thoracic spine should be in a neutral position, and the most painful movements are done last. Refer to Table 7–2 for muscles of the thoracic spine, their actions and innervation.

SPECIAL TESTS

If the examiner suspects a problem with movement of the spinal cord, any of the tests that stretch the cord may be performed. These include the *straight leg test* and *Kernig's sign* (see Chapter 8, "The Lumbar Spine"). Either neck flexion from above or straight leg raise from below will stretch the spinal cord.

The following two tests should be performed only if the examiner feels they are relevant.

Passive Scapular Approximation

The patient lies prone while the examiner passively approximates the scapulae by lifting the shoulder up and back. Pain in the scapular area is indicative of a T1 or T2 nerve root problem on the side where the pain is being experienced.[10]

First Thoracic Nerve Root Stretch

The patient abducts the arm to 90° and flexes the pronated forearm to 90°. No symptoms should appear in this position. The patient then fully flexes the elbow, putting the hand behind the neck. This action stretches the ulnar nerve and T1 nerve root. Pain into the scapular area or arm is indicative for a positive test.[10]

REFLEXES AND CUTANEOUS DISTRIBUTION

Within the thoracic spine there is a great deal of overlap in dermatomes (Fig. 7–27). The dermatomes tend to follow the ribs, and the absence of only one dermatome may lead to no loss in sensation at all. Pain may be referred to the thoracic spine from various abdominal organs (Fig. 7–28 and Table 7–3). Although there are no reflexes to test in conjunction with the thoracic

Table 7–2. Muscles of the Thorax and Abdomen: Their Action and Innervation in the Thoracic Spine

Action	Muscles Involved	Innervation
Flexion of thoracic spine	1. Rectus abdominis	T6–T12
	2. External abdominal oblique (both sides acting together)	T7–T12
	3. Internal abdominal oblique (both sides acting together)	T7–T12, L1
Extension of thoracic spine	1. Spinalis thoracis	T1–T12
	2. Iliocostalis thoracis (both sides acting together)	T1–T12
	3. Longissimus thoracis (both sides acting together)	T1–T12
	4. Semispinalis thoracis (both sides acting together)	T1–T12
	5. Multifidus (both sides acting together)	T1–T12
	6. Rotatores (both sides acting together)	T1–T12
	7. Interspinalis	T1–T12
Rotation and side flexion of thoracic spine	1. Iliocostalis thoracis (to same side)	T1–T12
	2. Longissimus thoracis (to same side)	T1–T12
	3. Intertransverse (to same side)	T1–T12
	4. Internal abdominal oblique (to same side)	T7–T12, L1
	5. Semispinalis thoracis (to opposite side)	T1–T12
	6. Multifidus (to opposite side)	T1–T12
	7. Rotatores (to opposite side)	T1–T12
	8. External abdominal oblique (to opposite side)	T7–T12
	9. Transversus abdominis (to opposite side)	T7–T12, L1
Elevation of ribs	1. Scalenus anterior (1st rib)	C4–C6
	2. Scalenus medius (1st rib)	C3–C8
	3. Scalenus posterior (2nd rib)	C6–C8
	4. Serratus posterior superior (2nd to 5th ribs)	2–5 intercostal
	5. Iliocostalis cervicis (1st to 6th rib)	C6–C8
	6. Levatores costarum (all ribs)	T1–T12
	7. Pectoralis major (if arm fixed)	Lateral pectoral (C6, C7)
		Medial pectoral (C7, C8, T1)
	8. Serratus anterior (lower ribs if scapula fixed)	Long thoracic (C5, C6, C7)
	9. Pectoralis minor (2nd to 5th ribs if scapula fixed)	Lateral pectoral (C6, C7)
		Medial pectoral (C7, C8)
	10. Sternocleidomastoid (if head fixed)	Accessory C2, C3

Table continued on opposite page

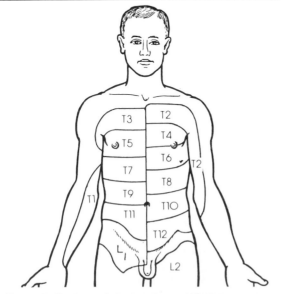

Figure 7–27. The cutaneous areas (dermatomes) supplied by the thoracic nerve roots (After Foerster). By comparing both sides the degree of overlapping and the area of exclusive supply of any individual nerve root may be estimated. (Adapted from Williams, P., and R. Warwick (eds.): Gray's Anatomy, 36th British ed. Philadelphia, W. B. Saunders, 1980, p. 1116.)

spine, the examiner would be wise to test the lumbar reflexes: (1) L3, the patellar reflex; (3) L5, the medial hamstrings reflex; and (3) S1, the Achilles reflex as pathology in the thoracic spine can affect these reflexes.

JOINT PLAY MOVEMENTS

The joint play movements performed on the thoracic spine are specific ones that were developed by Maitland.[11] The following movements should be performed, with the examiner noting any decreased range of motion, muscle spasm, pain, or difference in end feel that would normally be tissue stretch:

1. Posteroanterior central vertebral pressure (PACVP).

2. Posteroanterior unilateral vertebral pressure (PAUVP).

3. Transverse vertebral pressure (TVP).

4. Rib springing.

For the first three movements, the patient lies prone. The examiner palpates the thoracic spi-

Table 7–2. Muscles of the Thorax and Abdomen: Their Action and Innervation in the Thoracic Spine *Continued*

Action	Muscles Involved	Innervation
Depression of ribs	1. Serratus posterior inferior (lower 4 ribs)	T9–T12
	2. Iliocostalis lumborum (lower 6 ribs)	L1–L3
	3. Longissimus thoracis	T1–T12
	4. Rectus abdominis	T6–T12
	5. External abdominal oblique (lower 5 to 6 ribs)	T7–T12
	6. Internal abdominal oblique (lower 5 to 6 ribs)	T7–T12, L1
	7. Transversus abdominal (all acting depress lower ribs)	T7–T12, L1
	8. Quadratus lumborum (12th rib)	T12, L1–L4
	9. Transversus thoracis	T1–T12
Approximation of ribs	1. Iliocostalis thoracis	T1–T12
	2. Intercostals (internal and external)	1–11 intercostal phrenic
	3. Diaphragm	
Inspiration	1. External intercostals	1–11 intercostal
	2. Transverse thoracis (sternocostalis)	1–11 intercostal
	3. Diaphragm	Phrenic
	4. Sternocleidomastoid	Accessory C2, C3
	5. Scalenus anterior	C4–C6
	6. Scalenus medius	C3–C8
	7. Scalenus posterior	C6–C8
	8. Pectoralis major	Lateral pectoral (C5, C6); Medial pectoral (C7, C8, T1)
	9. Pectoralis minor	Lateral pectoral (C6, C7); Medial pectoral (C7, C8)
	10. Serratus anterior	Long thoracic (C5, C6, C7)
	11. Latissimus dorsi	Thoracodorsal (C6, C7, C8)
	12. Serratus posterior superior	2–5 intercostal
	13. Iliocostalis thoracis	T1–T12
Expiration	1. Internal intercostals	1–11 intercostal
	2. Rectus abdominis	T6–T12
	3. External abdominal oblique	T7–T12
	4. Internal abdominal oblique	T7–T12, L1
	5. Iliocostalis lumborum	L1–L3
	6. Longissimus	T1–L3
	7. Serratus posterior inferior	T9–T12
	8. Quadratus lumborum	T12, L1–L4

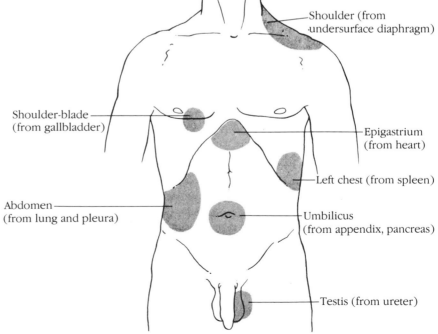

Figure 7–28. Referred pain in the thorax and chest. (From Judge, R. D., et al.: Clinical Diagnosis: A Physiological Approach. Boston, Little, Brown & Co., 1982, p. 285.)

Table 7–3. Differences in Pain Perception

Structure	Effective Stimulus†	Conscious Pain Perception
Skin	Discrete touch, prick, heat, cold	Precisely localized, superficial, burning sharp
Chest wall (muscles, ribs, ligaments, parietal pleura)	Movement, deep pressure	Intermediate in localization and depth; aching, sharp, or dull
Thoracic viscera	Ischemia, distension, muscle spasm	Vague, diffuse, deep, aching, usually dull

*From Levene, D. L.: Chest Pain: An Integrated Diagnostic Approach. Philadelphia, Lea & Febiger, 1977.
†The effectiveness of all stimuli is heightened by the presence of inflammation.

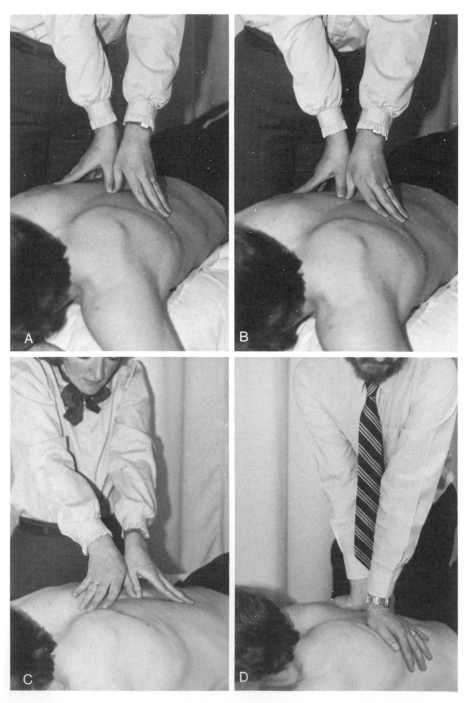

Figure 7–29. Hand, finger, and thumb position for joint play movements. (*A*) Posteroanterior central vertebral pressure. (*B*) Posteroanterior unilateral vertebral pressure. (*C*) Transverse vertebral pressure. (*D*) Rib springing (prone).

nous processes, starting at C6 and working down to L1 or L2.

Posteroanterior Central Vertebral Pressure (PACVP)

The examiner's hands, fingers, and thumb are positioned as in Figure 7–29A. The examiner then applies a pressure to the spinous process through the thumbs, pushing the vertebra forward. Care must be taken when applying the pressure to do it slowly with careful control so that one can "feel" the movement, which is minimal. This "springing test" may be repeated several times to determine the quality of the movement. Each spinous process is done in turn, starting at C6 and working down to L1 or L2. When doing this test, the examiner must keep in mind the fact that the thoracic spinous processes are not always at the level of the same vertebral body. For example, the spinous processes of T1, T2, T3, and T12 are at the same level as the T1, T2, T3, and T12 vertebral bodies and the spinous processes of T7, T8, T9, and T10 are at the same level as the T8, T9, T10, and T11 vertebral bodies, respectively.

Posteroanterior Unilateral Vertebral Pressure (PAUVP)

The examiner's fingers are moved laterally away from the tip of the spinous process so that the thumbs rest on the lamina or transverse process of the thoracic vertebra (Figs. 7–29B and 7–30). The same anterior springing pressure is applied as in the PACVP technique. Again, each vertebra is done in turn. Both sides should be examined and compared. It must be remembered that in the thoracic area, the spinous process is not necessarily at the same level as the transverse process on the same vertebra. For example, T9 spinous process is at the level of T10 transverse process. Therefore, it is necessary to move the fingers up and out from the tip of T9 spinous process to the T9 transverse process, which is at the level of the T8 spinous process. This difference does not hold true for the entire thoracic spine.

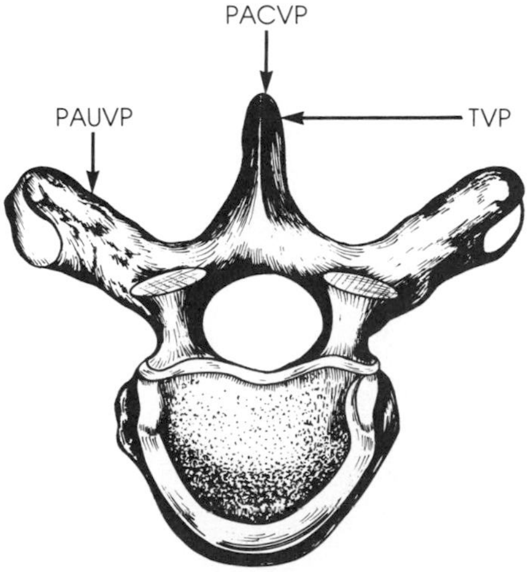

Transverse Vertebral Pressure (TVP)

The examiner's fingers are placed along the side of the spinous process, as shown in Figure 7–29C. The examiner then applies a transverse springing pressure to the side of the spinous process, feeling for the quality of movement. As previously, each vertebra is assessed in turn starting at C6 and working down to L1 or L2. Pressure should be applied to both sides of the spinous process to compare the movement.

Similar procedures to the three mentioned here may also be applied to the cervical and lumbar spines.

Rib Springing

The patient lies prone or on the side while the examiner's hands are placed around the posterolateral aspect of the rib cage (Fig. 7–29D). The examiner's hands are at approximately 45° to the vertical axis of the patient's body. The examination begins at the top of the rib cage and extending inferiorly springing the ribs by pushing in with the hands on each side in turn. The amount and quality of movement occurring on both sides should be noted. If one rib appears hypo- or hypermobile relative to the others being tested, it can be tested individually.

PALPATION

As with any palpation technique, the examiner is looking for any tenderness, muscle spasm, temperature alterations, swelling, or other signs that may indicate disease. Palpation should begin on the anterior chest wall, move around the lateral chest wall, and finish with the posterior structures (Fig. 7–31). Palpation is usually done with the patient sitting, although it may be done combining the supine and prone lying positions. At the same time, the thorax may be divided into sections (Fig. 7–32) to give some idea, in charting, where the pathology is suspected.

Figure 7–30. Direction of pressure during joint play movements. PACVP = Posteroanterior central vertebral pressure; PAUVP = posteroanterior unilateral vertebral pressure; TVP = transverse vertebral pressure.

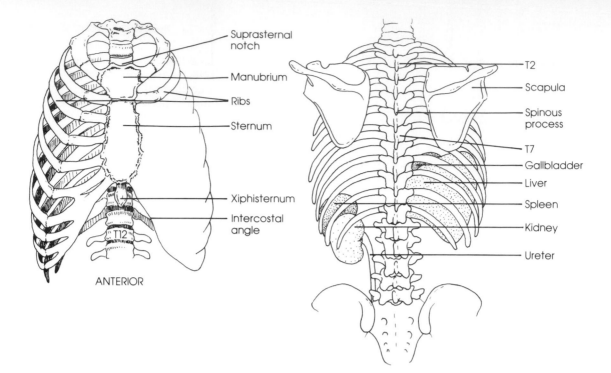

Figure 7–31. Landmarks of the thoracic spine.

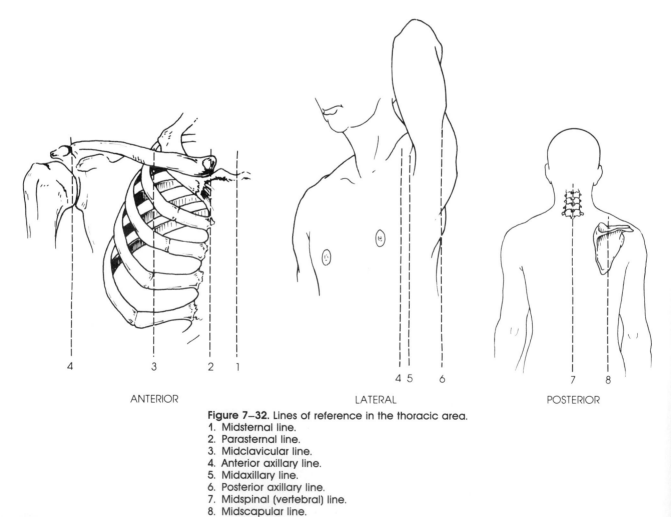

Figure 7–32. Lines of reference in the thoracic area.
1. Midsternal line.
2. Parasternal line.
3. Midclavicular line.
4. Anterior axillary line.
5. Midaxillary line.
6. Posterior axillary line.
7. Midspinal (vertebral) line.
8. Midscapular line.

Anterior Aspect

Anteriorly, the following structures should be palpated:

Sternum. In the midline of the chest, the manubrium sternum, body of the sternum, and xiphoid process should be palpated for any abnormality or tenderness.

Ribs and Costal Cartilage. Adjacent to the sternum, the examiner should palpate the sternocostal and costochondral articulations, noting any swelling, tenderness, or abnormality. These "articulations" are sometimes sprained or subluxed, or a costochondritis *(Tietze syndrome)* may be evident. The ribs should be palpated as they extend around the chest wall, with any potential pathology or crepitations (e.g., subcutaneous emphysema) noted.

Clavicle. The clavicle should be palpated along its length for abnormal bumps (callus) or tenderness.

Abdomen. The abdomen should be palpated for tenderness or other signs indicating pathology. The palpation is done in a systematic fashion, using the fingers of one hand to feel the tissues while the other hand may be used to apply pressure. Palpation is carried out to a depth of 1 to 3 cm to reveal areas of tenderness and abnormal masses. Palpation is usually carried out using the quadrant or the nine-region system (Fig. 7–33).

Posterior Aspect

The examiner then moves to the posterior aspect of the chest wall to complete the palpation.

Scapula. The medial, lateral and superior borders of the scapula should be palpated for any swelling or tenderness. The scapula normally extends from the spinous process of T2 to that of T7. After the borders of the scapula have been palpated, the examiner palpates the posterior surface of the scapula. Structures palpated will be the supraspinatus and infraspinatus muscles and the spine of the scapula.

Spinous Processes of the Thoracic Spine. In the midline, posteriorly the examiner may palpate the thoracic spinous processes for abnormality. The examiner then moves laterally about 2 to 3 cm to palpate the thoracic facet joints. As a result of the overlying muscles, it is usually very difficult to palpate these joints, although the examiner may be able to palpate for muscle spasm and tenderness in the area. Muscle spasm may also

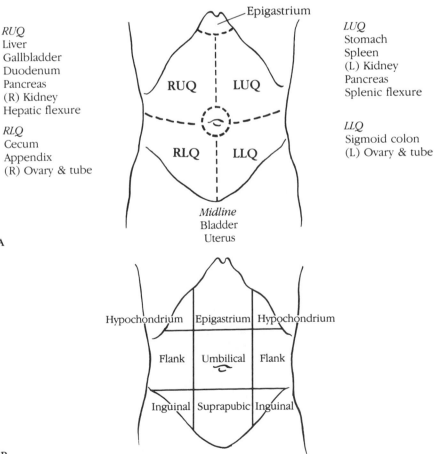

RUQ
Liver
Gallbladder
Duodenum
Pancreas
(R) Kidney
Hepatic flexure

RLQ
Cecum
Appendix
(R) Ovary & tube

LUQ
Stomach
Spleen
(L) Kidney
Pancreas
Splenic flexure

LLQ
Sigmoid colon
(L) Ovary & tube

Figure 7–33. Superficial topography of the abdomen. *(A)* Four-quadrant system. *(B)* Nine-region system. (From Judge, R. D., et al.: Clinical Diagnosis: A Physiological Approach. Boston, Little, Brown & Co., 1982, p. 284.)

A

B

be elicited if some internal structures are injured. For example, pathology affecting the following structures can cause muscle spasm in the surrounding area:

1. *Gallbladder.* Spasm on the right side in the area of the eighth and ninth costal cartilages.

2. *Spleen.* Spasm at the level of ribs 9, 10, and 11 on the left side.

3. *Kidneys.* Spasm at the level of ribs 11 and 12 on both sides at the level of the L3 vertebra. Evidence of positive findings with no comparable history of musculoskeletal origin could poten-

tially lead the examiner to believe the problem was not of a musculoskeletal origin.

RADIOLOGY OF THE THORACIC SPINE

Anteroposterior (A-P) View. With this view (Fig. 7–34), the examiner should note:

1. Any wedging of the vertebrae.
2. Whether the disc spaces appear normal.
3. Whether the ring epiphysis, if present, is normal.

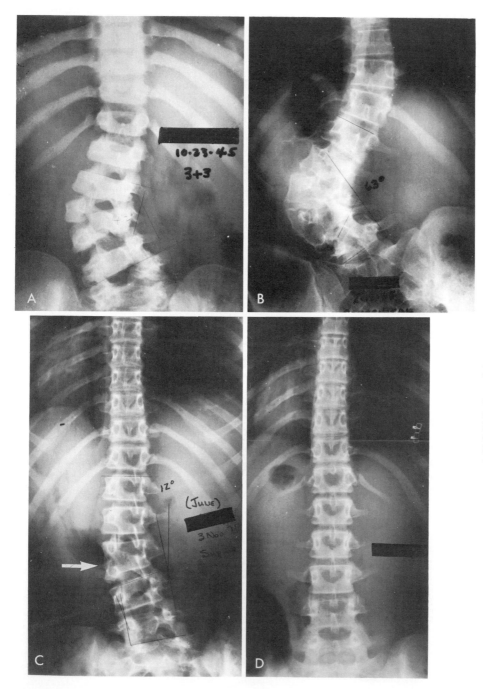

Figure 7–34. Structural scoliosis caused by congenital defect. (*A*) Left midlumbar and right lumbosacral hemivertebra in a 3-year-old child (example of hemimetameric shift). (*B*) A first cousin also demonstrates a midlumbar hemivertebra as well as asymmetric development of the upper sacrum. (*C*) This girl has a semisegmented hemivertebra in the midlumbar spine with a mild 12-degree curve. (*D*) Her identical twin sister showed no congenital anomalies of the spine. (From Moe, J. H., et al.: Scoliosis and Other Spinal Deformities. Philadelphia, W. B. Saunders Co., 1978, p. 134.)

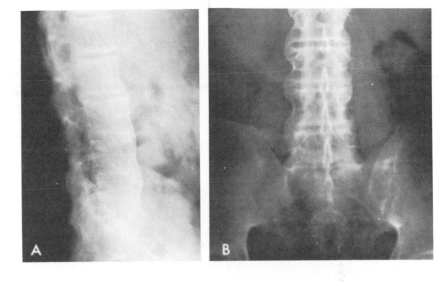

Figure 7–35. Ankylosing spondylitis of spine. Note the bamboo effect on the anteroposterior view and bony encasement of vertebral bodies on the lateral view. (From Gartland, J. J.: Fundamentals of Orthopedics. Philadelphia, W. B. Saunders Co., 1979.)

4. Whether there is a "bamboo" spine that is indicative of ankylosing spondylitis (Fig. 7–35).

5. Any scoliosis (Fig. 7–36).

6. Malposition of heart and lungs.

7. Normal symmetry of the ribs.

Lateral View. The examiner should note:

1. A normal mild kyphosis.

2. Any wedging of the vertebrae, which may be an indication of structural kyphosis resulting from conditions such as Scheuermann's disease or wedge fracture (Fig. 7–37).

3. Whether the disc spaces appear normal.

4. Whether the ring epiphysis, if present, is normal.

5. Whether there are any *Schmorl's nodes* (herniation of the intervertebral disc into the vertebral body).

6. Angle of the ribs.

7. Any osteophytes.

Measurement of Spinal Curvature for Scoliosis. With the *Cobb method* (Fig. 7–38), an anteroposterior view is used.[5] A line is drawn parallel to the superior cortical plate of the proximal end vertebrae and to the inferior cortical

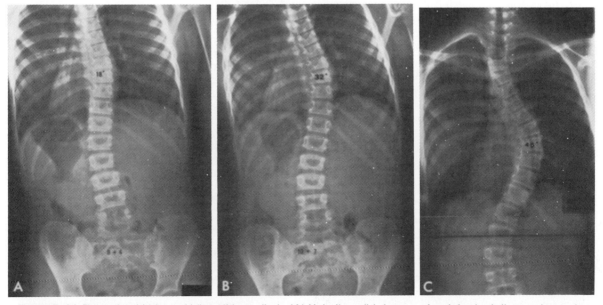

Figure 7–36. The natural history of idiopathic scoliosis. (*A*) Note the mild degree of vertebral rotation and curvature and the imbalance of the upper torso. (*B*) Note the rather dramatic increase in curvature and the increased rotation of the apical vertebrae one year later. (*C*) Further progression of the curvature has occurred, and the opportunity for brace treatment has been missed. (From Bunnell, W. P.: Orthop. Clin. North Am. 10:817, 1979.)

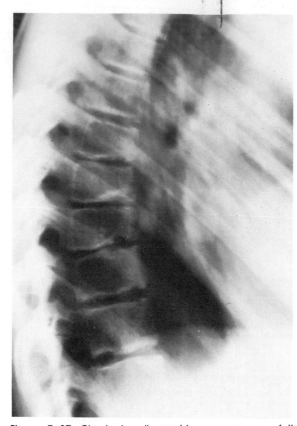

Figure 7–37. Classical radiographic appearance of the spine in a patient with Scheuermann's disease. Note the wedged vertebra, Schmorl's nodules, and marked irregularity of the vertebral end-plates. (From Moe, J. H.: Scoliosis and Other Spinal Deformities. Philadelphia, W. B. Saunders Co., 1978, p. 32.)

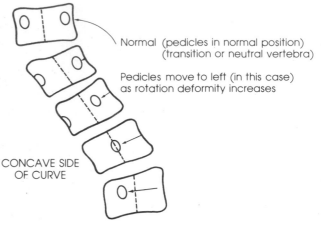

Normal (pedicles in normal position) (transition or neutral vertebra)

Pedicles move to left (in this case) as rotation deformity increases

CONCAVE SIDE OF CURVE

Figure 7–39. Rotation of vertebra seen in scoliosis. On x-ray the pedicles will appear to be "off center" as the curve progresses.

plate of the distal end vertebra. A perpendicular line is erected to each of these lines, and the angle of intersection of the perpendicular lines is the angle of the spine curve resulting from scoliosis.

The rotation of the vertebrae may also be estimated from an anteroposterior view (Fig. 7–39). This estimation is best done by the *pedicle method*, in which the examiner determines the relation of the pedicles to the lateral margin of the vertebral bodies. The vertebra is in neutral when the pedicles are equal distances from the lateral margin of the peripheral bodies. If rotation is evident, the pedicles will appear to move laterally toward the concavity of the curve.

Précis of the Thoracic Spine Assessment

History
Observation
Examination
  Active movements
    Forward flexion
    Extension
    Side flexion (left and right)
    Rotation (left and right)
    Costovertebral expansion
    Rib motion
  Passive movements
    Forward flexion
    Extension
    Side flexion (left and right)
    Rotation (left and right)
  Resisted isometric movements (as in Passive movements)
  Special tests
  Reflexes and cutaneous distribution
  Joint play movements
    Posteroanterior central vertebral pressure
    Posteroanterior unilateral vertebral pressure
    Transverse vertebral pressure
    Rib springing
  Palpation
  X-ray viewing

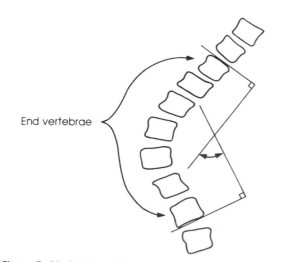

End vertebrae

Figure 7–38. Cobb method of measuring scoliotic curve.

Following any assessment, the patient should always be warned of the possibility of exacerbation of symptoms as a result of examination.

REFERENCES

CITED REFERENCES

1. Williams, P., and R. Warwick (eds.): Gray's Anatomy, 36th British ed. Philadelphia, W. B. Saunders Co., 1980.
2. MacConaill, M. A., and J. V. Basmajian: Muscles and Movements—A Basis for Human Kinesiology. Baltimore, The Williams and Wilkins Co., 1969.
3. Mitchell, F. L., P. S., Moran, and N. A. Pruzzo: An Evaluation and Treatment Manual of Osteopathic Muscle Energy Procedures. Valley Park, Mo., Mitchell, Moran and Pruzzo, Assoc., 1979.
4. Wiles, P., and R. Sweetnam: Essentials of Orthopaedics. London, J. A. Churchill, 1965.
5. Heim, H. A.: Scoliosis. Clinical Symposia 25:1–32, 1973.
6. Keim, H. A.: The Adolescent Spine. New York, Springer-Verlag, 1982.
7. Sutherland, I. D.: Funnel chest. J. Bone Joint Surg. 40B:244, 1958.
8. McKenzie, R.A.: The Lumbar Spine: Mechanical Diagnosis and Therapy. Waikanae, New Zealand, Spinal Publications Ltd., 1981.
9. Stoddard, A.: Manual of Osteopathic Technique. London, Hutchinson Medical Publications, 1959.
10. Cyriax, J.: Textbook of Orthopaedic Medicine, 1: Diagnosis of Soft Tissue Lesions. London, Bailliere Tindall, 1982.
11. Maitland, G. D.: Vertebral Manipulation. London, Butterworths, 1973.

GENERAL REFERENCES

Adams, J. C.: Outline of Orthopaedics. London, E & S Livingstone, 1968.
American Orthopaedic Association: Manual of Orthopaedic Surgery. Chicago, 1972.
Beetham, W. P., H. F. Polley, C. H. Slocumb, and W. F. Weaver: Physical Examination of the Joints. Philadelphia, W. B. Saunders Co., 1965.
Bourdillon, J. R.: Spinal Manipulation, 3rd ed. New York, Appleton-Century-Crofts, 1982.
Bradford, D. S.: Juvenile kyphosis. Clin. Orthop. Relat. Res. 128:45, 1977.
Brashear, H. R., and R. B. Raney: Shand's Handbook of Orthopaedic Surgery. St. Louis, C. V. Mosby Co., 1978.
Bunnell, W. P.: Treatment of idiopathic scoliosis. Orthop. Clin. North Am. 10:813, 1979.
Cailliet, R.: Scoliosis: Diagnosis and Management. Philadelphia, F. A. Davis Co., 1975.
Drummond, D. S., E. Rogala, and J. Gurr: Spinal deformity: Natural history and the role of school screening. Orthop. Clin. North Am. 10:751, 1979.
Gartland, J. J.: Fundamentals of Orthopaedics. London E & S Livingstone, 1968.
Goldstein, L. A., and T. R. Waugh: Classification and terminology of scoliosis. Clin. Orthop. Relat. Res. 93:10, 1973.

Gregersen, G.G. and D. B. Lucas: An in vivo study of the axial rotation of the human thoracolumbar spine. J. Bone Joint Surg., 49A:247, 1967.
Grieve, G. P.: Common Vertebral Joint Problems. New York, Churchill Livingstone, 1981.
Grieve, G. P.: Mobilization of the Spine. New York, Churchill Livingstone, 1979.
Hollingshead, W. H., and D. R. Jenkins: Functional Anatomy of the Limbs and Back. Philadelphia, W. B. Saunders Co., 1981.
Hoppenfeld, S.: Physical Examination of the Spine and Extremities. New York, Appleton-Century-Crofts, 1976.
James, J. J. P.: The etiology of scoliosis. J. Bone Joint Surg. 52B:410, 1970.
Judge, R. D., G. D. Zuidema, and F. T. Fitzgerald: Clinical Diagnosis: A Physiologic Approach. Boston, Little, Brown and Co., 1982.
Kapandji, I. A.: The Physiology of the Joints, vol. III: The Trunk and Vertebral Column. New York, Churchill Livingstone, 1974.
Levene, D. L.: Chest Pain: An Integrated Diagnostic Approach. Philadelphia, Lea & Febiger, 1977.
Liebgott, B.: The Anatomical Basis of Dentistry. Philadelphia, W.B. Saunders Co., 1982.
Maigne, R.: Orthopaedic Medicine: A New Approach to Vertebral Manipulation. Springfield, Ill., Charles C Thomas, 1972.
Moe, J. H., R. B. Winter, D. S. Bradford, and J. F. Lonstein: Scoliosis and Other Spinal Deformities. Philadelphia, W. B. Saunders Co., 1978.
Moll, J. H., and V. Wright: Measurement of spinal movement. In Jayson, M. (ed.): Lumbar Spine and Back Pain. New York, Grune & Stratton, Inc., 1976.
Moll, J. M. H., and V. Wright: An objective clinical study of chest expansion. Ann. Rheum. Dis. 31:1–8, 1972.
Nash, C. L., and J. H. Moe: A study of vertebral rotation. J. Bone Joint Surg. 52A:223, 1969.
O'Donoghue, D. H.: Treatment of Injuries to Athletes, 4th ed. Philadelphia, W. B. Saunders Co., 1984.
Papaioannu, T., I. Stokes, and J. Kenwright: Scoliosis associated with limb length inequality. J. Bone Joint Surg. 64A:59, 1982.
Rothman, R. H., and F. A. Simeone: The Spine. Philadelphia, W. B. Saunders Co., 1982.
Simmons, E. H.: Kyphotic deformity of the spine in ankylosing spondylitis. Clin. Orthop. Relat. Res. 128:65, 1977.
Sturrock, R. D., J. A. Wojtulewski, and F. D. Hart: Spondylometry in a normal population and in ankylosing spondylitis. Rheumatol. Rehabil. 12:135, 1973.
Tsou, P. M.: Embryology of congenital kyphosis. Clin. Orthop. Relat. Res. 128:18, 1977.
Tsou, P. M., A. Yau, and A. R. Hodgson: Embryogenesis and prenatal development of congenital vertebral anomalies and their classification. Clin. Orthop. Relat. Res. 152:211, 1980.
White, A. A.: Kinematics of the normal spine as related to scoliosis. J. Biomech. 4:405, 1971.
Whiteside, T. E.: Traumatic kyphosis of the thoracolumbar spine. Clin. Orthop. Relat. Res. 128:78, 1977.
Wyke, B.: Morphological and functional features of the innervation of the costovertebral joints. Folia Morphol. 23:296, 1975.

8

Lumbar Spine

Back pain is one of the great afflictions of mankind today. Almost anyone born today in Europe or North America has a great chance of suffering a disabling back injury regardless of occupation.

The lumbar spine furnishes support for the upper body and transmits weight of the upper body to the pelvis and lower limb. Because of the strategic location of the lumbar spine, the examiner must remember that this structure should be included in any examination of the spine as a whole in terms of posture or in any examination of the hip and/or sacroiliac joints. Unless there is a definitive history of trauma, it is difficult to determine whether an injury originates in the lumbar spine, sacroiliac joints or hip joints; thus, all three should be examined in a sequential fashion.

Applied Anatomy

There are five pairs of, or ten, facet joints in the lumbar spine. These diarthrodial joints consist of superior and inferior facets and a capsule. The facets are located on the vertebral arches. Injury, degeneration, or trauma may lead to *spondylosis* (degeneration of the intervertebral disc), *spondylolysis* (a defect in the pars interarticularis of the arch), or *spondylolisthesis* (a forward displacement of one vertebra over another). The superior facets, or articular processes, face medially and backward and are generally concave; the inferior facets face laterally and forward and are convex. There are, however, abnormalities, or *tropisms*, that can occur in the shape of the facets, especially at the L5-S1 level (Fig. 8–1).

These posterior, apophyseal, or facet joints direct the movement that occurs in the lumbar spine. Because of the shape of the facets, rotation in the lumbar spine is minimal and is accomplished only by a shearing force. Side flexion, extension, and flexion can occur in the lumbar spine, but the direction of movement is controlled by the facet joints. The close packed position of the facet joints in the lumbar spine is extension. Normally, the facet joints are not the weight-bearing type; with increased extension, however, they begin to have a weight-bearing function. The resting position is midway between flexion and

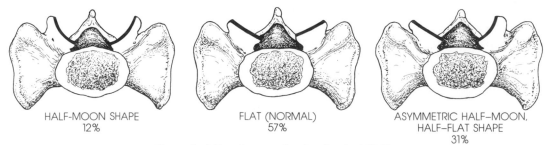

HALF-MOON SHAPE
12%

FLAT (NORMAL)
57%

ASYMMETRIC HALF-MOON, HALF-FLAT SHAPE
31%

Figure 8–1. Facet anomalies (tropisms) at L5-S1.

extension. The capsular pattern is side flexion and rotation, equally limited followed by extension. The examiner may find, however, that if only one facet joint in the lumbar spine has a capsular restriction, the amount of observable restriction will be minimal. The first sacral segment is usually included when one talks about the lumbar spine, and it is at this joint where the fixed segment of the sacrum joins with the mobile segments of the lumbar spine. In some cases, the S1 segment may be mobile. This occurrence is called *lumbarization* of S1, resulting in a sixth "lumbar" vertebra. At other times, the fifth lumbar segment may be fused to the sacrum or ilium, resulting in a *sacralization* of that vertebra. Sacralization results in four mobile lumbar vertebrae.

The intervertebral discs make up approximately 20 to 25 per cent of the total length of the vertebral column. With age, this percentage will decrease as a result of disc degeneration and loss of hydrophilic action in the disc. The *annulus fibrosus*, the outer laminated portion of the disc, is made up of three zones:

1. The outer zone is made up of fibrocartilage, classified as *Sharpey's fibers*, attaching to the outer or peripheral aspect of the vertebral body. The number of cartilage cells present in the fibrous strands increases with depth.

2. The intermediate zone is made up of another layer of fibrocartilage.

3. The inner zone is made up primarily of fibrocartilage, with the largest number of cartilage cells.[1]

The annulus fibrosus is made up of 20 concentric collar-like rings of collagenous fibers that criss-cross each other to increase their strength and to accommodate torsion movements.[2] The nucleus pulposus is well developed in the cervical and lumbar spine. Initially, at birth, it is made up of a hydrophilic mucoid tissue that is gradually replaced by fibrocartilage. With increasing age, the nucleus pulposus more and more resembles the annulus fibrosus. The water-binding capacity of the disc decreases with age, and degenerative changes begin to occur in the spine after the second decade. (As mentioned, the degeneration of the intervertebral disc is called spondylosis.) Initially, the disc contains approximately 85 to 90 per cent water, but the amount decreases to 65 per cent with age.[3] As well, it contains a high portion of mucopolysaccharides, which cause the disc to act as an incompressible fluid. However, these mucopolysaccharides decrease with age and are replaced with collagen. The nucleus pulposus lies slightly posterior to the center of rotation of the disc in the lumbar spine.

The shape of the disc corresponds to that of the body to which it is attached, adhering to the bodies by the cartilaginous end plate. The end plate consists of thin layers of cartilage covering the inferior and superior surfaces of the vertebral bodies. The cartilaginous end plates are approximately 1 mm thick and allow fluid to move between the disc and the vertebral body. The discs are primarily avascular, with only the periphery receiving a blood supply. The rest of the disc receives nutrition by means of diffusion primarily through the cartilaginous end plate. Until the age of 8, the intervertebral discs have some vascularity; however, this vascularity decreases with age.

Usually, the intervertebral disc has no nerve supply, although the peripheral posterior aspect of the annulus fibrosus may be innervated by a few nerve fibers from the sinuvertebral nerve.[4, 5] The lateral aspects of the disc are innervated peripherally by the branches of the anterior rami and gray rami communicantes. The pain-sensitive structures around the intervertebral disc are the anterior longitudinal ligament, posterior longitudinal ligament, vertebral body, nerve root, and cartilage of the facet joint.

With the movement of fluid vertically through the cartilaginous end plate, the pressure of the disc is decreased as an individual approaches the natural lordotic posture in the lumbar spine. Direct vertical pressure on the disc can cause the disc to push fluid into the vertebral body. If the pressure is great enough, defects may occur in the cartilaginous end plate, resulting in *Schmorl's nodes*, which are herniations of the nucleus pulposus into the vertebral body. An adult is usually 1 to 2 cm taller in the morning than in the evening. This change is due to the fluid movement in and out of the disc during the day through the cartilaginous end plate. This fluid shift acts as a safety valve to protect the disc.

If there is an injury to the disc, four problems can result. There may be a *protrusion of the disc*, in which the disc bulges posteriorly without rupturing the annulus fibrosus. In the case of a *disc prolapse*, only the outermost fibers of the annulus fibrosus contain the nucleus. A *disc extrusion* means that the annulus fibrosus is perforated and discal material (part of nucleus pulposus) moves into the epidural space (Fig. 8–2). The fourth problem is a *sequestrated disc*, or a formation of discal fragments from the annulus fibrosus and nucleus pulposus outside the disc proper.[6]

Within the lumbar spine, different postures can increase the pressure on the intervertebral disc (Fig. 8–3). This information is based on the work of Nachemson,[7, 8] who performed studies of intradiscal pressure changes in the L3 disc with changes in posture. In regard to these figures, the pressure in the standing position is classified as the norm, and the values given are increases above this norm that occur with the change in

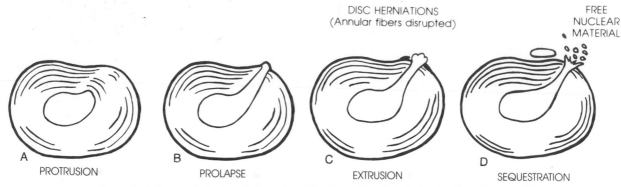

DISC HERNIATIONS
(Annular fibers disrupted)

FREE NUCLEAR MATERIAL

A PROTRUSION   B PROLAPSE   C EXTRUSION   D SEQUESTRATION

Figure 8–2. Types of disc herniations. (Modified from MacNab, I.: Backache. Baltimore, The Williams and Wilkins Co., 1977. p. 94.)

posture. For example, the following actions increase the pressure in the L3 intervertebral disc by the following amounts:

1. Coughing or straining, 5 to 35 per cent.
2. Laughing, 40 to 50 per cent.
3. Walking, 15 per cent.
4. Side bending, 25 per cent.
5. Small jumps, 40 per cent.
6. Bending forward, 150 per cent.
7. Rotation, 20 per cent.
8. Lifting a 20-kg weight with the back straight and knees bent, 73 per cent.

9. Lifting a 20-kg weight with the back bent and knees straight, 169 per cent.

Generally, the L5-S1 segment is the most common site of problems in the vertebral column because this joint bears more weight than any other vertebral joint. The center of gravity passes directly through this vertebra, which is of benefit because it may decrease the shearing stresses to this segment. There is a transition from the mobile segment, L5, to the stable or fixed segment of the sacrum, which can increase the stress on this area. Because the angle between L5 and S1 is

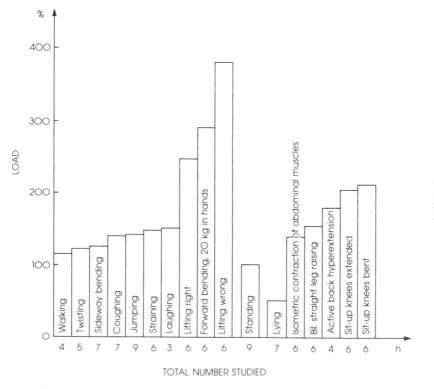

Figure 8–3. Mean change in load on L3 disc compared with upright standing. (From Nachemson, A., and C. Elfstrom. Scand. J. Rehabil. Med., Suppl. 1, 1970, p. 31.)

greater than between the other vertebrae, it has a greater chance of stress being applied to it. Another factor increasing the stress on this area is the greater amount of movement, relatively, which occurs at this level, compared with other levels of the lumbar spine.

Patient History

In addition to the general questions asked in Chapter 1, the following information should be ascertained:

1. What is the patient's usual activity or pastime?

2. What kind of activity originally caused the back pain? Often, lifting is a common cause of low back pain. This fact is not surprising, when one considers the forces exerted on the lumbar spine and disc. For example, a 77-kg man lifting a 91-kg weight approximately 36 cm from the intervertebral disc exerts a force of 940 kg on that disc. The force exerted on the disc can be calculated roughly by saying it is approximately ten times the weight being lifted. Pressure on the intervertebral discs varies, depending on the position of the person. From the work of Nachemson,[7, 8] it has been shown that pressure on the disc can be decreased by increasing the *supported* inclination of the back rest (for example, an angle of 130° decreases the pressure on the disc by 50 per cent). Using the arms for support can also decrease the pressure on the disc. When one is standing, the disc pressure is about 35 per cent of the pressure in the relaxed sitting position. The examiner should also keep in mind that stress on the lower back tends to be 15 to 20 per cent higher in men than in women because men are taller and their weight is distributed higher in the body.

3. Where are the sites and boundaries of pain? Have the patient point to the location(s).

4. Is there any radiation of pain? It is helpful for the examiner to remember this and correlate it with dermatome findings when evaluating sensation.

5. Is the pain deep? Superficial? Shooting? Burning? Aching?

6. Is there paresthesia (pins and needles) or anesthesia? A sensation or lack of sensation may be experienced if there is pressure on a nerve root. Paresthesia occurs if pressure is relieved from a nerve trunk. Does the patient experience any paresthesia or tingling and numbness in the extremities, perineal (saddle) area, or pelvic area? Abnormal sensations in the perineal (saddle) area often have associated micturition (urination) problems. The examiner must remember that the adult spinal cord ends at the bottom of the L1 vertebra and becomes the cauda equina within the spinal column. The nerve roots extend in such a way that it is rare for the disc to pinch on the nerve root of the same level. For example, the L5 nerve root is more likely to be compressed by the L4 intervertebral disc than the L5 intervertebral disc (Fig. 8–4). Seldom is the nerve root compressed by the disc at the same level except when the protrusion is more lateral.

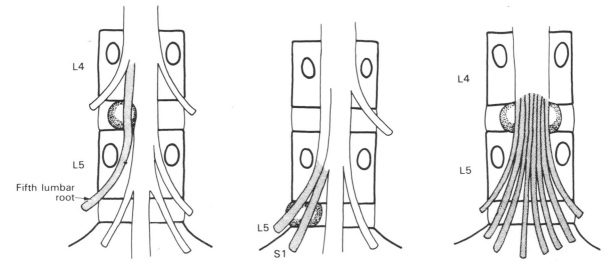

Figure 8–4. Possible effects of disc herniation. (*A*) A herniation of the disc between L4 and L5 will compress the fifth lumbar root. (*B*) A large herniation of the L5-S1 disc will compromise not only the nerve root crossing it (the first sacral nerve root) but also the nerve root emerging through the same foramen (the fifth lumbar nerve root). (*C*) A massive central sequestration of the disc at the L4-5 level will involve all the nerve roots in the cauda equina and may result in bowel and bladder paralysis. (From MacNab, I.: Backache. Baltimore, The Williams and Wilkins Co., 1977, pp. 96–97.)

7. Which activities aggravate the pain? Is there anything in the patient's lifestyle that increases the pain?

8. Which activities ease the pain?

9. Is the pain improving? Worsening? Staying the same?

10. What about the patient's sleeping position? Is there any problem sleeping? What type of mattress is used (hard, soft)?

11. Does the patient have any difficulty with micturition? If so, the examiner should proceed with caution because the condition may involve more than the lumbar spine. Conversely, this symptom may result from a disc protrusion or spinal stenosis with minimal or no back pain or sciatica. A disc derangement may cause total urinary retention; chronic, long-standing partial retention; vesicular irritability; or the loss of desire or awareness of the necessity to void.

12. Is there any increase in pain with coughing? Sneezing? Deep breathing? Laughing? All of these actions increase the *intrathecal pressure* (the pressure inside the covering of the spinal cord).

13. Are there any postures or actions that specifically increase or decrease the pain or cause difficulty?[9, 10] For example, if sitting increases the pain and other symptoms, the examiner could suspect that sustained flexion is causing mechanical deformation of the spine. If sitting decreases the pain and other symptoms, sustained flexion is decreasing the mechanical deformation. If standing increases pain and other symptoms, the examiner might suspect that extension, especially relaxed standing, is the cause. If walking increases pain and other symptoms, extension is probably causing the mechanical deformation because walking accentuates extension. If lying (especially prone) increases pain and other symptoms, extension may be the cause. Persistent pain or progressive increase in pain in the supine position would lead the examiner to suspect neurogenic or space-occupying lesions, such as infection or tumors. It must be remembered that pain may radiate to the lumbar spine from a pathologic condition in other areas as well as from direct mechanical problems. For example, tumors of the pancreas refer pain to the low back. Stiffness and/or pain after rest may be indicative of ankylosing spondylitis or Scheuermann's disease. Pain from mechanical breakdown tends to increase with activity and decrease with rest. Discogenic pain increases if a patient holds one posture (especially flexion) for a long period. Pain arising from the spine almost always is influenced by posture and movement.

14. Is the pain altered by changing posture?[10] For example, does the pain increase or decrease when the patient goes from a standing to sitting position? The normal lumbosacral angle while standing is 140°, the sacral angle is 30° (Fig. 8–5), and the normal pelvic angle is 30°. The pelvis

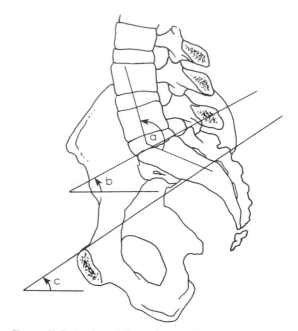

Figure 8–5. Angles of the spine and sacrum. a = Lumbosacral angle (normal = 140°); b = sacral angle (normal = 30°); c = pelvic angle (normal = 30°).

is the key to proper back posture. In order for the pelvis to "sit" properly on the femora, the abdominal, hip flexor, hip extensor, and back extensor muscles must be strong, supple, and balanced. Any deviation in the normal alignment should be noted and recorded.

15. Is the pain worse in the morning? Evening? As the day goes on? Is the pain better as the day goes on? For example, osteoarthritis of the facet joints leads to morning stiffness, which in turn is relieved by activity.

16. Which movements hurt? Which movements are stiff? The examiner must help the patient differentiate between true pain and discomfort that is due to stretching. *Postural* or *static muscles* tend to respond to pathology by tightness in the form of spasm or adaptive shortening; *dynamic* or *phasic muscles* tend to respond by atrophy. For example, the iliopsoas muscle will adaptively shorten, but the abdominal muscles will weaken in certain pathologic conditions. Does the patient describe a painful arc of movement on forward or side flexion? If so, it may indicate a disc protrusion with a nerve root riding over the bulge.[10]

17. Is the patient taking any medication? For example, long-term use of steroid therapy can lead to osteoporosis.

18. What is the patient's sex? Lower back pain has a higher incidence in females.

19. What is the patient's occupation? Back pain tends to be greater in individuals with strenuous occupations. For example, truck drivers and warehouse workers have a very high incidence of back injury.

Observation

The patient must be suitably undressed. Males must be only in shorts, and females, only in a bra and shorts. When doing the observation, the examiner should note the willingness of the patient to move and the pattern of movement. The patient should be observed first standing, then sitting. The examiner should note the following:

Body Type. There are three general body types:

1. *Ectomorphic.* Thin body build, characterized by relative prominence of structures developed from the embryonic ectoderm.

2. *Mesomorphic.* Muscular or sturdy body build, characterized by relative prominence of structures developed from the embryonic mesoderm.

3. *Endomorphic.* Heavy (fat) body build, characterized by relative prominence of structures developed from the embryonic endoderm.

Gait. Does the gait appear to be normal when the patient walks into the area, or is it altered in some way? If it is altered, the examiner must take time to find out whether the problem is in the limb or whether the gait is altered to relieve symptoms elsewhere.

Attitude. Is the patient tense? Bored? Lethargic? What is the appearance of the individual? Healthy-looking? Emaciated? Overweight?

Total Spinal Posture. The patient should be examined in the habitual relaxed posture that is usually adopted. The patient should be observed anteriorly, laterally, and posteriorly (Fig. 8–6). Anteriorly the head should be straight "on the shoulders" and the nose in line with the manubrium sternum and xiphisternum or umbilicus. The shoulders and clavicles should be level and equal, although the dominant side may be slightly lower. The waist angles should be equal. The arbitrary "high" point on each iliac crest should be the same height on both sides. The anterior superior iliac spines should be level on each side. The patella should point straight ahead. The lower limbs should be straight and not in genu varum or genu valgum. The heads of the fibulae should be level. The medial malleoli should be level, as should the lateral malleoli. The medial longitudinal arches of the feet should be evident, and the feet should angle out equally. The arms should be an equal distance from the trunk and equally medially or laterally rotated. Any protrusion or depression of the sternum, ribs, or costocartilage as well as any bowing of bones should be noted. The bony or soft-tissue contours should be equal on both sides.

From the side, the examiner should look at the head to ensure that the ear lobe is in line with the tip of the shoulder (acromion process) and the arbitrary high point of the iliac crest. Each

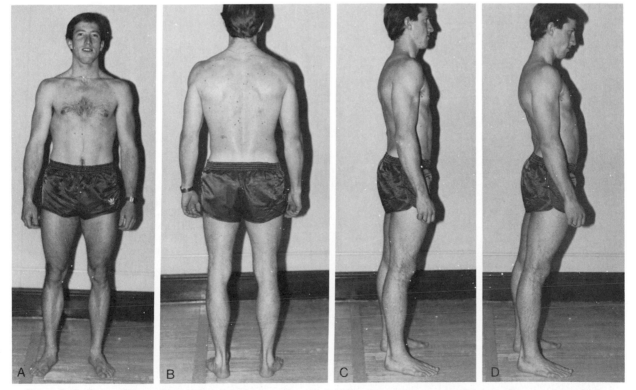

Figure 8–6. Views of the patient in the standing position. (*A*) Anterior view. (*B*) Posterior view. (*C*) Lateral view. (*D*) Lateral view with excessive lordosis.

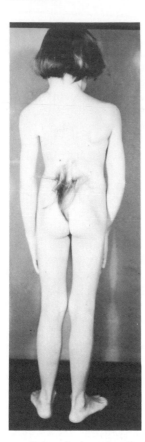

Figure 8–7. Congenital scoliosis and a diastematomyelia in a 9-year-old girl. This type of hairy patch strongly indicates a congenital maldevelopment of the neural axis. (From Rothman, R. H., and F. A. Simeone: The Spine. Philadelphia, W. B. Saunders Co., 1982, p. 371.)

segment of the spine should have a normal curve. Are any of the curves exaggerated or decreased? Is lordosis present? Kyphosis? Do the shoulders droop forward? Are the knees straight, flexed, or in recurvatum (hyperextended)?

From behind, the examiner should note the level of the shoulders, the spines of the scapula, and inferior angles; any deformities (such as a Sprengel's deformity) should also be noted. Any lateral spinal curve (scoliosis) should be noted (Fig. 8–7). The waist angles should be equal from the posterior aspect, as they were from the anterior aspect. The posterior superior iliac spines should be level. The examiner should note how the posterior superior iliac spine relates to the anterior superior iliac spine (higher or lower?). The gluteal folds and knee joints should be level. The Achilles tendons and heels should appear to be straight. The examiner should note whether there is any protrusion of the ribs or any bowing of bones. Does the pelvic angle appear to be normal? Any deviation in the normal spinal postural alignment should be noted and recorded. The various possible sources of pathology are discussed in Chapter 14, "Assessment of Posture."

Markings. A "faun's beard" (tuft of hair) may indicate a spina bifida occulta or diastematomyelia (Fig. 8–7).[11] "Café au lait" spots may indicate neurofibromatosis or collagen disease (Fig. 8–8). Unusual skin markings or the presence of skin lesions in the midline may lead the examiner to consider the possibility of underlying neural and mesodermal anomalies.

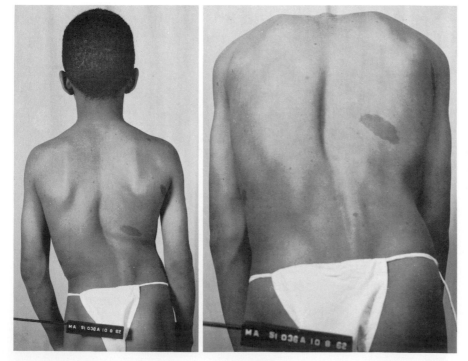

Figure 8–8. Neurofibromatosis with scoliosis. Note the café-au-lait spots on the right side of the trunk. (From Tachdjian, M. O.: Pediatric Orthopedics. Philadelphia, W. B. Saunders Co., 1972, p. 540.)

Step Deformity. A step deformity in the lumbar spine may indicate a spondylolisthesis.

Examination

The examiner must remember that a complete examination of the lumbar spine and lower limb is to be performed. Many of the symptoms that occur in the lower limb may originate in the lumbar spine. Unless there is a history of definitive trauma to a peripheral joint, a screening examination must accompany assessment of that joint to rule out problems within the lumbar spine.

ACTIVE MOVEMENTS

Active movements are performed with the patient standing (Fig. 8–9). The examiner is looking for differences in range of movement and the patient's willingness to do the movement. The range of motion taking place during the active movement is normally the summation of the movements of the whole lumbar spine, not just movement at one level. The most painful movements are done last.

While the patient is doing the active movements, the examiner must remember to look for limitation of movement and its possible causes, such as pain, spasm, stiffness, or blocking. As the patient reaches the full range of active movement, passive overpressure may be applied—but only if the active movement appears to be full and pain-free. The overpressure must be applied with extreme care because the upper body weight is already being applied to the lumbar joints by virtue of the position and gravity.

The greatest motion in the lumbar spine occurs between L4 and L5 and between L5 and S1. There is a considerable individual variability in the range of motion of the lumbar spine (Fig. 8–10).[12–16] In reality, little obvious movement occurs in the lumbar spine as a result of shape of the facet joints, tightness of the ligaments, intervertebral discs, and size of the vertebral bodies. The following active movements are carried out in the lumbar spine:

1. Forward flexion (40 to 60°).
2. Extension (20 to 35°).
3. Side flexion (left and right) (15 to 20°).
4. Rotation (left and right) (3 to 18°).

For *flexion* (forward bending), the maximum of range of motion is 40 to 60°. The examiner must ensure that the movement is occurring in the lumbar spine and not in the hips or thoracic spine. It must be remembered that an individual can touch the toes even if no movement occurs in the spine. On forward flexion, the lumbar curve should normally go from its normal lordotic curvature to at least a straight or slightly flexed curve (Fig. 8–11). If it does not do this, there is probably some hypomobility in the lumbar spine. As with the thoracic spine, the examiner may use a tape measure to obtain the distance of the increase in spacing of the spinous processes on forward flexion. Normally, the tape should increase 7 to 8 cm in length if the measurement is taken between the T12 spinous process and S1 (Fig. 8–9A, B). The examiner should note how far forward the patient is able to bend (i.e., to the mid-thigh, knees, mid-tibia, or floor) and compare this finding with the "straight leg raising" tests, since straight leg raising, especially bilaterally, is essentially the same, except that it is a movement occurring from below upward instead of from above downward.

Extension (backward bending) is normally limited to 20 to 35° in the lumbar spine. While performing the movement, the patient is asked to place the hands in the small of the back to help stabilize the back.

Lateral flexion is approximately 15 to 20° in the lumbar spine. The patient is asked to run the hand down the side of the leg and not to bend forward or backward while performing the movement. The examiner can then "eyeball" the movement and compare the movement to the left and right. One may also measure the distance from the fingertips to the floor on both sides and note any differences. As the patient side flexes, the examiner should watch the lumbar curve. (Normally, the lumbar curve should form a smooth curve on side flexion and there should be no obvious angulation at only one level.) If angulation does occur, it may indicate hypomobility or hypermobility at one level of the lumbar spine.

Rotation in the lumbar spine is normally 3 to 18° to the left and right and is accomplished by a shearing movement of the lumbar vertebrae on each other. Although the patient is usually in the standing position, it may be done sitting to eliminate pelvic and hip movement. If the patient stands, the examiner must take care to watch for this accessory movement and try to eliminate it as much as possible by stabilizing the pelvis.

If a movement such as side flexion toward the painful side alters the symptoms, (1) the lesion is intra-articular because the muscles and ligaments on that side are relaxed or (2) a disc protrusion, if present, is lateral to the nerve root, increasing the pain. If a movement such as side flexion away from the painful side alters the symptoms, (1) the lesion may be articular or muscular in origin or (2) a disc protrusion, if present, is medial to the nerve root (Fig. 8–12).

McKenzie advocates repeating the active movements, especially flexion and extension, ten times

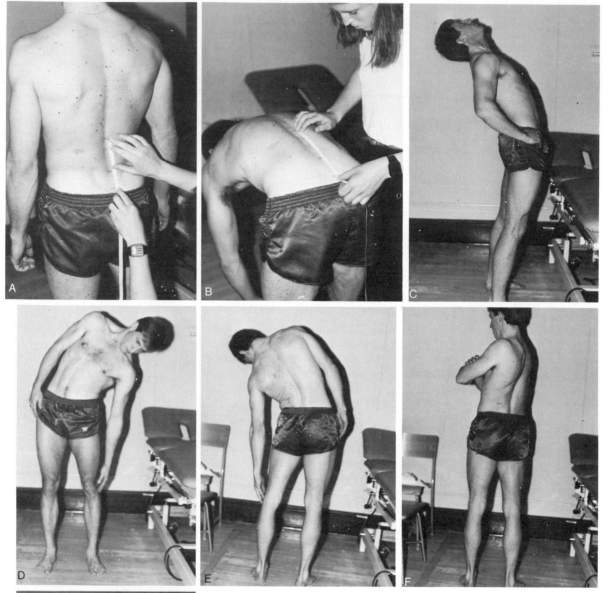

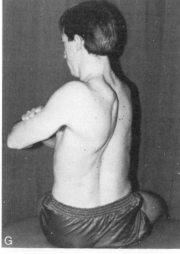

Figure 8–9. Active movements of the lumbar spine. (*A* and *B*) Measuring forward flexion using tape measure. (*C*) Extension. (*D*) Side flexion (anterior view). (*E*) Side flexion (posterior view). (*F*) Rotation (standing). (*G*) Rotation (sitting).

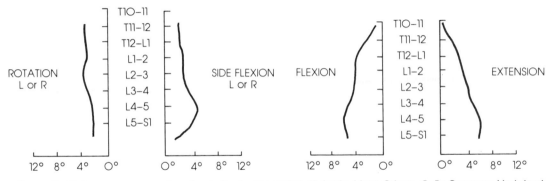

Figure 8–10. Average range of motion in the lumbar spine. (Adapted from Grieve, G. P.: Common Vertebral Joint Problems. New York, Churchill Livingstone, 1981.)

Figure 8–11. On forward flexion, the lumbar curve should normally flatten or go into slight flexion as shown.

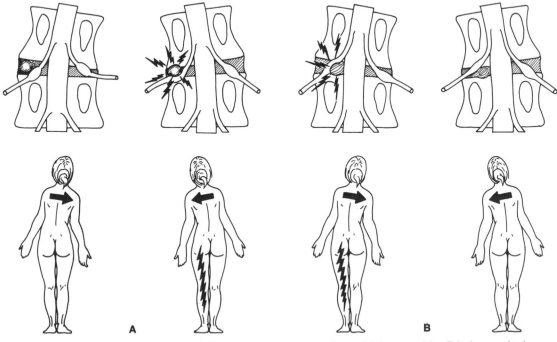

Figure 8–12. Patients with herniated disc disease may sometimes list to one side. This is a voluntary or involuntary mechanism to alleviate nerve root irritation. The list in some patients is toward the side of the sciatica; in others it is toward the opposite side. A reasonable hypothesis suggests that when the herniation is lateral to the nerve root (*A*), the list is to the side opposite the sciatica because a list to the same side would elicit pain. Conversely, when the herniation is medial to the nerve root (*B*), the list is toward the side of the sciatica because tilting away would irritate the root and cause pain. (From White, A. A., and M. M. Panjabi: Clinical Biomechanics of the Spine. Philadelphia, J. B. Lippincott, 1978, p. 299.)

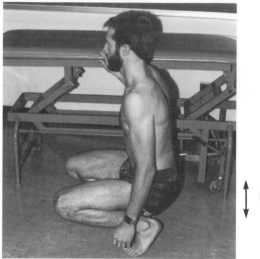

Figure 8–13. Quick test.

BOUNCE

While the patient is standing, a "quick test" may be done (Fig. 8–13). The patient squats down as far as possible, bouncing two or three times and returning to the standing position. This action will quickly test the ankles, knees, and hips for any pathologic condition. If the patient can fully squat and bounce without any signs and symptoms, these joints in all probability are free of pathology related to the complaint. It must be remembered that this test should be used only with caution and should not be done with patients suspected of having arthritis in the lower limb joints, with pregnant patients, or with older individuals who exhibit weakness and hypomobility. If this test is done and is negative, there is no need to test the peripheral joints in the lying position.

The patient is then asked to balance on one leg and to go up and down on the toes four or five times. While the patient does this, the examiner should watch for a Trendelenburg sign (Fig. 8–14). A positive sign may be due to a weak gluteus medius muscle or a coxa vara. If the patient is unable to complete the movement by going up and down on the toes, the examiner might suspect an S1 nerve root lesion. Both legs are tested.

McKenzie advocates doing flexion movement in the supine lying position as well.[9] In the standing position, flexion will take place from above downward so that pain at the end of the range of motion indicates L5-S1 being affected. In

to see whether the movement increases or decreases the symptoms.[9] He also advocates a side gliding movement in which the head and feet remain in position and the patient shifts the pelvis to the left and to the right.

If the examiner finds that side flexion and rotation have been equally limited followed by extension, a capsular pattern may be suspected. A capsular pattern in one lumbar segment, however, may be difficult to detect.

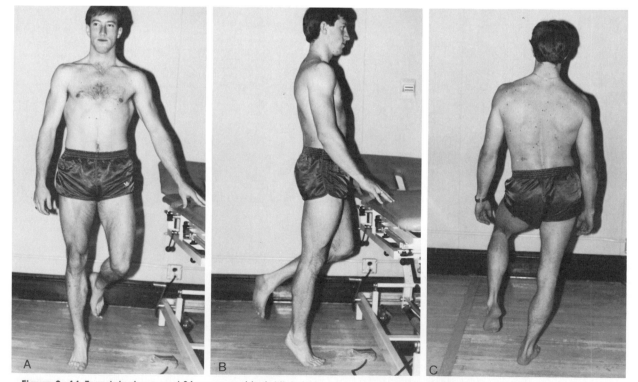

Figure 8–14. Trendelenburg and S1 nerve root test. (A) Anterior view, negative test. (B) Side view, negative test. (C) Posterior view, positive test.

the supine lying position, with the knees being lifted to the chest, flexion takes place from below upward so that pain at the beginning of movement indicates L5-S1 being affected. It must also be remembered that greater stretch is placed on L5-S1 in the lying position.

PASSIVE MOVEMENTS

In the lumbar spine, passive movements are very difficult to perform because of the weight of the body. As previously stated, if active movements are full and pain-free, overpressure can be attempted with care. The normal end feels of the lumbar spine are:
1. Flexion—tissue stretch.
2. Extension—tissue stretch.
3. Side flexion—tissue stretch.
4. Rotation—tissue stretch.

In actuality, it is safer to check the end feel of the individual vertebra in the lumbar spine when doing the joint play movements of the lumbar spine. The end feel will be the same, but the examiner will have better control of the patient and will be less likely to overstress the joints.

RESISTED ISOMETRIC MOVEMENTS

The patient is seated. These tests are the same movements as were done actively (Fig. 8–15):
1. Forward flexion.
2. Extension.
3. Side flexion (left and right).
4. Rotation (left and right).

The contraction must be resisted and isometric so that no movement occurs (Fig. 8–16). Because of the strength of the trunk muscles, the examiner should say: "Don't let me move you," so that minimal movement occurs. The examiner tests the various movements, as shown in Figure 8–16. The lumbar spine should be in a neutral position, and the painful movements should be done last. The examiner should keep in mind that strong abdominals help to reduce the load on the lumbar spine by about 30 per cent and on the thoracic spine by about 50 per cent as a result of the increased intrathoracic and intra-abdominal pressures caused by the contraction of these muscles. Table 8–1 lists the muscles acting on the lumbar vertebrae.

PERIPHERAL JOINTS

Once the resisted isometric movements have been completed, if the examiner did not use the "quick test" for peripheral joints or is unsure of the findings, the peripheral joints should be quickly scanned to rule out obvious pathology in the extremities. Any deviation from normal could lead the examiner to do a detailed examination of that joint. The following joints are scanned.[17]

Sacroiliac Joints. With the patient standing, the examiner palpates the posterior superior iliac spine on one side with one thumb and one of the sacral spines with the other thumb. The patient then flexes the hip on that side, and the examiner notes whether the posterior superior iliac spine drops as it normally should on the movement or whether it elevates, indicating fixation of the sacroiliac joint on that side (Fig. 8–17). The examiner then compares the other side. The examiner next places one thumb on one of the patient's ischial tuberosities and one thumb on the sacral apex. The patient is then asked to flex the hip on that side again. If the movement is normal, the

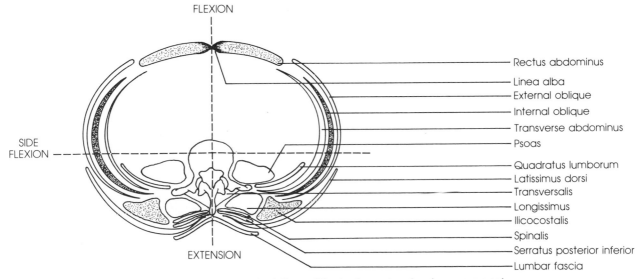

Figure 8–15. Diagram of relations of the lumbar spine showing movement.

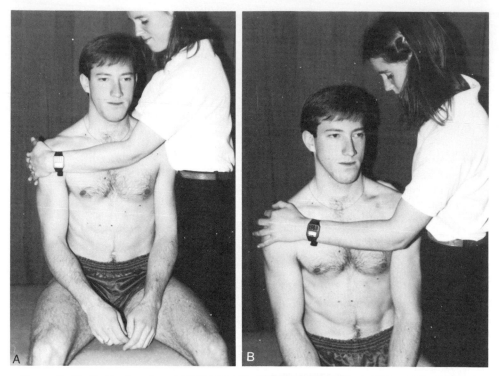

Figure 8–16. Positioning for resisted isometric movements of the lumbar spine. (A) Flexion, extension, and side flexion. (B) Rotation to right.

thumb on the ischial tuberosity will move laterally. If the sacroiliac joint on that side is fixed, the thumb will move up. The other side is then tested for comparison.

Hip Joints. These joints are actively moved through as full a range of motion of flexion, extension, abduction, adduction, and medial and lateral rotation as possible. Any pattern of restriction or pain should be noted. As the patient flexes the hip, the examiner may palpate the ilium, sacrum, and lumbar spine to determine when, during flexion, movement begins at the sacroiliac joint on that side and at the lumbar spine. Both sides should be compared.

Table 8–1. Muscles of the Lumbar Spine: Their Action and Innervation

Action	Muscles Involved	Innervation
Forward flexion	1. Psoas major	L1, L2, L3
	2. Rectus abdominis	T6–T12
	3. External abdominal oblique	T7–T12
	4. Internal abdominal oblique	T7–T12, L1
	5. Transversus abdominis	T7–T12, L1
Extension	1. Latissimus dorsi	Thoracodorsal (C6, C7, C8)
	2. Erector spinae	L1, L2, L3
	3. Transversospinalis	L1–L5
	4. Interspinales	L1–L5
	5. Quadratus lumborum	T12, L1–L4
Side flexion	1. Latissimus dorsi	Thoracodorsal (C6, C7, C8)
	2. Erector spinae	L1, L2, L3
	3. Transversospinalis	L1–L5
	4. Intertransversarii	L1–L5
	5. Quadratus lumborum	T12, L1–L4
	6. Psoas major	L1, L2, L3
	7. External abdominal oblique	T7–T12
Rotation*	—	—

*Very little rotation occurs in the lumbar spine because of the shape of the facet joints. Any rotation would be due to a shearing movement. If shear does occur, the transversospinal muscles would be responsible for the movement.

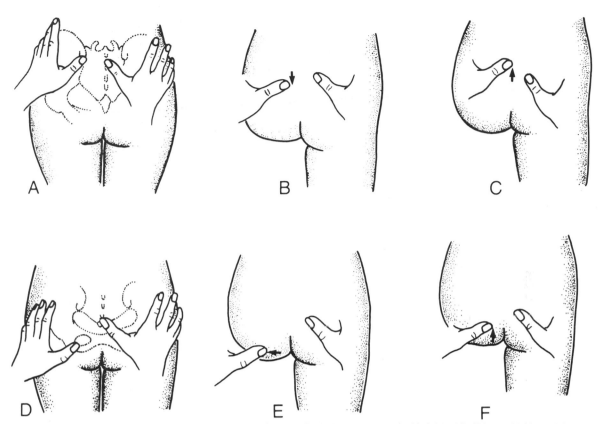

Figure 8–17. Tests to demonstrate left sacroiliac fixation. Tests for upper part of joint in (A), (B), and (C) and for lower part in (D), (E), and (F). (A) The examiner places the left thumb on the posterior superior iliac spine and the right thumb over one of the sacral spinous processes. (B) When movement is normal, the examiner's left thumb moves downward as the patient raises the left leg. (C) When the joint is fixed, the examiner's left thumb moves upward as the patient raises the left leg. (D) The examiner places the left thumb over the ischial tuberosity and the right thumb over the apex of the sacrum. (E) When movement is normal, the examiner's left thumb moves laterally as the patient raises the left leg. (F) When the joint is fixed, the examiner's left thumb moves slightly upward as the patient raises the left leg. (From Kirkaldy-Willis, W. H.: Managing Low Back Pain. New York, Churchill Livingstone, 1983, p. 94.)

Knee Joints. The patient actively moves the knee joints through as full range of flexion and extension as possible. Any restriction of movement or abnormal signs and symptoms should be noted.

Foot and Ankle Joints. Plantar flexion, dorsiflexion, supination, and pronation of the foot and ankle, as well as the flexion and extension of the toes, are actively performed through a full range of motion. Again, any alteration in signs and symptoms should be noted.

MYOTOMES

Having completed the scanning examination of the peripheral joints, the examiner next tests muscle power and possible neurologic weakness (Table 8–2).[17]

With the patient lying supine, the myotomes are tested by assessing the following resisted isometric movements (Fig. 8–18):

1. Hip flexion tests the L2 myotome.

2. Knee extension tests the L3 myotome.
3. Ankle dorsiflexion tests the L4 myotome.
4. Toe extension tests the L5 myotome.
5. Ankle plantar flexion tests the S1 myotome.
6. Ankle eversion tests the S1 myotome.

It should be remembered that the examiner has previously tested the S1 myotome with the patient standing and has tested for the positive Trendelenburg sign; thus these movements are repeated here only if the examiner is unsure of the result and wants to test again. The ankle movements should be tested with the knee flexed about 30°, especially if the patient complains of sciatic pain. The extended knee will increase the stretch on the sciatic nerve and may result in false signs, such as weakness that is due to pain rather than weakness that is due to pressure on the nerve root.

With the patient lying prone the following resisted isometric movements may be tested:

1. Hip extension tests the S1 myotome.
2. Knee flexion tests the S1 and S2 myotomes.

Table 8–2. Lumbar Root Syndromes

Root	Dermatome	Muscle Weakness	Reflexes Affected	Paresthesias
L1	Back, over trochanter, groin	None	None	Groin, after holding posture, which causes pain
L2	Back, front of thigh to knee	Psoas, hip adductors	None	Occasionally front of thigh
L3	Back, upper buttock, front of thigh and knee, medial lower leg	Psoas, quadriceps—thigh wasting	Knee jerk sluggish, PKB positive, pain on full SLR	Inner knee, anterior lower leg
L4	Inner buttock, outer thigh, inside of leg, dorsum of foot, big toe	Tibialis anterior, extensor hallucis	SLR limited, neck-flexion pain, weak or a bent knee jerk; side flexion limited	Medial aspect of calf and ankle
L5	Buttock, back and side of thigh, lateral aspect of leg, dorsum of foot, inner half of sole and first, second, and third toes	Extensor hallucis, peroneal, gluteus medius, ankle dorsiflexor, hamstrings—calf wasting	SLR limited to one side, neck-flexion pain, ankle jerk decreased, crossed-leg raising—pain	Lateral aspect of leg, medial three toes
S1	Buttock, back of thigh, and lower leg	Calf and hamstrings, wasting of gluteals, peroneals, plantar flexors	SLR limited	Lateral two toes, lateral foot, lateral leg to knee, plantar aspect of foot
S2	Same as S1	Same as S1 except peroneals	Same as S1	Lateral leg, knee, heel
S3	Groin, inner thigh to knee	None	None	None
S4	Perineum, genitals, lower sacrum	Bladder, rectum	None	Saddle area, genitals, anus, impotence, massive posterior

*Manipulation and traction are contraindicated if S4 or massive posterior displacement causes bilateral sciatica and S3 pain.
Abbreviations: PKB = Prone knee bendings; SLR = straight leg raise.

If the patient is in extreme pain, these last myotomes should be tested only after all tests in the supine lying position have been completed. This action will cut down on the amount of movement the patient has to do, decreasing the discomfort. Ideally, all testing in the standing position should be performed, following by sit-

ting, then supine lying, side lying, and finally prone lying. This procedure is shown in the précis at the end of the chapter.

When testing myotomes (Table 8–3), the examiner should place the test joint(s) in a neutral or resting position and then apply a resisted isometric pressure. The contraction should be

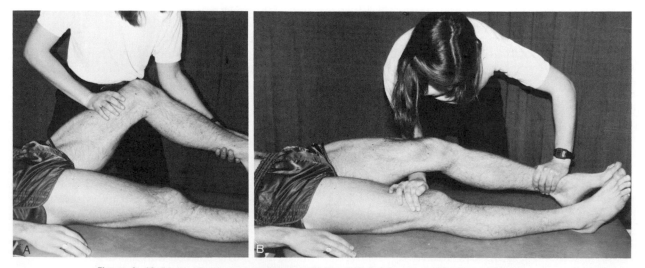

Figure 8–18. Positioning to test myotomes. (A) Hip flexion (L2). (B) Knee extension (L3).

Illustration continued on opposite page

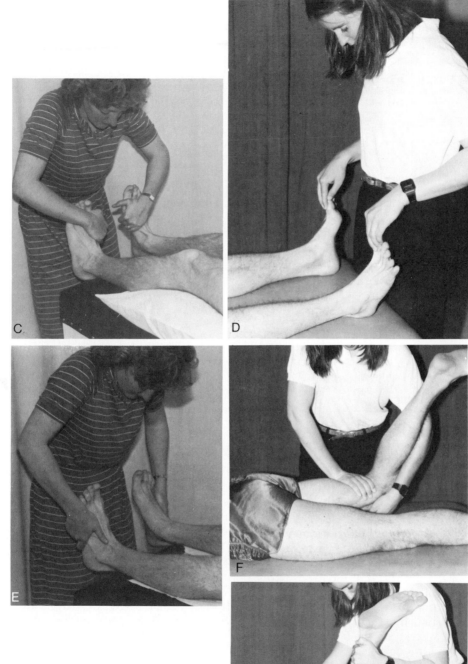

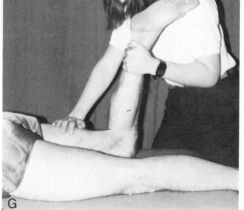

Figure 8–18 *Continued.* (*C*) Foot dorsiflexion (L4). (*D*) Extension of big toe (L5). (*E*) Ankle eversion (S1). (*F*) Hip extension (S1). (*G*) Knee flexion (S1, S2).

Table 8–3. Myotomes of the Lower Limb

Nerve Root	Test Action	Muscles
L1–L2	Hip flexion	Psoas, iliacus, sartorius, gracilis, pectineus, adductor longus, adductor brevis
L3	Knee extension	Quadriceps, adductor longus, magnus and brevis
L4	Ankle dorsiflexion	Tibialis anterior, quadriceps, tensor fasciae latae, adductor magnus, obturator externus, tibialis posterior
L5	Toe extension	Extensor hallucis longus, extensor digitorum longus, gluteus medius and minimus, obturator internus, semimembranosus, semitendinosus, peroneus tertius, popliteus
S1	Ankle plantar flexion Ankle eversion Hip extension Knee flexion	Gastrocnemius, soleus, gluteus maximus, obturator internus, piriformis, biceps femoris, semitendinosus, popliteus, peroneus longus and brevis, extensor digitorum brevis
S2	Knee flexion	Biceps femoris, piriformis, soleus, gastrocnemius, flexor digitorum longus, flexor hallucis longus, intrinsic foot muscles
S3		Intrinsic foot muscles (except abductor hallucis), flexor hallucis brevis, flexor digitorum brevis, extensor digitorum brevis

held for at least 5 seconds to show any weakness. When feasible, the examiner should test both sides simultaneously to provide a comparison. The simultaneous bilateral comparison is not possible for movements involving the hip and knee joints so both sides must be done individually. The examiner should not apply pressure over the joints because this action may mask symptoms or the true problem.

Hip flexion (L2 myotome) is tested by flexing the patient's hip to 30 to 40°. The examiner then applies a resisted force into extension proximal to the knee while ensuring that the heel of the patient's foot is not resting on the bed. The other side is then tested for comparison. To prevent excessive stress on the lumbar spine, the examiner must ensure that the patient does not increase the lumbar lordosis while doing the test.

To test *knee flexion* or the L3 myotome, the examiner flexes the patient's knee to 25 to 35° and then applies a resisted flexion force at the mid-shaft of the tibia. The other side is tested for comparison.

Ankle dorsiflexion (L4 myotome) is tested by asking the patient to place the feet at 90° relative to the leg. The examiner applies a resisted force to the dorsum of each foot and compares both sides. *Ankle plantar flexion* (S1 myotome) is compared in a similar fashion but the resistance is applied to the sole of the foot. As a result of the strength of the plantar flexor muscles, it is better to test this myotome with the patient standing. The patient slowly moves up and down on the toes of each foot in turn, and the examiner compares the differences as previously described. Ankle eversion (S1 myotome) is tested with the patient in the same starting position, and the examiner applies a force into inversion.

Toe extension (L5 myotome) is tested with the patient holding both large toes in a neutral position. The examiner applies resistance to the nails of both toes and compares both sides. It is imperative that the resistance is isometric so that the amount of force in this case is less than that applied during knee extension, as an example.

Hip extension (S1 myotome) is tested with the patient lying prone. The knee is flexed to 90°. The examiner then lifts the patient's thigh slightly off the bed while stabilizing the leg. A downward force is applied to the patient's posterior thigh with one hand while the other hand ensures that the patient's thigh is not resting on the bed.

Knee flexion (S1 and S2 myotomes) is tested in the same position with the knee flexed to 90°. An extension isometric force is applied just above the ankle. Although it is possible to test both knee flexors at the same time, it is not advisable to do this because the stress on the lumbar spine may be too great.

SPECIAL TESTS

When the special tests for the lumbar spine are performed, it is essential that the first two tests always be done. The other tests need only be done if the examiner feels that they are relevant.

Straight Leg Raising Test

Also known as *Lasègue's test* (Fig. 8–19), the straight leg raising test is done by the examiner with the patient completely relaxed.[18–25] It is a passive test, and each leg is tested individually. With the patient in the supine position, the hip medially rotated and the knee extended, the examiner flexes the hip until the patient complains of pain or tightness. The examiner then slowly and carefully drops the leg back slightly until there is no pain or tightness. The patient is then asked to flex the neck so the chin is on his chest; in some cases, if the patient has limited neck movement, the examiner may dorsiflex the patient's foot; or both actions may be done simultaneously. The neck flexion movement has also been called *Hyndman's sign* or *Brudzinski's sign*. Pain that increases with neck flexion, ankle dorsiflexion, or both indicates stretching of the dura mater of the spinal cord. Pain that does not increase with neck flexion may indicate the hamstring area (tight hamstrings) or the lumbosacral or sacroiliac joints. A *unilateral straight leg raise* is full at 70°; that is, the nerves are completely stretched, primarily the L5, S1, and S2 nerve roots, having an excursion of about 2 to 6 mm.[23] Thus, pain after 70° is probably joint pain from the lumbar area or sacroiliac joints (Fig. 8–20). The examiner should compare both legs for any difference.

The examiner should then test both legs simultaneously *(bilateral straight leg raise)* as in Figure 8–21. This test must be done with care, since the examiner is lifting the weight of both lower limbs. With the patient relaxed in the supine position and knees extended, the examiner lifts both of the patient's legs by flexing the hips until the patient complains of pain or tightness. If the test causes pain before 70°, the lesion is probably in the sacroiliac joints; if the test causes pain after 70°, the lesion is probably in the lumbar spine.

When doing the unilateral straight leg test, 80 to 90° of hip flexion is normal. If one leg is lifted and the patient complains of pain on the opposite side, it is an indication of a space-occupying lesion (e.g., a herniated disc). This finding indicates the opposite (good) leg, showing a positive test, and may be called the well leg raise test of Fajersztajn (Fig. 8–22), a prostrate leg raise test, sciatic phenomenon, or the cross-over sign.[23, 27, 28] It is usually indicative of a rather large intervertebral disc protrusion usually medial to the nerve root.[23] The test causes stretching of the ipsilateral as well as the contralateral nerve root, pulling laterally on the dural sac.

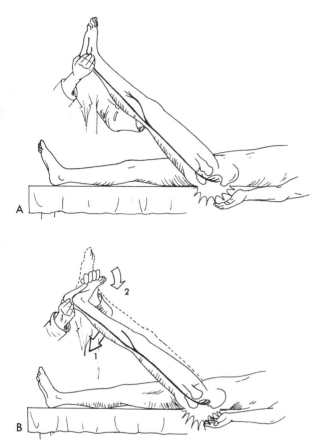

Figure 8–19. Straight leg raising. (*A*) Radicular symptoms are precipitated on the left with the straight leg raised. (*B*) The leg is lowered slowly until pain is relieved. The foot is then dorsiflexed, causing a return of symptoms; this indicates a positive test. (From Reilly, B. M.: Practical Strategies in Outpatient Medicine. Philadelphia, W. B. Saunders Co., 1984, p. 10.)

Figure 8–20. Dynamics of single straight leg raising test. (Modified from Fahrni, W. H.: Can. J. Surg. *9*:44, 1966.)

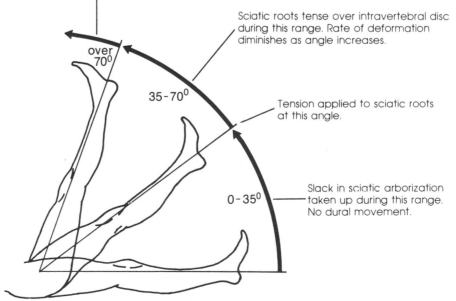

Practically no further deformation of roots occurs during further straight leg raising. Pain is probably joint pain.

Sciatic roots tense over intravertebral disc during this range. Rate of deformation diminishes as angle increases.

over 70°

35-70°

Tension applied to sciatic roots at this angle.

0-35°

Slack in sciatic arborization taken up during this range. No dural movement.

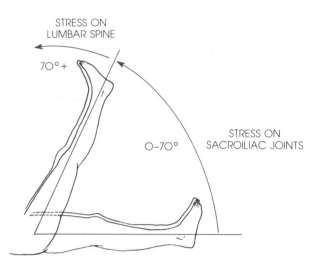

Figure 8–21. Dynamics of the bilateral straight leg raise.

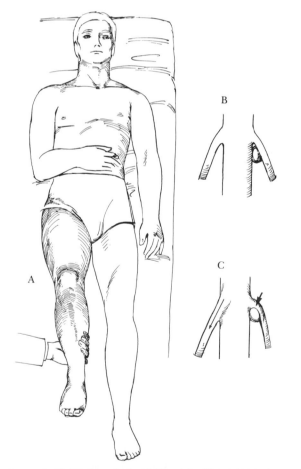

Figure 8–22. Well leg test of Fajersztajn. Movement of nerve roots when the leg on the opposite side is raised. (A) When the leg is raised on the unaffected side, the roots on the opposite side slide slightly downward and toward the midline. (B) In the presence of a disc lesion, this movement increases the root tension. (From DePalma, A. F., and R. H. Rothman: The Intervertebral Disc. Philadelphia, W. B. Saunders Co., 1970.)

During the unilateral straight leg test, tension develops in a sequential manner. It first develops in the greater sciatic foramen, followed by tension over the ala of the sacrum. Next, as the nerve crosses over the pedicle, tension develops in this area. Finally, tension occurs in the intervertebral foramen. The test will cause traction on the sciatic nerve, lumbosacral nerve roots and dura mater. Adhesions within these areas may be due to herniation of the intervertebral disc or to extradural or meningeal irritation. Pain that is felt by the patient comes from the dura mater, nerve root, adventitial sheath of the epidural veins, or the synovial facet joints. The test is positive if pain extends from the back down into the leg in the sciatic nerve distribution.

A *central protrusion* of an intervertebral disc will lead to pain primarily in the back; a *protrusion in the intermediate area* will cause pain in the posterior aspect at the lower limb and low back; a *lateral protrusion* will cause posterior leg pain primarily.

Prone Knee-Bending Test

The patient lies prone while the examiner passively flexes the knee as far as possible so that the patient's heel rests against the buttock.[29] At the same time, the examiner should ensure that the patient's hip is not rotated. If the examiner is unable to flex the patient's knee past 90° because of a pathologic condition, the test may be done by passive extension of the hip while the knee is flexed as much as possible. Unilateral pain in the lumbar area may indicate an L2 or L3 nerve root lesion (Fig. 8–23). The test also stretches the femoral nerve. Pain in the anterior thigh indicates tight quadriceps muscles. The flexed knee position should be maintained for 45 to 60 seconds.

Schober Test

The Schober test may be used to measure the amount of flexion occurring in the lumbar spine. To do this, a point is marked midway between the "dimples of the pelvis," which is the level of S2; then points 0.5 cm below and 10 cm above that level are marked. The distance between the three points is measured, the patient is asked to flex forward, and the distance is remeasured. The difference between the two measurements is an indication of the amount of flexion occurring in the lumbar spine.

Babinski Test

The examiner runs a pointed object along the plantar aspect of the patient's foot.[30] A positive

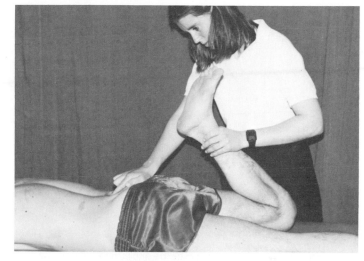

Figure 8–23. Prone knee bending test. Examiner is pointing to where one would expect pain in the lumbar spine with a positive test.

Babinski test suggests an upper motor neuron lesion and is shown by extension of the big toe and abduction (splaying) of the other toes. In an infant up to a few weeks of age, a positive test is normal. The test is often performed to determine pathologic reflexes.

Oppenheim Test

The examiner runs a fingernail along the crest of the patient's tibia.[30] A negative Oppenheim test is indicated by no reaction or no pain. A positive test is indicated by a positive Babinski sign and suggests an upper motor neuron lesion.

Hoover Test

The patient is in the lying position. The examiner places one hand under each calcaneus while the patient's legs remain relaxed on the bed (Fig. 8–24).[31–33] The patient is then asked to lift one leg off the bed, keeping the knees straight, as in an active straight leg raise. If the patient does not lift the leg or if the examiner does not feel pressure under the opposite calcaneus, the patient is probably not really trying or may be a malingerer. However, if the lifted limb is weaker, pressure under the normal heel will increase because of the increased effort to lift the weak leg. Both sides are compared for differences.

Kernig/Brudzinski Test

The patient is in the supine position with the hands cupped behind the head (Fig. 8–25).[26, 34–36] The patient is instructed to flex the head onto the chest. The extended leg is raised actively by flexing the hip until pain is felt. The patient then flexes the knee, and the pain will disappear. The

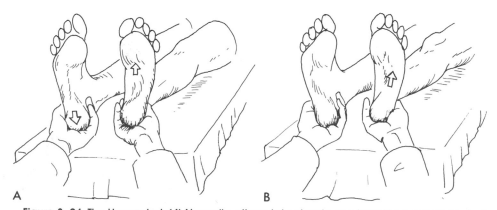

Figure 8–24. The Hoover test. (*A*) Normally, attempts to elevate one leg will be accompanied by downward pressure by the opposite leg. (*B*) When the "weak" leg attempts to elevate but the opposite (asymptomatic) leg does not "help," at least some of the weakness is probably feigned. (From Reilly, B. M.: Practical Strategies in Outpatient Medicine. Philadelphia, W. B. Saunders Co., 1984, p. 52.)

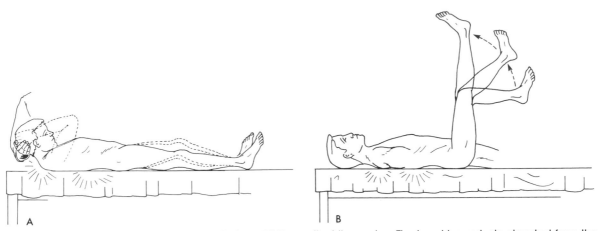

Figure 8-25. Brudzinski's (*A*) and Kernig's (*B*) signs. (*A*) The patient lies supine. The head is passively elevated from the table by the examiner. The patient complains of neck and low back discomfort and attempts to relieve the meningeal irritation by involuntary flexion of the knees and hips. (*B*) The patient lies supine with the hip and knee flexed. The knee is then gradually extended. Complaints of pain in the lower back, neck, and/or head are suggestive of meningeal irritation. (From Reilly, B. M.: Practical Strategies in Outpatient Medicine. Philadelphia, W. B. Saunders Co., 1984, p. 177.)

mechanics of the Kernig/Brudzinski test are similar to those of the straight leg raise test, except that the movements are done actively by the patient. Pain is a positive sign and may indicate meningeal irritation, nerve root involvement, or dural irritation. The neck flexion aspect of the test was originally described by Brudzinski and the hip flexion component by Kernig. The two parts of the test may be done individually, in which case they are described as the test of the original author (i.e., Brudzinski's sign or Kernig's sign).

Naffziger Test

The patient lies supine while the examiner gently compresses the jugular veins (which lie beside the carotid artery) for approximately 10 seconds (Fig. 8–26). The patient's face will flush. The patient is then asked to cough. If coughing causes pain in the low back, the spinal theca is being compressed, thus leading to an increase in intrathecal pressure. The theca is the covering (pia mater, arachnoid mater, and dura mater) around the spinal cord.

Valsalva Maneuver

The seated patient is asked to take a breath, hold it, and then to bear down as if evacuating the bowels (Fig. 8–27). If pain increases, it is an indication of increased intrathecal pressure. The symptoms may be accentuated by having the patient first flex the hip to a position just short of pain.[23]

Femoral Nerve Traction Test

The patient lies on the unaffected side with the unaffected limb flexed slightly at the hip and knee (Fig. 8–28).[37] The patient's back should be straight and not hyperextended. The patient's head should also be slightly flexed. The examiner grasps the patient's affected or painful limb and extends the knee while gently extending the hip approximately 15°. The patient's knee is then

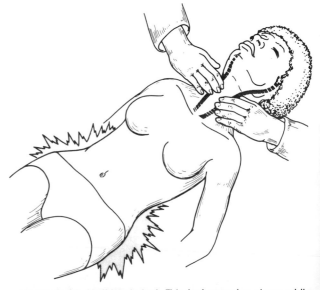

Figure 8-26. Naffziger's test. This test may be done while the patient is standing or lying down. The test is based on the hypothesis that bilateral jugular compression increases cerebral spinal fluid pressure. The pressure increase in the subarachnoid space in the root canal may cause back or leg pain by irritating a local mechanical or inflammatory condition. (From White, A. A., and M. M. Panjabi: Clinical Biomechanics of the Spine. Philadelphia, J. B. Lippincott, 1978, p. 299.)

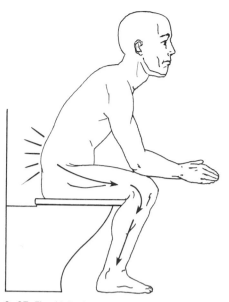

Figure 8–27. The Valsalva maneuver. Increased intrathecal pressure leads to symptoms in the sciatic nerve distribution in a positive test.

flexed on the affected side; this further stretches the femoral nerve. Pain will radiate down the anterior thigh if the test is positive.

This is a traction test for the nerve roots at the midlumbar area (L2, L3, and L4). As with the straight leg raise, there may be a contralateral positive test as well. Pain in the groin and hip that radiates along the anterior medial thigh indicates an L3 nerve root problem; pain extending to the mid-tibia indicates an L4 nerve root problem.

Stoop Test

The stoop test is done to assess neurogenic intermittent claudication to determine whether a relationship exists between neurogenic symptoms, posture, and walking.[38] When the patient

walks briskly for 1 minute pain will ensue in the buttock and lower limb within 50 meters of beginning. To relieve the pain, the patient flexes forward. These symptoms may also be relieved when the patient is sitting and forward flexing. If flexion does not relieve the symptoms, the test is negative. Extension may also be used to bring the symptoms back.

Gluteal Skyline Test

The patient is relaxed in a prone position with the head straight and arms by the sides.[39] The examiner stands at the patient's feet and observes the buttocks from the level of the buttocks. The affected gluteus maximus muscle will be flat as a result of atrophy. The patient is asked to contract the gluteals. The affected side may show less contraction, or may be atonic and remain flat. If this occurs, the test is positive and may indicate damage to the inferior gluteal nerve or pressure on the L5, S1, and/or S2 nerve roots.

"Bowstring" Test (Cram Test or Popliteal Pressure Sign)

The examiner carries out a straight leg raise test and pain results (Fig. 8–29).[6, 40] The knee is slightly flexed (20°), reducing the symptoms; the thigh remains in the same position. Thumb or finger pressure is then applied to the popliteal area to re-establish the painful radicular symptoms. The test is an indication for tension or pressure on the sciatic nerve.

The Sitting Root Test

The patient sits with a flexed neck. The knee is actively extended while the hip remains flexed

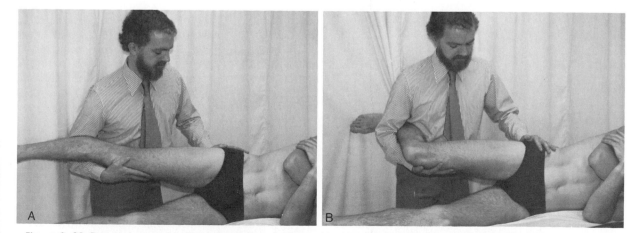

Figure 8–28. Femoral nerve traction test. (A) Step 1: Hip and knee extended. (B) Step 2: Hip extended and knee flexed.

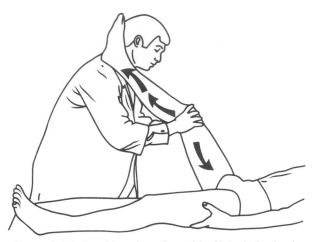

Figure 8–29. Bowstring sign. (From MacNab, I.: Backache. Baltimore, The Williams and Wilkins Co., 1977, p. 175.)

at 90°. Increased pain indicates tension on the sciatic nerve.

Sciatic Tension Test

The patient is instructed to sit with the back straight and with no twisting and is then told not to move but to support or brace himself with his arms.[41] The knee of the affected limb is passively extended to the point of pain, is lowered slightly below the point of pain, and is held clasped between the examiner's knees while the examiner presses the fingers of both hands into the popliteal space. Pain resulting from these maneuvers indicates a positive test and pressure or tension on the sciatic nerve. The test is similar to the Bowstring test.

Yeomans' Test

The patient lies prone while the examiner stabilizes the pelvis and extends each of the patient's hips in turn with the knees extended. The examiner then extends both of the patient's legs in turn with the knees flexed. In both cases, the patient remains passive. A positive test is indicated by pain in the lumbar spine during both parts of the test.

Flip Sign

While the patient is sitting, the examiner extends the patient's knee and looks for symptoms. The patient is then placed supine, and a unilateral straight leg test is performed. For the sign to be positive, both tests must cause pain in the sciatic nerve distribution. If only one test is positive, the examiner should be suspicious of problems in the lower lumbar spine. This is a combination of the classical Lasègue test and the sitting root test.

Sign of the Buttock

The patient lies supine,[17] and the examiner performs a passive unilateral straight leg test. If there is unilateral restriction, the examiner then flexes the knee to see whether hip flexion increases. If the problem is in the lumbar spine, hip flexion will increase. This finding indicates a negative sign of the buttock test. If hip flexion does not increase when the knee is flexed, it is a positive sign of the buttock test and indicates disease in the buttock, such as a bursitis, tumor, or abscess. The patient should also exhibit a noncapsular pattern of the hip.

REFLEXES AND CUTANEOUS DISTRIBUTION

Following the special tests, the following reflexes should be checked for differences between the two sides (Fig. 8–30):
1. Patellar (L3).
2. Achilles (S1).
3. Medial hamstrings (L5).
4. Lateral hamstrings (S1).

The deep tendon reflexes are tested with a reflex hammer, and the patient's muscles and tendons are relaxed. The patellar and Achilles reflexes may be done with the patient sitting or lying, and the hammer strikes the tendon directly. To test the patellar reflex, the knee should be flexed to 30° (supine lying) or 90° (sitting). For the Achilles reflex, the ankle should be at 90° or slightly dorsiflexed. To test the hamstrings reflex (semitendinosus and biceps femoris) the examiner places the thumb over the tendon and taps the thumbnail to elicit the reflex. Again, the knee should be slightly flexed to peform the test.

It is also important to check the dermatome patterns of the nerve roots as well as the peripheral sensory distribution of the peripheral nerves (Table 8–4 and Fig. 8–31). (It should be remembered that dermatomes will vary from person to person, and the accompanying representations are estimations only.) The examiner tests for sensation by running relaxed hands over the back, abdomen, and lower limbs, (front, sides, and back), being sure to cover all aspects of the leg and foot. If any difference is noted between the sides during this "sensation scan," the examiner may then use a pinwheel, pin, cotton ball and/or brush to map out the exact area of sensory difference to determine the nerve or nerve root affected.

One must remember that neurogenic intermittent claudication may cause the reflexes to be

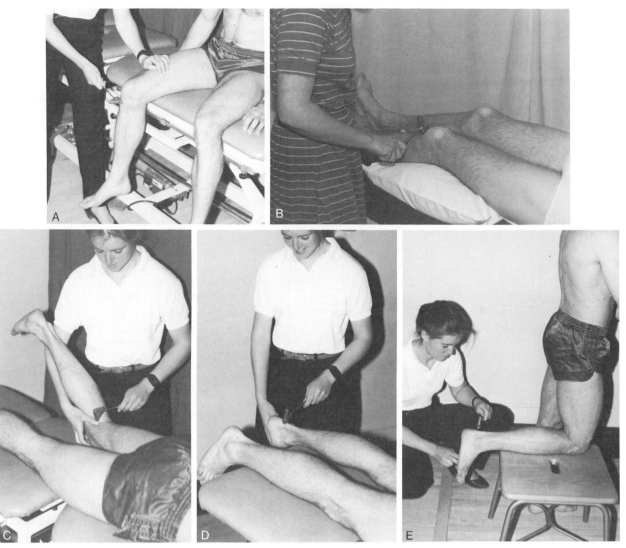

Figure 8–30. Reflexes of the lower limb. (*A*) Patellar (L3) in sitting position. (*B*) Patellar (L3) in lying position. (*C*) Medial hamstrings (L5) in prone lying position. (*D*) Achilles (S1) in prone position. (*E*) Achilles (S1) in kneeling position.

absent shortly after exercise (Table 8–5).[42, 43] If neurogenic intermittent claudication is suspected, it is necessary to do the reflexes immediately because reflexes may return within 1 to 3 minutes after stopping the activity.

Another reflex that may be tested is the *superficial cremasteric reflex,* which occurs in males only (Fig. 8–32). The patient lies supine while the examiner strokes the inner side of the upper thigh with a pointed object. The test is negative if the scrotal sac on the tested side pulls up. Absence or reduction of both superficial reflexes suggests an upper motor neuron lesion. A unilateral absence suggests a lower motor neuron lesion between L1 and L2. Absences have increased significance if they are associated with increased deep tendon reflexes.[44]

Two other superficial reflexes are the *superficial abdominal reflex* (Fig. 8–33) and the *superficial anal reflex.* To test the superficial abdominal reflex, the examiner, using a pointed object, strokes each quadrant of the abdomen of the supine patient in a triangular fashion around the umbilicus. Absence of the reflex indicates an upper motor neuron lesion, whereas unilateral absence indicates a lower motor neuron lesion from T7 to L2, depending on where the absence is noted as a result of the segmental innervation.

The examiner tests the superficial anal reflex by touching the perianal skin. A negative test is shown by contraction of the external and anal sphincter muscles (S2 to S4).

Finally, the examiner should perform one or more of the pathologic reflex tests used to determine upper motor lesions or pyramidal tract disease, such as the Babinski or Oppenheim test previously described. The presence of these reflexes indicates the possible presence of disease, whereas their absence reflects the normal situation.

Table 8–4. Peripheral Nerve Lesions*

Nerve (Root Derivation)	Sensory Supply	Sensory Loss	Motor Loss	Reflex Change	Lesion
Lateral cutaneous nerve of thigh (L2, 3)	Lateral thigh	Lateral thigh; often intermittent	None	None	Lateral inguinal entrapment
Posterior cutaneous nerve of thigh (S1, S2)	Posterior thigh	Posterior thigh	None (N.B. Sciatic nerve often involved, too)	None	Local (buttock) trauma Pelvic mass Hip fracture
Saphenous branch of femoral nerve (L2, 3, 4)	Anteromedial knee and medial leg	Medial leg	None (N.B. Positive Tinel sign 5–10 cm above medial femoral epicondyle of knee)	None	Local trauma Entrapment above medial epicondyle
Obturator nerve (L2, 3, 4)	Medial thigh	Often none ± medial thigh	Thigh adduction	None	Pelvic mass?
Femoral nerve (L2, 3, 4)	Anteromedial thigh and leg	Anteromedial thigh and leg	Knee extension ± hip flexion	Diminished knee jerk	Retroperitoneal or pelvic mass Femoral artery aneurysm (or puncture) Diabetic mononeuritis
Sciatic nerve (L4, 5; S1)	Anterior and posterior leg Sole and dorsum of foot	Entire foot	Foot dorsiflexion Foot inversion ± plantar flexion ± knee flexion	Diminished ankle jerk	Pelvic mass Hip fracture Pyriform entrapment Misplaced buttock injection
Peroneal nerve (division of sciatic)	Anterior leg, dorsum of foot	None or dorsal foot	Foot dorsiflexion, inversion, and eversion (N.B. Positive Tinel sign at lateral fibular neck)	None	Entrapment pressure at neck of fibula Rarely, diabetes, vasculitis, leprosy

*From Reilly, B. M.: Practical Strategies in Outpatient Medicine, Philadelphia, W. B. Saunders Co., 1984, p. 32.

Table 8–5. Differential Diagnosis of Intermittent Claudication

	Vascular	Neurogenic
Pain	Related to exercise; occurs at various sites simultaneously	Related to exercise; sensations spread from area to area
Pulse	Absent after exercise	Present after exercise
Protein content of cerebrospinal fluid	Normal	Raised
Sensory change	Variable	Follows more specific dermatomes

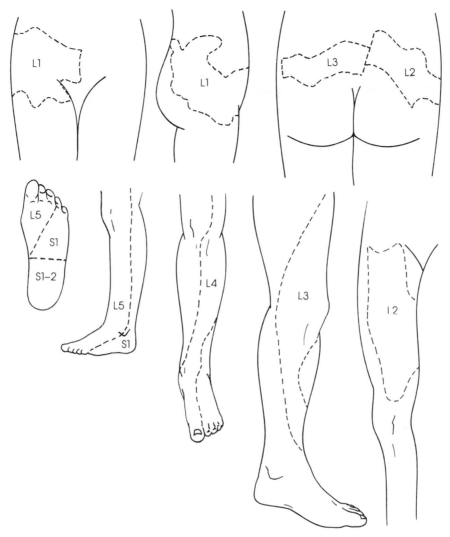

Figure 8–31. Lumbar dermatomes.

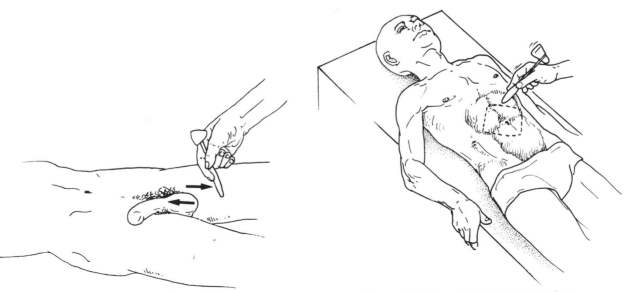

Figure 8–32. Cremasteric reflex.

Figure 8–33. Superficial abdominal reflex.

JOINT PLAY MOVEMENTS

The joint play movements take special importance in the lumbar spine because they are used to determine the end feel of joint movement as well as the presence of joint play. The following joint play movements should be performed, with any decreased range of motion, pain, or difference in end feel noted:

1. Flexion, extension, and side flexion.
2. Posteroanterior central vertebral pressures.
3. Posteroanterior unilateral vertebral pressures.
4. Transverse vertebral pressures.

Flexion, Extension, and Side Flexion

Flexion is accomplished with the patient in the side lying position. The examiner flexes both of the patient's hips to the chest with the knees bent. While palpating between the spinous processes

Figure 8–34. Joint play movements of the lumbar spine. (*A*) Flexion. (*B*) Posteroanterior central vertebral pressure. (*C*) Posteroanterior unilateral vertebral pressure. (*D*) Transverse vertebral pressure.

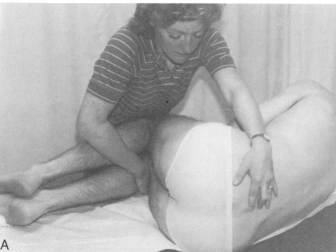

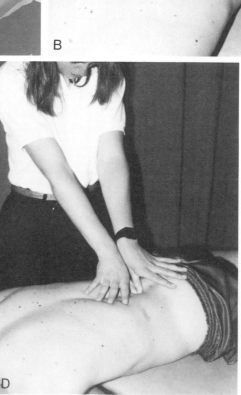

A

B

C

D

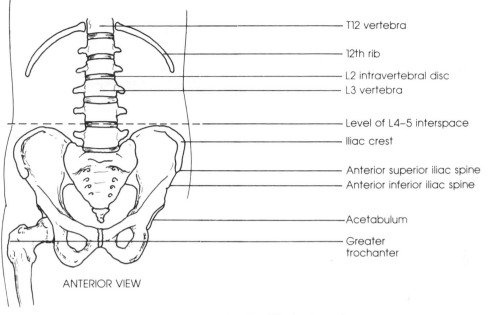

Figure 8–35. Bony landmarks of the lumbar spine.

of the lumbar vertebrae with one hand (one finger on spinous process, one finger above, and one finger below the process), the examiner passively flexes and releases the patient's hips; the examiner's body weight is used to cause the movement. The examiner should feel the spinous processes "gap" or move apart on flexion. If this gapping does not occur between two spinous processes or if it is excessive relative to the other gapping movements, the segent is either hypomobile or hypermobile, respectively.

Extension and *side flexion* are tested in a similar fashion, except that the movement is passive extension or passive side flexion rather than passive flexion.

Central, Unilateral, and Transverse Vertebral Pressures (PACVP, PAUVP, and TVP)

To perform the last three joint play movements, the patient lies prone.[45] The lumbar spinous processes are palpated beginning at L5 and working up to L1.

The examiner positions the hands, fingers, and thumbs as shown in Figure 8–34 to perform *posteroanterior central vertebral pressure.* Pressure is applied through the thumbs, with the vertebra being pushed anteriorly. The examiner must take care to apply the pressure slowly and carefully so that the "feel" of movement can be recognized. In reality, the movement is minimal. This "springing test" may be repeated several times to determine the quality of the movement.

To perform *posteroanterior unilateral vertebral pressure,* the examiner moves the fingers laterally away from the tip of the spinous process so the thumbs rest on the lamina or transverse process of the lumbar vertebra. The same anterior "springing" pressure is applied as in the central pressure technique. Both sides should be evaluated and compared.

To perform *transverse vertebral pressure,* the examiner's fingers are placed along the side of the spinous process of the lumbar spine (Fig. 8–34). The examiner then applies a transverse springing pressure to the side of the spinous process, feeling for the quality of movement. Pressure should be applied to both sides of the spinous process to compare the quality of movement.

PALPATION

If the examiner, having completed the scanning examination of the lumbar spine, decides that the problem is in another joint, palpation should be left until the joint is completely examined. However, when palpating the lumbar spine, any tenderness, altered temperature, muscle spasm, or other signs and symptoms that may indicate the source of pathology should be noted. If the problem is suspected to be in the lumbar spine area, palpation should be carried out in a systematic fashion, starting on the anterior aspect and working around to the posterior aspect.

Anterior Aspect

Anteriorly with the patient lying supine, the following structures are palpated (Fig. 8–35):

Umbilicus. The umbilicus lies at the level of

the L3-L4 disc space and is the point of intersection of the "lines" that divide the abdomen into quadrants. It is also the point at which the aorta divides into the common iliac arteries. With some individuals, the examiner may be able to palpate the anterior aspect of L4, L5, and S1 vertebrae along with the discs and anterior longitudinal ligament. The abdomen may also be carefully palpated for symptoms arising from internal organs. For example, the appendix is palpated in the right lower quadrant and the liver is palpated in the right upper quadrant; the kidneys are located in the left and right upper quadrants; and the spleen is found in the left upper quadrant.

Inguinal Area. The inguinal area is located between the anterior superior iliac spine (ASIS) and the symphysis pubis. Carefully, the examiner should palpate for symptoms of a hernia, abscess, infection (lymph nodes), or other pathologic condition in the area.

Iliac Crest. The examiner palpates the iliac crest from the anterior superior iliac spine posteriorly, looking for any symptoms (e.g., hip pointer or apophysitis).

Symphysis Pubis. The symphysis pubis is palpated with the examiner using both thumbs. Standing at the patient's side, the examiner pushes both thumbs down onto the symphysis pubis so that the thumbs rest on the superior aspect of the pubis bones (see Figure 9–4). In this way, one can ensure that the two pubic bones are level at the joint. The symphysis pubis may also be palpated for any tenderness (e.g., osteitis pubis).

Posterior Aspect

The patient is then asked to lie prone, and the following structures are palpated posteriorly (Fig. 8–36):

Spinous Process of the Lumbar Spine. The examiner palpates a point in the midline, which is on a line joining the high point of the two iliac crests. This point is the L4-L5 interspace. Moving down to the first hard mass, the fingers will rest on the spinous process of L5. Moving toward the head, the interspaces and spinous process of the remaining lumbar vertebrae can be palpated. In addition to looking for tenderness, muscle spasm, and other signs of pathology, the examiner should watch for signs of a spondylolisthesis, which is most likely to occur at L4-L5 or L5-S1. A visible or palpable dip from one spinous process to another may be evident, depending on the type of spondylolisthesis present. Absence of a spinous process may be seen in spina bifida. If the examiner moves laterally 2 to 3 cm from the spinous processes, the fingers will rest over the lumbar facet joints. These joints should also be palpated for signs of pathology. Because of the depth of these joints, the examiner may have difficulty palpating them. However, pathology in this area will result in spasm of the overlying paraspinal muscles, which should be palpated at the same time.

Sacrum, Sacral Hiatus, and Coccyx. If the examiner returns to the spinous process of L5 and moves caudally, the fingers will rest on the sacrum. Like the lumbar spine, the sacrum has spi-

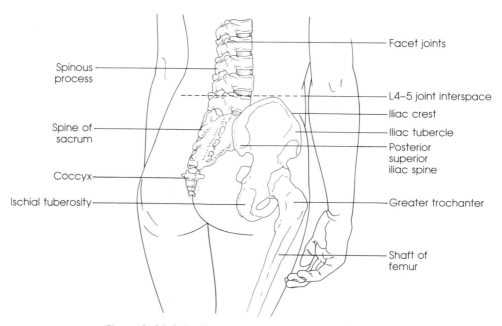

Figure 8–36. Palpation of the posterior lumbar spine.

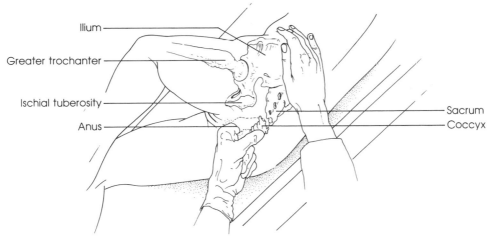

Ilium

Greater trochanter

Ischial tuberosity

Anus

Sacrum

Coccyx

Figure 8–37. Palpation of the coccyx.

nous processes, but they are much harder to distinguish because there is no interposing soft-tissue spaces between them. The S2 spinous process is at the level of a line joining the two posterior superior iliac spines ("posterior dimples"). Moving distally, the examiner's fingers may palpate the sacral hiatus, which is the caudal portion of the sacral canal. It has an inverted "U" shape and lies approximately 5 cm above the tip of the coccyx. The two bony prominences on either side of the hiatus are called the *sacral cornua* (see Figure 9–25). As the examiner's fingers move further distally, they will eventually rest on the posterior aspect of the coccyx. Proper palpation of the coccyx requires a rectal examination using a surgical rubber glove (Fig. 8–37). The index finger is lubricated and inserted into the anus while the patient's sphincter muscles are relaxed. The finger is inserted as far as possible and then rotated so that the pulpy surface rests against the anterior surface of the coccyx. The examiner then places the thumb of the same hand against the posterior aspect of the sacrum. In this way, the coccyx can be moved back and forth. Any major tenderness (e.g., coccydynia) should be noted.

Iliac Crest, Ischial Tuberosity, and Sciatic Nerve. Beginning at the posterior superior iliac spines, the examiner moves along the iliac crest, palpating for signs of pathology. Then, moving slightly distally, the examiner palpates the gluteal muscles for spasm, tenderness, or the presence of abnormal nodules. Just under the gluteal folds, the examiner should palpate the ischial tuberosities on both sides for any abnormality. As the examiner moves laterally, the greater trochanter of the femur is palpated. It is often easier to palpate if the hip is flexed to 90°. Palpating midway between the ischial tuberosity and the greater trochanter, the examiner may be able to

palpate the sciatic nerve. Deep to the gluteal muscles, the piriformis muscle should also be palpated for potential pathology. This muscle is in a line, dividing the posterior superior iliac spine of the pelvis/greater trochanter of the femur and the anterior superior iliac spine of the pelvis/ischial tuberosity of the pelvis.

RADIOLOGY OF THE LUMBAR SPINE [46–53]

Anteroposterior View. With this view (Fig. 8–38), the examiner should note the following:

1. Shape of the vertebrae.

2. Any wedging of the vertebrae, possibly from fracture (Fig. 8–39).

3. Disc spaces. Do they appear normal or are there height decreases, as is seen in spondylosis?

4. Any vertebral deformity, such as a hemivertebra or other anomalies (Figs. 8–40 and 8–41).

5. The presence of a bamboo spine, as seen in ankylosing spondylosis.

6. Any evidence of lumbarization of S1, in which case S1 becomes mobile, making the S1-2 the first mobile segment rather than L5-S1. Lumbarization is seen in 2 to 8 per cent of the population (Fig. 8–42).

7. Any evidence of sacralization of L5, in which case L5 becomes fused to the sacrum or pelvis, making the L4-5 level the first mobile segment rather than L5-S1. This anomaly is seen in 3 to 6 per cent of the population (Fig. 8–43).

8. Any evidence of spina bifida occulta, seen in 6 to 10 per cent of the population (Fig. 8–44).

Lateral View. With this view (Fig. 8–45), the examiner should note the following:

1. Any evidence of spondylolysis or spondylolisthesis, which is seen in 2 to 4 per cent of the

Text continued on page 208

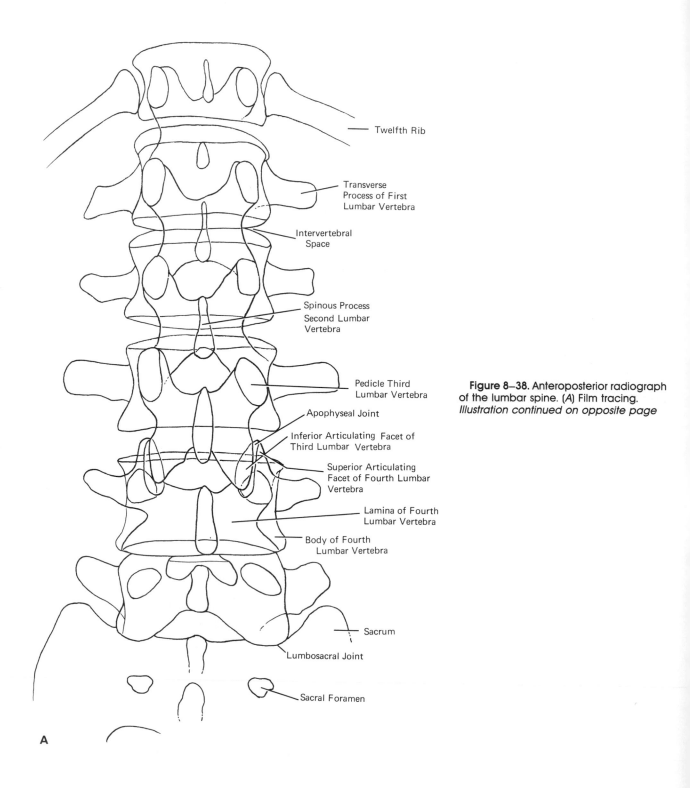

Twelfth Rib

Transverse Process of First Lumbar Vertebra

Intervertebral Space

Spinous Process Second Lumbar Vertebra

Pedicle Third Lumbar Vertebra

Apophyseal Joint

Inferior Articulating Facet of Third Lumbar Vertebra

Superior Articulating Facet of Fourth Lumbar Vertebra

Lamina of Fourth Lumbar Vertebra

Body of Fourth Lumbar Vertebra

Sacrum

Lumbosacral Joint

Sacral Foramen

A

Figure 8–38. Anteroposterior radiograph of the lumbar spine. (*A*) Film tracing. *Illustration continued on opposite page*

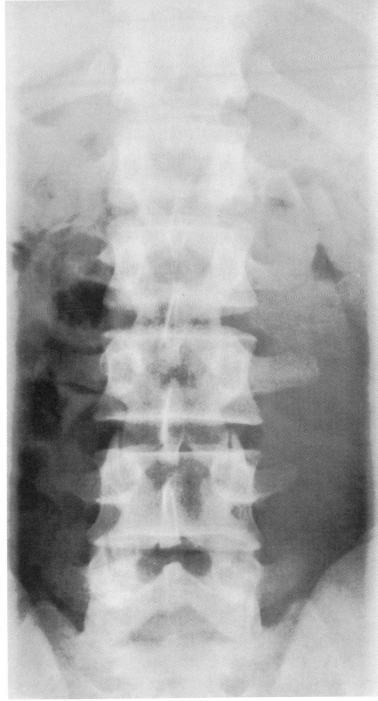

B

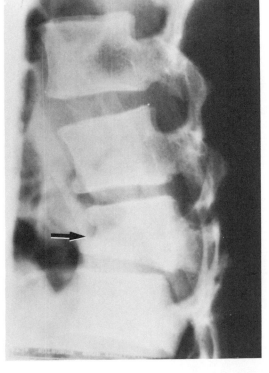

Figure 8–38 *Continued.* (*B*) Radiograph. (From Finneson, B. E.: Low Back Pain. Philadelphia, J. B. Lippincott, 1973, pp. 52–53.)

Figure 8–39. Wedging of a vertebral body.

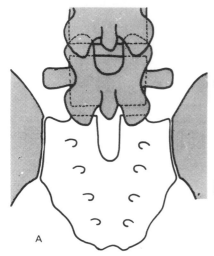

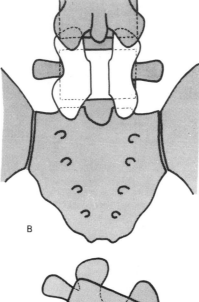

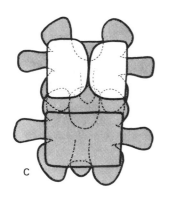

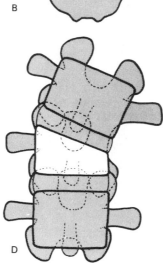

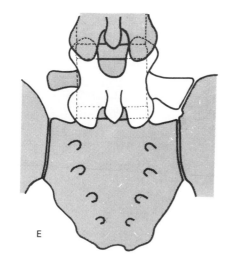

Figure 8–40. Diagrammatic representation of the x-ray appearance of common anatomic anomalies in the lumbosacral spine. (*A*) Spina bifida occulta, S1. (*B*) Spina bifida, L5. (*C*) Anterior spina bifida ("butterfly vertebra"). (*D*) Hemivertebra. (*E*) Iliotransverse joint.

Illustration continued on opposite page

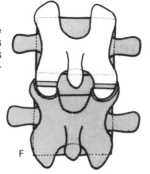
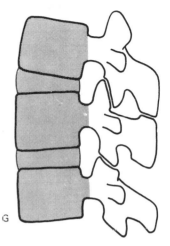

Figure 8–40 *Continued.* (*F*) Ossicles of Oppenheimer. These are free ossicles seen at the tip of the inferior articular facets and are usually found at the level of L3. (*G*) "Kissing" spinous processes. (From MacNab, I.: Backache. Baltimore, The Williams and Wilkins Co., 1977, pp. 14–15.)

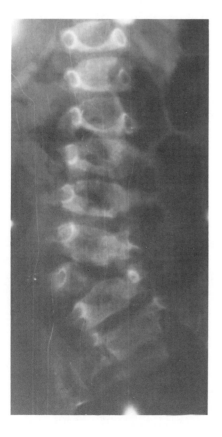

Figure 8–41. Hemivertebra shown on an anteroposterior radiograph.

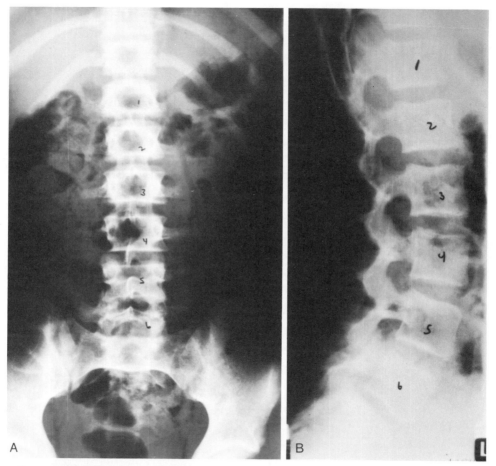

Figure 8–42. Lumbarization of the S1 vertebra seen on anteroposterior (*A*) and lateral (*B*) radiographs.

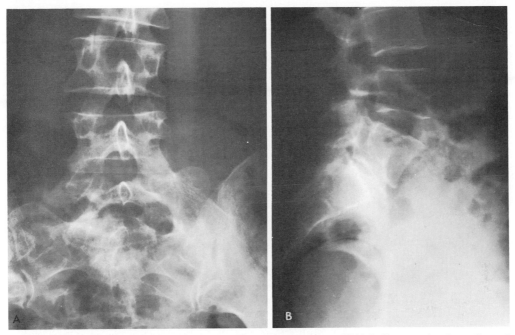

Figure 8–43. Unilateral sacralization of the fifth lumbar vertebra. (*A*) Note the massive formation of sacral ala on the left side with relatively normal transverse process on the right (anteroposterior view). (*B*) Lateral view showing the very narrow disc space and the massive arches. (From O'Donoghue, D. H.: Treatment of Injuries to Athletes, 4th ed. Philadelphia, W. B. Saunders Co., 1984, p. 403.)

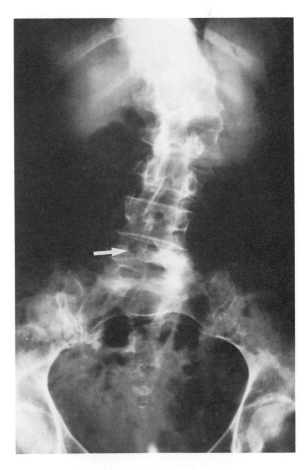

Figure 8–44. Spina bifida occulta, anteroposterior view.

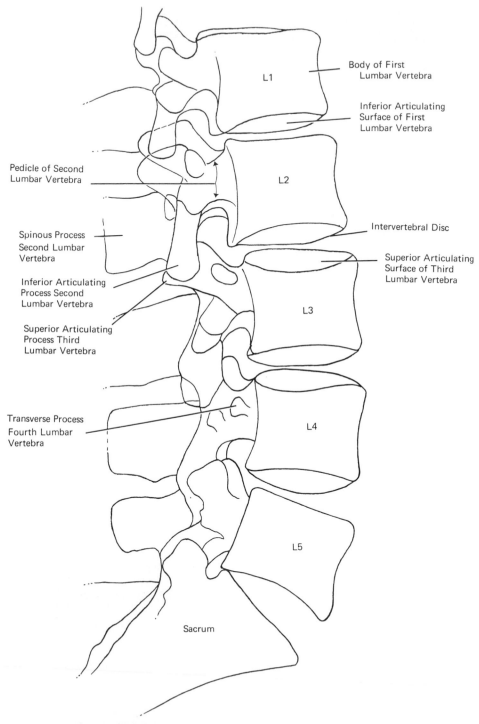

Body of First
Lumbar Vertebra

Inferior Articulating
Surface of First
Lumbar Vertebra

Pedicle of Second
Lumbar Vertebra

Intervertebral Disc

Spinous Process
Second Lumbar
Vertebra

Superior Articulating
Surface of Third
Lumbar Vertebra

Inferior Articulating
Process Second
Lumbar Vertebra

Superior Articulating
Process Third
Lumbar Vertebra

Transverse Process
Fourth Lumbar
Vertebra

Sacrum

L1

L2

L3

L4

L5

Figure 8–45. Lateral radiograph of the lumbar spine. (A) Film tracing.
Illustration continued on opposite page

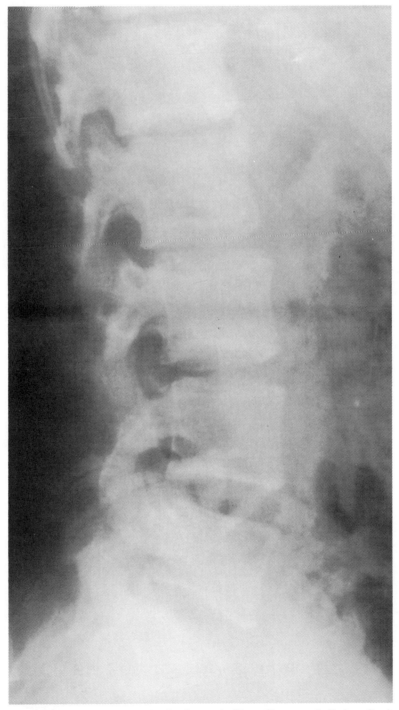

Figure 8–45 *Continued.* (*B*) Radiograph. (From Finneson, B. E.: Low Back Pain. Philadelphia, J. B. Lippincott, 1973, pp. 54, 55.)

population (Fig. 8–46). The degree of slipping can be graded as shown in Figure 8–47.

2. A normal lordosis.

3. Any wedging of the vertebrae.

4. Normal disc spacing.

5. Any osteophyte formation or traction spurs (Fig. 8–48).[53] Traction spurs indicate an unstable lumbar intervertebral segment. A traction spur occurs approximately 1 mm away from the disc border; an osteophyte occurs at the discal border with the vertebral body.

Oblique View. With the oblique view (Fig. 8–49), the examiner should look for any evidence of spondylolisthesis (sometimes referred to as a "Scotty dog decapitated") or spondylolysis (sometimes referred to as a "Scotty dog with a collar") (Fig. 8–50).

Myelogram. A myelogram can confirm the presence of a protruding intervertebral disc, a tumor, or spinal stenosis (Figs. 8–51 through 8–53). The examiner must be careful of the side effects of myelograms, which include headache, stiffness, low back pain, cramps, or paresthesia in the lower limbs. Although side effects do occur, no permanent injury has ever been noted.

Computed Tomography. A computed tomographic (CT) scan may be used to delineate a fracture or to show the presence of spinal stenosis, caused by protrusion or a tumor (Figs. 8–54 and 8–55).

Text continued on page 216

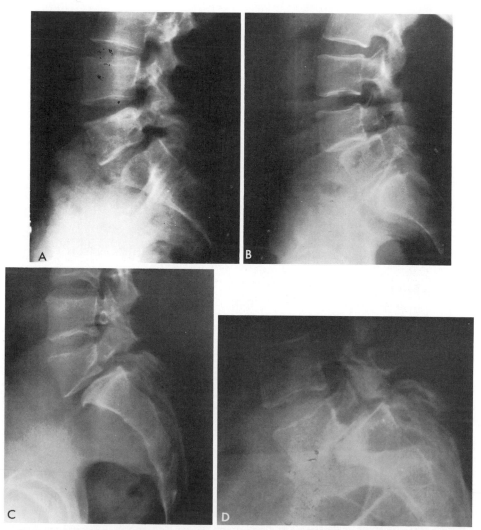

Figure 8–46. Spondylolisthesis. (*A*) Grade 1. The arch defect in L-5 with mild forward displacement of L-5 on S-1. Backache but no gross disability. (*B*) Grade II. Note more forward slipping between L-4 and L-5 with collapse of the intervertebral disc. Definite symptomatic back with restriction of motion, muscle spasm, and curtailment of activities. (*C*) Grade III. More extensive slipping combined with a wide separation at the arch defect, and degenerative changes of the disc. Grossly symptomatic. (*D*) Grade IV. Vertebra slipped forward over halfway. Severe disability. (From O'Donoghue, D. H.: Treatment of Injuries to Athletes, 4th ed. Philadelphia, W. B. Saunders Co., 1984, p. 402.)

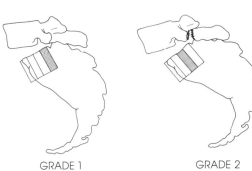
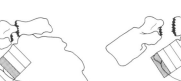
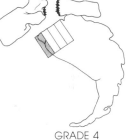

NORMAL   GRADE 1   GRADE 2

Figure 8–47. Meyerding grading system for slipping in spondylolisthesis.

GRADE 3   GRADE 4

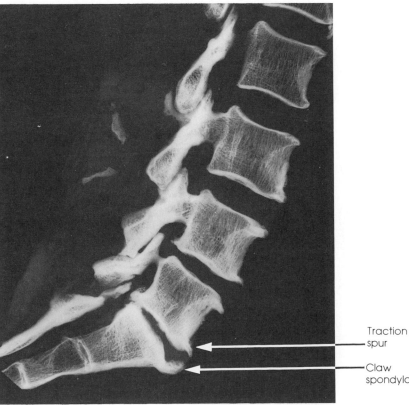

Traction spur

Claw spondylophyte

Figure 8–48. Lateral radiograph of a thin-slice pathologic section of lumbar spine. Note traction spur and claw spondylophyte. (From Rothman, R. H., and F. A. Simeone: The Spine. Philadelphia, W. B. Saunders Co., 1982, p. 512.)

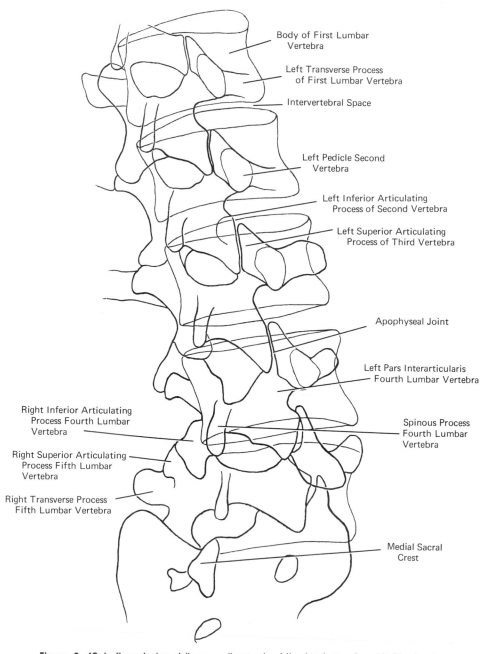

Figure 8–49. Left posterior oblique radiograph of the lumbar spine. (*A*) Film tracing.
Illustration continued on opposite page

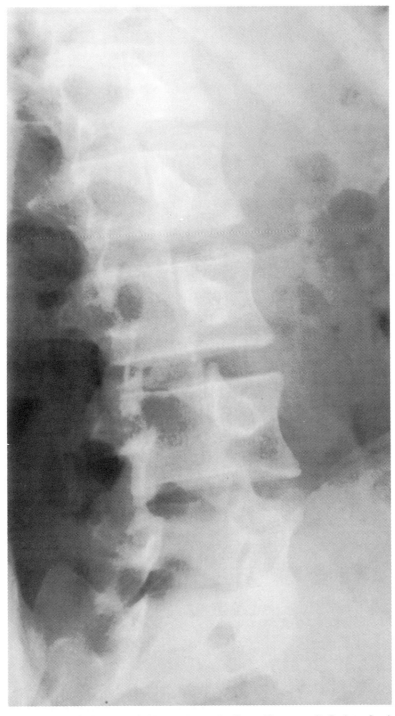

Figure 8–49 *Continued.* (*B*) Radiograph. (From Finneson, B. E.: Low Back Pain. Philadelphia, J. B. Lippincott, 1973, pp. 56, 57.)

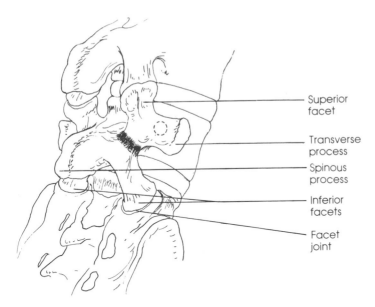

Superior
facet

Transverse
process

Spinous
process

Inferior
facets

Facet
joint

A SPONDYLOLYSIS
"Scotty dog with collar"

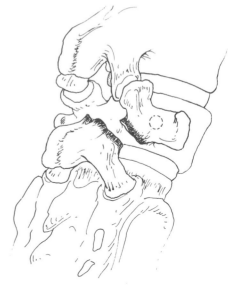

SPONDYLOLISTHESIS
"Scotty dog decapitated"

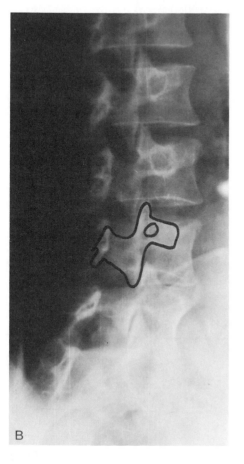

B

Figure 8–50. (*A*) Diagrammatic representation (posterior oblique view) illustrating spondylolysis and spondylolisthesis. (*B*) Posterior oblique film showing "Scotty dog."

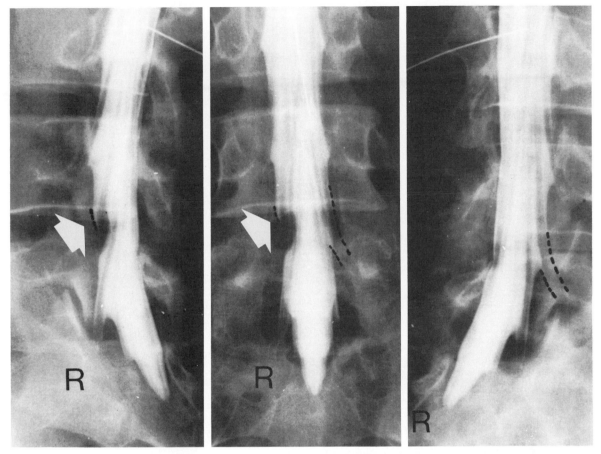

Figure 8–51. Metrizamide myelogram illustrating herniated disc at L4-5 on the right. Note amputation of the nerve root sleeve and indentation of the dural sac. (From Rothman, R. H., and F. A. Simeone. The Spine. Philadelphia, W. B. Saunders Co., 1982, p. 550.)

Figure 8–52. Oil myelograms show the characteristic appearance of chronic disc degeneration and spinal stenosis with diffuse posterior bulging of the annulus and osteophyte formation. (A) There is symmetric wasting of the dye column in the anteroposterior view. Note the hour-glass configuration. (B) Indentation of the dye column of the annulus anteriorly and the buckled ligamentum flavum and facet joints posteriorly (lateral view). (From Rothman, R. H., and F. A. Simeone: The Spine. Philadelphia, W. B. Saunders Co., 1982, p. 553.)

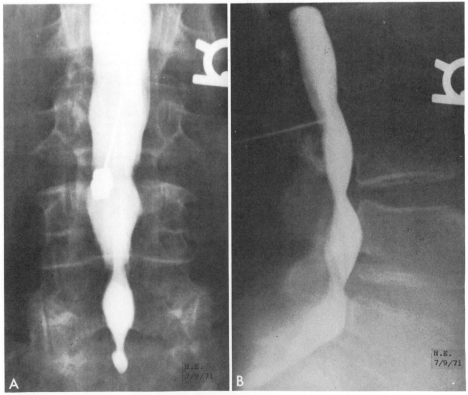

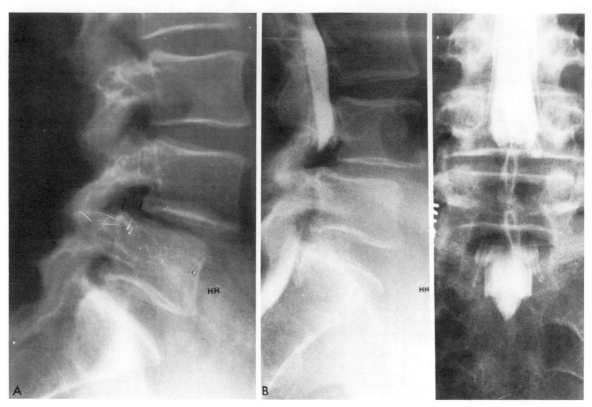

Figure 8–53. Metrizamide myelogram shows stenotic block at the L4-5 level as a result of degenerative spondylolisthesis and spinal stenosis at the L4-5 level. (*A*) Note the 4-mm anterior migration of L4 on L5 caused by the degenerative spondylolisthesis. (*B*) The extensive block on the myelogram is due to spinal stenosis. (From Rothman, R. H., and F. A. Simeone: The Spine. Philadelphia, W. B. Saunders Co., 1982, p. 553.)

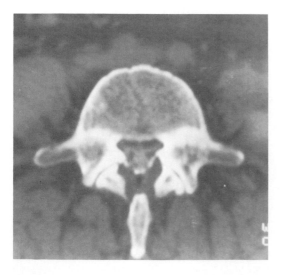

Figure 8–54. CT scan showing facet joints.

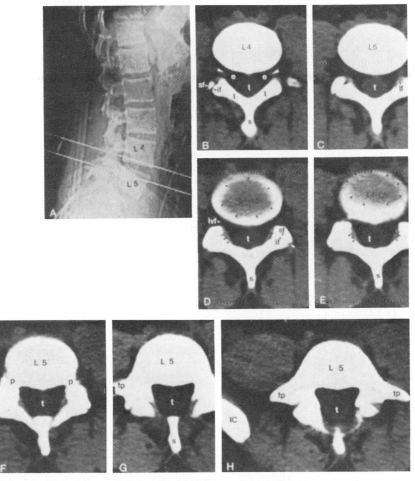

Figure 8–55. Soft tissue detail of the L4-L5 intervertebral disc space.

(*A*) Lateral digital scout view obtained through the lumbosacral spine. The upper and lower scan limits through L4-L5 region are designated with an electronic cursor. Scan collimation is 5 mm thick; incrementation is 3 mm (2 mm overlap).

(*B*) Axial CT section of L4. The L4 root ganglia and spinal nerves are seen within the intervertebral foramina (*white arrowheads*) surrounded by abundant epidural fat (e). The thecal sac (t) is bounded anterolaterally by fat in the lateral recess. The posterior arch of L4 consists of inferior facets (if), laminae (l), and spinous process (s). The superior facet of L5 (sf) is just visible.

(*C*) The next-lower axial section demonstrates the L4-L5 facet articulations. The ligamentum flavum (lf) is contiguous with the facet joint capsule. Again, the thecal sac (t) is readily apparent; it is slightly higher in density than the adjacent epidural fat. Note that without subarachnoid contrast media the intrathecal contents cannot be discerned.

(*D*) Axial CT section at the L4-L5 disk space. The disk (*multiple black arrowheads*) is a region of central hypodensity surrounded by the cortical margin of L4. The posterior arch of L4 projects below the disc level. The intervertebral foramina (ivf) have begun to close. The cartilaginous articular surfaces (*white arrowhead*) between superior (sf) and inferior (if) facets are poorly demonstrated with these window settings. The ligamentum flavum (*double black arrowheads*) is noted medial to the facet joints (t = thecal sac; s = spinous process.)

(*E*) The next inferior CT section demonstrates the disc (*multiple arrowheads*) positioned somewhat more anteriorly, marginated posteriorly at this level by the posterosuperior cortical rim of the L5 body. The ligamentum flavum (*double arrowheads*) normally maintains a flat medial surface adjacent to the thecal sac (t). The posterior arch of L4 and its spinous process (s) are still in view.

(*F*) Axial CT section through the L5 body at the level of the pedicles (p). The canal now completely encloses the thecal sac (t).

(*G*) Immediately below, only the spinous process (s) of the posterior arch of L4 is visible. The transverse process (tp) of L5 is noted. (t = thecal sac.)

(*H*) At the level of the iliac crest (IC), the posterior arch of L5 (*small arrowheads*) has just begun to form. The transverse process (tp) are quite large at this level. (t = thecal sac.)

(From Le Masters, D. L., and R. L. Dowart: High-resolution, cross-sectional computed tomography of the normal spine. Orthop. Clin. North Am. *16*:359, 1985.)

Précis of the Lumbar Spine Assessment*

History (sitting)
Observation (standing)
Examination
  Active movements (standing)
    Forward flexion
    Extension
    Side flexion (left and right)
    Rotation (left and right)
    Quick test
    Trendelenburg and S1 nerve root test
  Passive movements (only with care and caution)
  Peripheral joint scan (standing)
    Sacroiliac joints
  Resisted isometric movements (sitting)
    Forward flexion
    Extension
    Side flexion (left and right)
    Rotation (left and right)
  Peripheral joint scan (supine lying)
    Hip joints (flexion, extension, abduction, adduction, and medial and lateral rotation)
    Knee joints (flexion and extension)
    Ankle joints (dorsiflexion and plantar flexion)
    Foot joints (supination, pronation)
    Toe joints (flexion, extension)
  Myotomes (supine lying)
    Hip flexion (L2)
    Knee extension (L3)
    Ankle dorsiflexion (L4)
    Toe extension (L5)
    Ankle eversion and/or plantar flexion (S1)
  Special tests (supine lying)
  Reflexes and cutaneous distribution (anterior and side aspects)
  Palpation (supine lying)
  Joint play movements
    Flexion (side lying)
    Posteroanterior central vertebral pressure (prone lying)
    Posteroanterior unilateral vertebral pressure (prone lying)
    Transverse vertebral pressure (prone lying)
  Myotomes (prone lying)
    Hip extension (S1)
    Knee flexion (S1, S2)
  Special tests (prone lying)
  Reflexes and cutaneous distribution (prone lying) (posterior aspect)
  Palpation (prone lying)
  X-ray viewing

Following any examination, the patient should always be warned of the possibility of exacerbation of symptoms as a result of the assessment.

---

*This précis shows an order that will limit the amount of movement that the patient has to do but that will ensure that all necessary structures are tested.

REFERENCES

CITED REFERENCES

1. Kramer, J.: Intervertebral Disk Diseases: Causes, Diagnosis, Treatment and Prophylaxis. Chicago, Year Book Medical Publishers, 1981.
2. Farfan, H. F.: Mechanical Disorders of the Low Back. Philadelphia, Lea & Febiger, 1973.
3. Coventry, M. B., R. K. Ghormley, and J. W. Kernohan: The intervertebral disc: Its microscopic anatomy and pathology. Part I—anatomy, development and physiology; Part II—changes in the intervertebral disc concomitant with age; Part III—pathological changes in the intervertebral disc. J. Bone Joint Surg. 27:105 (Part I), 233 (Part II), 460 (Part III), 1945.
4. Bogduk, N.: The innervation of the lumbar spine. Spine 8:286, 1983.
5. Edgar, M. A., and J. A. Ghadially: Innervation of the lumbar spine. Clin. Orthop. Relat. Res. 115:35, 1976.
6. Macnab, I.: Backache. Baltimore, The Williams and Wilkins Co., 1977.
7. Nachemson, A., and J. M. Morris: In vivo measurements of intradiscal pressure. J. Bone Joint Surg. 46A:1077, 1964.
8. Nachemson, A., and C. Elfstrom: Intravital dynamic pressure measurements in lumbar discs. Scand. J. Rehabil. Med. (Suppl. 1), 1970.
9. McKenzie, R. A.: The Lumbar Spine: Mechanical Diagnosis and Therapy. Waikanae, New Zealand, Spinal Publications Ltd., 1981.
10. Stoddard, A.: Manual of Osteopathic Practice. New York, Harper & Row, 1970.
11. Matson, D. D., R. P. Woods, J. B. Campbell, and F. D. Ingraham: Diastematomyelia (congenital clefts of the spinal cord). Pediatrics 6:98, 1950.
12. Allbrook, D.: Movements of the lumbar spinal column. J. Bone Joint Surg. 39B:339, 1957.
13. Moll, J. M. H., and V. Wright: Normal range of spinal mobility: An objective clinical study. Ann. Rheum. Dis. 30:381, 1971.
14. Moll, J., and V. Wright: Measurement of spinal movement. In Jayson, M. (ed.): The Lumbar Spine and Back Pain. New York, Grune & Stratton, Inc., 1976.
15. Pennal, G. F., G. S. Conn, G. McDonald, et al.: Motion studies of the lumbar spine. J. Bone Joint Surg. 54B:442, 1972.
16. Tanz, S. S.: Motion of the lumbar spine: A roentgenologic study. Am. J. Roentgenol. 69:399, 1953.
17. Cyriax, J.: Textbook for Orthopaedic Medicine, vol. I: Diagnosis of Soft Tissue Lesions. London, Bailliere Tindall, 1975.
18. Breig, A., and J. D. G. Troup: Biomechanical considerations in straight-leg-raising test: Cadaveric and clinical studies of the effects of medical hip rotation. Spine 4:242, 1979.
19. Charnley, J.: Orthopedic signs in the diagnosis of disc protrusion with special reference to the straight-leg-raising test. Lancet 1:156, 1951.
20. Edgar, M. A., and W. M. Park: Induced pain patterns on passive straight-leg-raising in lower lumbar disc protrusion. J. Bone Joint Surg. 56B:658, 1974.
21. Fahrni, W. H.: Observations on straight-leg-raising with special reference to nerve root adhesions. Can. J. Surg. 9:44, 1966.
22. Goddard, B. S., and J. D. Reid: Movements induced by straight-leg-raising in the lumbo-sacral roots, nerves, and plexus and in the intrapelvic section of the sciatic nerve. J. Neurol. Neurosurg. Psychiatry 28:12, 1965.
23. Scham, S. M., and T. K. F. Taylor: Tension signs in lumbar disc prolapse. Clin. Orthop. Relat. Res. 75:195, 1971.

24. Urban, L. M.: The straight-leg-raising test: A review. J. Orthop. Sports Phys. Ther. 2:117, 1981.
25. Wilkins, R. H., and I. A. Brody: Lasègue's sign. Arch. Neurol. 21:219, 1969.
26. Wartenberg, R.: The signs of Brudzinski and of Kernig. J. Pediatr. 37:679, 1950.
27. Hudgins, W. R.: The crossed-straight-leg-raising test. N. Engl. J. Med. 297:1127, 1977.
28. Woodhall, R., and G. J. Hayes: The well-leg-raising test of Fajersztajn in the diagnosis of ruptured lumbar intervertebral disc. J. Bone Joint Surg. 32A:786, 1950.
29. Herron, L. D., and H. C. Pheasant: Prone knee–flexion provocative testing for lumbar disc protrusion. Spine 5:65, 1980.
30. Dommisse, G. F., and L. Grobler: Arteries and veins of the lumbar nerve roots and cauda equina. Clin. Orthop. Relat. Res. 115:22, 1976.
31. Archibald, K. C., and F. Wiechec: A reappraisal of Hoover's test. Arch. Phys. Med. Rehabil. 51:234, 1970.
32. Arieff, A. J., E. I. Tigay, J. F. Kurtz, and W. A. Larmon: The Hoover sign: An objective sign of pain and/or weakness in the back or lower extremities. Arch. Neurol. 5:673, 1961.
33. Hoover, C. F.: A new sign for the detection of malingering and functional paresis of the lower extremities. J.A.M.A. 51:746, 1908.
34. Brody, I. A., and R. H. Williams: The signs of Kernig and Brudzinski. Arch. Neurol. 21:215, 1969.
35. Brudzinski, J.: A new sign of the lower extremities in meningitis of children (neck sign). Arch. Neurol. 21:217, 1969.
36. Kernig, W.: Concerning a little noted sign of meningitis. Arch. Neurol. 21:216, 1969.
37. Dyck, P.: The femoral nerve traction test with lumbar disc protrusion. Surg. Neurol. 6:163, 1976.
38. Dyck, P.: The stoop-test in lumbar entrapment radiculopathy. Spine 4:89, 1979.
39. Katznelson, A., J. Nerubay, and A. Level: Gluteal skyline (G. S. L.): A search for an objective sign in the diagnosis of disc lesions of the lower lumbar spine. Spine 7:74, 1982.
40. Cram, R. H.: A sign of sciatic nerve root pressure. J. Bone Joint Surg. 35B:192, 1953.
41. Deyerle, W. M., and V. R. May: Sciatic tension test. South. Med. J. 49:999, 1956.
42. Dyck, P., H. C. Pheasant, J. B. Doyle, and J. J. Reider: Intermittent cauda equina compression syndrome. Spine 2:75, 1977.
43. Joffe, R., A. Appleby, and V. Arjona: Intermittent ischemia of the cauda equina due to stenosis of the lumbar canal. J. Neurol. Neurosurg. Psychiatry 29:315, 1966.
44. Hoppenfeld, S.: Physical Examination of the Spine and Extremities. New York, Appleton-Century-Crofts, 1976.
45. Maitland, G. D.: Examination of the lumbar spine. Aust. J. Phys. Ther. 17:5, 1971.
46. Fullenlove, T. M., and A. J. Williams: Comparative roentgen findings in symptomatic and asymptomatic back. Radiology 68:572, 1957.
47. Gillespie, H. W.: The significance of congenital lumbosacral abnormalities. Br. J. Radiol. 22:270, 1949.
48. Magora, A., and A. Schwartz: Relation between the low back pain syndrome and x-ray findings. Scand. J. Rehabil. Med. 10:135, 1978.
49. Southworth, J. D., and S. R. Bersack: Anomalies of the lumbosacral vertebrae in five hundred and fifty individuals without symptoms referable to the low back. Am. J. Roentgenol. 64:624, 1950.
50. Tulsi, R. S.: Sacral arch defect and low backache. Australas. Radiol. 18:43, 1974.
51. Willis, T. A.: An analysis of vertebral anomalies. Am. J. Surg. 6:163, 1929.
52. Willis, T. A.: Lumbosacral anomalies. J. Bone Joint Surg. 41A:935, 1959.
53. Macnab, I.: The traction spur: An indicator of segmental instability. J. Bone Joint Surg. 53A:663, 1971.

GENERAL REFERENCES

Adams, M. A., and W. C. Hutton: The mechanical function of the lumbar apophyseal joints. Spine 8:327, 1983.
Anderson, B. J. G., R. Ortengen, A. L. Nachemson, et al.: The sitting posture: An electromyographic and discometric study. Orthop. Clin. North Am. 6:105, 1975.
Brown, M. D.: Diagnosis of pain syndromes of the spine. Orthop. Clin. North Am. 6:233, 1975.
Carmichael, S. W., and S. L. Buckart: Clinical anatomy of the lumbosacral complex. Phys. Ther. 59:966, 1979.
Chadwick, P. R.: Examination, assessment and treatment of the lumbar spine. Physiotherapy 70:2, 1984.
Crock, H. V.: Normal and pathological anatomy of the lumbar spinal nerve root canals. J. Bone Joint Surg. 63B:487, 1981.
Crock, H. V., and H. Yoshizawa: The blood supply of the lumbar vertebral column. Clin. Orthop. Relat. Res. 115:6, 1976.
Crouch, J. E.: Functional Human Anatomy. Philadelphia, Lea & Febiger, 1972.
Crow, N. E.: The "normal" lumbosacral spine. Radiology 72:97, 1959.
Cyriax, J.: Examination of the spinal column. Physiotherapy 56:206, 1970.
Davies, E. M.: Backache and its treatment by active exercise. Physiotherapy 49:81, 1963.
Davis, P. R.: The mechanics and movements of the back in working situations. Physiotherapy 53:44, 1967.
Dixon, A. St.: Diagnosis of low back pain: Sorting the complainers. In Jayson, M. (ed.): The Lumbar Spine and Back Pain. New York, Grune & Stratton, Inc., 1976.
Dohrmann, G. J., and W. J. Nowack: The upgoing great toe. Optimal method of elicitation. Lancet 1:339, 1973.
Dommisse, G. F., and L. Grobler: Arteries and veins of the nerve roots and cauda equina. Clin. Orthop. Relat. Res. 115:22, 1976.
Edgelow, P. I.: Physical examination of the lumbosacral complex. Phys. Ther. 59:974, 1979.
Finneson, B. E.: Low Back Pain. 2nd ed. Philadelphia, J. B. Lippincott Co., 1981.
Floman, Y., S. W. Wiesel, and R. H. Rothman: Cauda equina syndrome presenting as a herniated lumbar disc. Clin. Orthop. Relat. Res. 147:234, 1980.
Forst, J. J.: Contribution to the clinical study of sciatica. Arch. Neurol. 21:220, 1969.
Friberg, O.: Clinical symptoms and biomechanics of lumbar spine and hip joint in leg length inequality. Spine 8:643, 1983.
Gartland, J. J.: Fundamentals of Orthopedics. Philadelphia, W. B. Saunders Co., 1979.
Golub, B. S., and B. Silverman: Transforaminal ligaments of the lumbar spine. J. Bone Joint Surg. 51A:947, 1969.
Grieve, G. P.: Common Vertebral Joint Problems. New York, Churchill Livingstone, 1981.
Grieve, G. P.: Mobilization of the Spine. New York, Churchill Livingstone, 1979.
Gutrecht, J. A., P. A. Espinosa, and P. J. Dyck: Early descriptions of common neurologic signs. Mayo Clin. Proc. 43:807, 1968.
Hall, G. W.: Neurologic signs and their discoveries. J.A.M.A. 95:703, 1930.
Helfet, A. J., and Lee, D. M.: Disorders of the Lumbar Spine. Philadelphia, J. B. Lippincott Co., 1978.
Hirsch, C., R. O. Ingelmark, and M. Miller: The anatomical bases for low back pain. Acta Orthop. Scand. 33:1–17, 1963.

Hollinshead, W. H., and D. B. Jenkins: Functional Anatomy of the Limbs and Back. Philadelphia, W. B. Saunders Co., 1981.

Jackson, H. C., R. K. Winkelmann, and W. H. Bickel: Nerve endings in the human lumbar spinal column and related strucures. J. Bone Joint Surg. 48A:1272, 1966.

Jayson, M.: The Lumbar Spine and Back Pain. New York, Grune & Stratton, 1976.

Jensen, G. M.: Biomechanics of the lumbar intervertebral disk: A review. Phys. Ther. 60:765, 1980.

Jonck, L. M.: The mechanical disturbances resulting from lumbar disc space narrowing. J. Bone Joint Surg. 43:362, 1961.

Kapandji, L. A.: The Physiology of Joints, vol. 3: The Trunk and Vertebral Column. New York, Churchill Livingstone, 1974.

Keim, H. A.: Low back pain. Clin. Symp. 26:2, 1974.

Keim, H. A.: The Adolescent Spine. New York, Springer-Verlag, 1982.

Kirkaldy-Willis, W. H.: Diagnosis and treatment of lumbar spinal stenosis. American Academy of Orthopedic Surgeons Symposium on the Lumbar Spine. St. Louis, C. V. Mosby Co., 1976.

Kirkaldy-Willis, W. H.: Managing Low Back Pain. New York, Churchill Livingstone, 1983.

Kirkaldy-Willis, W. H.: The relationship of structural pathology to the nerve root. Spine 9:49, 1984.

Koreska, J., D. Robertson, R. H. Mills, D. A. Gibson, and A. M. Albisser: Biomechanics of the lumbar spine and its clinical significance. Orthop. Clin. North Am. 8:121, 1977.

Lamb, D. W.: The neurology of spinal pain. Phys. Ther. 59:971, 1979.

Lucas, D. B.: Mechanics of the spine. Hospital for Joint Diseases (New York Bulletin) 31:115, 1970.

Maigne, R.: Orthopaedic Medicine: A New Approach to Vertebral Manipulation. Springfield, Ill., Charles C Thomas, 1972.

McRae, R.: Clinical Orthopaedic Examination. New York, Churchill Livingstone, 1976.

Mitchell, F. L., P. S. Moran, and N. A. Pruzzo: An Evaluation and Treatment Manual of Osteopathic Muscle Energy Procedures. Valley Park, Mo., Mitchell, Moran and Pruzzo, 1979.

Morris, J. M.: Biomechanics of the spine. Arch. Surg. 107:418, 1973.

Murphy, R. W.: Nerve roots and spinal nerves in degenerative disc disease. Clin. Orthop. Relat. Res. 129:46, 1977.

Nachemson, A.: Towards a better understanding of low back pain: A review of the mechanics of the lumbar disc. Rheumatol. Rehabil. 14:129, 1975.

O'Donoghue, D. H.: Treatment of Injuries to Athletes, 4th ed. Philadelphia, W. B. Saunders Co., 1984.

Paris, S. V.: Anatomy as related to function and pain. Orthop. Clin. North Am. 14:475, 1983.

Ramsey, R. H.: The anatomy of the ligamentum flava. Clin. Orthop. Relat. Res. 44:129, 1966.

Reilly, B. M.: Practical Strategies in Outpatient Medicine. Philadelphia, W. B. Saunders Co., 1984.

Rose, K., and P. Balasubramaniam: Nerve root canals in the lumbar spine. Spine 9:16, 1984.

Rothman, R. H., and F. A. Simeone: The Spine. Philadephia, W. B. Saunders Co., 1982.

Rydevik, B., M. D. Brown, and G. Lundberg: Pathoanatomy and pathophysiology of nerve root compression. Spine 9:7, 1984.

Seimen, L. P.: Low Back Pain: Clinical Diagnosis and Management. Norwalk, Conn., Appleton-Century-Crofts, 1983.

Selby, D. K.: When to operate and what to operate on. Orthop. Clin. North Am. 14:577, 1983.

Snook, S. H.: Low back pain in industry. American Academy of Orthopaedic Surgeons Symposium on Idiopathic Low Back Pain, pp. 23–38, St. Louis, C. V. Mosby Co., 1982.

Tachdjian, M. O.: Pediatric Orthopedics. Philadelphia, W. B. Saunders Co., 1972.

White, A. A., and M. M. Panjabi: Clinical Biomechanics of the Spine. Philadelphia, J. B. Lippincott Co., 1978.

Wiesel, S. W., P. Bernini, and R. H. Rothman: The Aging Lumbar Spine. Philadelphia, W. B. Saunders Co., 1982.

Williams, P. L., and Warwick, R. (eds.): Gray: Anatomy, 36th British ed. Philadelphia, W. B. Saunders Co., 1980.

Yong-Hing, K., and W. H. Kirkaldy-Willis: The pathophysiology of degenerative disease of the lumbar spine. Orthop. Clin. North Am. 14:491, 1983.

9

Pelvic Joints

The *sacroiliac joints* are the "key" of the arch between the two pelvic bones; with the *symphysis pubis,* they help to transfer the weight from the spine to the lower limbs. This triad of joints also acts as a buffer to decrease the force of jars and bumps to the spine and upper body from the lower limb's contact with the ground. Because of this shock-absorbing function, the structure of the sacroiliac and symphysis pubis joints is different from most joints that are assessed. Assessment of the sacroiliac joints and symphysis pubis should be included in the examination of the lumbar spine and/or hips if there is no direct trauma to either one of these joints. Normally, a comprehensive examination is not made of the sacroiliac joints until examination of the lumbar spine and/or hip has been completed. If both of these joints are examined and the problem still seems to be present and remain undiagnosed, an examination of the pelvic joints should be initiated.

Applied Anatomy

The sacroiliac joints are part synovial and part syndesmosis. A syndesmosis is a type of fibrous joint in which the intervening fibrous connective tissue forms an interosseous membrane or ligament. The synovial portion of the joint is C-shaped with the convex iliac surface of the "C" facing anteriorly and inferiorly. Kapandji[1] states that the greater or more acute the angle of the

"C," the more stable the joint and the less the likelihood of a lesion to the joint. The sacral surface is slightly concave.

The size, shape, and roughness of the articular surfaces vary greatly among individuals. In the child, these surfaces are smooth. In the adult, they become irregular depressions and elevations that fit into one another; by so doing, they restrict movement at the joint and add strength to the joint for transferring weight from the lower limb to the spine. The articular surface of the ilium is covered with fibrocartilage; the articular surface of the sacrum is covered with hyaline cartilage, which is three times thicker than that of the ilium. In older persons, part of the joint surfaces may be obliterated by adhesions.

The sacroiliac joints, although relatively mobile in young people, become progressively stiffer as age progresses. In some cases, ankylosis results. It must be remembered that the movements occurring in the sacroiliac and symphysis pubis joints are small in relation to the movements in the spinal joints.

The symphysis pubis is a cartilaginous joint. There is a disc of fibrocartilage between the two joint surfaces called the *interpubic disc.*

The sacroiliac joints and symphysis pubis have no muscles that control their movements directly. However, they are influenced by the action of the muscles moving the lumbar spine and hip because many of these muscles attach to the sacrum and pelvis.

The *sacrococcygeal joint* is usually a fused line

219

(symphysis) united by a fibrocartilaginous disc. It is found between the apex of the sacrum and the base of the coccyx. Occasionally the joint is freely movable and is synovial. With advanced age, the joint may fuse and be obliterated.

Patient History

In addition to the general questions asked in Chapter 1, the following information should be ascertained:

1. What is the patient's usual activity or pastime?

2. Where is the pain, and does it radiate? With a lesion of the sacroiliac joint, pain tends to be unilateral and can be referred to the posterior thigh, iliac fossa, and buttock on the affected side.

3. When does the pain occur? Pain that is due to sacroiliac joint problems is usually felt when turning in bed, getting out of a bed, or stepping up with the affected leg. Often the pain is constant and unrelated to position. Symphysis pubis pain tends to be localized and increases with any movement involving the adductor or rectus abdominus muscles.

4. Does the patient have or feel any weakness in the lower limb? Neurologic deficit in the limbs can be present if the sacroiliac joint is affected.

5. Has there been a recent pregnancy? Sprain of the sacroiliac ligaments can be the result of increased laxity of the ligaments caused by hormonal changes. It may take 3 or 4 months or longer for the ligaments to return to their "normal" state following a pregnancy.

6. Has the patient had any recent falls, twists, or strains? These movements increase the chance of sacroiliac joint sprains.

7. What is the patient's habitual working stance? Is a great deal of sitting or twisting involved?

8. Does the patient have a past history of rheumatoid arthritis, Reiter's disease, or ankylosing spondylitis? Each of these conditions can involve the sacroiliac joints.

Observation

The patient must be suitably undressed. For the sacroiliac joints to be observed properly, the patient is often required to be nude from the midchest to the toes. If the patient wishes to wear shorts, they must be rolled down as far as possible so that the sacroiliac joints are visible. The patient stands and is viewed from the front, side, and back. The examiner should note the following:

1. Whether posture and gait are normal. If *contranutation*[2] occurs at the sacroiliac joint (which indicates an anterior torsion of the joint on that side), the lower limb on that side will in all probability be medially rotated. Contranutation occurs when the anterior superior iliac spine (ASIS) is lower and the posterior superior iliac spine (PSIS) is higher on that particular side.[2] A painful sacroiliac joint may cause reflex inhibition of the gluteus medius, leading to a Trendelenburg gait or lurch. *Nutation*[2] is the backward rotation of the ilium on the sacrum (Fig. 9–1). If nutation occurs only on one side, the ASIS is higher and the PSIS is lower on that side.[2] Nutation occurs when a person goes into a "pelvic

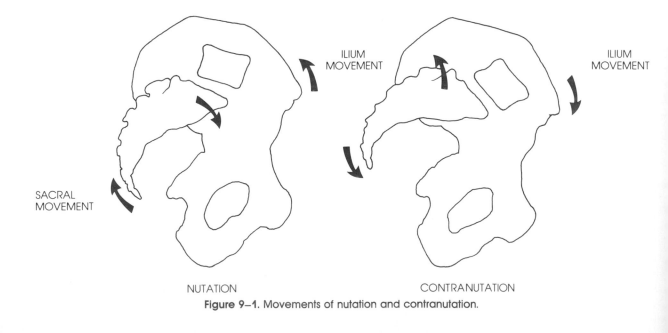

ILIUM MOVEMENT

SACRAL MOVEMENT

NUTATION

ILIUM MOVEMENT

CONTRANUTATION

Figure 9–1. Movements of nutation and contranutation.

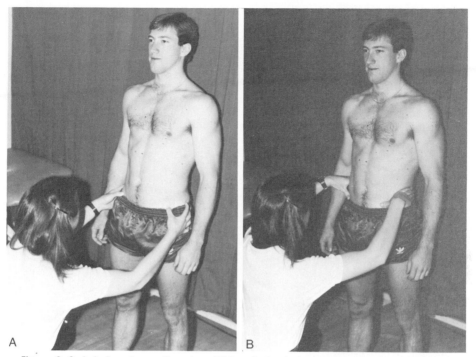

Figure 9–2. Anterior observation view. (A) Level of anterior superior iliac spines. (B) Level of iliac crests.

tilt'' position. Contranutation occurs when a person goes into a ''lordotic'' or ''anterior pelvic tilt'' position.

2. Whether the anterior superior iliac spines are level when viewed anteriorly (Fig. 9–2). On the affected side, they tend to be higher and slightly forward. The examiner must remember this difference, if present, when the patient is viewed from behind (Fig. 9–3). If the ASIS and PSIS on one side are higher than the ASIS and PSIS on the other side, this indicates an upslip of the ilium on the sacrum on the high side or a short leg.[3] If the ASIS is higher on one side and the PSIS is lower at the same time, it indicates a torsion of the sacrum on that side.[3] This torsion may result in a spinal scoliosis and/or an apparent altered leg length.

3. Whether both pubic bones are level at the symphysis pubis. The examiner tests for level equality by placing one finger or thumb on the superior aspect of each pubic bone and comparing the height (Fig. 9–4). If the ASIS on one side is higher, the pubic bone on that side is suspected to be higher and can be confirmed by this procedure, indicating a backward torsion problem on that side. This procedure is usually done with the patient lying supine.

4. Whether the patient stands with equal weight on both feet, favors one leg, or has a lateral pelvic tilt. This finding may indicate pathology or a short leg.

5. Whether the anterior superior iliac spines are equidistant from the center line of the body.

6. What type of pelvis the patient has. Gynecoid and android types are the most common (as described in Table 9–1 and Figure 9–5).

7. Whether the sacrovertebral or lumbosacral angle is normal (140°).

8. Whether the pelvic angle or inclination is normal (30°).

9. Whether the sacral angle is normal (30°) (Fig. 9–6).

10. Whether the iliac crests are level. Leg length may alter the height.

11. Whether the posterior superior iliac spines are level.

12. Whether the buttock contours or gluteal folds are normal. The painful side will often be flatter if there is loss of tone in the gluteus maximus muscle.

13. Whether there is any unilateral or bilateral spasm of the erector spinae muscles.

14. Whether the ischial tuberosities are level. If one tuberosity is higher, it may indicate an upslip of the ilium on the sacrum on that side.[3]

15. Whether there is excessive lumbar lordosis. Forward or backward sacral torsion may increase or decrease the lordosis.

16. Whether the posterior superior iliac spines are equidistant from the center line of the body.

17. Whether the sacral sulci are equal. If one is deeper, it may indicate a sacral torsion.

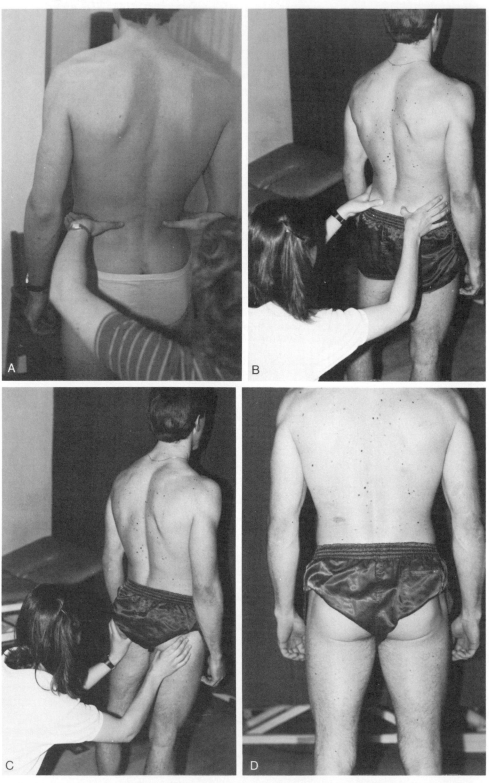

Figure 9–3. Posterior observational view. (*A*) Level of iliac crests. (*B*) Level of posterior superior iliac spines. (*C*) Level of ischial tuberosities. (*D*) Level of gluteal folds.

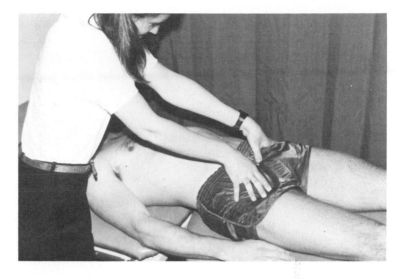

Figure 9–4. Determining level of pubic bones.

Table 9–1. A Comparison of the Two Most Common Types of Pelvis Seen in Males and Females

Feature	Gynecoid	Android
Inlet	Round	Triangular
Sacrosciatic notch	Average size	Narrow
Sacrum	Average	Forward
Subpubic arch	Inclination well curved	Inclination straight

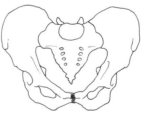

A

Pelvic inlet

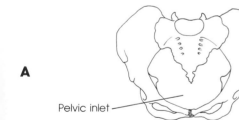

B

Sacrosciatic notch

Ischial spine

Figure 9–5. Gynecoid (predominantly female) and android (primarily male) pelvises. (*A*) Anterosuperior view. (*B*) Lateral view. (*C*) Anterior view of the pubis ischium.

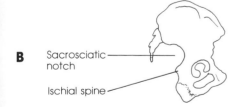

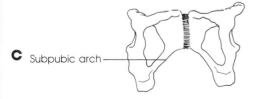

C Subpubic arch

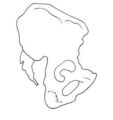

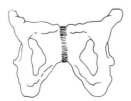

GYNECOID   ANDROID

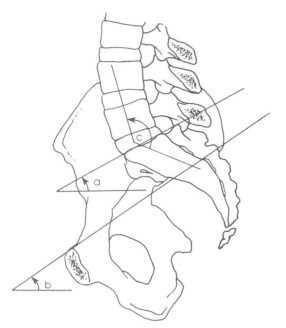

Figure 9–6. Angles of the pelvic joints. a) Pelvic angle (normal = 30°). b) Sacral angle (normal = 30°). c) Lumbosacral angle (normal = 140°).

18. Whether the feet face forward to the same degree. Often the affected limb will be medially rotated. With spasm of the piriformis muscle, the limb would be laterally rotated on the affected side.

Examination

When assessing the pelvic joints, the examiner should first assess the lumbar spine and hip unless the history definitely indicates one of the pelvic joints.

The lumbar spine and hip can, and frequently do, refer pain to the sacroiliac joint area. Because the sacroiliac joints are partly a syndesmosis, movement at these joints is minimal compared with the other peripheral joints. It should also be remembered that any condition altering the position of the sacrum relative to the ilium will cause a corresponding change in position of the symphysis pubis.

ACTIVE MOVEMENTS

The sacroiliac joints do not have muscles directly controlling their movement, as do other peripheral joints. However, because contraction of the muscles of the other joints may stress these joints or the symphysis pubis, the examiner must be careful during the active or resisted isometric movements of other joints and be sure to ask the patient about the exact location of the pain on each movement. For example, resisted abduction of the hip can cause pain in the sacroiliac joint on the same side if it is injured because the gluteus medius muscle pulls the ilium away from the sacrum when it contracts strongly. As well, side flexion to the same side increases the shearing stress to the sacroiliac joint on that side.

The sacroiliac joints move in a "nodding" fashion of anteroposterior rotation. The sacrum moves forward on the ilia when one changes from a standing to lying position or when one flexes the trunk. The opposite occurs for movements in the opposite direction. Normally, the posterior superior iliac spines approximate when one stands and separate when one lies prone. When one stands on one leg, the pubic bone on the supported side moves forward in relation to the pubic bone on the opposite side as a result of rotation at the sacroiliac joint.

The examiner looks for unequal movement, loss of movement (hypomobility), tissue contracture, tenderness, inflammation, or hypermobility. The following active movements should be carried out with the patient standing:

1. Forward flexion of the spine (40 to 60°).
2. Extension of the spine (20 to 35°).
3. Rotation of the spine (left and right) (3 to 18°).
4. Side flexion of the spine (left and right) (15 to 20°).
5. Flexion of the hip (110 to 120°).
6. Abduction of the hip (30 to 50°).
7. Adduction of the hip (30°).
8. Extension of the hip (0 to 15°).
9. Medial rotation of the hip (30 to 40°).
10. Lateral rotation of the hip (40 to 60°).

The movements of the spine put a stress on the sacroiliac joints as well as the lumbar and lumbosacral joints. Forward flexion movement while standing tests the movement of the ilia on the sacrum.

The hip movements performed are also affected by sacroiliac lesions. As the patient flexes each hip maximally, the examiner should observe the range of motion present, the pain produced, and the movement of the posterior superior iliac spines. The examiner first notes whether the posterior superior iliac spines are level before the patient flexes the hip (Fig. 9–7A). Normally, flexion of the hip with the knee flexed to 90° causes the sacroiliac joint on that side to drop or move caudally relative to the other sacroiliac joint. If this drop does not occur, it may indicate hypomobility on the flexed side. The examiner can also test this movement by placing one thumb over the PSIS and the other thumb over the spinous process of S2.

Following the test, the examiner places one thumb over the lowest sacral spinous process palpable and the other thumb over the PSIS. The

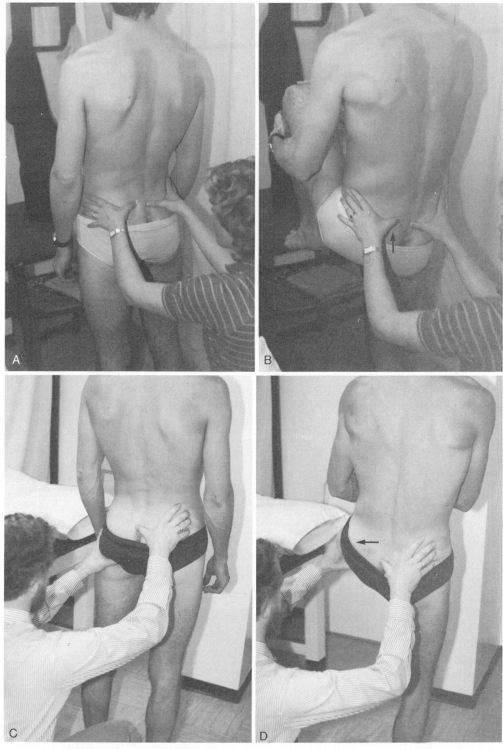

Figure 9–7. Active movements demonstrating how to show hypomobility of the sacroiliac joints. (*A*) Starting position for sacral spine and posterior superior iliac spine. (*B*) Hip flexion (tight sacroiliac joint illustrated. Ilium does not drop). (*C*) Starting position for sacral spine and ischial tuberosity. (*D*) Hip flexion. Ischeal tuberosity moves laterally as one would normally expect.

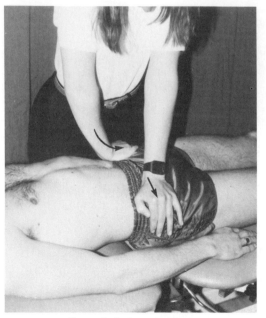

Figure 9–8. Gapping test.

patient is again asked to flex the hip with the knee flexed as far as possible (Fig. 9–7B). The examiner should normally note a downward movement of the thumb over the PSIS relative to the other thumb in the normal sacroiliac joint. In the hypomobile sacroiliac joint, this thumb would remain in the same position relative to the other thumb or would move up cranially. Both sides are compared. The examiner then leaves the one thumb over the sacral spinous process and moves the other thumb over the ischial tuberosity (Fig. 9–7C). The patient is again asked to flex the hip as far as possible. In the normal sacroiliac joint, the thumb over the ischial tuberosity will move laterally (Fig. 9–7D). With a fixed joint, the thumb

will move superiorly or toward the head (cephalad). Again, both sides are compared.

PASSIVE MOVEMENTS

The passive movements carried out on the pelvic joints are also in reality stress tests that assess the ligaments as well as the joints themselves. The following stress tests should be performed:

1. *Gapping test.* The patient lies supine while the examiner applies crossed-arm pressure to the anterior superior iliac spines (Fig. 9–8). The examiner pushes down and out with the arms. The test is positive only if unilateral gluteal or posterior leg pain is produced, indicating a sprain of the anterior sacroiliac ligaments. Care must be taken when performing this test. The examiner's hands pushing against the ASIS can elicit pain, since the soft tissue between the examiner's hands and the patient's pelvis is being compressed. These ligaments may also be stressed by lateral rotation of the hip to the extreme and resisted adduction of the thighs. This second test would be done with the patient prone.

2. *Approximation test.* The patient is in the side lying position while the examiner's hands are placed over the upper part of the iliac crest, pressing toward the floor (Fig. 9–9). The movement causes forward pressure on the sacrum. Increased feeling of pressure in the sacroiliac joints indicates a possible sacroiliac lesion and/or a sprain of the posterior sacroiliac ligaments.

3. *"Squish" test.* With the patient supine (Fig. 9–10), the examiner places both hands on the patient's anterior superior iliac spines and iliac crests and pushes down and in at a 45° angle. This movement will test the posterior sacroiliac ligaments. A positive test is indicated by pain.

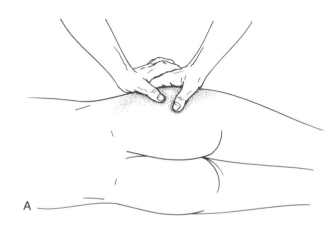

Figure 9–9. Approximation test. (*A*) Posterior view. (*B*) Anterior view.

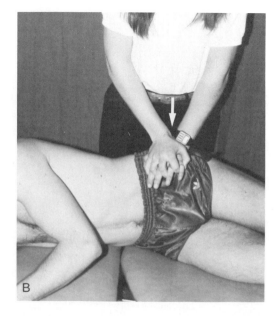

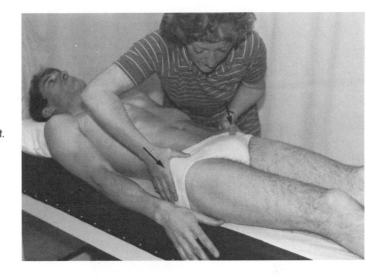

Figure 9–10. "Squish" test.

4. *Sacroiliac rocking ("knee-to-shoulder") test.* The patient is in a supine position (Fig. 9–11). The examiner flexes the patient's knee and hip fully and then adducts the hip. The sacroiliac joint is "rocked" by flexion and adduction of the patient's hip. To do the test properly, the knee is moved toward the patient's opposite shoulder. Pain in the sacroiliac joints indicates a positive test. Care must be taken because the test places a great deal of stress on the hip and sacroiliac joints. While performing the test, the examiner may palpate the sacroiliac joint on the test side to feel for a slight amount of movement that normally would be present.

5. *Sacral apex pressure (prone springing) test.* The patient lies in a prone position on a firm surface while the examiner places the base of the hand at the apex of the patient's sacrum (Fig. 9–12). Pressure is then applied to the apex of the sacrum, causing a shear of the sacrum on the ilium. The test may indicate a sacroiliac joint problem if pain is produced over the joint. The test causes a rotational shift of the sacroiliac joints.

RESISTED ISOMETRIC MOVEMENTS

As previously stated, there are no specific muscles acting directly on the sacroiliac joints and symphysis pubis. However, contraction of adjacent muscles can stress these joints. The patient is in a supine position, and the following resisted isometric movements are tested:

1. Foward flexion of spine (the abdominals stress the symphysis pubis).

2. Flexion of hip (the iliacus stresses the sacroiliac joint).

3. Abduction of hip (the gluteus medius stresses the sacroiliac joint).

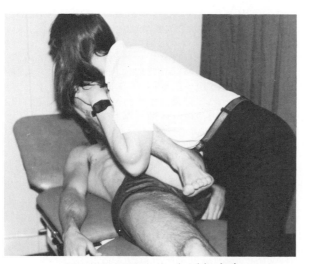

Figure 9–11. Knee-to-shoulder test.

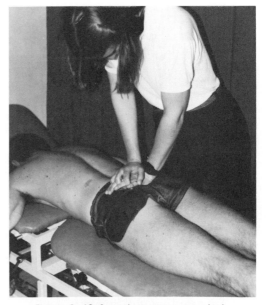

Figure 9–12. Sacral apex pressure test.

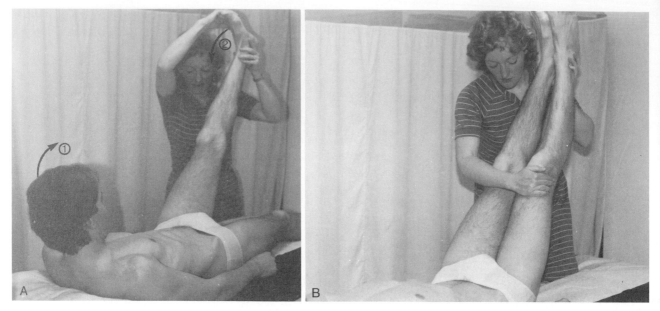

Figure 9–13. Straight leg test. (*A*) Unilateral. (1, 2, or both may be done). (*B*) Bilateral.

4. Adduction of hip (the adductors stress the symphysis pubis).

5. Extension of hip (the gluteus maximus stresses the sacroiliac joints).

SPECIAL TESTS

When examining the sacroiliac joints, the examiner should always do the following five tests:

Straight Leg Raising (Lasègue's) Test

Although the Lasègue sign is primarily considered a test of the lumbar spine, this test also places a stress on the sacroiliac joints. With the patient in supine position (Fig. 9–13), the examiner passively flexes the patient's hip with the knee extended. Pain occurring after 70° is indicative of joint pain. If the examiner then does a passive bilateral straight leg raise in a similar fashion, pain occurring before 70° is usually indicative of sacroiliac joint problems. A greater description of the straight leg raise test is given in Chapter 8.

Sign of the Buttock Test

With the patient supine, the examiner performs a passive unilateral straight leg test as done previously (Fig. 9–14). If restriction is found on one side, the examiner flexes the patient's knee to see whether flexion of the hip increases. If the problem is in the lumbar spine, hip flexion will increase. This finding indicates a negative sign of the buttock test. If hip flexion does not increase when the knee is flexed, it is a positive sign of the buttock test and indicates pathology in the buttock such as a bursitis, tumor, or abscess. The patient would also exhibit a noncapsular pattern of the hip.

Leg Length Test

The leg length test, described in detail in chapter 10 ("The Hip"), should always be performed if the examiner suspects a sacroiliac joint lesion. Nutation (backward rotation) of the ilium on the sacrum will result in a decrease in leg length, as will contranutation (anterior rotation) on the opposite side. If the iliac bone on one side of the symphysis pubis is lower, the leg on that side will usually be shorter. True leg length is measured by having the patient in a supine position with the anterior superior iliac spines level and the patient's lower limbs perpendicular to the line joining the anterior superior iliac spines (Fig. 9–15). Using a flexible measuring tape, the examiner obtains the distance from the ASIS to the medial or lateral malleolus on the same side. The measurement is repeated on the other side, and the results are compared. A difference of 1 to 1.3 cm is considered normal.

Piedallu's Sign

The patient is asked to sit on a hard, flat surface (Fig. 9–16). This position keeps the muscles (such as the hamstrings) from affecting the pelvic flexion symmetry and increases stability of the ilia.

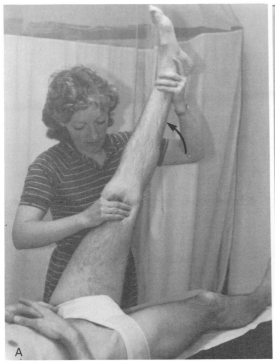

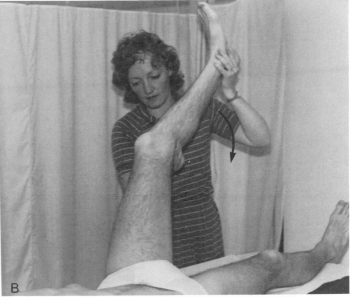

Figure 9–14. Sign of the buttock test. (*A*) Step 1. Flex hip with knee straight until resistance or pain felt. (*B*) Step 2. Once resistance or pain is felt, flex knee to see if further hip flexion can be achieved.

In effect, it is a test of the sacrum on the ilia. The examiner finds the posterior superior iliac spines and compares their height. If one PSIS, usually the painful one, is lower than the other, the patient is asked to forward flex while remaining seated. If the lower PSIS becomes the higher one on forward flexion, the test is positive and it is that side that is affected. Because the affected joint does not move properly and is hypomobile, it goes from a low to a high position. It indicates an abnormality in the torsion movement at the sacroiliac joint.

Trendelenburg's Test or Sign

The patient is standing (Fig. 9–17) and is asked to stand or balance first on one leg and then the other leg. While the patient is balancing on one leg, the examiner watches the movement of the pelvis. If the pelvis on the side of the stance leg rises, the test is considered negative. If the pelvis on the side of the stance leg falls, the test is considered positive and is an indication of weakness or instability of the hip abductor muscles, primarily the gluteus medius.

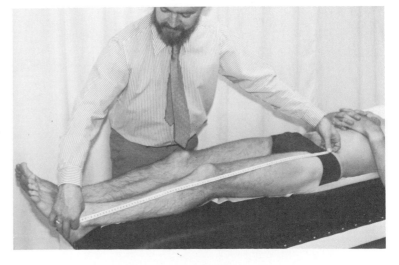

Figure 9–15. Measuring leg length.

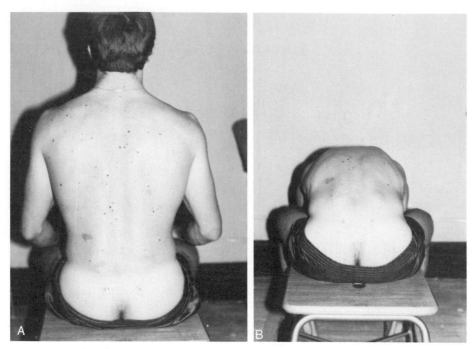

Figure 9–16. Piedallu's sign. The negative test is shown.

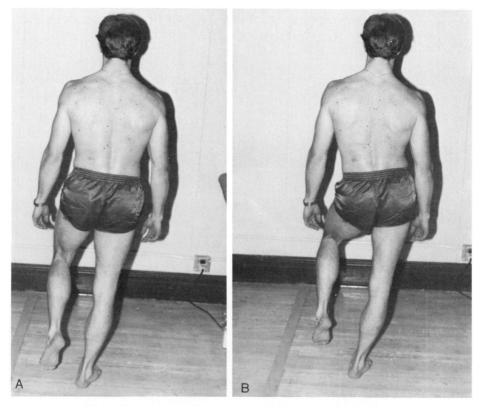

Figure 9–17. Trendelenburg negative (*A*) and positive (*B*) test.

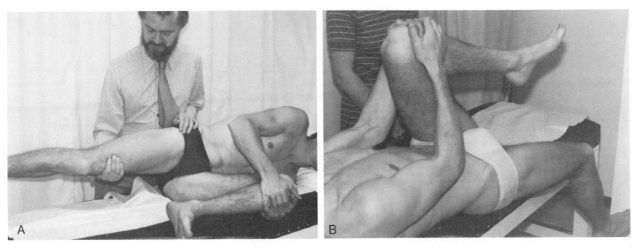

Figure 9–18. Gaenslen's test. (A) Method 1. Examiner extends test leg. (B) Method 2. Test leg is extended over edge of table.

Additional Tests

If the examiner feels the remaining special tests have relevance, they should also be performed.

Gaenslen's Test. The patient lies on the side with the upper leg hyperextended at the hip (Fig. 9–18). The patient holds the lower leg flexed against the chest. The examiner stabilizes the pelvis while extending the hip of the uppermost leg, which is the test leg. Pain indicates a positive test. The pain may be due to an ipsilateral sacroiliac joint lesion, hip pathology, or an L4 nerve root lesion.

The Gaenslen test is sometimes done in the supine position, but this position may limit the amount of hyperextension available. The patient is positioned so that the test hip extends beyond the edge of the table. The patient draws both legs up onto the chest and then slowly lowers the test leg down into extension. The other leg is tested in a similar fashion for comparison. Pain in the sacroiliac joints is indicative of a positive test.

Laguere's Sign. The patient lies in a supine position (Fig. 9–19). The examiner then flexes, abducts and laterally rotates the patient's hip, applying an overpressure at the end of the range of motion. The examiner must stabilize the pelvis on the opposite side by holding the opposite ASIS down. Pain in the sacroiliac joint on that side constitutes a positive test. This test should be performed with caution for patients with hip pathology, as hip pain may ensue.

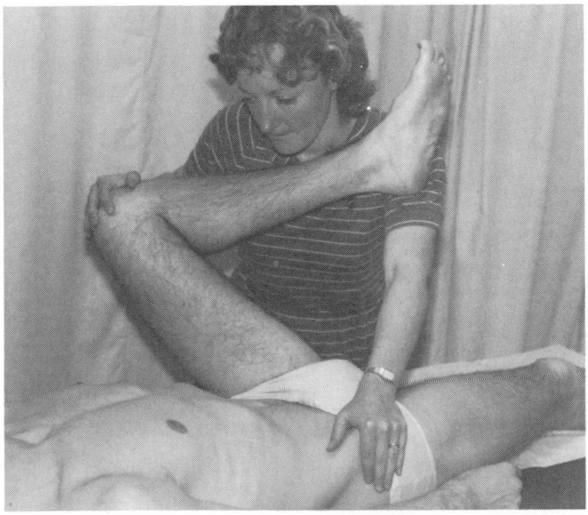

REFLEXES AND CUTANEOUS DISTRIBUTION

There are no reflexes to test for the pelvic joints. However, the examiner must be aware of the dermatomes from the sacral nerve roots (Fig. 9–20). Pain may be referred to the sacroiliac joints from the lumbar spine and the hip (Fig. 9–21). As well, the sacroiliac joint may refer pain to these same structures or along the courses of the superior gluteal and obturator nerves.

JOINT PLAY MOVEMENTS

The joint play movements are minimal for the sacroiliac joints and are similar to the passive movements, in that they are stress tests. The following joint play movements are performed (Fig. 9–22):

1. Cephalad movement of the sacrum/caudal movement of the ilium (left and right).

2. Cephalad movement of the ilium/caudal movement of the sacrum (left and right).

3. Anterior movement of the sacrum on the ilium.

To test all the movements, the patient is in the

Figure 9–19. Laguere's sign.

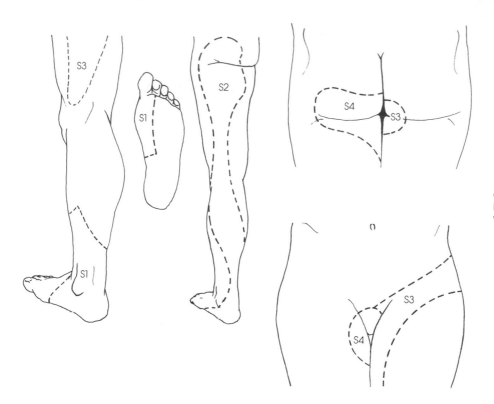

Figure 9–20. Posterior sacral dermatomes. The representation in the lower right is an anterior view.

prone position. For the first and second joint play movements, the examiner places the heel of one hand over the iliac crest and the heel of the other hand over the apex of the sacrum. The ilium is pushed down or caudally with one hand while the sacrum is pushed up or cephalad with the other hand. The test is repeated for the other ilium (Fig. 9–22A). The examiner should "feel" only minimal movement and no pain if the joint is normal. In an affected sacroiliac joint, there is usually pain over the joint and little or no movement. This positioning tests for cephalad movement of the sacrum and caudal movement of the ilium.

To test caudal movement of the sacrum and cephalad movement of the ilium, the examiner places the heel of one hand over the base of the sacrum and the heel of the other hand over the ischial tuberosity (Fig. 9–22B). The examiner then pushes the pelvis cephalad and the sacrum caudally. The test is repeated with the other half of the pelvis being moved. The movement and amount of pain are compared.

The anterior movement of the sacrum on the ilium is tested with the patient lying prone (Fig. 9–22C). The examiner places the heel of one hand over the sacrum and places the other hand under the iliac crest in the area of the ASIS on one side.

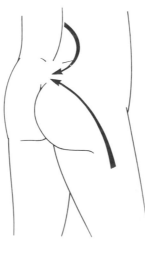

Figure 9–21. Referred pain from sacroiliac joint (*A*) to sacroiliac joint (*B*).

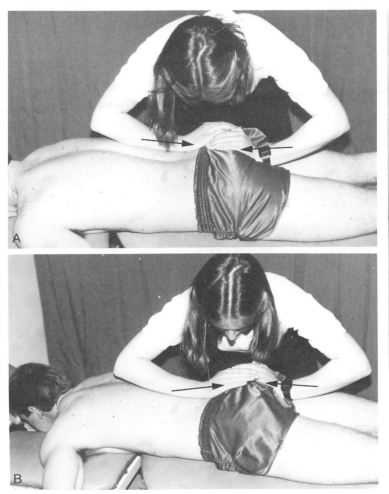

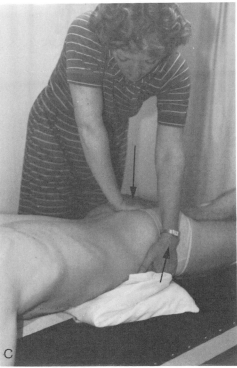

Figure 9–22. Joint play movements of the sacroiliac joints. (A) Cephalad movement of sacrum/caudal movement of ilium. (B) Cephalad movement of ilium/caudal movement of sacrum. (C) Anterior movement of sacrum on ilium (left side demonstrated).

The hand is then pushed down on the sacrum while the other hand lifts up. The process is repeated on the other side, and the results compared.

PALPATION

Because many structures are included in the assessment of the pelvic joints, palpation of this area is extensive, beginning on the anterior aspect and concluding posteriorly. While palpating, the examiner should note any tenderness, muscle spasm, or other signs that may indicate the source of pathology.

Anterior Aspect

The following structures should be carefully and thoroughly palpated (Fig. 9–23).

Iliac Crest and Anterior Superior Iliac Spine. The palpating fingers are placed on the iliac crests on both sides and gently moved anterior until each ASIS is reached. The inguinal ligament attaches to the ASIS and runs down and medially to the symphysis pubis.

McBurney's Point and Baer's Point. The examiner may then draw an imaginary line from the right ASIS to the umbilicus. *McBurney's point* lies along this line about one third the distance from the ASIS and is especially tender in the presence of acute appendicitis. Baer's point is located in the right iliac fossa anterior to the right sacroiliac joint and slightly medial to McBurney's point. It is tender in the presence of infection or when there are sprains of the right sacroiliac ligament and indicates spasm and tenderness of the iliacus muscle.

Lymph Nodes, Symphysis Pubis (Pubic Tubercles), Greater Trochanter of the Femur, Trochanteric Bursa, Femoral Triangle, and Surrounding Musculature. The examiner then returns to the ASIS and gently palpates the length of the inguinal ligament, feeling for any tenderness or swelling of the *lymph nodes* or possible inguinal hernia. At the distal end of the inguinal ligament, the examiner will come to the *pubic tubercles,*

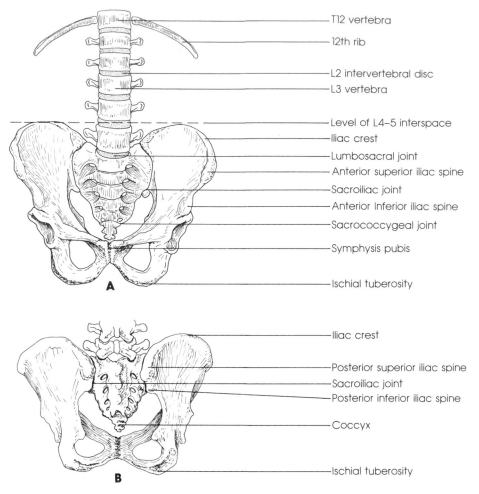

Figure 9–23. Landmarks of the sacroiliac joints and symphysis pubis. (*A*) Anterior view. (*B*) Posterior view.

which should be palpated for tenderness or signs of pathology.

The examiner then places the thumbs over the pubic tubercles and moves the fingers laterally until they feel the bony *greater trochanter of the femur*. The trochanters are usually level. The *trochanteric bursa* lies over the greater trochanter and is palpable only if it is swollen.

Returning to the ASIS, the examiner can move on to palpate the *femoral triangle*, which has as its boundaries the inguinal ligament superiorly, the adductor longus muscle medially, and the sartorius muscle laterally. It is in the superior aspect of the triangle that the examiner palpates for swollen lymph nodes. The femoral pulse can be palpated deeper in the triangle. Although almost impossible to palpate, the femoral nerve lies lateral to the artery while the femoral vein lies medial to it. The psoas bursa may also be palpated within the femoral triangle, but only if it is swollen. Before moving on to the posterior structures, the examiner should ascertain whether the adjacent *musculature*—the abductor, flexor, and ad-

ductor muscles—show any indication of pathology.

Posterior Aspect

To complete the posterior palpation, the patient lies in the prone position. The following structures should be palpated.

Iliac Crest and Posterior Superior Iliac Spine. Again, the examiner places the fingers on the iliac crest and moves posteriorly until they rest on the PSIS, which is at the level of the S2 spinous process. On many individuals, "dimples" indicate the position of the PSIS.

Ischial Tuberosity. If the examiner then moves distally from the PSIS and down to the level of the gluteal folds, the ischial tuberosities may be palpated. It is important that they be palpated because the hamstring muscles attach here and the bony prominences are what one "sits on."

Sacral Sulcus and Sacroiliac Joints. Returning to the PSIS as a starting point, the examiner should palpate slightly below it on the sacrum

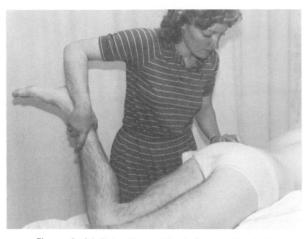

Figure 9–24. Palpation of the left sacroiliac joint.

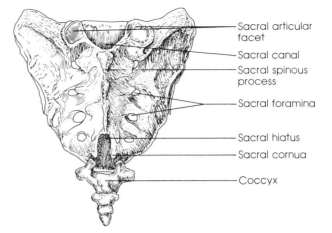

Figure 9–25. Posterior view of the sacrum and coccyx.

adjacent to the ilium. (This area is sometimes referred to as the *sacral sulcus.*) The depth on the right and left sides should be compared. If one side is deeper than the other, sacral torsion or rotation on the ilium about the horizontal plane is indicated.

If the examiner then moves slightly medially and distal to the PSIS, the fingers will rest adjacent to the *sacroiliac joints.* To palpate these joints, the patient's knee is flexed to 90° and the hip is passively medially rotated while the examiner palpates the sacroiliac joint on the same side (Fig. 9–24). The procedure is repeated on the other side and both are compared.

Sacrum, Lumbosacral Joint, Coccyx, Sacral Hiatus, Sacral Cornua, and Sacrotuberous and Sacrospinal Ligaments. The examiner again returns to the PSIS and moves to the midline of the *sacrum,* where the S2 spinous process can be palpated.

Moving superiorly two spinous processes, the fingers now rest on the spinous process of L5. As a check, the examiner may look to see if the fingers rest just below a horizontal line drawn from the high point of the iliac crests. This horizontal line will normally pass through the interspace between L4 and L5. Having found the L5 spinous process, the examiner then palpates between the spinous processes of L5 and S1, feeling for signs of pathology at the *lumbosacral joint.* Moving laterally approximately 2 to 3 cm, the fingers will lie over the lumbosacral facet joints, which are not palpable. However, the overlying structures may be palpated for tenderness or spasm, which may indicate pathology of these joints or related structures. In a similar fashion, the spinous processes and facet joints of the other lumbar spines and intervening structures can be palpated.

The examiner then returns to the S2 spinous process or tubercle. Carefully palpating further distally, just prior to the coccyx, the examiner may be able to palpate the *sacral hiatus* lying in the midline. If the fingers are moved slightly laterally, the *sacral cornua,* which are the distal aspect of the sacrum, may be palpated (Fig. 9–25).

To palpate the *coccyx* properly, the examiner

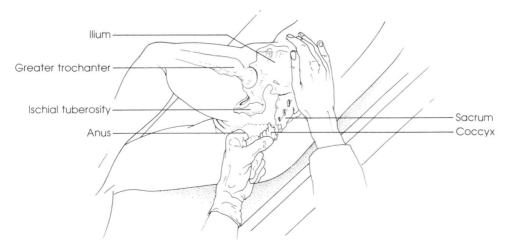

Figure 9–26. Palpation of the coccyx.

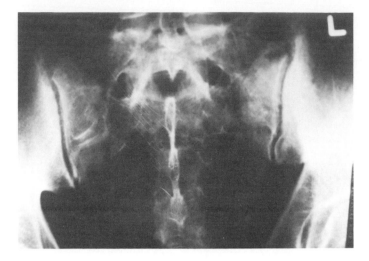

Figure 9–27. Anteroposterior radiograph of the sacroiliac joint.

Figure 9–28. Fusion of sacroiliac joint spaces in the late stage of sacroiliitis of ankylosing spondylitis. The sclerosis has resorbed, and there is slight narrowing of the left hip joint. (From Rothman, R. H., and F. A. Simeone: The Spine. Philadelphia, W. B. Saunders Co., 1982, p. 921.)

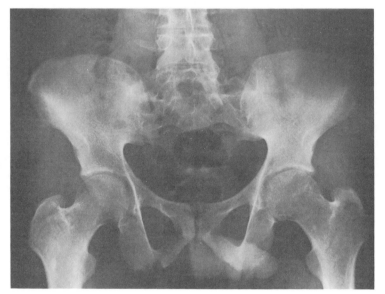

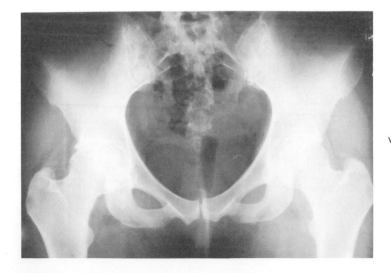

Figure 9–29. Anteroposterior radiograph of the pelvis. Note higher left pubic bone.

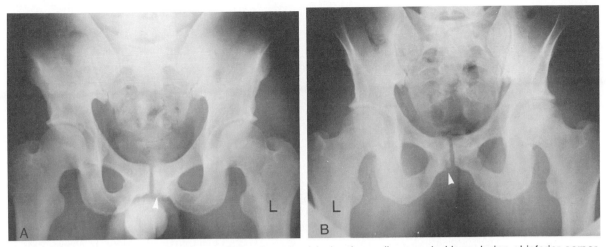

Figure 9–30. Osteitis pubis. (*A*) Anteroposterior view of pelvis showing well-concealed bony lesion at inferior corner of left pubis at the symphysis. (*B*) Posteroanterior view of pelvis. Bony fragment well delineated in this view. (From Wiley, J. J.: Am. J. Sports Med. *11*:361, 1983.)

performs a rectal examination (Fig. 9–26). A rubber glove is put on and the index finger lubricated. The index finger is then carefully pushed into the rectum as the patient relaxes the sphincter muscles. The index finger then palpates the anterior surface of the coccyx while the thumb of the same hand palpates its posterior aspect. While holding the coccyx between the finger and thumb, the examiner is able to move it back and forth, rocking it at the sacrococcygeal joint. Normally, this action should not cause pain.

The examiner then returns to the PSIS. Moving straight down or distally from the PSIS, the fingers will follow the path of the *sacrotuberous ligament*, which should be palpated for tenderness. Slightly more than halfway between the PSIS and ischial tuberosity and slightly medially, the examiner will pass over the *sacrospinous ligament*, which is deep to the sacrotuberous ligament. Tenderness in this area may indicate pathology of this ligament.

ROENTGENOGRAMS OF THE SACROILIAC JOINTS AND SYMPHYSIS PUBIS

With the *anteroposterior view* (Fig. 9–27), the examiner should look for or note:

1. Ankylosis of sacroiliac joints (e.g., ankylosing spondylitis) (Fig. 9–28).

2. Possible displacement of one sacroiliac joint and/or the symphysis pubis (Fig. 9–29).

3. Demineralization, sclerosis, or periosteal reaction of one or both pubic bones at the symphysis pubis (e.g., osteitis pubis) (Fig. 9–30).

4. Any fracture.

5. Relation of the sacrum to the ilium.

Précis of the Pelvic Joints Assessment*

History (sitting)
Observation (standing)
Examination
  Active movements (standing)
    Flexion of the spine
    Extension of the spine
    Rotation of the spine (left and right)
    Side flexion of the spine (left and right)
    Flexion of the hip
    Abduction of the hip
    Adduction of the hip
    Extension of the hip
    Medial rotation of the hip
    Lateral rotation of the hip
  Special tests (standing)
  Special tests (sitting)
  Passive movements (supine)
    Gapping test
    "Squish" test
    Rocking ("Knee to-shoulder") test
    Sacral apex pressure test
  Resisted isometric movements (supine)
    Forward flexion of the spine
    Flexion of the hip
    Abduction of the hip
    Adduction of the hip
    Extension of the hip
  Special tests (supine)
  Passive movements (side lying) (approximation test)
  Reflexes and cutaneous distribution (supine, then prone)

*This précis shows an order that will limit the amount of movement or changes in position that the patient has to do but that will ensure that all necessary structures are tested.

Passive movements (prone) (sacral apex pressure test)

Special tests (prone)

Joint play movements (prone)

Cephalad movement of the sacrum/caudal movement of the ilium

Cephalad movement of the ilium/caudal movement of the sacrum

Palpation (prone, then supine)

X-ray viewing

As previously stated, assessment of the sacroiliac joints and symphysis pubis is only done after an assessment of the lumbar spine and hips unless there has been specific trauma to the sacroiliac joints or symphysis pubis. Thus, completing the examination of the sacroiliac joints and symphysis pubis may involve only passive movements, special tests, joint play movements, and palpation, since the other tests would have been completed when assessing the other joints.

Following any examination, the patient should always be warned of the possibility of exacerbation of symptoms as a result of the assessment.

REFERENCES

Cited References

1. Kapandji, L. A.: The Physiology of the Joints, vol. III: The Trunk and Vertebral Column. New York, Churchill Livingstone, 1974.
2. Maigne, R.: Orthopaedic Medicine: A New Approach to Vertebral Manipulation. Springfield, Ill., Charles C Thomas, 1972.
3. Mitchell, F. L., P. S. Moran, and N. A. Pruzzo: An Evaluation and Treatment Manual of Osteopathic Muscle Energy Procedures. Valley Park, Mo., Mitchell, Moran and Pruzzo, 1979.

General References

Bourdillon, J. F.: Spinal Manipulation, 3rd ed. New York, Appleton-Century-Crofts, 1982.

Bowen, V., and J. D. Cassidy: Macroscopic and microscopic anatomy of the sacroiliac joint from embryonic life until the eighth decade. Spine 6:620, 1981.

Brooke, R.: The sacro-iliac joint. J. Anat. 58:299, 1924.

Cohen, A. S., J. M. McNeill, E. Calkins, et al.: The "normal" sacroiliac joint. Analysis of 88 sacroiliac roentgenograms. Am. J. Roentgenol. 100:559, 1967.

Cyriax, J.: Textbook of Orthopaedic Medicine, vol. 1: Diagnosis of Soft Tissue Lesions. London, Bailliere Tindall, 1975.

Finneson, B. E.: Low Back Pain. Philadelphia, J. B. Lippincott Co., 1981.

Frigerio, N. A., R. R. Stowe, and J. W. Howe: Movement of the sacroiliac joint. Clin. Orthop. Relat. Res. 100:370, 1974.

Gray, H.: Sacro-iliac joint pain: The finer anatomy. New International Clinics 2:54, 1938.

Grieve, G. P.: Mobilization of the Spine. New York, Churchill Livingstone, 1979.

Grieve, G. P.: The sacro-iliac joint. Physiotherapy, 62:382, 1976.

Grieve, G. P.: Common Vertebral Joint Problems. New York, Churchill Livingstone, 1981.

Hanson, P. G.: M. Angevine, and J. H. Juhl: Osteitis pubis in sports activities. Physician Sportsmed 6:111, 1978.

Hollinshead, W. H., and D. R. Jenkins: Functional Anatomy of the Limbs and the Trunk and Vertebral Column. New York, Churchill Livingstone, 1981.

Kirkaldy-Willis, W. H.: Managing Low Back Pain. New York, Churchill Livingstone, 1983.

Klinefelter, F. W.: Osteitis pubis. Am. J. Roentgenol. 63:368, 1950.

Macnab, I.: Backache. Baltimore, Williams & Wilkins Co., 1977.

McRae, R.: Clinical Orthopedic Examination. New York, Churchill Livingstone, 1976.

Pitkin, H. C., and H. C. Pheasant: Sacrathrogenetic telalgia: A study of referred pain. J. Bone Joint Surg. 18:111, 1936.

Reilly, B. M.: Practical Strategies in Outpatient Medicine. Philadelphia, W. B. Saunders Co., 1984.

Rothman, R. H., and F. A. Simeone: The Spine. Philadelphia, W. B. Saunders Co., 1982.

Rudge, S. R., A. J. Swannell, D. H. Rose, and J. H. Todd: The clinical assessment of sacro-iliac joint involvement in ankylosing spondylitis. Rheumatol. Rehabil. 51:15, 1982.

Stoddard, A.: Manual of Osteopathic Practice. New York, Harper & Row, 1970.

Stoddard, A.: Manual of Osteopathic Technique. Atlantic Highlands, N. J., Humanities Press, 1969.

Wiley, J. J.: Traumatic osteitis pubis: The gracilis syndrome. Am. J. Sports Med. 11:360, 1983.

Williams, P. L., and Warwick, R.: Gray's Anatomy, 36th British ed. Philadelphia, W. B. Saunders Co., 1980.

Willis, T. A.: Lumbosacral anomalies. J. Bone Joint Surg. 41A:935, 1959.

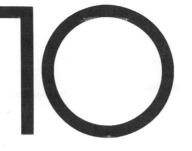

The Hip

The hip joint is one of the largest and most stable joints in the body. If it is injured or if it exhibits pathology, the lesion is usually immediately perceptible during walking. Because pain from the hip can be referred to the sacroiliac joint or the lumbar spine, it is imperative, unless there is evidence of direct trauma to the hip, that these joints be examined along with the hip.

gruous, providing maximum surface contact. The maximum contact brings the load per unit area down to a tolerable level. An example of the forces involved in the hip are as follows:

1. Standing—one third of the body weight.
2. Standing on one limb—2.4 to 2.6 times the body weight.
3. Walking—1.3 to 5.8 times the body weight.

Applied Anatomy

The hip joint is a multiaxial ball-and-socket joint that has maximum stability because of the deep insertion of the head of the femur into the acetabulum. It has a strong capsule and very strong muscles that control its actions. The acetabulum is formed by the fusion of the ilium, ischium, and pubis and is deepened by a labrum. The acetabulum opens outward, forward, and downward. It is half of a sphere, and the femoral head is two thirds of a sphere.

The joint has three degrees of freedom. The *resting position* of the hip is 30° of flexion, 30° of abduction, and slight lateral rotation. The *capsular pattern* of the hip is flexion, abduction, and medial rotation. These three movements will always be affected the most in a capsular pattern, but the order may be altered. For example, medial rotation may be most limited, followed by flexion and abduction. The *close packed position* of the joint is maximum extension, medial rotation, and abduction.

Under low loads, the joint surfaces are incongruous; under heavy loads, they become con-

Patient History

In addition to the general history questions presented in Chapter 1, the following information should be ascertained:

1. What is the patient's usual activity or pastime?
2. Is there any history of trauma to the joint?
3. What are the details of the present pain and other symptoms? Hip pain is felt mainly in the groin and frontal or medial side of the thigh. In this position, the pain may simulate L4 nerve root pain; thus the back should also be examined for problems. Hip pain may also be referred to the knee or back and may increase on walking.
4. Is the condition improving? Worsening? Staying the same?
5. Does any type of activity ease the pain or make it worse?
6. What is the age of the patient?
7. Are there any movements that the patient feels are weak or abnormal? For example, in *piriformis syndrome*, the sciatic nerve may be compressed, the piriformis muscle is tender, and hip abduction and lateral rotation are weak.

Observation

When the patient comes into the assessment area, the gait should be observed. If the hip is affected, the weight will be lowered carefully on the affected side and the knee will bend slightly to absorb the shock. The length of the step on the affected side will be shorter so that weight can be taken off the leg quickly. If the hip is stiff, the whole trunk and affected leg swing forward together. The different types of gait are discussed in greater detail in Chapter 13.

If the patient uses a cane, it should be held in the hand opposite the affected side to negate some of the force of gravity on the affected hip. The use of a cane can decrease the load on the hip up to 40 per cent.[1]

The patient should be standing and suitably undressed for the examiner to do a proper observation. The following are viewed from the front, side, and behind:

1. Posture.

2. Whether the patient can and/or will stand on both legs.

3. Whether the limb positions are equal and symmetric.

4. Any obvious shortening of a leg.

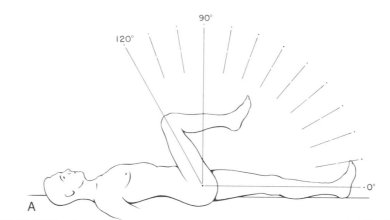

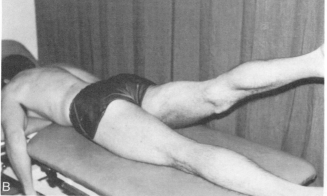

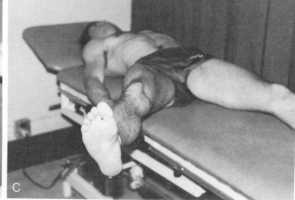

Figure 10–1. Active movements of the hip. (*A*) Flexion. (*B*) Extension. (*C*) Abduction. (*D*) Adduction.

Illustration continued on opposite page

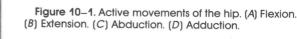

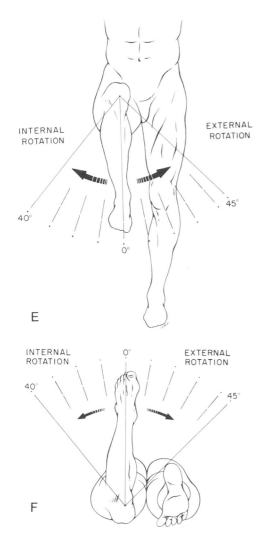

EXTERNAL
ROTATION

40°

45°

0°

E

INTERNAL
ROTATION

0°

EXTERNAL
ROTATION

40°

45°

F

Figure 10–1 *Continued.* (*E*) Rotation in the supine position. (*F*) Rotation in the prone position. (*A, E,* and *F* from Beetham, W. P., et al.: Physical Examination of the Joints. Philadelphia, W. B. Saunders Co., 1965, pp. 134, 137, 138.)

5. Color and texture of the skin.
6. Any scars or sinuses.
7. The patient's willingness to move.

Anterior View. The examiner should note any abnormality of the bony and soft-tissue contours. With many individuals, because of muscle bulk and other soft-tissue deposition, differences in these contours may be difficult to detect. The examiner must therefore look closely. The same is true for swelling. Swelling in the hip joint itself is virtually impossible to detect by observation, whereas swelling resulting from a psoas or trochanteric bursitis may be easily missed if the examiner is not careful.

Lateral View. When the patient is viewed from the side, the contour of the buttock should be observed for any abnormality. As well, a hip flexion deformity is best observed from this position. The examiner should take the time to compare both sides to note any subtle differences between them.

Posterior View. The position of the hip and the effect, if any, of this position on the spine should be noted. For example, a hip flexion contracture may lead to an increased lumbar lordosis. Any differences in bony and soft-tissue contours should again be noted.

Examination

When doing an examination of the hip, the examiner must keep in mind that pain may be referred to the hip from the sacroiliac joints and lumbar spine, and vice versa. Thus the examination may be an extensive one. If there is any doubt as to the location of the lesion, an assessment of the lumbar spine and sacroiliac joints should be performed. It is only through a careful examination of the three areas that the examiner is able to discern where the lesion lies.

As with any examination, the examiner should compare one side of the body with the other, noting any differences. This comparison is necessary because of the individual differences among normal people.

ACTIVE MOVEMENTS

The active movements are done in such a way that the most painful ones are done last. In order to keep movement of the patient to a minimum, some movements are tested in the supine position, others in the prone position. For ease of description, the movements will be described together. When examining the patient, however, the examiner should follow the order as stated in the précis at the end of the chapter.

The following movements should be actively completed in the hip region (Fig. 10–1):

1. Flexion (110 to 120°).
2. Extension (10 to 15°).
3. Abduction (30 to 50°).
4. Adduction (30°).
5. Lateral rotation (40 to 60°).
6. Medial rotation (30 to 40°).

Flexion of the hip is normally 110 to 120° with the knee flexed. The patient's knee is flexed during the test to prevent hamstring tightness from limiting movement.

Extension of the hip normally ranges from 0 to 15°. The patient is in the prone position, and the examiner must ensure that only hip movement is occurring. Patients will have a tendency to extend the lumbar spine, giving the appearance of increased hip extension. This lumbar extension should not be allowed to occur.

Hip abduction ranges from 30 to 50° and is tested with the patient supine. Before asking the patient to do the abduction or adduction movement, the examiner should ensure that the patient's pelvis is "balanced"—with the anterior superior iliac spines (ASIS) level and the legs perpendicular to a line joining the two ASIS. The patient is then asked to abduct one leg at a time without pelvic motion. Pelvic motion is detected by palpation of the ASIS and by telling the patient to stop the movement as soon as the ASIS on either side starts to move. When the patient abducts the leg, the opposite ASIS will move first; with an adduction contracture, this will occur earlier in the range of movement.

Hip *adduction* is normally 30° and is measured from the same starting position. The patient is asked to adduct one leg over the other resting leg while the examiner ensures that the pelvis does not move. When the patient adducts the leg, the ASIS on the same side will move first. This movement will occur earlier in the range of motion with an abduction contracture. Adduction may also be measured by asking the patient to abduct one leg and leave it abducted. The other leg is then tested for the amount of adduction present. The advantage of this method is that the test leg does not have to be flexed to clear the other leg before doing the adduction movement.

Rotation movements may be performed with the patient supine or prone. Medial rotation is normally 30 to 40° while lateral rotation ranges from 40 to 60°. In the supine position, the patient simply rotates the straight leg on a "balanced" pelvis. Turning the foot or leg outward tests lateral rotation; turning the foot or leg inward tests medial rotation. In another supine test (Fig. 10–1E), the patient is asked to flex both the hip and knee to 90°. When using this method, however, one must recognize that having the patient rotate the leg out tests medial rotation whereas the patient rotating the leg in tests lateral rotation. With the patient prone, the pelvis is "balanced" by aligning the legs at right angles to a line joining the posterior superior iliac spines (PSIS). The patient then flexes the knee to 90°. Again, medial rotation is being tested when the leg is rotated outward and lateral rotation is being tested when the leg is rotated inward (Fig. 10–1F). Usually, one of the last two methods is used to measure hip rotation, since it is easier to measure the angle when performing the test.

If the patient is able to do the preceding activities with little difficulty, the examiner may use a series of *functional tests* to see if increased intensity of activity produces pain or other symptoms. The functional activities in order of sequence are:

1. Squatting.
2. Going up and down stairs one at a time.
3. Crossing the legs so that the ankle of one foot rests on the knee of the opposite leg.
4. Going up and down stairs two or more at a time.
5. Running straight ahead.
6. Running and twisting.
7. Jumping.

These tests must be geared to the individual patient. Older individuals should not be expected to do the last four activities unless they have been doing these movements or similar ones in the recent past.

PASSIVE MOVEMENTS

If, during the active movements, the range of movement was not full and the examiner was unable to test end feel, passive movements should be performed to determine the end feel and passive range of motion. The passive movements are the same as the active movements. All the movements except extension can be tested in the supine lying position.

The capsular pattern of the hip is flexion, abduction, and medial rotation. These movements are always the ones most limited in a capsular pattern, although the order of restriction may vary. For example, medial rotation may be most limited, followed by flexion and abduction. The hip joint is the only joint to exhibit this altered pattern of the same movements.

The normal end feels the examiner should find on passive movements of the hip are as follows:

1. Flexion—tissue approximation or tissue stretch.
2. Extension—tissue stretch.
3. Abduction—tissue stretch.
4. Adduction—tissue approximation or tissue stretch.
5. Medial rotation—tissue stretch.

Intra-abdominal inflammation in the lower pelvis, as in the case of an abscess, may elicit pain on passive medial and lateral rotation of the hip when the patient is supine with the hip and knee at 90°.

During hip movements the pelvis should not move. Groin discomfort and a limited range of motion on medial rotation are good indications of hip problems.

RESISTED ISOMETRIC MOVEMENTS

The resisted isometric movements are done with the patient supine (Fig. 10–2). Because the hip muscles are very strong, the examiner should position the patient's hip properly and say to the patient: "Don't let me move your hip," to ensure that the movement is isometric. By carefully not-

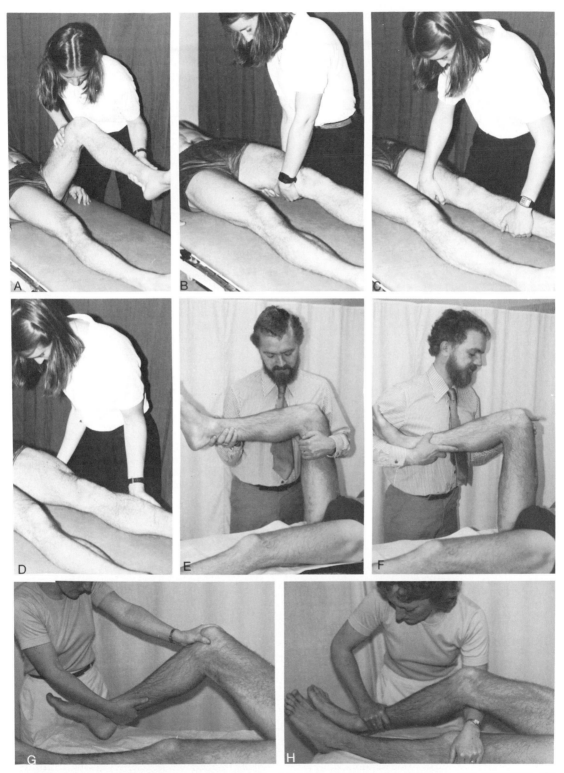

Figure 10–2. Resisted isometric movements about the hip. (*A*) Flexion. (*B*) Extension. (*C*) Adduction. (*D*) Abduction. (*E*) Medial rotation. (*F*) Lateral rotation. (*G*) Knee flexion. (*H*) Knee extension.

ing which movements cause pain or show weakness when doing the tests isometrically, the examiner should be able to determine which muscle if any, is at fault. For example, the gluteus maximus is the only muscle that is involved in all of the following movements: extension, adduction, and lateral rotation. As with active movements, the most painful movements are performed last.

The movements tests isometrically are:
1. Flexion of the hip.
2. Extension of the hip.
3. Abduction of the hip.
4. Adduction of the hip.
5. Medial rotation of the hip.
6. Lateral rotation of the hip.
7. Flexion of the knee.
8. Extension of the knee.

Resisted isometric flexion and extension of the knee must be performed because there are two joint muscles (hamstrings, rectus femoris) that act over the knee as well as the hip. The examiner must be aware that intra-abdominal inflammation in the area of the psoas muscle may elicit pain on resisted hip flexion. The pain from intra-abdominal inflammation will not present in a subacute infection or with a rigid abdominal wall. Refer to Table 10–1 for the muscles that act on the hip.

Table 10–1. Muscles of the Hip: Their Action, Innervation, and Nerve Root Deviation

Action	Muscle Involved	Innervation	Nerve Root Deviation
Flexion of hip	1. Psoas	L1, L2, L3	L1, L2, L3
	2. Iliacus	Femoral	L2, L3
	3. Rectus femoris	Femoral	L2, L3, L4
	4. Sartorius	Femoral	L2, L3
	5. Pectineus	Femoral	L2, L3
	6. Adductor longus	Obturator	L2, L3, L4
	7. Adductor brevis	Obturator	L2, L3, L5
	8. Gracilis	Obturator	L2, L3
Extension of hip	1. Biceps femoris	Sciatic	L5, S1, S2
	2. Semimembranosus	Sciatic	L5, S1, S2
	3. Semitendinosus	Sciatic	L5, S1, S2
	4. Gluteus maximus	Inferior gluteal	L5, S1, S2
	5. Gluteus medius (posterior part)	Superior gluteal	L5, S1
	6. Adductor magnus (ischiocondylar part)	Sciatic	L2, L3, L4
Abduction of hip	1. Tensor fasciae latae	Superior gluteal	L4, L5
	2. Gluteus minimus	Superior gluteal	L5, S1
	3. Gluteus medius	Superior gluteal	L5, S1
	4. Gluteus maximus	Inferior gluteal	L5, S1, S2
	5. Sartorius	Femoral	L2, L3
Adduction of hip	1. Adductor longus	Obturator	L2, L3, L4
	2. Adductor brevis	Obturator	L2, L3, L4
	3. Adductor magnus (ischiofemoral portion)	Obturator	L2, L3, L4
	4. Gracilis	Obturator	L2, L3
	5. Pectineus	Femoral	L2, L3
Medial rotation of hip	1. Adductor longus	Obturator	L2, L3, L4
	2. Adductor brevis	Obturator	L2, L3, L4
	3. Adductor magnus	Obturator and sciatic	L2, L3, L4 L2, L3, L4
	4. Gluteus medius (anterior part)	Superior gluteal	L5, S1
	5. Gluteus minimus (anterior part)	Superior gluteal	L5, S1
	6. Tensor fasciae latae	Superior gluteal	L4, L5
	7. Pectineus	Femoral	L2, L3
	8. Gracilis	Obturator	L2, L3
Lateral rotation of hip	1. Gluteus maximus	Inferior gluteal	L5, S1, S2
	2. Obturator internus	N. to obturator internus	L5, S1
	3. Obturator externus	Obturator	L3, L4
	4. Quadratus femoris	N. to quadratus femoris	L5, S1
	5. Piriformis	L5, S1, S2	L5, S1, S2
	6. Gemellus superior	N. to obturator internus	L5, S1
	7. Gemellus inferior	N. to quadratus femoris	L5, S1
	8. Sartorius	Femoral	L2, L3
	9. Gluteus medius (posterior part)	Superior gluteal	L5, S1

SPECIAL TESTS

Only those tests which the examiner feels are necessary should be performed.

Sign of the Buttock

The patient lies in a supine position, and the examiner performs a straight leg raise test. If there is limitation on the straight leg raise, the examiner then flexes the patient's hip with the knee flexed. If there is a combination of restriction with knee straight and flexed, the lesion is in the buttock and not in the hip, sciatic nerve, or hamstring muscles. There may also be some limited trunk flexion. A cause of this problem is a bursitis, a neoplasm, or an abscess in the buttock.

True Leg Length

Before any measuring is done, the examiner must set the pelvis square, level, or "balanced" with the lower limbs. *Balanced* means that the ASIS are in a straight line and the lower limbs perpendicular to that line.[2-4] The legs should be 15 to 20 cm apart and parallel to each other (Fig. 10–3). If the legs are not placed in proper relation to the pelvis, apparent shortening of the limb may occur. The lower limbs must be placed in comparable positions relative to the pelvis because abduction of the hip brings the medial malleolus closer to the ASIS on that side and adduction of the hip takes the medial malleolus further from the ASIS on that side. If one hip is fixed in abduction or adduction, the good hip should be adducted or abducted an equal amount.

In North America, leg length measurement is usually taken to the medial malleolus; however, these values may be altered by muscle wasting or obesity. Measuring to the lateral malleolus is less likely to be affected by this technique. To obtain the leg length, the examiner measures from the ASIS to the lateral malleolus. The flat metal end of the tape measure is placed immediately distal to the ASIS and pushed up against it. The thumb then presses the tape end firmly against the bone, giving rigid fixation of the tape measure against the bone. The index finger of the other hand is placed immediately distal to the lateral malleolus and pushed against it. The thumbnail is brought down against the tip of the index finger so that the tape measure is pinched between them. A slight difference, up to 1 to 1.5 cm, is considered normal; however, it can still cause symptoms.

If one leg is shorter than the other (Fig. 10–4), the examiner can determine where the difference is by measuring:

1. From the iliac crest to the greater trochanter of the femur for coxa vara.

2. From the greater trochanter of the femur to the knee joint line on the lateral aspect for femoral shaft shortening.

3. From the knee joint line on the medial side to the medial malleolus for the tibial shaft shortening.

Apparent or functional shortening (Fig. 10–5) of the leg is evident if the patient has a lateral pelvic tilt when the measurement is taken. When measuring apparent leg length shortening, the examiner obtains the distance from the tip of the xiphisternum or umbilicus to the medial malleolus. Values obtained by these measurements may be affected by muscle wasting, obesity, and asymmetric position of xiphisternum or umbilicus.

The neck-shaft angle of the femur (Fig. 10–6) is between 150° and 160° at birth and decreases to between 120° and 135° in the adult (Fig. 10–7). If this angle is less than 120° in an adult, it is known as *coxa vara*; if greater than 135° in the adult, the condition is called *coxa valga*.

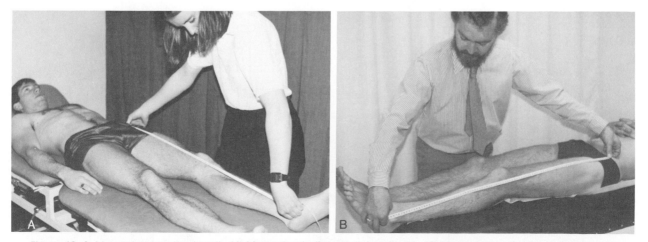

Figure 10–3. Measuring true leg length. (A) Measuring to the medial malleolus. (B) Measuring to the lateral malleolus.

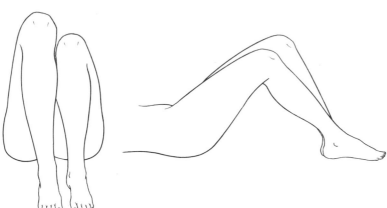

LEFT SHORTENED
TIBIA

RIGHT SHORTENED
FEMUR

Figure 10–4. Leg length discrepancy.

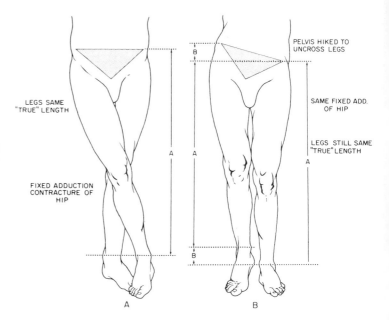

LEGS SAME
"TRUE" LENGTH

FIXED ADDUCTION
CONTRACTURE OF
HIP

PELVIS HIKED TO
UNCROSS LEGS

SAME FIXED ADD.
OF HIP

LEGS STILL SAME
"TRUE" LENGTH

A

B

Figure 10–5. Functional shortening. (From the American Orthopaedic Association: Manual of Orthopaedic Surgery. Chicago, 1972, p. 45.)

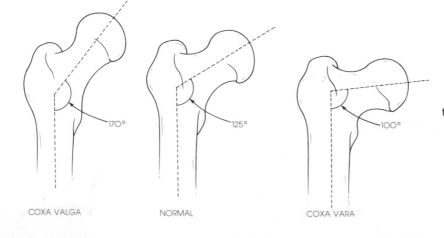

170°

125°

100°

COXA VALGA

NORMAL

COXA VARA

Figure 10–6. Neck-shaft angles of the femur in adults.

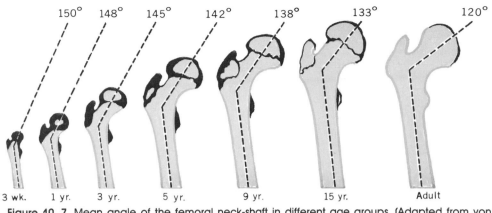

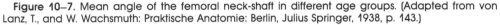

Figure 10–7. Mean angle of the femoral neck-shaft in different age groups. (Adapted from von Lanz, T., and W. Wachsmuth: Praktische Anatomie: Berlin, Julius Springer, 1938, p. 143.)

Adduction Contracture Test

The patient lies supine with the anterior superior iliac spines level. If a contracture is present, the affected leg will form an angle of less than 90° with the line joining the two anterior superior iliac spines. If the examiner then attempts to "balance" the lower limb with the pelvis, the pelvis will shift up on the affected side or down on the unaffected side and balancing will not be possible. This type of contracture can lead to functional shortening of the limb rather than true shortening.

Abduction Contracture Test

The patient lies in the supine position with each ASIS level. If a contracture is present, the affected leg will form an angle of more than 90°, with a line joining each ASIS. If the examiner then attempts to balance the lower limb with the pelvis, the pelvis will shift down on the affected side or up on the unaffected side and balancing will not be possible. This can lead to functional shortening of the limb rather than true shortening.

Nélaton's Line

Nélaton's line is an imaginary line drawn from the ischial tuberosity of the pelvis to the ASIS of the pelvis on the same side (Fig. 10–8).[5] If the greater trochanter of the femur is palpated well above the line, it is an indication of a dislocated hip or coxa vara. Both sides should be compared.

Bryant's Triangle

With the patient lying supine, the examiner drops an imaginary perpendicular line from the ASIS of the pelvis to the examination table.[5] A second imaginary line is projected up from the tip of the greater trochanter of the femur to meet the first line at a right angle (Fig. 10–9). This line is measured and both sides are compared for coxa vara, dislocated hip, and so on. This measurement can be done on radiographs, in which case the lines may be drawn on the radiograph.

Thomas Test

The Thomas test is used to assess a hip flexion contracture, the most common contracture of the hip. The patient lies supine while the examiner ensures that excessive lordosis is not evident. In most cases with tight hip flexors, it will be. The examiner flexes one of the patient's hips bringing the knee to the chest to flatten out the lumbar spine and the patient holds the flexed hip against

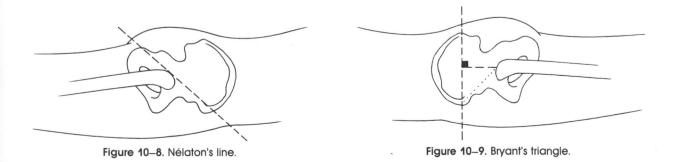

Figure 10–8. Nélaton's line.

Figure 10–9. Bryant's triangle.

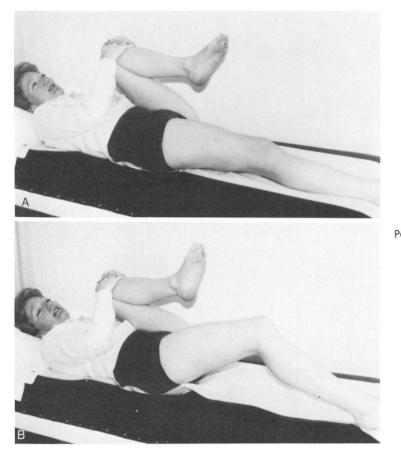

Figure 10–10. Thomas test. (*A*) Negative test. (*B*) Positive test.

the chest. If there is no flexion contracture, the hip being tested (the straight leg) will remain on the treatment table. If a contracture is present, the patient's straight leg will rise off the bed, indicating a positive sign (Fig. 10–10). The angle of contracture can be measured. If the lower limb is pushed down onto the table the patient may exhibit an increased lordosis; again, this would indicate a positive test.

Rectus Femoris Contracture (Method 1)

The patient lies supine with the knees bent over the end or edge of a treatment table. The patient flexes one knee onto the chest and holds it (Fig. 10–11). The angle of the other knee should remain at 90° when the hip is flexed to the chest. If it does not (i.e., the test knee extends slightly),

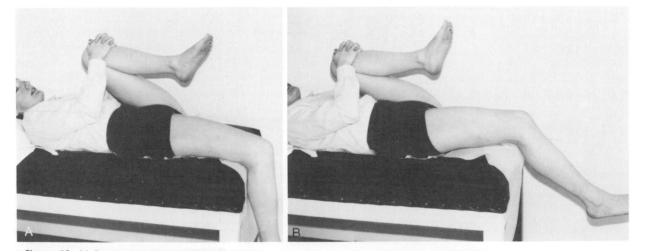

Figure 10–11. Rectus femoris contracture. (*A*) The movement leg is brought to the chest with the test leg bent over the end of the examining table (negative test). (*B*) The right knee extends, indicating a positive test.

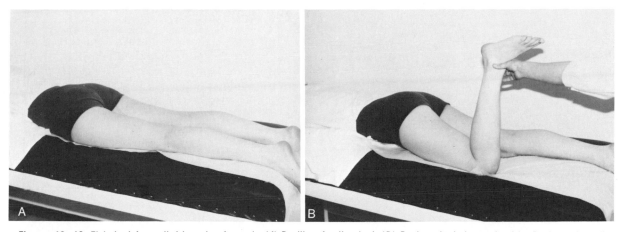

Figure 10–12. Ely's test for a tight rectus femoris. (*A*) Position for the test. (*B*) Posture test shown by hip flexion when the knee is flexed.

a contracture is probably present. The examiner may attempt to passively flex the knee to see whether it will remain at 90° of its own volition. The examiner should always palpate for muscle tightness when doing any contracture test. If there is no palpable tightness, the probable cause of restriction is tight joint structures (e.g., the capsule). Both sides should be tested and compared.

Ely's Test (Test for Tight Rectus Femoris—Method 2)

The patient lies prone, and the examiner passively flexes the patient's knee (Fig. 10–12).[6] On flexion of the knee, the patient's hip on the same side will spontaneously flex, indicating that the rectus femoris muscle is tight on that side and that the test is positive. Both sides should be tested and compared.

Ober's Test

Ober's test assesses tensor fasciae latae (iliotibial band) contracture (Fig. 10–13).[7] The patient is in the sidelying position with the lower leg flexed at the hip and knee for stability. The examiner then passively abducts and extends the patient's upper leg with the knee straight or flexed to 90°. The examiner slowly lowers the upper limb and if a contracture is present, it will remain abducted and will not fall to the bed. When doing this test, it is important to extend the hip slightly so that the iliotibial band passes over the greater trochanter of the femur. To do this, the examiner stabilizes the pelvis at the same time to stop the pelvis from "falling backwards." Ober originally described the test with the knee flexed.[7] However, the iliotibial band has a greater stretch placed on it when the knee is extended.

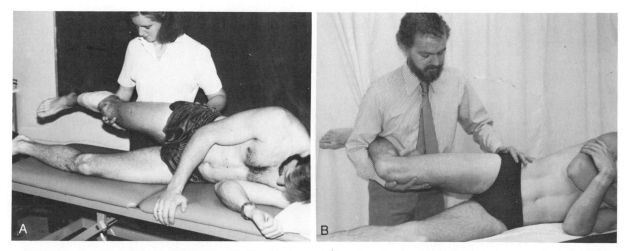

Figure 10–13. Ober's test. (*A*) Knees straight. The hip is passively extended by the examiner to ensure that the tensor fasciae latae runs over the greater trochanter. A positive test is indicated when the leg remains abducted while the patient's muscles are relaxed. (*B*) Knee flexed.

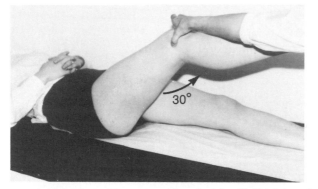

Figure 10-14. Noble compression test for iliotibial band friction syndrome. The patient extends the knee. The examiner is indicating where pain will be felt.

Noble Compression Test

This test is used to determine whether iliotibial band friction syndrome exists near the knee (Fig. 10–14).[8] The patient lies in a supine position, and the knee is flexed to 90° accompanied by hip flexion. The examiner then applies pressure with the thumb to the lateral femoral epicondyle or 1 to 2 cm proximal to it. While maintaining the pressure, the patient's knee is slowly extended. At about 30° of flexion (0° being a straight leg), the patient will complain of severe pain over the lateral femoral condyle; this indicates a positive test. The patient will say it is the same pain that accompanies activity (e.g., running).

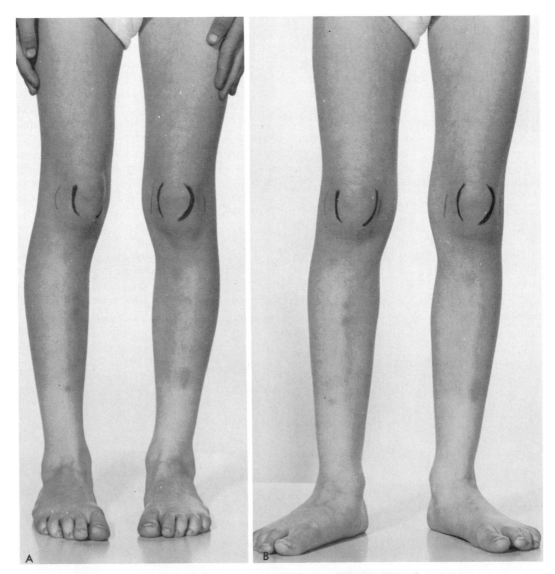

Figure 10-15. Clinical appearance of excessive femoral torsion in a girl. (*A*) With the knees in full extension and the feet aligned (pointing straight forward), the legs appear bowed and the patellae face inward (squinting patella). (*B*) Upon lateral rotation of the hips so that the patellae are facing to the front, the feet and legs point outward and the bowleg appearance is corrected. (From Tachdjian, M. O.: Pediatric Orthopedics. Philadelphia, W. B. Saunders Co., 1972, p. 1453.)

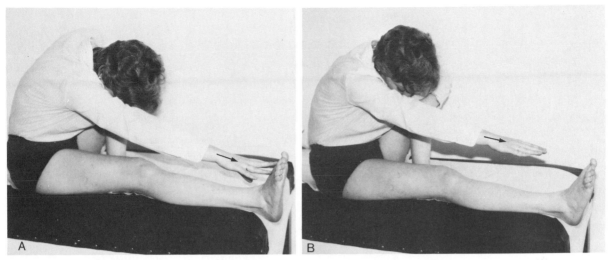

Figure 10–16. Test for hamstring tightness (Method 1). (*A*) Negative test. (*B*) Positive test.

Rotational Deformities

The patient lies supine with the lower limbs straight while the examiner looks at the patellae.[9] If the patellae face in ("squinting" patellae), it is an indication of medial rotation of the femur or tibia. If the patellae face up and out away from each other ("frog's eye" or "grasshopper eye" patellae), it is an indication of lateral rotation of the femur or tibia. If the tibia is affected, the feet will face in ("pigeon toe") for medial rotation and face out more than 10° for excessive lateral rotation of the tibia (Fig. 10–15). Normally, the feet angle out 5 to 10° for better balance.

Hamstrings Contracture Test (Method 1)

The patient is instructed to sit with one knee flexed against the chest to stabilize the pelvis and the other knee extended (Fig. 10–16). The patient then attempts to flex the trunk and touch the toes of the extended lower limb (test leg) with the fingers. The test is then repeated on the other side. A comparison is made between the two sides. Normally, an individual should be able to at least touch the toes while keeping the knee extended. If the patient is unable to do so, it is an indication of tight hamstrings on the straight leg.

Figure 10–17. Tripod sign.

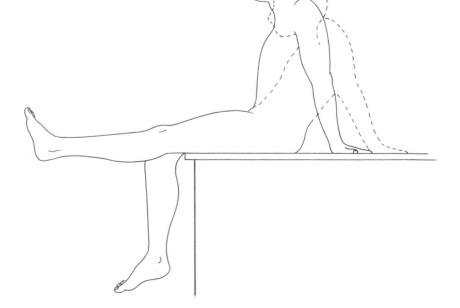

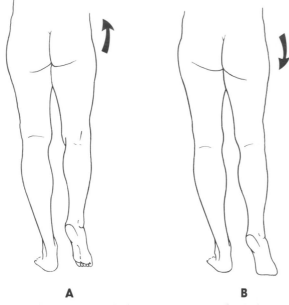

Figure 10–18. Trendelenburg sign. (*A*) Negative test. (*B*) Positive test.

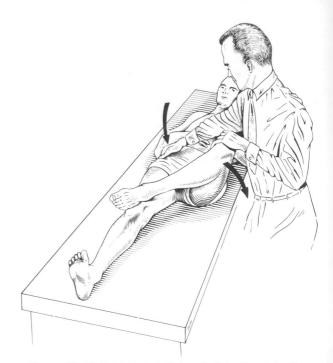

Figure 10–19. Patrick's test (Faber test) for the detection of limitation of motion in the hip. (From Beetham, W. P., et al.: Physical Examination of the Joints. Philadelphia, W. B. Saunders Co., 1965, p. 139.)

Tripod Sign (Hamstrings Contracture Method 2)

The patient is seated with both knees flexed to 90° over the edge of the examining table (Fig. 10–17).[10] The examiner then passively extends one knee. If the hamstring muscles on that side are tight, the patient will extend the trunk to relieve the tension in the hamstring muscles. The leg is returned to its starting position and the other leg is tested. A comparison of the two legs is made. Extension of the spine is indicative of a positive test. The examiner must be aware that nerve root problems (stretching of the sciatic nerve) can cause a similar positive sign.

Trendelenburg Test

This test assesses stability of the hip and the ability of the hip abductors to stabilize the pelvis on the femur. The patient is asked to stand on one lower limb. Normally the pelvis on the opposite side should rise. This finding indicates a negative test (Fig. 10–18). If, when the patient is asked to stand on the affected leg, the pelvis on the opposite side drops, it indicates a positive test. The test should always be performed on the

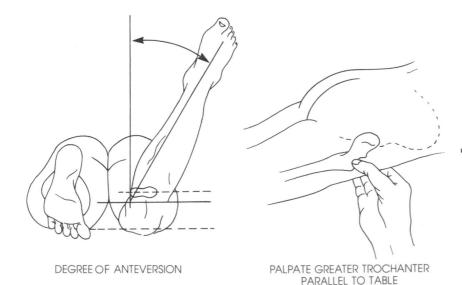

DEGREE OF ANTEVERSION

PALPATE GREATER TROCHANTER PARALLEL TO TABLE

Figure 10–20. Craig test for femoral anteversion.

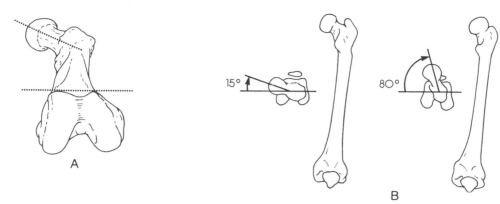

Figure 10–21. Anteversion of the hip. (*A*) Femoral anteversion angle. (From the American Orthopaedic Association: Manual of Orthopaedic Surgery. Chicago, 1972, p. 105.) (*B*) Normal angle. (*C*) Excessive angle.

sound side first so that the patient understands what to do. If the pelvis drops on the opposite side, it indicates a weak gluteus medius or an unstable hip on the affected side.

Patrick's Test ("Faber" Test)

The patient lies supine, and the examiner places the patient's test leg so that the foot of the test leg is on the top of the opposite knee (Fig. 10–19). The examiner then slowly lowers the test leg in abduction toward the examining table. A negative test is indicated by the test leg falling to the table or being at least parallel with the opposite leg. A positive test is indicated by the test leg remaining above the opposite straight leg. If positive, the test indicates that (1) the hip joint may be affected, there may be iliopsoas spasm, or the sacroiliac joint may be affected. "Faber"—*f*lexion, *ab*duction and *e*xternal *r*otation—is the position of the hip when the patient begins the test.

Craig Test

The Craig test measures femoral anteversion, or forward torsion (Fig. 10–20). Anteversion of the

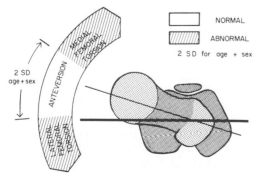

Figure 10–22. Axial view of right femur showing approximately normal range of anteversion and torsional deformity beyond. (From Staheli, L. T.: Orthop. Clin. North Am. *11*:40, 1980.)

hip is the angle the femoral neck makes with the femoral condyles (Fig. 10–21). It is the degree of forward projection of the femoral neck from the coronal plane of the shaft (Fig. 10–22). It decreases with age. For example, at birth the mean angle is about 30° and in the adult the mean average is 8 to 15° (Fig. 10–23). Increased anteversion will lead to squinting patellae and toeing-in. Excessive anteversion is twice as common in girls as in boys. A common clinical finding of excessive anteversion is excessive medial hip rotation and decreased lateral rotation. In *retroversion*, the plane of the femoral neck rotates

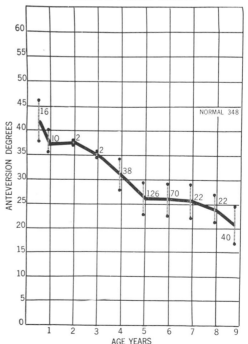

Figure 10–23. The degree of normal femoral torsion in relation to age. Solid lines represent the mean; vertical lines represent standard deviation. (From Crane, L.: J. Bone Joint Surg. *41-A*:423, 1959.)

backward in relation to the coronal condylar plane.[5, 9, 11, 12]

For the Craig test, the patient lies in a prone position with the knee flexed to 90°. The examiner palpates the posterior aspect of the greater trochanter of the femur. The hip is then passively medially and laterally rotated until the greater trochanter is parallel with the examining table or until it reaches its most lateral position. The degree of anteversion can then be estimated, based on the angle of the lower leg with the vertical. The test is also called the *Ryder method* for measuring anteversion or retroversion.

Ortolani's Sign

The Ortolani test can determine whether an infant has a congenital dislocation of the hip (Fig. 10–24A and B).[9] With the infant in the supine position, the examiner flexes the hips and grasps

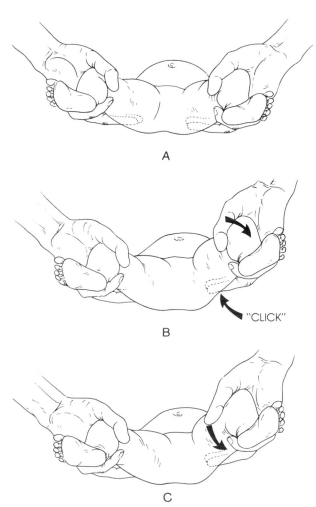

"CLICK"

Figure 10–24. Ortolani's sign and Barlow's test. In the newborn, both hips can be equally flexed, abducted, and externally rotated without producing a "click." (*A*) Normal. (*B*) Ortolani's sign or first part of Barlow's test. (*C*) Barlow's test, second part.

the legs so that the thumbs are against the inside of the knee and thigh and the fingers are placed along the outside of the thigh to the buttock. With gentle traction, the thighs are abducted and pressure is applied against the greater trochanters of the femur. Resistance will begin to be felt to abduction and lateral rotation at about 30 to 40°. The examiner may feel a "click," "clunk," or "jerk," which indicates a positive test and that the hip has reduced; it will be found that increased abduction of the hip will be obtained. The femoral head has slipped over the acetabular ridge into the acetabulum and normal abduction of 70 to 90° can then be obtained.

This test is valid only for the first few weeks after birth and only for dislocated and lax hips, not for dislocations that are difficult to reduce. The examiner should take care to feel the quality of the click. Soft clicks may occur without dislocation and are thought to be due to the iliofemoral ligament clicking over the anterior surface of the head of the femur as it is laterally rotated. Soft clicking usually occurs without the prior resistance that is seen with dislocations. By repeated rotation of the hip, the exact location of the click can be palpated. However, Ortolani's test should not be repeated too often because it could potentially lead to damage of the articular cartilage of the femoral head.

Barlow's Test

Barlow's test is a modification of Ortolani's test[9] (Fig. 10–24A–C). The infant lies supine with the legs facing the examiner. The hips are flexed to 90°, and the knees are fully flexed. Each hip is evaluated individually while the other hand steadies the opposite femur and pelvis. The examiner's middle finger of each hand is placed over the greater trochanter, and the thumb is placed adjacent to the inner side of the knee and thigh opposite the lesser trochanter. The hip is taken into abduction while the examiner's middle finger applies forward pressure behind the greater trochanter. If the femoral head slips forward into the acetabulum with a click, clunk, or jerk, the test is positive, indicating that the hip was dislocated. This part of the test is identical to Ortolani's test. The examiner then uses the thumb to apply pressure backward and outward on the inner thigh. If the femoral head slips out over the posterior lip of the acetabulum and then reduces again when pressure is removed, the hip is classified as "unstable." The hip is not dislocated, but is dislocatable. The procedure is repeated for the other hip.

This test may be used for infants up to 6 months of age. It should not be repeated too often because it may result in a dislocated hip as well as articular damage to the head of the femur.

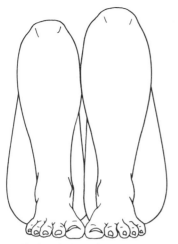

Figure 10–25. Galeazzi's sign (Allis' test).

Galeazzi's Sign (Allis' Test)

The Galeazzi test is good for assessing unilateral congenital dislocation of the hip only and may be used in children from 3 to 18 months of age. The child lies in a supine position with the knees flexed and the hips flexed to 90°. A positive test is indicated by one knee being higher than the other (Fig. 10–25).

Telescoping Sign

The telescoping sign is evident in children who have a dislocated hip. The child lies supine. The examiner flexes the knee and hip to 90°. The femur is then pushed down into the treatment table. The femur and leg are then lifted up and away from the table (Fig. 10–26). With the normal hip, it will be found that little movement occurs with this action. With the dislocated hip, however, there will be a lot of relative movement. This excessive movement is called *telescoping* or *pistoning*.

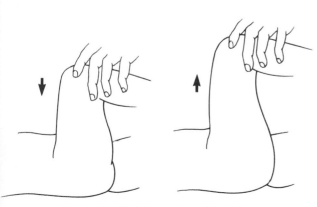

Figure 10–26. Telescoping of the hip.

REFLEXES AND CUTANEOUS DISTRIBUTION

There are no reflexes about the hip that can be easily evaluated. However, the examiner should assess the normal dermatome patterns of the nerve roots (Fig. 10–27) as well as the cutaneous distribution of the peripheral nerves (Fig. 10–28). For example, in a condition called *meralgia paresthetica*, there is pressure placed on the lateral cutaneous nerve of the thigh, running in the fascia near the ASIS as it passes under the inguinal ligament. There will be an alteration in sensation and possibly painful skin in the area supplied by the nerve. Since dermatomes vary from person to person, the accompanying diagrams are estimations only. Testing for altered sensation is performed by running the relaxed hands and fingers over the pelvis and legs anteriorly, posteriorly, and laterally. Any difference in sensation should be noted and can be mapped out more exactly using a pinwheel, pin, cotton batten, and/or brush.

True hip pain is usually referred to the groin, but it may also be referred to the ankle, knee, lumbar spine, and sacroiliac joints (Fig. 10–29).

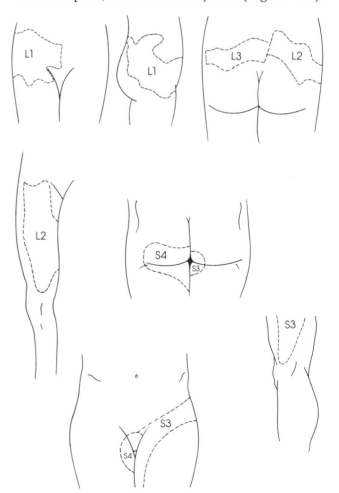

Figure 10–27. Dermatomes about the hip. One side only is illustrated.

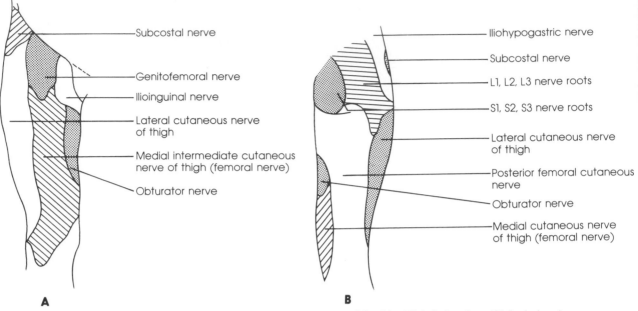

Figure 10–28. Sensory distribution of peripheral nerves about the hip. (*A*) Anterior view. (*B*) Posterior view.

The knee, sacroiliac joints, and lumbar spine may refer pain to the hip as well.

JOINT PLAY MOVEMENTS

The joint play movements are completed with the patient in the supine position. The examiner should attempt to compare the amount of available movement on both sides. Small differences may be difficult to detect because of the large muscle bulk in the area.

The joint play movements performed at the hip are shown in Figure 10–30:

1. Caudal glide of the femur (long leg traction or long axis extension).

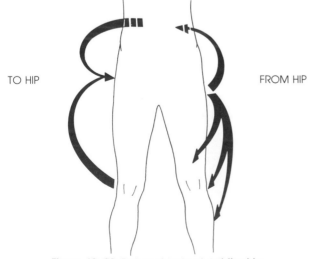

Figure 10–29. Referred pain about the hip.

2. Compression.
3. Lateral distraction.
4. Quadrant test.[23]

Caudal Glide

The examiner places both hands around the patient's leg slightly above the ankle. The examiner then leans back, applying a long axis extension to the entire lower limb. Part of the movement will occur in the knee. If one suspects some pathology in the knee or the knee is stiff, both hands should be placed around the thigh just proximal to the knee and again traction force applied (Fig. 10–30A). The first method enables the examiner to apply a greater force. During the movement, any telescoping or excessive movement occurring in the hip should be noted.

Compression

The examiner places the patient's knee in the resting position, then applies a compressive force to the hip through the longitudinal axis of the femur by pushing through the femoral condyles.

Lateral Distraction

The examiner applies the lateral distraction force to the hip by placing a wide strap around the leg as high up in the groin as possible. The strap is then wrapped around the examiner's buttocks. The examiner leans back, using the

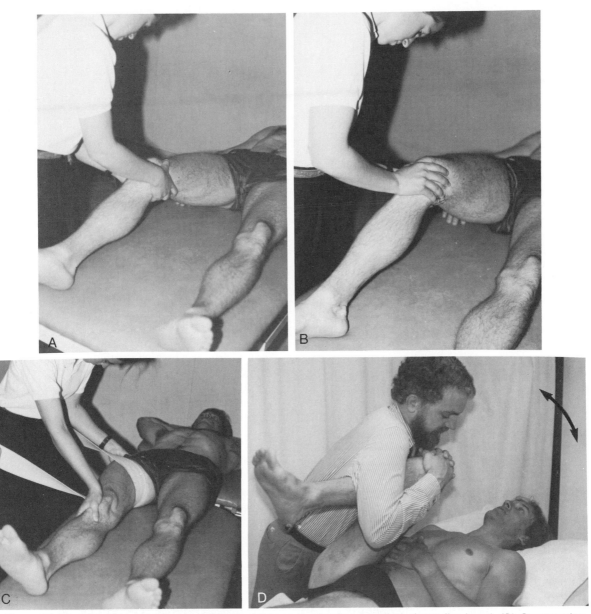

Figure 10–30. Joint play movements of the hip. (*A*) Long leg traction (applied above the knee). (*B*) Compression. (*C*) Lateral distraction. (*D*) Quadrant test.

buttocks to apply the distractive force to the hip. The proximal hand is used to palpate hip movement while the distal hand prevents abduction of the leg and hence torque to the hip.

Quadrant Test

The examiner flexes and adducts the patient's hip so that the hip faces the patient's opposite shoulder and resistance to the movement is felt. While slight resistance is being maintained, the patient's hip is taken into abduction while maintaining flexion in an arc of movement. As the movement is performed, the examiner should look for any irregularity in the movement (e.g., "bumps"), pain, or patient apprehension, which may give an indication of where the pathology is occurring in the hip.[13]

PALPATION

During palpation of the hip and associated muscles, the examiner should note any tenderness, temperature, muscle spasm, or other signs and symptoms that may indicate the source of disease.

Anterior Aspect

Anteriorly, the following structure should be palpated as shown in Figure 10–31.

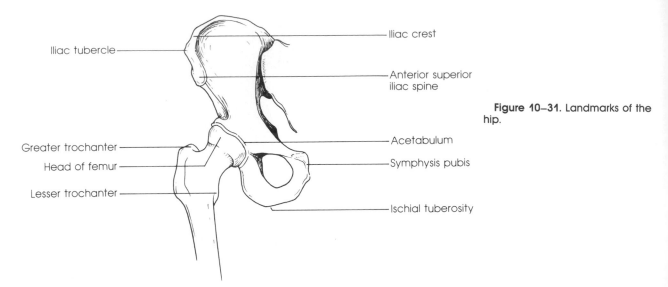

Iliac tubercle

Iliac crest

Anterior superior iliac spine

Figure 10–31. Landmarks of the hip.

Greater trochanter

Head of femur

Lesser trochanter

Acetabulum

Symphysis pubis

Ischial tuberosity

Iliac Crest, Greater Trochanter, and Anterior Superior Iliac Spine. The iliac crests are easily palpated and should be level. The crest should be palpated for any tenderness because several muscles insert into this structure. In athletes, a condition called a "hip pointer" may be located on the iliac crest. This occurs from a strain of the muscles that insert into the crest or from a contusion of the same muscles where they insert. During palpation along the lateral aspect of the crest, the iliac tubercle will be felt. The examiner then moves anteriorly to the ASIS. The greater trochanter, located approximately 10 cm distal to the iliac tubercle of the iliac crest, is palpated next. If the examiner's thumbs are placed over each ASIS, the fingers will naturally lie along the lateral aspects of the thigh and the greater trochanter on each side can be felt with the fingers. If the trochanteric bursa is swollen, it may also be palpated over the greater trochanter.

Inguinal Ligament, Femoral Triangle, Hip Joint, and Symphysis Pubis. The examiner's fingers are placed on the ASIS. Palpation gently continues along the inguinal ligament to the pelvic tubercles (symphysis pubis), with the examiner noting any signs of pathology (Fig. 10–32). The psoas bursa, if swollen, is usually palpable over the inguinal ligament at its midpoint. Moving distal to the inguinal ligament, the examiner palpates the femoral triangle, the boundaries of which are the inguinal ligament (superiorly), the sartorius muscle (laterally), and the adductor longus muscle (medially). Within the femoral triangle, the examiner may palpate swollen lymph glands (Fig. 10–33) and the femoral artery. The femoral nerve lies lateral to the artery and the femoral vein lies medial to the artery, but neither of these structures is easily palpated. At this stage, the examiner may decide to palpate for an inguinal hernia in the male. The head of the femur is then palpated. Although the hip joint is deep

and not easily palpable, the surrounding structures may show signs of pathology. The head of the femur is 1 to 2 cm below the middle one third of the inguinal ligament and is found on a horizontal line running halfway between the pubic tubercle and the greater trochanter.

The examiner concludes the anterior palpation by palpating the hip flexor, adductor, and abductor muscles for signs of pathology.

Posterior Aspect

The patient is then asked to lie prone so that the following structures can be palpated.

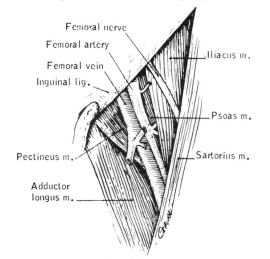

Femoral nerve

Femoral artery

Femoral vein

Inguinal lig.

Iliacus m.

Psoas m.

Pectineus m.

Sartorius m.

Adductor longus m.

Figure 10–32. Femoral triangle. Note compartment formed by the inguinal ligament above, the iliopsoas laterally, adductors medially, the compartment housing the femoral artery, vein and nerve. The sartorius and rectus attach to the anterosuperior spine whereas the adductor muscles attach along the pubic ramus. Note also how the psoas and iliacus blend to form the iliopsoas tendon, which attaches to the lesser trochanter of the femur. Modified from Ancon, B. J.: Atlas of Human Anatomy. Philadelphia, W. B. Saunders Co., 1963, p. 583.

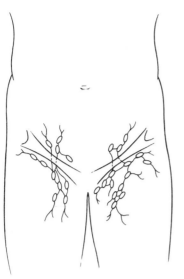

Figure 10–33. Lymph glands in the groin area.

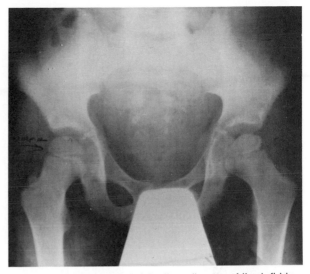

Figure 10–34. Legg-Calvé-Perthes disease of the left hip.

Iliac Crest, Posterior Superior Iliac Spine, Ischial Tuberosity, and Greater Trochanter. The examiner begins posterior palpation by following the iliac crests, which are easily palpable, posteriorly to the PSIS. On most individuals, each PSIS is evident by overlying skin dimples. As the examiner moves caudally, the ischial tuberosities, which are at about the level of the gluteal folds, may be felt. If the ischial bursa is swollen, it is sometimes palpable over the ischial tuberosities. The tuberosities should also be palpated for possible tenderness of the hamstrings muscle insertions. Laterally the posterior aspect of the greater trochanter is felt. If the distance between the ischial tuberosity and greater trochanter is divided in half, the fingers will lie over the sciatic nerve as it enters the lower limb. Normally, the nerve is not palpable. The examiner then palpates upward from the midpoint to see whether there is any tenderness of the hip lateral rotators, especially the piriformis muscle. In addition, the gluteal and hamstring muscle bellies should be palpated for signs of pathology.

Sacroiliac, Lumbosacral, and Sacrococcygeal Joints. If the examiner suspects pathology in these joints, they should be palpated. A detailed description of their palpation is given in Chapters 8 (lumbar spine) and 9 (pelvic joints).

RADIOLOGY OF THE HIP

Anteroposterior View

The examiner should compare both hips, noting the following features:

1. Joint spaces.
2. Presence of any bone disease (i.e., Legg-Calvé-Perthes disease, bony cysts, or tumors) (Fig. 10–34).
3. Neck-shaft angle. The examiner should note whether the angle is normal or whether the patient exhibits a coxa vara or coxa valga.
4. Shape of the femoral head.
5. Presence of osteophytes.
6. Whether *Shenton's line* is normal. Normally, Shenton's line is curved, drawn along the medial curved edge of the femur, continuing upward in a smooth arc along the inferior edge of the pubis (Fig. 10–35). If the head of the femur is dislocated or fractured, two lines form two separate arcs, indicating a broken line. A broken Shenton's line is diagnostic.
7. Any evidence of fracture or dislocation (Fig. 10–36). Is the pelvic ring intact, or has it been disrupted? Disruption of the pelvic ring indicates severe injury.

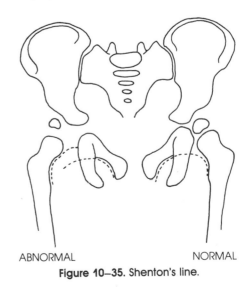

ABNORMAL   NORMAL

Figure 10–35. Shenton's line.

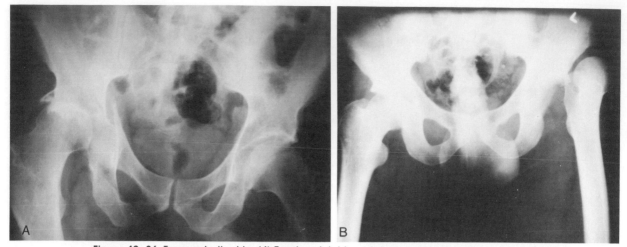

Figure 10–36. Trauma to the hip. (*A*) Fractured right acetabulum. (*B*) Dislocated left femur.

8. Pelvic distortion.

9. Whether Hilgenreiner's and Perkin's lines are within normal limits. *Hilgenreiner's line* is horizontal, drawn between the inferior parts of the ilium. *Perkin's line* is vertical, drawn through the upper outer point of the acetabulum (Fig. 10–37). Normally, the developing femoral head or ossification center of the femoral head lies in the inner distal quadrant formed by the two lines. If the ossification center lies in the upper outer quadrant, the finding is indicative of a dislocation. In the newborn, the ossification center is not visible (Fig. 10–38).

10. Whether the femoral head and acetabulum are normal on both sides. In congenital dislocation of the hip, both structures may show dysplasia and the acetabular index on the affected side may be greater than the normal 30°. The *acetabular index* is determined by first drawing Hilgenreiner's line. An intersecting line is drawn from the lateral to medial edges of the acetabulum, and the angle formed by the two lines is called the acetabular index, or *Hilgenreiner's angle* (Table 10–2). The greater the slope angle, the less stable the femoral head in the acetabulum.

11. "Sagging rope" sign. With Legg-Calvé-

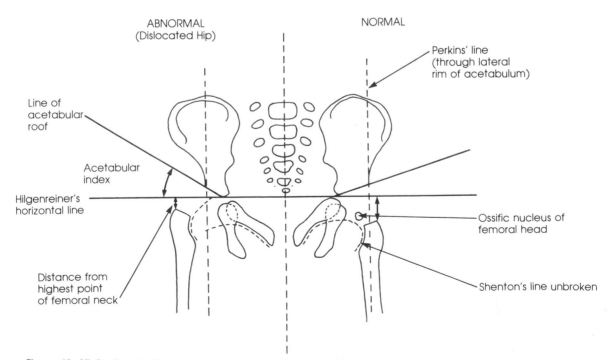

Figure 10–37. Radiologic findings in congenital dislocation of the hip compared with normal findings in a 12- to 15-month-old child. Acetabular index: normal = 30°; in newborn = 27.5°. If the ossific nucleus of the femoral head is present, it should sit in the inner lower quadrant.

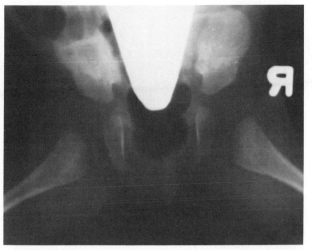

Figure 10–38. Radiograph of the hip in the newborn. Ossification of the femoral head has not yet developed.

Perthes disease, only the head of the femur is affected. If avascular necrosis of a developing femoral head occurs, the "sagging rope" sign may be seen (Fig. 10–39). The sign indicates damage to the growth plate with marked metaphyseal reaction. Its presence indicates a severe disease process.

12. "Teardrop" sign. Migration of the femoral head upward in relation to the pelvis due to degeneration as seen in osteoarthritis may be detected by the "teardrop" sign (Fig. 10–40). The teardrop is visible at the base of the pubic bone, extending vertically downward to terminate in a round teardrop, or head. The x-ray beam must be centered relative to the pelvis. A line is drawn between the two teardrops and is extended to the femoral heads on both sides. The examiner can then measure from the teardrop to the femoral head. A difference of greater than 10 mm between the two sides indicates significant migration of the head of the femur. Serial films or films taken over a period of time will often show a progression of the migration.

Lateral View

The examiner looks for any pelvic distortion or any slipping of the femoral head, as might be seen in slipped capital femoral epiphysis. The lateral view will be the first by which slipping may be seen.

Table 10–2. Average Values of Hilgenreiner Angle (Acetabular Index)

	Newborn	Six Months	One Year
Male	26°	20°	20°
Female	28°	22°	20°

Arthrogram

Although arthrograms are not routinely done on the hip, they may be done if the hip will not reduce following a dislocation (Fig. 10–41). The arthrogram will indicate a possible *inverted limbus* (infolding of a meniscus-like structure), or it may indicate an "hourglass" configuration from a contracted capsule.

"Head at Risk" Signs

With Legg-Calvé-Perthes disease, the examiner should note the radiologic head at risk signs on an anteroposterior film:
1. Cage's sign. This is a small osteoporotic segment on the lateral side of the epiphysis that appears translucent (Fig. 10–42).
2. Calcification lateral to the epiphysis (if collapse is occurring).
3. Lateral subluxation of the head (an increase in the inferomedial joint space).
4. Angle of the epiphyseal line (horizontal in this case).
5. Metaphyseal reaction.
Patients who exhibit three or more head at risk signs have a poor prognosis, and surgery is usually performed.

Signs of a Slipped Capital Femoral Epiphysis

With a slipped capital femoral epiphysis (Fig. 10–43), the following x-ray signs may be noted:
1. The epiphyseal line may widen.
2. Lipping or stepping may be seen, as occurs on lateral films.
3. The superior femoral neck line does not transect the overhanging ossified epiphysis as it does in the normal hip.
4. Shenton's line does not describe a continuous arch. (The line is also broken if the hip is dislocated or subluxed.)

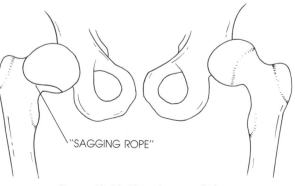

Figure 10–39. "Sagging rope" sign.

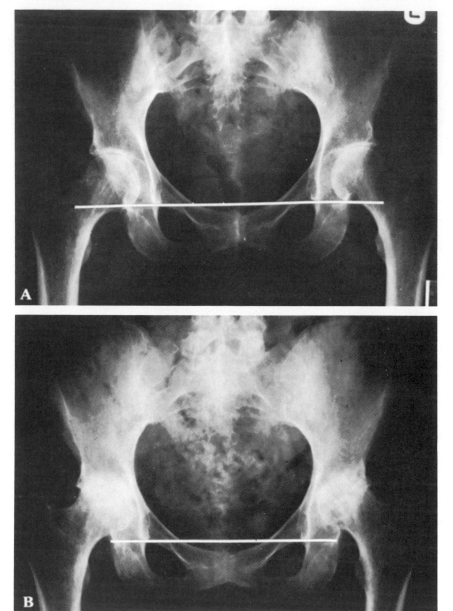

Figure 10–40. "Teardrop" sign. (*A*) A line has been drawn between the tips of the two "teardrops" and extended into the femoral neck. Osteoarthritis of both hip joints seems to be equal with equivalent narrowing of the joint space, but the left hip is already at a slightly higher level than the right in relation to the line. (*B*) Later, both hips have gradually moved upward as a result of loss of the bone at the apex of each femoral head. The left hip is now at a higher level than the right, confirming the original observation that the process of destruction in the left hip was ahead of that in the right. (From Greubel Lee, D. M.: Disorders of the Hip. Philadelphia, J. B. Lippincott, 1983, p. 61.)

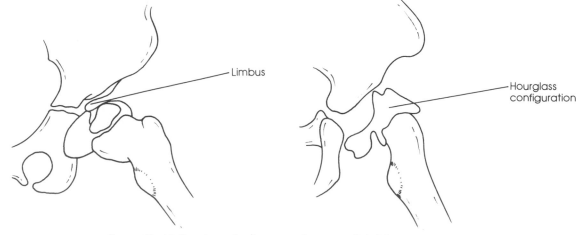

Figure 10–41. Drawings of arthrograms in congenital dislocation of the hip.

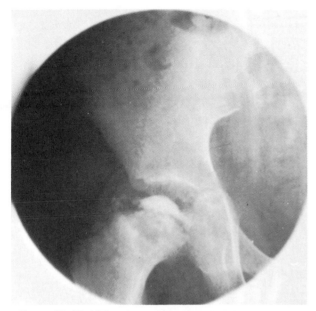

Figure 10–42. All the signs of the "head at risk" are present: lateral subluxation, abnormal direction of the growth plates, Cage's sign, lateral calcification, and irregularity of the epiphysis. (From Greubel Lee, D. M.: Disorders of the Hip. Philadelphia, W. B. Saunders Co., 1983, p. 146.)

In addition to a slipped capital femoral epiphysis causing a coxa vara, fractures and congenital malformations may lead to the same deformity (Figs. 10–44 and 10–45).

Précis of the Hip Assessment*

History
Observation
Examination
    Active movements (supine)
        Active hip flexion
        Active hip abduction
        Active hip adduction
        Active hip lateral rotation
        Active hip medial rotation
    Passive movements (supine) (as in Active movements, if necessary)
    Resisted isometric movements (supine)
        Hip flexion
        Hip extension

*The precis is shown in an order that will limit the amount of movement which the patient has to do, but will ensure all the necessary structures are tested.

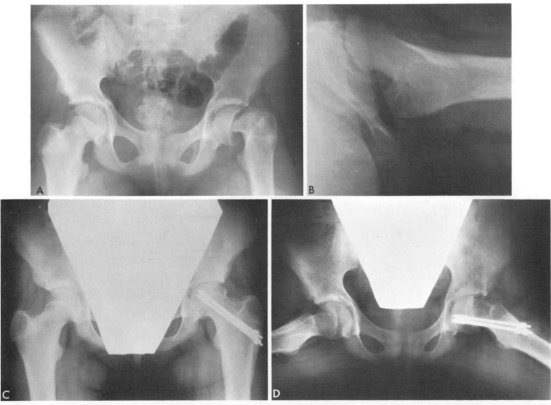

Figure 10–43. Acute slipped femoral epiphysis in a 14-year-old boy. Following a fall, the patient complained of severe pain in the left groin and anterior thigh and was unable to bear weight on left lower limb.

(A, B). Preoperative roentgenograms show the severe slip on the left. He was placed in bilateral split Russell traction with internal rotation straps on the left thigh and leg. Gradually, within a period of three to four days, the slip was reduced.

(C, D) Postoperative roentgenograms approximately 6 months later show closure of epiphyseal plate and normal position of femoral head. The hip had full range of motion.

(From Tachdjian, M. O.: Pediatric Orthopedics. Philadelphia, W. B. Saunders Co., 1972, p. 470.)

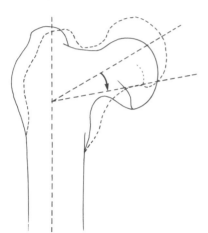
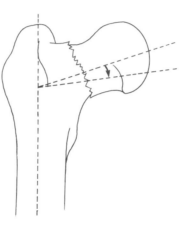
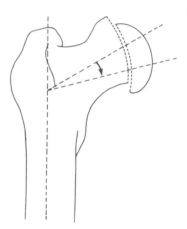

CONGENITAL

FRACTURE

SLIPPED CAPITAL
FEMORAL EPIPHYSIS

Figure 10–44. Some causes of coxa vara.

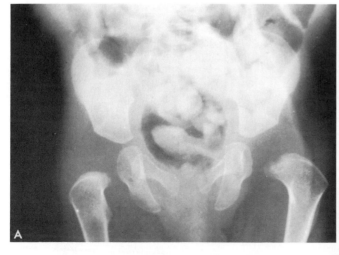

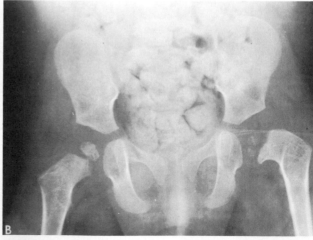

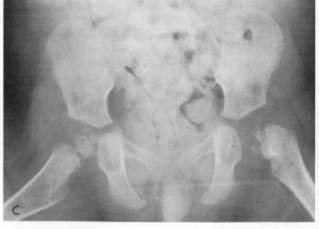

Figure 10–45. Congenital coxa vara of the left hip in an infant. (*A*) Anteroposterior roentgenograms of both hips at 3 months of age, taken because of limited abduction of left hip and suspicion of congenital hip dislocation. It was interpreted to be normal. (*B, C*) Roentgenograms of the hips of same patient at one year of age when he started walking with a painless gluteus medius lurch on the left. Varus deformity of the left hip is evident.

(From Tachdjian, M. O.: Pediatric Orthopedics. Philadelphia, W. B. Saunders Co., p. 183.)

Hip adduction
Hip abduction
Hip medial rotation
Hip lateral rotation
Knee flexion
Knee extension
Special tests (supine)
Reflexes and cutaneous sensation (supine)
Joint play movements (supine)
    Caudal glide
    Compression
    Lateral distraction
    Quadrant test
Palpation (supine)
Active movement (prone)
    Hip extension
Passive movement (prone)
    Hip extension
Resisted isometric movements (prone)
    Hip medial rotation (if not previously done)
    Hip lateral rotation (if not previously done)
    Knee flexion (if not previously done)
    Knee extension (if not previously done)
Special tests (prone and side lying)
Reflexes and cutaneous sensation (prone)
Palpation (prone)
X-ray viewing

When the rest of the examination is completed, the examiner can ask the patient to perform the appropriate functional tests.

Following any examination, the patient should always be warned of the possibility of exacerbation of symptoms as a result of assessment.

REFERENCES

CITED REFERENCES

1. Brand R. A., and R. D. Crowinshield: The effect of cane use on hip contact force. Clin. Orthop. Relat. Res. 147:181, 1980.
2. Clarke, G. R.: Unequal leg length: An accurate method of detection and some clinical results. Rheumatol. Phys. Med. 11:385, 1972.
3. Fisk, J. W., and M. L. Balgent: Clinical and radiological assessment of leg length. N. Z. Med. J. 81:477, 1975.
4. Woerman, A. L., and S. A. Binder-Macleod: Leg-length discrepancy assessment: Accuracy and precision in five clinical methods of evaluation. J. Orthop. Sports Phys. Ther. 5:230, 1984.
5. Adams, M. C.: Outline of Orthopaedics. London, E & S Livingstone, 1968.
6. Gruebel-Lee, D. M., Disorders of the Hip. Philadelphia, J. B. Lippincott Co., 1983.
7. Ober, F.B.: The role of the iliotibial and fascia lata as a factor in the causation of low-back disabilities and sciatica. J. Bone Joint Surg. 18:105, 1936.
8. Noble, H. B., M. R. Hajek, and M. Porter: Diagnosis and treatment of iliotibial band tightness in runners. Physician Sportsmedicine 10:67, 1982.
9. Tachdjian, M. O.: Pediatric Orthopedics. Philadelphia, W. B. Saunders Co., 1972.
10. American Orthopaedic Association: Manual of Orthopaedic Surgery. Chicago, 1972.
11. Crane, L.: Femoral torsion and its relation to toeing-in and toeing-out. J. Bone Joint Surg. 41A:421, 1959.
12. Staheli, L. T.: Medial femoral torsion. Orthop. Clin. North Am. 11:39, 1980.
13. Maitland, G. D.: The Peripheral Joints: Examination and Recording Guide. Adelaide, Australia, Virgo Press, 1973.

GENERAL REFERENCES

Beetham, W. P., H. F. Polley, C. H. Slocumb, and W. F. Weaver: Physical Examination of the Joints. Philadelphia, W. B. Saunders Co., 1965.
Chung, S. M. K.: Hip Disorders in Infants and Children. Philadelphia, Lea & Febiger, 1981.
Crock, H. V.: An atlas of the arterial supply of the head and neck of the femur in man. Clin. Orthop. Relat. Res. 152:17, 1980.
Crouch, J. E.: Functional Human Anatomy. Philadelphia, Lea & Febiger, 1973.
Cyriax, J.: Textbook of Orthopaedic Medicine, volume 1. Diagnosis of Soft Tissue Lesions. London, Bailliere Tindall, 1975.
Debrunner, H. N.: Orthopaedic Diagnosis. London, E & S Longman Group Ltd., 1973.
Grieve, G. P.: The hip. Physiotherapy 57:212, 1971.
Hoaglund, F. T., A. C. Yau, and W. L. Wong: Osteoarthritis of the hip and other joints in southern Chinese in Hong Kong. J. Bone Joint Surg. 55A:545, 1973.
Hoaglund, F. T., and W. D. Low: Anatomy of the femoral neck and head, with comparative data from Caucasians and Hong Kong Chinese. Clin. Orthop. Relat. Res. 152:10, 1980.
Hollinshead, W. H., and D. B. Jenkins: Functional Anatomy of the Limbs and Back. Philadelphia, W. B. Saunders Co., 1969.
Hoppenfeld, S.: Physical Examination of the Spine and Extremities. New York, Appleton-Century-Crofts,, 1976.
Judge, R. D., G. D. Zuidema, and F. T. Fitzgerald: Clinical Diagnosis: A Physiological Approach. Boston, Little, Brown and Co., 1982.
Kapandji, I. A.: The Physiology of the Joints, vol. II. Lower Limb. New York, Churchill Livingstone, 1970.
Kaltenborn, F. M.: Mobilization of the Extremity. Oslo, Olaf Norlis Bokhandel, 1980.
McRae, R.: Clinical Orthopaedic Examination. New York, Churchill Livingstone, 1976.
Moseley, C. F.: The biomechanics of the pediatric hip. Orthop. Clin. North Am. 11:39, 1980.
O'Donoghue, D. H.: Treatment of Injuries to Athletes, 4th ed. Philadelphia, W. B. Saunders Co., 1984.
Radin, E. L.: Biomechanics of the hip. Clin. Orthop. Relat. Res. 152:28, 1980.
Williams, P. L., and Warwick, P. (eds.): Gray's Anatomy, 36th British ed. Philadelphia, W. B. Saunders Co., 1980.

11

The Knee

The knee joint is particularly susceptible to traumatic injury because it is located at the ends of two long lever arms—the tibia and the femur. The joint depends on the ligaments and muscles that surround it for its strength and stability and not on its bony configuration.

Because the knee joint depends on its ligaments to such a great extent, it is imperative that the ligaments be tested during the examination of the knee. Thus, the assessment of the knee varies slightly from the norm in that the ligamentous tests are not included under special tests but are given a separate section of their own. This change ensures that the ligaments are always included in the examination of the knee.

The knee is a complicated area to assess, and the examiner must take time to ensure that all the relevant structures are tested. It must also be remembered that beause the lumbar spine, hip, and ankle may refer pain to the knee, these joints must be assessed if it appears that other joints may be involved.

Applied Anatomy

The *tibiofemoral joint* is the largest joint in the body. It is a modified hinge joint having two degrees of freedom. The *synovium* around the joint is extensive and communicates with many of the bursae and pouches around the knee joint. Although the synovial membrane "encapsules" the whole knee joint, its distribution within the knee is such that the *cruciate ligaments*, which run from the middle of the tibial plateau to the intercondylar area of the femur, are extrasynovial. ("Cruciate" means that the ligaments cross each other.)

The articular surfaces of the tibia and femur are not congruent. This lack of congruency enables the two bones to move different amounts guided by the muscles and ligaments. The two bones approach congruency in full extension, which is the close packed position. Kaltenborn[1] has stated that the close packed position includes full lateral rotation of the tibia as well. The lateral femoral condyle projects anteriorly more than the medial femoral condyle to help prevent lateral dislocation of the patella. In females, this enlargement is important because of the female's broader pelvis and the increased inward angle of the femur, which allow the femoral condyles to be parallel with the ground (Fig. 11–1). The resting position of the joint is approximately 25° of flexion, and the capsular pattern is flexion more limited than extension.

The space between the two bones is partially filled by two menisci that are attached to the tibia to add congruency. The *medial meniscus* is a small part of a large circle (i.e., "C"-shaped) and is thicker posteriorly than anteriorly. The *lateral meniscus* is a large part of a small circle (i.e., "O"-shaped) and is generally of equal thickness throughout. Both menisci are thicker along the periphery and thinner on the inner margin.

During the movement from extension to flexion, both menisci move posteriorly, the lateral meniscus being displaced more than the medial meniscus. The menisci are avascular in their cartilaginous inner two thirds and are partly vascular and fibrous in their outer one third.[2] They are held in place by the coronary ligaments attaching to the tibia.

The menisci serve several functions in the knee. They aid in the lubrication and nutrition of the joint and act as shock absorbers, spreading the stress over the articular cartilage and decreasing

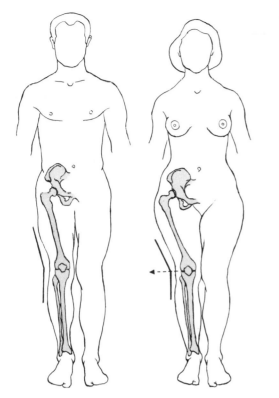

Figure 11–1. Q-angle differences in males and females. Note that because of the broader pelvis in the female, it is necessary for the femur to come inward at an increased angle in order to make the distal end of the condyles parallel with the ground. The quadriceps, patella, and patellar tendon make an angle centered at the patella. As the quadriceps contracts, the angle tends to straighten, which forces the patella laterally. (From O'Donoghue, D. H.: Treatment of Injuries to Athletes, 4th ed. Philadelphia, W. B. Saunders Co., 1984, p. 522.)

cartilage wear. They make the joint surfaces more congruent and improve weight distribution by increasing the area of contact between the condyles. The menisci reduce friction during movement and aid the ligaments and capsule in preventing hyperextension. The menisci prevent the joint capsule from entering the joint and participate in the "locking" mechanism of the joint by directing the movement of the femoral articular condyles. Because most recent literature indicates that removal of the total meniscus can lead to early degeneration of the joint,[3, 4] most surgeons today remove only the torn portion of the meniscus rather than the entire structure.

Since the meniscus possesses no nerves, there is no pain when it is damaged unless the coronary ligaments have been damaged as well. Because the menisci are primarily avascular, especially in the inner two thirds, there is seldom bloody effusion in injury; however, there may be synovial effusion. It is because of the poor blood supply that they have is a low regeneration potential.

The lateral meniscus is not as firmly attached to the tibia as the medial meniscus and is thus less prone to injury. The coronary ligaments tend to be longer on the lateral aspect, and the horns of the lateral meniscus are closer together. The lateral meniscus has an excursion of 10 mm; the medial meniscus, 2 mm.

The *patellofemoral joint* is a modified plane joint, the lateral articular surface of the patella being wider. The patella contains the thickest layer of cartilage in the body. It has five facets, or ridges—superior, inferior, lateral, medial, and odd. It is the "odd" facet that is most frequently the first part of the patella to be affected in chondromalacia patellae (i.e., premature degeneration of the patellar cartilage).

During the movement from flexion to extension, different parts of the patella articulate with the femoral condyles (Fig. 11–2).[5, 6] For example, the odd facet does not come into contact with the femoral condyles until at least 135° of flexion is reached. Incorrect alignment or malalignment of the patellar movement over the femoral condyles can lead to patellofemoral arthralgia. The capsule of this joint is continuous with the capsule of the tibiofemoral joint.

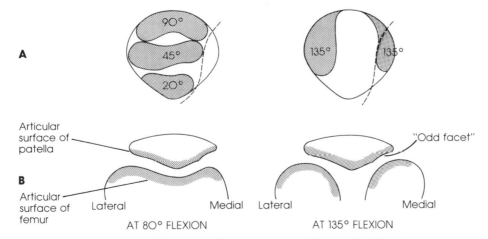

Figure 11–2. (*A*) Area of contact of the patella during different degrees of flexion. (*B*) Articulation between patella and femur.

The *patella* improves the efficiency of extension during the last 30° of extension (that is, 30° to 0° of extension with the straight leg being 0°), since it holds the quadriceps tendon away from the axis of movement. The patella also functions as a guide for the quadriceps tendon, decreases friction of the quadriceps mechanism, controls capsular tension in the knee, acts as a bony shield for the cartilage of the femoral condyles, and improves the esthetic appearance of the knee.

The *superior tibiofibular joint* is a plane synovial joint between the tibia and the head of the fibula. Movement occurs in this joint with any activity involving the ankle. Hypomobility at this joint can lead to pain in the knee area on activity because the fibula can bear up to one sixth of the body weight. In about 10 per cent of the population, the capsule of this joint is continuous with that of the tibiofemoral joint.

Patient History

In addition to the general history questions outlined in Chapter 1, the following information should be ascertained:

1. What is the patient able or unable to do functionally? Is there disability on running, cutting, pivoting, twisting, climbing, or descending stairs?

2. Is there any pain? If so, where? What type is it? Is it diffuse? Aching? Retropatellar? Aching pain may indicate degenerative changes, whereas sharp, "catching" pain usually indicates a mechanical problem. Arthritic pain is more likely to be associated with stiffness in the morning and to ease with activity. Pain at rest is not usually mechanical in origin.

3. Is there any "clicking," or was there a "pop" when the injury occurred? A distinct pop may indicate an anterior cruciate ligament tear or osteochondral fracture.

4. Does the knee "give way" or catch? This finding usually indicates instability in the knee.

5. Do certain positions or activities have an increased or decreased effect on the pain the patient experiences? Which activities produce pain? How much activity is needed to produce pain? Which positions or activities ease the pain? Does the pain go away when activity ceases? The examiner must take note of constant pain that is unrelated to activity, time, or posture, since it is usually indicative of serious pathology such as a tumor.

6. Is the gait normal?

7. Has the knee been injured before, or does it have any feeling of weakness?

8. How did the accident occur? Was it due to trauma, such as a direct or indirect blow? Was the patient bearing weight at the time of injury? From which direction did the injuring force come (i.e., what is the mechanism of injury)? For example, meniscal injuries, especially on the medial

Table 11–1. Mechanisms of Injury to the Knee and Possible Structures Injured†

Mechanism of Injury	Structure Possibly Injured
Varus or valgus contact without rotation	1. Collateral ligaments 2. Epiphyseal fracture 3. Patellar dislocation or subluxation
Varus or valgus contact with rotation	1. Collateral and cruciate ligaments 2. Collateral ligaments and patellar dislocation of subluxation 3. Meniscus tear
Blow to patellofemoral joint, fall on flexed knee, foot dorsiflexed	Patellar articular injury or osteochondral fracture
Blow to tibial tubercle, fall on flexed knee, foot plantar flexed	Posterior cruciate ligament
Anterior blow to tibia, resulting in knee hyperextension	1. Anterior cruciate ligament 2. Anterior and posterior cruciate ligament
Noncontact hyperextension Noncontact deceleration	Anterior cruciate ligament Anterior cruciate ligament
Noncontact deceleration, with tibial medial rotation *or* femoral lateral rotation on fixed tibia	Anterior cruciate ligament
Noncontact, quickly turning one way with tibia rotated in opposite direction	Patellar dislocation or subluxation
Noncontact, rotation with varus or valgus loading	Meniscus injury
Noncontact, compressive rotation	1. Meniscus injury 2. Osteochondral fracture

*Adapted from Clancy, W. G.: Evaluation of acute knee injuries. American Association of Orthopedic Surgeons, Symposium on Sports Medicine: The Knee. St. Louis, C. V. Mosby, 1985.

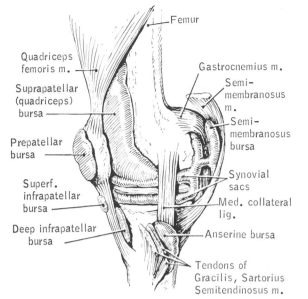

Figure 11–3. The bursae about the knee (medial aspect). (From O'Donoghue, D. H.: Treatment of Injuries to Athletes, 4th ed. Philadelphia, W. B. Saunders Co., 1984, p. 466.)

side, occur as a result of torsion injury that combines compression and rotation.

9. Does the joint swell? Often there may be no swelling in the knee following severe injury. This lack of swelling occurs because with a severe injury the fluid extravasates into the soft tissues surrounding the joint; also, a number of structures around the knee joint are avascular and can be injured without bloody swelling. Synovial swelling, however, may occur 8 to 24 hours after the injury. Any swelling caused by blood will begin to occur almost immediately. Localized swelling may be due to an inflamed bursa (Fig. 11–3).

10. Is there any grating on movement or clicking in the knee? Grating or clicking may be due to degeneration or to one structure snapping over another.

11. What type of shoes does the person wear? Shoes with negative heels (e.g., "earth" shoes) can often increase the incidence of chondromalacia patellae.

Observation

For a proper observation, the patient must be suitably undressed so that the examiner can observe the posture of the spine as well as the hips, knees, and ankles. Initially, the examiner should note whether the patient puts weight on the affected limb or whether the patient stands with only a slight amount of weight on the affected side. In addition to the common observational items mentioned in Chapter 1, the examiner should look for the following alterations about the knee.

Anterior View, Standing

From the anterior aspect (Fig. 11–4), the examiner should note any genu varum (*bowleg*) or genu valgum (*knock-knee*) (Fig. 11–5). It should be remembered that although in adults the legs should be straight, in the child the normal development of the knee is from genu varum to straight, to genu valgum to straight. Initially, a child's lower limbs are in genu varum until about 18 or 19 months when they straighten. The knee then goes into genu valgum until about 3 or 4 years of age (Fig. 11–6). The limbs should again be straight by age 6 and remain that way.

To observe genu varum and valgum, the patient is positioned so that the patellae face forward and the medial aspect of the knees and medial malleoli of both limbs are as close together as possible. If the knees touch and the ankles do not, the patient has a genu valgum. A distance of 9 to 10 cm between the ankles is considered excessive. If the ankles touch and the knees do not, the patient has a genu varum. On x-ray studies, the normal femoral-tibial shaft angle is about 6° (Fig. 11–7).

The patient is asked to extend the knees to see if the movement can be performed and what effect it has on the knee. Both knees should extend equally. If not, something must be limiting the

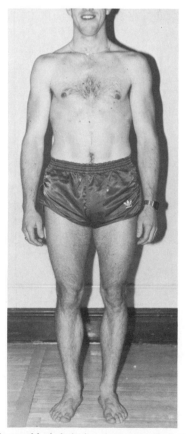

Figure 11–4. Anterior view of lower limb.

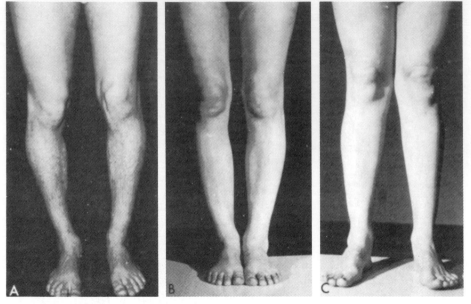

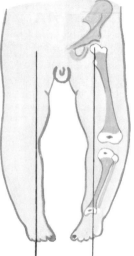
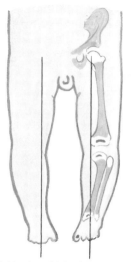
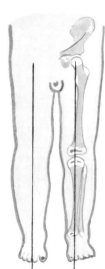

Figure 11–5. Genu varum and genu valgum. (A) Tibia vara of proximal third. Genu varum deformity located mainly in proximal tibia. Along with external tibial torsion and internal femoral torsion, this gives "bandy-legged" appearance. (B) Genu varum of entire lower extremities. (C) Genu valgum deformity of both lower extremities. (From Hughston, J. C., et al.: Patellar Subluxation and Dislocation. Philadelphia, W. B. Saunders Co., 1984, p. 221.)

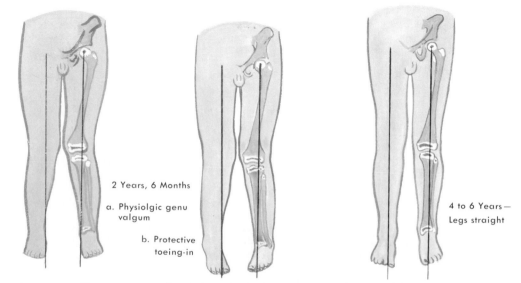

Newborn—Moderate genu varum

6 Months—Minimal genu varum

1 Year, 7 Months—Legs straight

2 Years, 6 Months

a. Physiolgic genu valgum

b. Protective toeing-in

4 to 6 Years— Legs straight

Figure 11–6. Physiologic evolution of lower limb alignment at various ages in infancy and childhood. (From Tachdjian, M. O.: Pediatric orthopedics. Philadelphia, W. B. Saunders Co., 1972, p. 1463.)

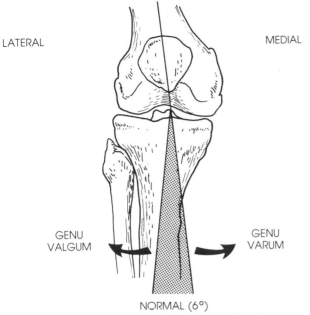

Figure 11–7. Normal femoral-tibia shaft angle.

LATERAL

MEDIAL

GENU
VALGUM

GENU
VARUM

NORMAL (6°)

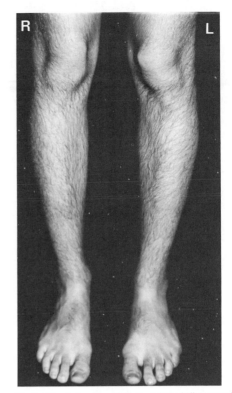

R   L

Figure 11–9. "Squinting" patellae, especially prominent on the patient's left knee. Both patellae point inward in a medial fashion, a sign of excessive femoral anteversion or increased femoral torsion. (From Carson, W. A., et al.: Clin. Orthop. Relat. Res. *185*:169, 1984.)

movement (e.g., swelling, loose body, or meniscus).

Is there any apparent swelling in the knees? If there is intracapsular swelling, or at least sufficient swelling, the knee will assume a position of 15 to 25° of flexion, which provides the synovial cavity with the maximum capacity to hold fluid. This position is also called the *resting position* of the knee.

Is the swelling intracapsular or extracapsular? Intracapsular swelling is evident over the whole joint; extracapsular swelling tends to be more localized. An example of extracapsular swelling is shown in Figure 11–8, which illustrates *prepatellar bursitis*.

The examiner should ask the patient to contract the quadriceps muscles to see whether there is

any visible wasting of the quadriceps muscles. The prominence of the vastus medialis is due to the obliquity of the distal fibers, the inferior position of its insertion, and the thinness of the fascial covering when compared with the other quadriceps muscles.

The position of the patella should be noted. A "squinting" patella may be indicative of medial femoral or lateral tibial torsion (Fig. 11–9). Any

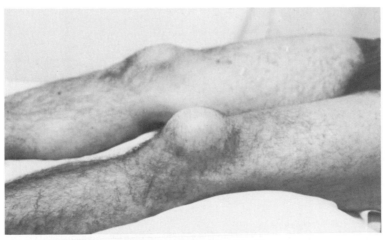

Figure 11–8. Prepatellar bursitis.

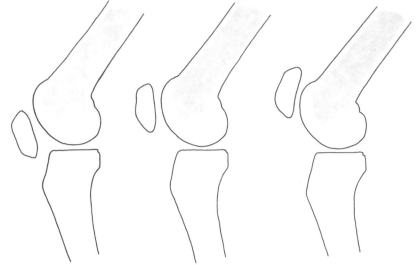

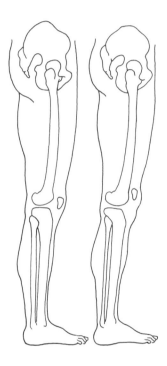

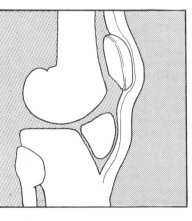

Patella Baja   Normal   Patella Alta

Figure 11–10. The normal patellar posture for exerting deceleration forces in the functional position of 45° of knee flexion places the patellar articular surface squarely against the anterior femur. A lower posture represents patellar baja. A higher posture represents patella alta. Patella alta makes the patella less efficient in exerting normal forces. (From Hughston, J. C., et al.: Patellar Subluxation and Dislocation. Philadelphia, W. B. Saunders Co., 1984, p. 8.)

Figure 11–11. "Camel" sign. Double hump seen from side caused by high-riding patella and uncovered infrapatellar fat pad. (From Hughston, J. C., et al.: Patellar Subluxation and Dislocation. Philadelphia, W. B. Saunders Co., 1984, p. 22.)

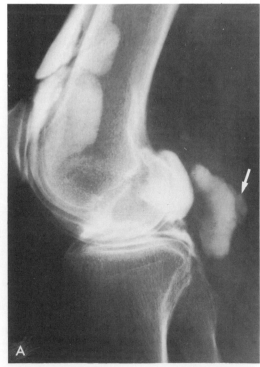

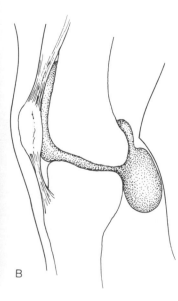

Figure 11–12. Popliteal (Baker's) cysts. (A) This 74-year-old man presented with the acute onset of calf pain and swelling without knee pain. The initial suspected diagnosis was popliteal thrombosis. A venogram was normal. An arthrogram reveals a collection of dye posterior to the joint space—the popliteal cysts (arrow). (From Reilly, B. M.: Practical Strategies in Outpatient Medicine. Philadelphia, W. B. Saunders Co., 1984, p. 231.) (B) Schematic diagram of Baker's cyst.

bruising or discoloration about the knee should also be noted as well as well as any scars or sinuses indicating recent injury or surgery.

Lateral View, Standing

The examiner then views the patient from both sides for comparison. It should be noted whether *genu recurvatum* (hyperextended knee) is present and whether one or both patellae are higher (*patella alta*) or lower (*patella baja*) than normal (Fig. 11–10). With an abnormally high patella, a "camel sign" may be present (Fig. 11–11). Because of the high patella (one "hump"), the infrapatellar fat pad (second "hump") becomes more prominent. This finding is especially noticeable in females. The patient should again extend the knees to see if the active range of motion is the same for both limbs. The examiner should note whether the patient stands "on the ligaments" with both legs completely extended or with the knees slightly flexed or unlocked. An individual with an excessive lordosis in the lumbar spine will often hyperextend the knees to compensate for the poor posture. This change may lead to posterior knee pain.

Posterior View, Standing

Next, the examiner views the patient from behind, looking for findings similar to those from the anterior aspect. In addition, one should look for abnormal swellings such as a popliteal (Baker's) cyst, i.e., herniation of synovial tissue through a weakening in the posterior capsule wall (Fig. 11–12).

Anterior and Lateral Views, Sitting

For the final part of the observation, the patient sits with the knees flexed to 90° and the feet non-weight-bearing or dangling free. The patient is observed from the front and side. In this position, the patella should face forward and should very nearly rest on the distal end of the femur. With patella alta, the patella will become more aligned with the anterior surface of the femur. If the patella is laterally displaced, or laterally displaced with a patella alta, the patella will take on the appearance of "frog's eyes" or "grasshopper eyes" (Fig. 11–13), meaning that the patellae face up and out, away from each other. Any bony enlargements such as those seen in Osgood-

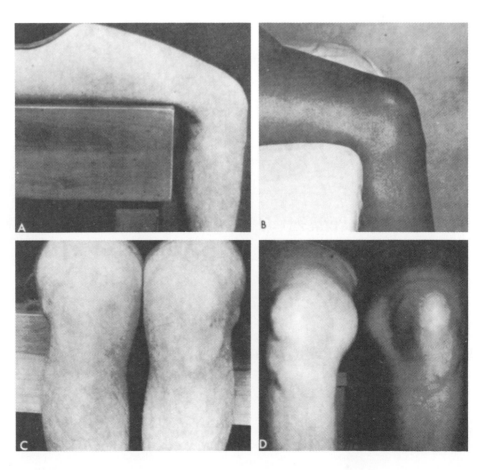

Figure 11–13. (A) Normal knee seen from side; patella faces straight ahead in line with femur. (B) Patella alta seen from side; patella points toward ceiling. (C) Normal patellae seen from front; patellae centered in outline of knees. (D) High and lateral posturing of patellae seen from front, giving "grasshopper eyes" or "frog's eyes" appearance. (From Hughston, J. C., et al.: Patellar Subluxation and Dislocation. Philadelphia, W. B. Saunders Co., 1984, p. 23.)

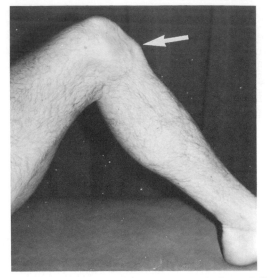

Figure 11–14. Osgood-Schlatter disease (enlarged tibial tuberosity).

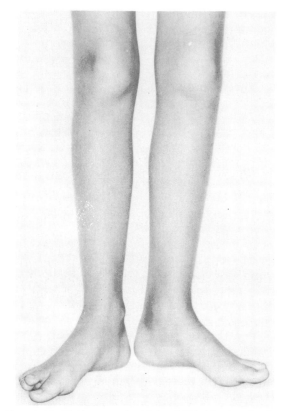

Figure 11–15. Exaggerated lateral tibial torsion. In stance, with the patellae facing straight forward, the feet point outward. (From Tachdjian, M. O.: Pediatric Orthopedics. Philadelphia, W. B. Saunders Co., 1972, p. 1461.)

Schlatter disease (i.e., an enlarged tibial tubercle) should be noted (Fig. 11–14).

In the same position, any tibial torsion should be noted (Fig. 11–15).[7, 8] If there is tibial torsion, it is medial torsion that is associated with genu varum. Genu valgum is associated with lateral tibial torsion. Normally, the forefoot points straight forward or slightly laterally. With medial tibial torsion, the feet point toward each other, resulting in a "pigeon-toed" foot deformity. These deformities can be exacerbated by habitual postures. The positions illustrated in Figures 11–16 and 11–17A cause problems only if they are employed habitually. Excessive tibial torsion can contribute to conditions such as chondromalacia patellae, patellofemoral instability, and fat pad entrapment. When standing, most people exhibit a lateral tibial torsion—the Fick angle (see Figure 12–3)—which increases as the child grows. It is

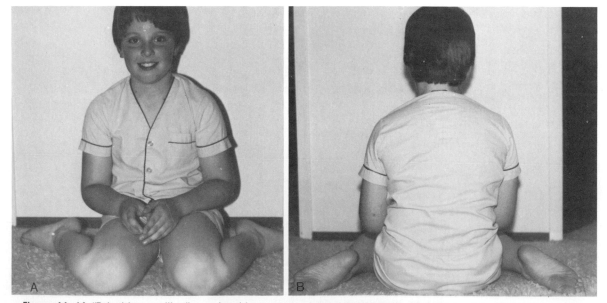

Figure 11–16. "Television position" may lead to excessive lateral tibial torsion. (A) Anterior view. (B) Posterior view.

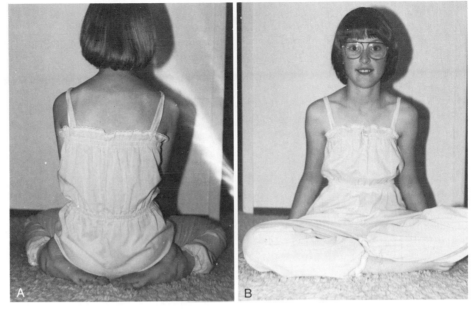

Figure 11–17. Medial tibial torsion. (*A*) Position to be avoided for preventing excessive medial tibial torsion. (*B*) Tailor position maintains normal medial tibial torsion.

approximately 5° in babies and up to 18° in adults. To test for tibial torsion, the examiner aligns the patient's straight legs (knees extended) so that the patellae face straight ahead. The examiner then looks at the feet to see at what angle they are relative to the shaft of the tibia.

Femoral torsion, or anteversion (discussed in Chapter 10), can also affect the position of the patella relative to the femur and tibia.

Examination

ACTIVE MOVEMENTS

Examination is performed <u>initially with the patient sitting, then lying</u>. During the active movements, the examiner should observe (1) the ex-

cursion of the patella to ensure that it tracks freely and smoothly; (2) the range of motion available; (3) whether pain occurs during the movement and, if so, where; and (4) what appears to be blocking limiting the movement. The active movements may be done in sitting or in a supine position, and, as always, the most painful movements should be done last (Fig. 11–18).

The active movements to be assessed for the knee are shown in Figure 11–19:

1. Flexion (0 to 135°).
2. Extension (0 to 15°).
3. Medial rotation of the tibia on the femur (20 to 30°).
4. Lateral rotation of the tibia on the femur (30 to 40°).

Full knee flexion is 135° (0° being straight knee). Active knee extension is approximately 0° but

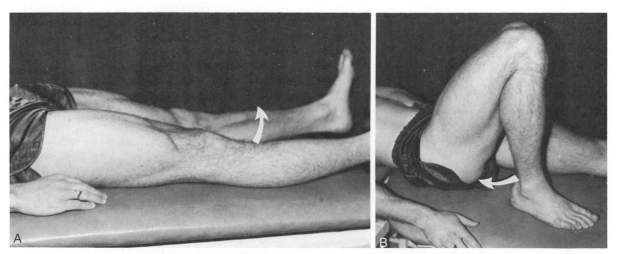

Figure 11–18. Active movements of the knee. (*A*) Extension. (*B*) Flexion.

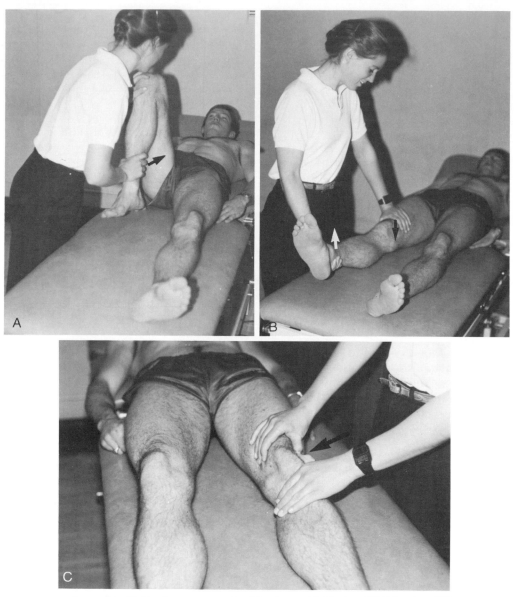

Figure 11–19. Passive movements of the knee. (*A*) Flexion. (*B*) Extension. (*C*) Patella (medially shown).

may be − 15°, especially in women who are more likely to have hyperextended knees (genu recurvatum). The knee extensor muscles develop the greatest force around the angle of 60°, and the knee flexor muscles develop their greatest force at the angles of 45° and 10°. To complete the last 15° of knee extension, a 60 per cent increase in force of the quadriceps muscles is required. The examiner should also watch for evidence of quadriceps lag, which is the result of the loss of mechanical advantage, muscle atrophy, decreasing power of the muscle as it shortens, adhesion formation, effusion, or reflex inhibition. The active medial rotation of the tibia on the femur should be 20 to 30°; active lateral rotation should be 30 to 40°.

If the preceding tests are performed with little difficulty, the examiner may put the patient through a series of *functional tests* to see if these sequential activities produce pain or other symptoms. The functional activities in order of sequence are:

1. Squatting. (Both knees should flex symmetrically.)
2. Squatting and bouncing at the end of the squat. (Again, both knees should act symmetrically.)
3. Going up and down stairs.
4. Running straight ahead.
5. Running and twisting.
6. Jumping.
7. Jumping and going into a full squat.

These functional activities, which are provided as examples, must be geared to the individual patient. Older individuals should not be expected to accomplish the last four movements unless they have, in the recent past, been doing these or similar activities.

PASSIVE MOVEMENTS

If, on active movements, the range of motion is full, overpressure may be gently applied to test the end feel of the various movements in the tibiofemoral joint. This action would preclude the need to do passive movements to the tibiofemoral joint. However, the examiner must do movements of the patella passively (Fig. 11–19).

At the tibiofemoral joint, the end feel of flexion is tissue approximation; the end feel of extension and medial and lateral rotation of the tibia on the femur is tissue stretch. It must be remembered that during the passive movement the examiner is also looking for a capsular pattern of the tibiofemoral joint. This pattern is more limitation of flexion than extension. Passive medial rotation of the tibia on the femur should be approximately 30° when the knee is flexed to 90°. Passive lateral rotation of the tibia on the femur at 90° of knee flexion should be 40°.

Passive medial and lateral movement of the patella is also carried out to determine its mobility and to compare it with the unaffected side. Normally, the patella should move half its width medially and laterally. The end feel of these movements is tissue stretch. Lateral displacement must be done with care, especially in patients who have experienced a dislocated patella.

The examiner must also ensure full and normal flexibility of the quadriceps, hamstring, and abductor and adductor muscles of the thigh as well as the gastrocnemius muscles (Fig. 11–20). Tightness of any of these structures can alter gait and postural mechanics, which may lead to pathology.

Tests for the hamstring, abductor, adductor, and rectus femoris muscles have been described in Chapter 10. A functional test for the quadriceps (described under Special Tests in this chapter) is a passive movement test (heel to buttock) for the femoral nerve. To test the gastrocnemius muscle, the examiner extends the patient's knee and, while holding it straight, dorsiflexes the patient's ankle. The examiner should be able to reach at least 90°, although 10 to 15° of dorsiflexion is more common.

RESISTED ISOMETRIC MOVEMENTS

For a proper test of the muscles, resisted and isometric movements must be done. The patient is in a supine position and performs the following movements (Fig. 11–21):
1. Flexion of the knee.
2. Extension of the knee.
3. Ankle plantar flexion.
4. Ankle dorsiflexion.

Ideally, these tests are performed with the joint in its resting position. Segal and Jacob[9] suggest testing the quadriceps muscle at 0°, 30°, 60°, and 90° while observing any abnormal tibial movement (e.g., ligament instability) or excessive pain from patellar compression (e.g., chondromalacia patellae). Refer to Table 11–2 for the muscles acting at the knee.

Although these movements are tested with the patient supine lying, the hamstrings are usually tested with the patient prone. If the knee is flexed to 90° and the heel is turned out, the greatest stress is placed on the lateral hamstring muscle (biceps femoris) with resisted knee flexion. If the heel is turned in, the greatest stress is placed on the medial hamstring (semimembranosus and semitendinosus) muscles.

LIGAMENT STABILITY

Because the knee, more than any other joint in the body, depends on its ligaments to maintain its integrity, it is imperative that the ligaments be tested. The ligaments of the knee joint act as primary stabilizers and guide the movement of the bones in proper relation to one another. There are several ligaments about the knee, but four deserve special mention (Fig. 11–22).

Collateral and Cruciate Ligaments

Collateral Ligaments. The *medial (tibial) collateral ligament* lies more posteriorly than ante-

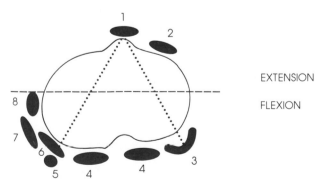

Figure 11–20. Movement diagram of the knee showing quadriceps hamstrings tripod. (*1*) Patellar tendon (quadriceps). (*2*) Iliotibial band. (*3*) Biceps femoris. (*4*) Gastrocnemius. (*5*) Semitendinosus. (*6*) Semimembranosus. (*7*) Gracilis. (*8*) Sartorius.

EXTENSION

FLEXION

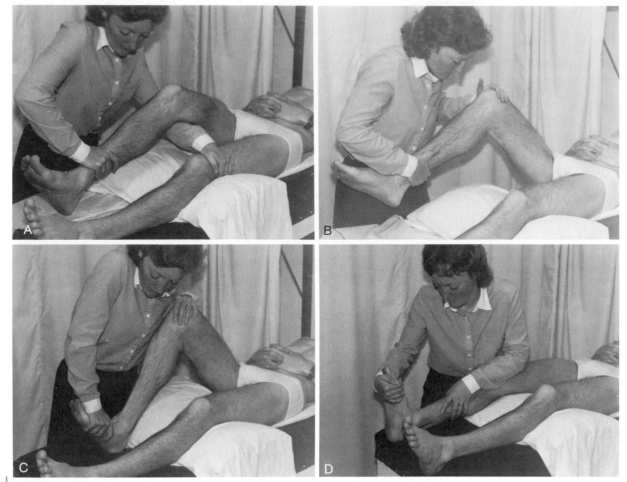

Figure 11-21. Resisted isometric movements of the knee. (*A*) Knee extension. (*B*) Knee flexion. (*C*) Ankle dorsiflexion. (*D*) Ankle plantar flexion.

Table 11-2. Muscles of the Knee: Their Actions, Nerve Supply, and Nerve Root Derivations

Action	Muscles Involved	Innervation	Nerve Root Derivation
Flexion of knee	1. Biceps femoris	Sciatic	L5, S1, S2
	2. Semimembranosus	Sciatic	L5, S1, S2
	3. Semitendinosus	Sciatic	L5, S1, S2
	4. Gracilis	Obturator	L2, L3
	5. Sartorius	Femoral	L2, L3
	6. Popliteus	Tibial	L4, L5, S1
	7. Gastrocnemius	Tibial	S1, S2
	8. Tensor fasciae latae (in 45–145° of flexion)	Superior gluteal	L4, L5
	9. Plantaris	Tibial	S1, S2
Extension of knee	1. Rectus femoris	Femoral	L2, L3, L4
	2. Vastus medialis	Femoral	L2, L3, L4
	3. Vastus intermedius	Femoral	L2, L3, L4
	4. Vastus lateralis	Femoral	L2, L3, L4
	5. Tensor fasciae latae (in 0–30° of flexion)	Superior gluteal	L4, L5
Medial rotation of flexed leg (non-weight-bearing)	1. Popliteus	Tibial	L4, L5
	2. Semimembranosus	Sciatic	L5, S1, S2
	3. Semitendinosus	Sciatic	L5, S1, S2
	4. Sartorius	Femoral	L2, L3
	5. Gracilis	Obturator	L2, L3
Lateral rotation of flexed leg (non-weight-bearing)	Biceps femoris	Sciatic	L5, S1, S2

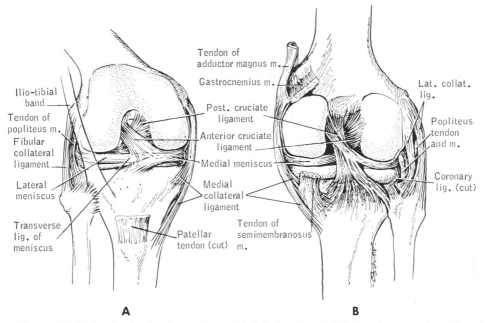

Tendon of adductor magnus m.

Gastrocnemius m.

Post. cruciate ligament

Anterior cruciate ligament

Medial meniscus

Medial collateral ligament

Tendon of semimembranosus m.

Patellar tendon (cut)

Transverse lig. of meniscus

Lateral meniscus

Lateral collat. lig.

Popliteus tendon and m.

Coronary lig. (cut)

Ilio-tibial band

Tendon of popliteus m.

Fibular collateral ligament

A

B

Figure 11–22. Anatomic drawings of knee. (*A*) Anterior view. Patellar tendon is sectioned and the patella reflected upward. Knee flexed. Note that the cruciate ligament rises in front of anterior tibial spine, not from it. Note also that the medial meniscus is firmly attached to the medial collateral ligament. (*B*) Posterior view, knee extended. Note that the posterior ligament has been removed. The two layers of the medial collateral ligament are shown diagrammatically, as is the tibial portion of the lateral collateral ligament. The posterior cruciate ligament rises behind the tibia, not on its upper surface. Observe the femoral attachment of the anterior cruciate ligament at the back of the notch. (From O'Donoghue, D. H.: Treatment of Injuries to Athletes, 4th ed. Philadelphia, W. B. Saunders Co., 1984, p. 477.)

riorly on the medial aspect of the tibiofemoral joint. It is made up of two layers, a superficial and a deep layer. The deep layer is a thickening of the joint capsule and blends with the *medial meniscus*. (It is sometimes called the *medial capsular ligament*.) The superficial layer is a strong, broad triangular strap. It starts distal to the adductor tubercle and extends to the medial surface of the tibia about 6 cm below the joint line. It blends with the posterior capsule and is separated from the capsule and medial meniscus by a bursa.

The entire medial collateral ligament is tight throughout the full range of motion, although there is a greater stress placed on different parts of the ligament as it goes through the range of motion because of the shape of the femoral condyles. All of its fibers are taut on full extension. In flexion, the anterior fibers are the most taut; in midrange, the posterior fibers are the most taut.[10]

The *lateral (fibular) collateral ligament* is round, lying under the tendon of the biceps femoris muscle. It too lies more posteriorly than anteriorly when the tibiofemoral joint is in extension. As the knee flexes, it does provide protection to the lateral aspect of the knee. It is not attached to the lateral meniscus, but is separated from it by a small fat pad.[10]

Cruciate Ligaments. The cruciate ligaments (which cross each other) are the primary rotary stabilizers of the knee.[11] These strong ligaments are named in relation to their attachment to the tibia and are intracapsular but extrasynovial. Each ligament has an anteromedial and a posterolateral portion. The *anterior cruciate ligament* also has an intermediate portion.

The anterior cruciate ligament extends superiorly, posteriorly, laterally, twisting on itself as it extends from the tibia to the femur. Its main functions are to prevent anterior movement of the tibia on the femur, to check external rotation of the tibia in flexion, and to a lesser extent, to check extension and hyperextension at the knee. It also helps to control the normal rolling and gliding movement of the knee. The anteromedial bundle is tight in both flexion and extension, whereas the posterolateral bundle is tight on extension. As a whole, the ligament has the least amount of stress on it between 30° and 60° flexion.[10, 12, 13]

The *posterior cruciate ligament* extends superiorly, anteriorly, medially from the tibia to the femur. This strong fan-shaped ligament, the stoutest ligament in the knee, is a primary stabilizer of the knee against posterior movement of the tibia on the femur, and it checks extension and

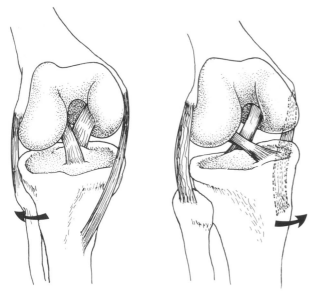

EXTERNAL ROTATION   INTERNAL ROTATION

Figure 11–23. Effect of tibial rotation on cruciate ligaments. *Left:* The collateral ligament is taut; the cruciate ligament is lax. *Right:* The collateral ligament is lax; the cruciate ligament is taut.

hyperextension. As well, the ligament helps to maintain rotary stability and functions as the knee's central axis of rotation. Along with the anterior cruciate ligament, it acts as a rotary guide to the "screwing home" mechanism of the knee.[10, 13]

As with the medial and lateral collateral ligaments, both cruciate ligaments are taut through the full range of motion, although the amount of tightness will vary throughout the range. For example, for the posterior cruciate ligament, the bulk of the fibers are tight at 30° flexion but the posterolateral fibers are loose in early flexion.

With lateral rotation of the tibia, both collateral ligaments become more taut and the cruciate ligaments become relaxed (Fig. 11–23). With medial rotation of the tibia, the reverse action occurs, the collateral ligaments becoming more relaxed and the cruciate ligaments becoming tighter.[10, 14]

Testing of Ligaments

When testing the ligaments of the knee, the examiner must watch for four one-plane instabilities and four rotational instabilities (Table 11–3). Thus, this section includes tests for:

1. One-plane medial instability.
2. One-plane lateral instability.
3. One-plane anterior instability.
4. One-plane posterior instability.

5. Anteromedial rotary instability.
6. Anterolateral rotary instability.
7. Posteromedial rotary instability.
8. Posterolateral rotary instability.

There are a number of tests for each type of instability. The examiner may use the one or two that obtain the best results. It is not essential to do all the tests discussed. The techniques chosen must be practiced diligently so that the examiner becomes proficient at doing them. Only with practice will the examiner be able to determine which structures are injured.

When testing for ligament stability of the knee, the examiner should keep the following in mind:

1. The normal knee is tested first, in order to establish a baseline as well as show the patient what to expect. This action helps to gain the patient's confidence by showing what the test involves.

2. The appropriate stress should be applied gently.

3. The stress is repeated several times and is increased to the point of pain to demonstrate maximum laxity without causing muscle spasm.

4. It is not only the degree of opening but also the quality of the opening (i.e., the end feel) that is of concern.

5. If the ligament is intact, there should be an abrupt stop or end feel when the ligament is stressed. A soft or indistinct end feel usually signifies ligamentous injury.

6. Ligaments of the knee tend to act in concert to maintain stability, and individual ligaments are difficult to isolate in terms of their function. Thus, more than one test may be found to be positive in assessments for the different instabilities. For example, a patient may exhibit a one-plane medial instability as well as an anteromedial and/or anterolateral rotary instability, depending on the severity of the injury to the various ligamentous structures.

7. Tests for ligament instability are more accurate for assessment of a chronic injury than for assessment of an acute injury in the unanesthetized knee because of the presence of muscle spasm and swelling in the acutely injured knee.

8. The muscles must be relaxed if the tests are to be valid.

Tests for One-Plane Medial Instability

The **abduction (valgus stress) test** is an assessment for one-plane (straight) medial instability, which means that the tibia moves away from the femur on the medial side (Fig. 11–24). The examiner applies a valgus stress (pushes the knee medially) at the knee while the ankle is stabilized in slight lateral rotation. The knee is first in full extension and then it is slightly flexed so that it is "unlocked" (20 to 30°).

If the test is positive (i.e., if the tibia moves away from the femur an excessive amount when a valgus stress is applied) when the knee is in extension, the following structures may have been injured to some degree:

1. Medial collateral ligament (superficial and deep fibers).
2. Posterior oblique ligament.
3. Posteromedial capsule.
4. Anterior cruciate ligament.
5. Posterior cruciate ligament.
6. Medial quadriceps expansion.
7. Semimembranosus muscle.

The examiner will usually find that one or more of the rotary tests is also positive. A positive finding on full extension is classified as a major disruption of the knee. If the examiner applies lateral rotation to the foot when performing the test in extension and finds excessive lateral rotation on the affected side, it is a sign of possible anteromedial rotary instability.

If the test is positive when the knee is flexed to 20 to 30°, the following structures may have been injured to some degree:

1. Medial collateral ligament.
2. Posterior oblique ligament.
3. Posterior cruciate ligament.

This part of the valgus stress test would be classified as the true test for one-plane medial instability.

If a stress radiograph is taken when the test is performed in full extension, a 5-mm opening is indicative of a grade 1 injury; up to 10 mm, a grade 2 injury; and over 10 mm, a grade 3 injury.[10, 15]

Tests for One-Plane Lateral Instability

The **adduction (varus stress) test** is an assessment for one-plane lateral instability (i.e., the tibia moves away from the femur an excessive amount on the lateral aspect of the leg). The examiner applies a varus stress (i.e., pushes the knee laterally) at the knee while the ankle is stabilized (Fig. 11–25). The test is first done in full extension and then in 20 to 30° of flexion.

If the test is positive (i.e., if the tibia moves away from the femur when a varus stress is applied) in extension the following structures may have been injured to some degree:

1. Fibular or lateral collateral ligament.
2. Posterolateral capsule.
3. Arcuate-popliteus complex.
4. Biceps femoris tendon.
5. Posterior cruciate ligament.
6. Anterior cruciate ligament.
7. Lateral gastrocnemius muscle.

The examiner will find that one or more rotary instability tests will usually be positive as well. A positive test is indicative of major instability of the knee.

If the test is positive when the knee is flexed 20 to 30° with lateral rotation of the tibia, the following structures may have been injured to some degree:

1. Lateral collateral ligament.
2. Posterolateral capsule.
3. Arcuate-popliteus complex.
4. Iliotibial band.
5. Biceps femoris tendon.

This part of the varus stress test is classified as the true test for one-plane lateral instability.

If a stress radiograph is taken when the test is performed in full extension, a 5-mm opening is indicative of a grade 1 injury; up to 8 mm, a grade 2 injury; and over 8 mm, a grade 3 injury, to the lateral ligaments of the knee.[10, 15]

Tests for One-Plane Anterior and One-Plane Posterior Instability

Lachman Test. The Lachman test is the best indicator for injury to the anterior cruciate ligament, especially the posterolateral band.[16] It is a test for one-plane anterior instability. The patient lies in a supine position with the involved leg beside the examiner. The examiner holds the patient's knee between full extension and 30° of flexion. The patient's femur is stabilized with one of the examiner's hands while the proximal aspect of the tibia is moved forward with the other hand (Fig. 11–26). A positive sign is indicated by a "mushy" or soft end feel when the tibia is moved forward on the femur and the interpatellar tendon slope disappears. A positive sign indicates that the following structures may have been injured to some degree:

1. Anterior cruciate ligament (especially the posterolateral bundle).
2. Posterior oblique ligament.
3. Arcuate-popliteus complex.

Posterior "Sag" Sign (Gravity Drawer Test). The patient lies supine with the hip flexed to 45° and the knee to 90°. In this position, the tibia will "drop back" or sag back on the femur if the posterior cruciate ligament is torn (Fig. 11–27). It is a test for one-plane posterior instability. The examiner must be careful because the position could result in a false-positive anterior drawer test for the anterior cruciate ligament if the sag remains unnoticed. If there is minimal or no swelling, the sag is quite evident because there is an obvious concavity distal to the patella. If the posterior sag sign is present, the following structures may have been injured to some degree:

1. Posterior cruciate ligament.

Table 11–3. Tests for Ligamentous Instability about the Knee

Instability	Tests Used to Determine Instability	Structures Injured to Some Degree If Test Positive*	Notes
One-plane medial (straight medial)	1. Abduction (valgus) stress with knee *in full extension*	1. Medial collateral ligament (superficial and deep fibers) 2. Posterior oblique ligament 3. Posteromedial capsule 4. Anterior cruciate ligament 5. Posterior cruciate ligament 6. Medial quadriceps expansion 7. Semimembranosus muscle	If either cruciate ligament torn (third-degree sprain) or stretched, rotary instability will also be evident
	2. Abduction (valgus) stress with knee *slightly flexed* (20–30°)	1. Medial collateral ligament (superficial and deep fibers) 2. Posterior oblique ligament 3. Posterior cruciate ligament	1. If posterior cruciate ligament torn (third-degree sprain), rotary instability will also be evident 2. Opening of 12–15° signifies injury to posterior cruciate ligament 3. If tibia externally rotated, stress is taken off posterior cruciate ligament 4. If tibia is internally rotated, stress is increased on cruciate ligaments while medial collateral ligament relaxes
One-plane lateral (straight lateral)	1. Adduction (varus) stress with knee *in full extension*	1. Lateral collateral liagment 2. Posterolateral capsule 3. Arcuate-popliteus complex 4. Biceps femoris tendon 5. Posterior cruciate ligament 6. Anterior cruciate ligament 7. Lateral gastrocnemius muscle	If either cruciate ligament is torn (third-degree sprain) or stretched, rotary instability will also be evident
	2. Adduction (varus) stress with knee *slightly flexed* (20–30°) and tibia *externally rotated*	1. Lateral collateral ligament 2. Posterolateral capsule 3. Arcuate-popliteus complex 4. Iliotibial band 5. Biceps femoris tendon	1. If tibia not externally rotated, maximum stress will not be placed on lateral collateral ligament 2. External rotation of tibia results in relaxation of both cruciate ligaments 3. With flexion, the iliotibial band lies over the center of the lateral joint line 4. If tibia is internally rotated, stress is increased on both cruciate ligaments while lateral collateral ligament relaxes
One-plane anterior	1. Lachman test (20–30° knee flexion)	1. Anterior cruciate ligament 2. Posterior oblique ligament 3. Arcuate-popliteus complex	1. Medial collateral ligament and iliotibial band lax in this position 2. Tests primarily posterolateral bundle of anterior cruciate ligament
	2. Anterior drawer sign (90° knee flexion)	1. Anterior cruciate ligament 2. Posterolateral capsule 3. Posteromedial capsule 4. Medial collateral ligament 5. Iliotibial band 6. Posterior oblique ligament 7. Arcuate-popliteus complex	1. Tests primarily anteromedial bundle of anterior cruciate ligament 2. If anterior cruciate ligament and medial or lateral structures torn (third-degree sprain) or stretched, rotary instability will also be evident
One-plane posterior	1. Posterior drawer sign (90° knee flexion) 2. Posterior sag sign	1. Posterior cruciate ligament 2. Arcuate-popliteus complex 3. Posterior oblique ligament 4. Anterior cruciate ligament	If posterior cruciate ligament and medial or lateral structures torn (third-degree sprain) or stretched, rotary instability will also be evident

Table continued on following page

Table 11-3. Tests for Ligamentous Instability about the Knee *(Continued)*

Instability	Tests Used to Determine Instability	Structures Injured to Some Degree If Test Positive*	Notes
Anteromedial rotary	Slocum test (foot laterally rotated 15°)	1. Medial collateral ligament (superficial and deep fibers) 2. Posterior oblique ligament 3. Posteromedial capsule 4. Anterior cruciate ligament	Test must *not* be done in extreme lateral rotation of tibia, since passive stabilizing will result from "coiling" to maximum rotation
Anterolateral rotary	1. Slocum test (foot medially rotated 30°) 2. Losee test 3. Jerk test of Hughston	1. Anterior cruciate ligament 2. Posterolateral capsule 3. Arcuate-popliteus complex 4. Lateral collateral ligament 5. Illiotibial band	1. Tests bring about anterior subluxation of tibia on femur, causing patient to experience "giving way" sensation 2. Slocum test must *not* be done in extreme medial rotation of tibia, since passive stabilization will result from "coiling" to maximum rotation
	1. Lateral pivot shift test of MacIntosh 2. Slocum's "ALRI" test 3. Crossover test 4. Flexion-rotation drawer test	1. Anterior cruciate ligament 2. Posterolateral capsule 3. Arcuate-popliteus complex 4. Lateral collateral ligament 5. Iliotibial band	Tests cause reduction of subluxed tibia on femur
Posteromedial rotary	Hughston's posteromedial drawer sign	1. Posterior cruciate ligament 2. Posterior oblique ligament 3. Medial collateral ligament (superficial and deep fibers) 4. Semimembranosus muscle 5. Posteromedial capsule 6. Anterior cruciate ligament	
Posterolateral rotary	1. Hughston's posterolateral drawer sign 2. Jakob test (reverse pivot shift maneuver) 3. External rotational recurvatum test	1. Posterior cruciate ligament 2. Arcuate-popliteus ligament 3. Lateral collateral ligament 4. Biceps femoris tendon 5. Posterolateral capsule 6. Anterior cruciate ligament	

*The amount of displacement will give an indication of how badly and how many of the structures are injured (i.e., first-, second-, or third-degree sprain).

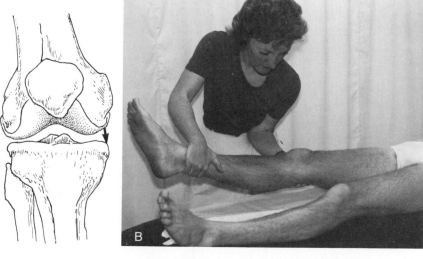

Figure 11-24. Abduction (valgus stress) test. (*A*) "Gapping" on the medial aspect of the knee. (*B*) Positioning for testing the medial collateral ligament (extended knee) is illustrated.

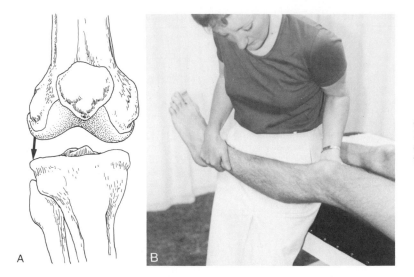

A

B

Figure 11–25. Adduction (varus stress) test. (A) One-plane lateral instability "gapping" on the lateral aspect. (B) Positioning for testing lateral collateral ligament (slightly flexed knee is illustrated).

2. Arcuate-popliteus complex.
3. Posterior oblique ligament.
4. Anterior cruciate ligament.

If it appears that the patient has a positive posterior sag sign, the patient should carefully extend the knee while the examiner holds the thigh in its present position. This action is sometimes called the *voluntary anterior drawer sign*. As the patient does this slowly, the tibial plateau will move or shift forward to its normal position, indicating that the tibia had been previously posteriorly subluxed on the femur.

Drawer Sign or Test. The drawer sign is a test for one-plane anterior and one-plane posterior instability.[17] The patient's knee is flexed to 90° and the hip to 45°. In this position, the anterior cruciate ligament is almost parallel with the tibial plateau. The patient's foot is held on the table by the examiner's body with the examiner sitting on the patient's forefoot and the foot in neutral ro-

tation. The examiner's hands are placed around the tibia to ensure that the hamstring muscles are relaxed (Fig. 11–28). The tibia is then drawn forward on the femur. The normal amount of movement that should be present is approximately 6 mm. This part of the test is an assessment for one-plane anterior instability. If the test is positive (that is, if the tibia moves forward more

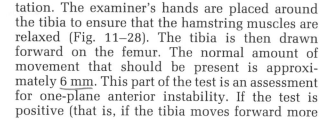

A

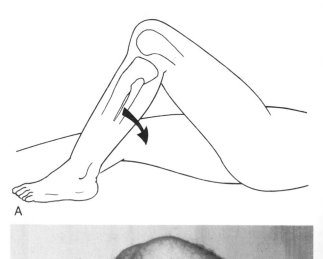

B

Figure 11–27. Sag sign. (A) Illustration of posterior sag sign. (B) Note profile of two knees; the left (nearer) sags backward compared with the normal right knee, indicating posterior cruciate defect. (From O'Donoghue, D. H.: Treatment of Injuries to Athletes, 4th ed. Philadelphia, W. B. Saunders Co., 1984, p. 450.)

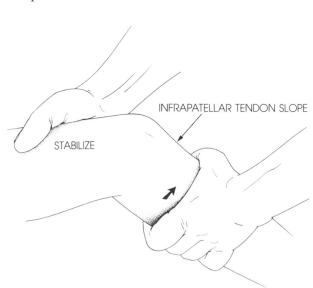

INFRAPATELLAR TENDON SLOPE

STABILIZE

Figure 11–26. Hand position for Lachman's test.

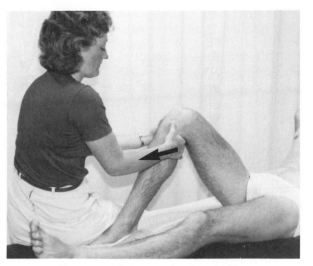

Figure 11–28. Position for drawer sign.

than 6 mm on the femur), the following structures may have been injured to some degree:

1. Anterior cruciate ligament (especially the anteromedial bundle).
2. Posterolateral capsule.
3. Posteromedial capsule.

4. Medial collateral ligament (deep fibers).
5. Iliotibial band.
6. Posterior oblique ligament.
7. Arcuate-popliteus complex.

When performing this test, the examiner must ensure that the posterior cruciate ligament is not torn or injured. If it has been torn, it will allow the tibia to drop back on the femur and when the examiner pulls the tibia forward, a large amount of movement will occur, giving a false-positive sign. (See Posterior "Sag" Sign earlier.)

Following the anterior movement of the tibia on the femur, the posterior movement of the tibia on the femur should be completed. In this part of the test, the tibia is pushed back on the femur. This phase is a test for one-plane posterior instability. If the test is positive, the following structures may have been injured to some degree:

1. Posterior cruciate ligament.
2. Arcuate-popliteus complex.
3. Posterior oblique ligament.
4. Anterior cruciate ligament.

With the drawer sign or test, if the anterior and/or posterior cruciate ligaments are torn (third-degree sprain), some rotary instability will be evident when the appropriate ligamentous tests are done (Fig. 11–29).

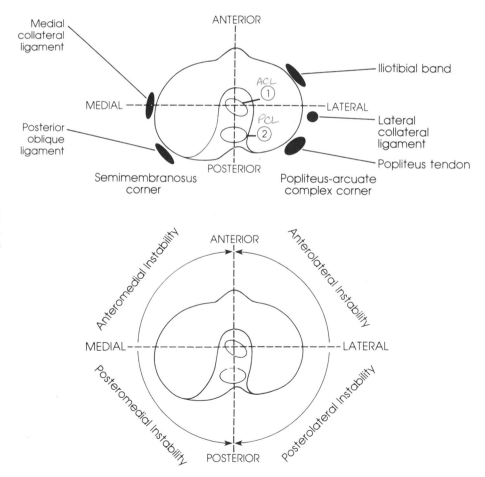

Figure 11–29. (A) Axes of the knee. 1 = Anterior cruciate ligament; 2 = posterior cruciate ligament. (B) Rotary instabilities of the knee.

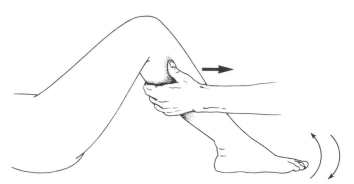

Figure 11–30. Slocum test.

Tests for Anteromedial and Anterolateral Rotary Instability

Slocum Test. The Slocum test assesses both anterior rotary instabilities.[18] The patient's knee is flexed to 80 or 90° and the hip to 45°. The foot is first placed in 30° medial rotation (Fig. 11–30). The examiner then sits on the patient's forefoot to hold the foot in position, draws the tibia forward, and if the test is positive, movement will occur primarily on the lateral side of the knee. This movement would be excessive relative to the good side and indicates anterolateral rotary instability. It indicates that the following structures may have been injured to some degree:

1. Anterior cruciate ligament.
2. Posterolateral capsule.
3. Arcuate-popliteus complex.
4. Lateral collateral ligament.

5. Posterior cruciate ligament.
6. Iliotibial band (tensor fasciae latae).

If the examiner finds anterolateral instability during this first position of the Slocum test, the second part of the test, which assesses antero-medial rotary instability in this position, is of less value.[19]

With the foot placed in 15° of lateral rotation, the tibia is drawn forward by the examiner. If the test is positive, the movement will occur primarily on the medial side of the knee. This movement would be excessive relative to the good side and would be indicative of anteromedial rotary instability. It indicates that the following structures may have been injured to some degree:

1. Medial collateral ligament (especially the superficial fibers, although the deep fibers may also be affected).
2. Posterior oblique ligament.
3. Posteromedial capsule.
4. Anterior cruciate ligament.

For the Slocum test, it is imperative that the examiner medially or laterally rotate the foot to the degrees shown. If the examiner rotates the tibia as far as it will go, the test will be negative because this action tightens up all the structures remaining.

If a stress radiograph is taken during the test, minimal or no movement indicates a negative test; 1 mm or less, a grade 1 injury; 1 to 2 mm, a grade 2 injury; and more than 2 mm, a grade 3 injury.[15]

The test may also be performed with the patient sitting with the knees flexed over the edge of the

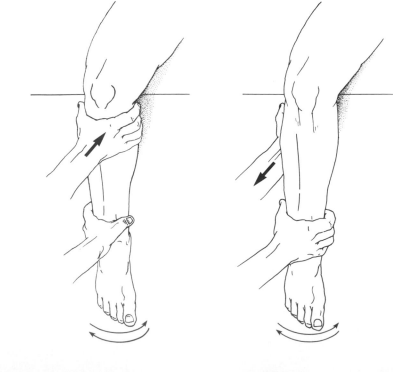

Figure 11–31. Slocum test with the patient in the sitting position.

treatment table (Fig. 11–31).[10] The examiner applies an anterior or posterior force while holding the foot medially or laterally rotated. If this procedure is used, the examiner must remember that the anterior force is testing for anterior rotary instability while the posterior force is testing for posterior rotary instability. (See Hughston's Posterolateral and Posteromedial Drawer Sign in the next section.) The examiner should note whether the movement is excessive on the medial or lateral side of the knee relative to the normal knee. Excessive movement indicates a positive test.

Lateral Pivot Shift Maneuver (Test of MacIntosh). This is the primary test used to assess anterolateral rotary instability of the knee (Fig. 11–32).[20–22] During this test, the tibia moves away from the femur on the lateral side and moves anteriorly in relation to the femur.

Normally, the knee's center of rotation changes constantly through its range of motion as a result of the shape of the femoral condyles, ligamentous restraint, and muscle tension. The path of movement of the tibia on the femur is described as a combination of rolling and sliding, with rolling predominating when the instant center is near the joint line and sliding predominating when the instant center shifts distally from the contact area. The MacIntosh test is a duplication of the anterior subluxation-reduction phenomenon that occurs during the normal gait cycle when the anterior cruciate ligament is torn. Thus, it illustrates a dynamic subluxation. This shift occurs between 20 and 40° of flexion (0° being the knee in the extended position). It is this phenomenon that gives the patient the clinical description of the feeling of the knee "giving way" (Fig. 11–33).

The patient lies supine with the hip flexed to 20° and relaxed in slight medial rotation (20°). The examiner holds the patient's foot with one

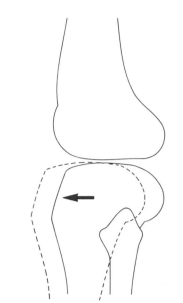

Figure 11–33. Anterior shift of the tibia during the lateral pivot shift test.

hand while the other hand flexes the knee slightly (5°). This is done by placing the heel of the hand behind the fibula over the lateral head of the gastrocnemius muscle with the tibia medially rotated, causing the tibia to sublux anteriorly (Fig. 11–34). As the knee approaches extension, the secondary restraints (hamstrings, lateral femoral condyle, and lateral meniscus) are less sufficient than in flexion. The examiner then applies a

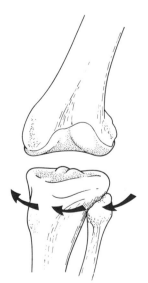

Figure 11–32. Anterolateral rotary instability.

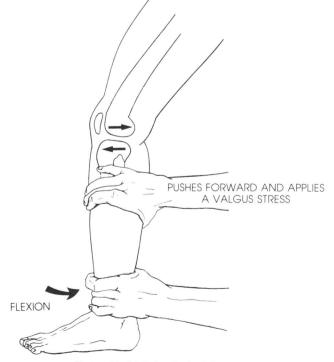

PUSHES FORWARD AND APPLIES A VALGUS STRESS

FLEXION

Figure 11–34. Lateral pivot shift test.

valgus stress to the knee while maintaining a medial rotation torque at the tibia at the ankle. If the leg is then flexed at about 30 to 40°, the tibia will reduce or jog backward and the patient will say that is what the "giving way" feels like, indicating a positive test. The reduction is due to the change in position of the iliotibial band moving from an extensor function to a flexor function, thus pulling the tibia back to its normal position. Kennedy advocated pushing on the fibula with the thumb when performing this maneuver.[15] If the test is positive, the following structures have been injured to some degree:

1. Anterior cruciate ligament.
2. Posterolateral capsule.
3. Arcuate-popliteus complex.
4. Lateral collateral ligament.
5. Iliotibial band.

Losee Test. The patient lies in a supine position and relaxed.[23] The examiner holds the patient's ankle and foot so that the leg is laterally rotated and braced against the abdomen. The knee is then flexed to 30°, and the examiner ensures that the hamstring muscles are relaxed (Fig. 11–35). The lateral rotation ensures that the subluxation of the knee is reduced at the beginning of the test. With the examiner's other hand positioned so that the fingers lie over the patella and the thumb is hooked behind the fibular head, a valgus force is applied to the knee; the examiner uses his abdomen as a fulcrum while extending the patient's knee and applying forward pressure behind the fibular head with the thumb. The valgus stress compresses the structures in the lateral compartment and makes the anterior subluxation, if present, more noticeable. At the same time, the foot and ankle are allowed to drift into medial rotation. If the foot and ankle are not allowed to rotate medially, the anterior subluxation of the lateral tibial plateau may be prevented. Just before full extension of the knee, there will be a "clunk" forward if the test is positive and the patient must recognize the movement as the instability that was previously experienced. This clunk means that the tibia has subluxed anteriorly and indicates injury to the same structures as did the pivot shift maneuver. The Losee test assesses anterolateral rotary instability.

Jerk Test of Hughston. This test is similar to the pivot shift maneuver; the positioning of the patient and the examiner are the same, except that the patient's hip is flexed to 45°. With this test,[24] the knee is first flexed to 90°. The leg is then extended, maintaining medial rotation and a valgus stress. At about 20 to 30° of flexion, the tibia will shift forward, causing a subluxation of the lateral tibial plateau with a "jerk" if the test is positive. If the leg is carried into further extension, it will spontaneously reduce. A positive jerk test shows the same structures injured as in the

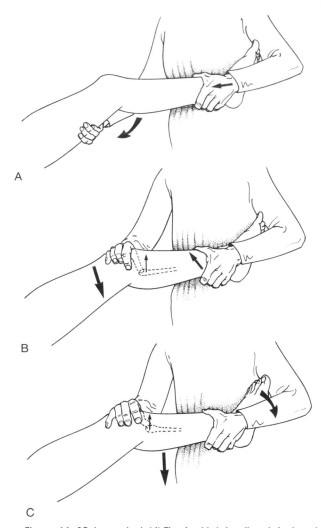

Figure 11–35. Losee test. (A) The foot is laterally rotated and cradled in examiner's hand; the abdomen is against the fibula; and the leg is flexed to relax the hamstrings. (B) The examiner's right thumb pushes the fibula forward while valgus stress is applied with the abdomen. (C) The patient's knee is extended while the foot is allowed to internally rotate; valgus stress is still applied and the fibula is pushed forward.

pivot shift maneuver and assesses anterolateral rotary instability. According to the literature,[10] this test is not as sensitive as the pivot shift test.

Slocum's "ALRI" Test. The Slocum ALRI test also assesses anterolateral rotary instability.[10, 19] The patient is in a side lying position (approximately 30° from supine). The bottom leg is the uninvolved leg. The knee of the uninvolved leg is flexed to add stability (Fig. 11–36). The foot of the test leg rests and is stabilized on the examining table with the patient's foot in medial rotation and the knee in extension and valgus. This position helps to eliminate the hip rotation during the test. The examiner applies a valgus stress to the knee while flexing the knee. The subluxation of the knee will reduce during this test between 25 and 45° of flexion if the test is positive. A

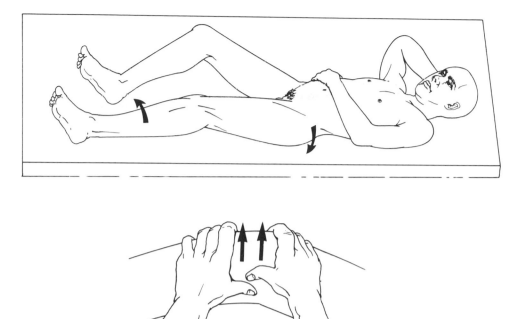

Figure 11-36. Slocum's anterolateral rotary instability (ALRI) test.

positive ALRI test indicates the same structures injured as in the pivot shift maneuver. The main advantage of this particular test is that it does aid in relaxation of the patient's hamstring muscles and is easier to perform on heavy or tense patients.

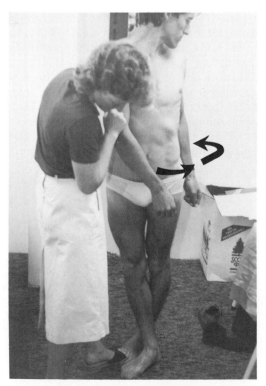

Figure 11-37. Crossover test.

Crossover Test. The patient is asked to cross the uninvolved leg in front of the test leg (Fig. 11-37). The examiner then carefully steps on the patient's involved foot to stabilize it and instructs the patient to rotate the upper torso away from the injured leg approximately 90° away from the fixed foot. When this position is achieved, the patient then contracts the quadriceps muscles, producing the same symptoms (and testing the same structures) as in the lateral pivot shift test. The crossover test assesses anterolateral rotary instability.

Flexion-Rotation Drawer Test. Described by Noyes,[25] this test is a modification of the pivot-shift test. The examiner flexes the patient's knee to 20 to 30° while maintaining the tibia in neutral rotation. The tibia is then pushed posteriorly as is done in a posterior drawer test. This posterior movement reduces the subluxation of the tibia, indicating a positive test for anterolateral rotary instability. If the tibia is alternately pushed posteriorly and released and the femur allowed to rotate freely, the reduction and subluxation will be seen and felt as the femur rotates medially and laterally.

Tests for Posterolateral and Posteromedial Rotary Instability

Hughston's Posterolateral and Posteromedial Drawer Sign. The patient lies in a supine position with the knee flexed to 80 to 90° and the hip to 45° (Fig. 11-38).[26] The examiner medially rotates

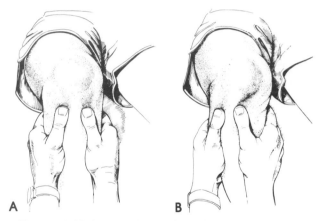

Figure 11–38. Posterolateral drawer test, anterior view. (A) Starting position for posterolateral drawer test. (B) Positive posterolateral drawer test with posterior and lateral rotation of the lateral tibial condyle. (From Hughston, J. C., and L. A. Norwood: Clin. Orthop. Relat. Res. *147*:83, 1980.)

the patient's foot slightly and sits on the foot to stabilize it. The examiner then pushes the tibia posteriorly. If the tibia moves or rotates posteriorly on the medial aspect an excessive amount relative to the normal knee, the test is positive and is indicative of posteromedial rotary instability. A positive test indicates that the following structures have probably been injured to some degree:

1. Posterior cruciate ligament.
2. Posterior oblique ligament.
3. Medial collateral ligament (superficial and deep fibers).
4. Semimembranous muscle.
5. Posteromedial capsule.
6. Anterior cruciate ligament.

The medial tibial tubercle will rotate posteriorly around the posterior cruciate ligament when the tibia is in mild medial rotation. If the posterior cruciate ligament is also torn, the posteromedial movement will be greater and the tibia will sublux posteriorly (Fig. 11–39).

The test may also be done in sitting with the knee flexed over the edge of the treatment table. The examiner pushes posteriorly while holding the leg in medial rotation, watching for the same excessive movement.

Posterolateral rotary instability may be tested in a similar fashion. The patient and examiner are in the same position, but the patient's foot is slightly laterally rotated. If, when the examiner pushes the tibia posteriorly, the tibia rotates posteriorly on the lateral side an excessive amount relative to the uninvolved leg, the test is positive for posterolateral rotary instability. The test will be positive only if the posterior cruciate ligament is torn. The examiner may palpate the fibula while doing the movement to feel for excessive movement. The test indicates that the following structures are probably injured to some degree:

1. Posterior cruciate ligament.
2. Arcuate-popliteus complex.
3. Lateral collateral ligament.
4. Biceps femoris tendon.
5. Posterolateral capsule.
6. Anterior cruciate ligament.

Jakob Test (Reverse Pivot Shift Maneuver). This is a test for posterolateral rotary instability.[10,][27] This test can be performed in two ways (Figs. 11–40 and 11–41).

Method 1. The patient stands and leans against a wall with the sound side adjacent to the wall and the body weight distributed equally on both feet. The examiner's hands are placed above and below the test knee and a valgus stress is exerted while flexion of the patient's knee is initiated. If, during this maneuver, there is a jerk in the knee or the tibia shifts posteriorly and the "giving way" phenomenon occurs, it indicates injury to the same structures as Hughston's posterolateral drawer sign.

Method 2. The patient lies in a supine position with the hamstring muscles relaxed. The examiner faces the patient and lifts the leg and supports it against the pelvis. The examiner's other hand supports the lateral side of the calf with the palm on the proximal fibula. The knee is flexed to 70

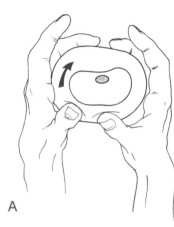

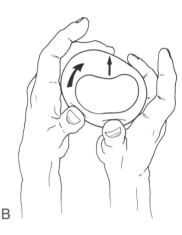

Figure 11–39. Posterolateral drawer test. If the posterior cruciate ligament is intact, the tibia will rotate posterolaterally as in *A*. If the posterior cruciate ligament is torn, the tibia will rotate posterolaterally and will sublux posteriorly (*B*).

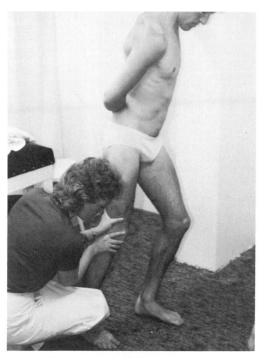

Figure 11–40. Jakob test. Method 1 showing valgus stress and flexion.

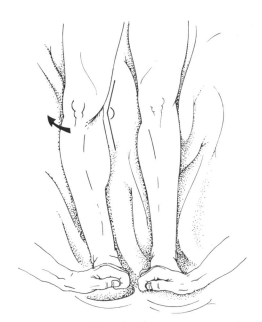

Figure 11–42. External rotational recurvatum test.

to 80° of flexion and the foot is laterally rotated, causing the lateral tibial plateau to sublux posteriorly (Fig. 11–41A). The knee is taken into extension by its own weight while the examiner leans on the foot to impart a valgus stress to the knee through the leg. As the knee approaches 20° of flexion, the lateral tibial tubercle will shift forward or anteriorly into the neutral rotation and reduce the subluxation, indicating a positive test

(Fig. 11–41B). The leg is then flexed again and the foot falls back into lateral rotation and posterior subluxation. This is a test for posterolateral rotary instability and is sometimes called the *reverse pivot shift test* (Fig. 11–41).

External Rotational Recurvatum Test. There are two methods for this test:

Method 1. The patient lies in a supine position with the lower limbs relaxed. The examiner gently grasps the big toe of both feet and lifts both feet off the examining table (Fig. 11–42).[26] The patient is told to keep the quadriceps muscles relaxed. While elevating the legs, the examiner

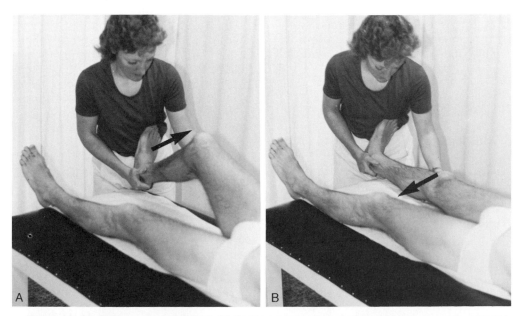

Figure 11–41. Reverse pivot shift test. (*A*) Position causes lateral tibial tubercle to sublux. (*B*) This position causes lateral tibial tubercle to reduce.

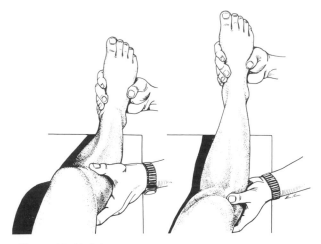

Figure 11–43. External recurvatum test (Method 2). The test is begun by holding the knee in flexion (left). As the knee is slowly extended, the hand at the knee will feel the external rotation and recurvatum at the posterolateral aspect of the knee. (From Hughston, J. C., and L. A. Norwood: Clin. Orthop. Relat. Res. *147*:86, 1980.)

watches the tibial tuberosities. For the test to be positive, the affected knee will go into relative hyperextension on the lateral aspect, with the tibia and tibial tuberosity rotating laterally. The affected knee will have the appearance of a relative genu varum. It is a test for posterolateral rotary instability in extension and assesses the same structures previously mentioned.

Method 2. The patient lies in a supine position and the examiner's hand holds the patient's heel or foot and flexes the knee to 30 to 40° (Fig. 11–43).[26] The examiner's other hand holds the posterolateral aspect of the patient's knee, which is being slowly extended. With the hand on the knee, the examiner will feel the relative hyperextension and lateral rotation occurring in the injured limb as opposed to the uninjured limb. This is a test for posterolateral rotary instability and assesses the same structures as previously mentioned.

SPECIAL TESTS

Tests for Meniscus Injury

Although there are several tests for a meniscus injury, none can be considered definitive without

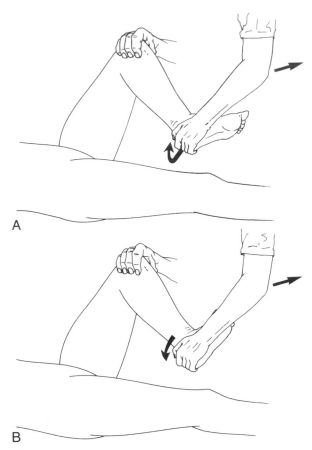

A

B

Figure 11–44. McMurray test (Method 2). (*A*) Lateral meniscus. (*B*) Medial meniscus.

considerable experience of the examiner. Because the menisci are avascular and have no nerve supply, an injury to the meniscus can potentially result with no pain or swelling, making diagnosis even more difficult.

McMurray Test. The patient lies in the supine position with the knee completely flexed (the heel to the buttock).[28] The examiner then medially rotates the tibia (Fig. 11–44). If there is a loose fragment of the lateral meniscus, this action will cause a snap or click which is often accompanied by pain. By repeatedly changing the amount of flexion, the examiner can test the entire posterior aspect of the meniscus from the posterior horn to the middle segment. The anterior half of the meniscus is not as easily tested because the pressure on the meniscus is not as great. To test the

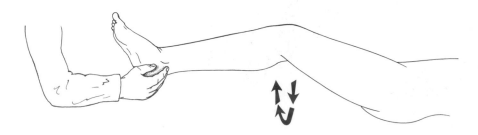

Figure 11–45. Bounce home test.

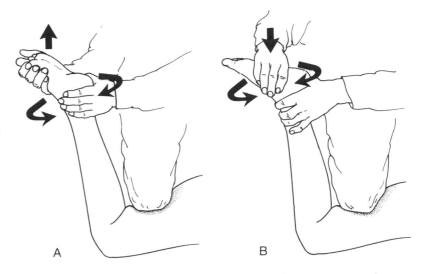

Figure 11–46. Apley's test. (*A*) Distraction. (*B*) Compression.

medial meniscus, the examiner performs the same procedure but with the knee laterally rotated.

The test may be modified by medially rotating the tibia and extending the knee and by moving through the full range of motion to test the lateral meniscus. The process is repeated several times. The tibia is then laterally rotated and the process repeated to test the medial meniscus. Both methods are described by McMurray.[28]

"Bounce Home" Test. The patient lies supine and the heel of the patient's foot is cupped in the examiner's hand (Fig. 11–45). The patient's knee is completely flexed, and the knee is passively allowed to extend. If extension is not complete or has a rubbery end feel ("springy block"), there is something blocking full extension. The most likely cause of a block is a torn meniscus.

O'Donoghue's Test. Having complained of pain along the joint line, the patient is asked to lie supine. The examiner flexes the knee to 90°, rotates it medially and laterally twice, and then fully flexes and rotates it both ways again. A positive sign is indicated by increased pain on rotation in either or both positions and is indicative of capsular irritation or a meniscus tear.

Apley's Test. The patient lies in a prone position with the knee flexed to 90°. The patient's thigh is then anchored to the bed by the examiner's knee (Fig. 11–46). The examiner medially and laterally rotates the tibia, combined first with distraction, noting any restriction or discomfort. The process is repeated using compression instead of distraction. If rotation plus distraction is more painful, the lesion is probably ligamentous. If the rotation plus compression is more painful, the lesion is probably a meniscus injury.

Modified Helfet Test.[29] In the normal knee, the tibial tuberosity is in line with the midline of the patella when the knee is flexed to 90°. When the knee is extended, however, the tibial tubercle is in line with the lateral border of the patella (Fig.

11–47). If this change does not occur with the change in movement, rotation is blocked, indicating injury to the meniscus or a possible cruciate injury.

Test for a Retreating or Retracting Meniscus. The patient sits on the edge of the examining table or lies in a supine position with the knee flexed to 90°.[29] The examiner places one finger over the joint line of the patient's knee anterior to the medial collateral ligament where the curved margin of the medial femoral condyle approaches the tibial tuberosity (Fig. 11–48). The patient's leg and foot are then passively laterally rotated and the meniscus will normally disappear. The leg is medially and laterally rotated several times. The knee must be flexed and the muscles relaxed to do the test. If the meniscus does not disappear, a torn meniscus may be present, since rotation of the tibia is not occurring. The examiner must palpate carefully because a distinct structure is difficult to palpate. If the examiner medially and

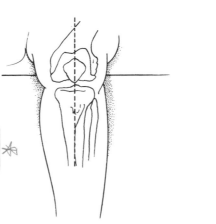

FLEXED KNEE   EXTENDED KNEE

Figure 11–47. Modified Helfet test (negative test shown).

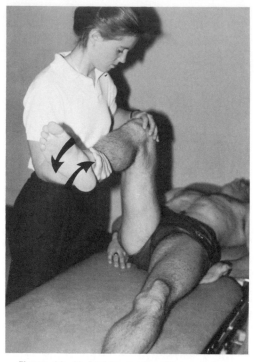

Figure 11–48. Test for a retreating meniscus.

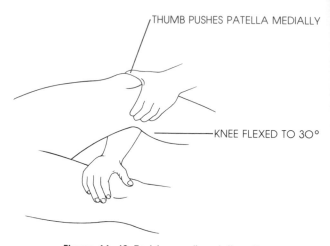

Figure 11–49. Test for mediopatellar plica.

laterally rotates the unaffected leg several times first, the meniscus will be felt pushing against the finger on medial rotation and disappear on lateral rotation.

Steinman's Tenderness Displacement Test. The Steinman sign is indicated by point tenderness and pain on the joint line that appears to move anteriorly when the knee is extended and moved posteriorly when the knee is flexed. It is indicative of a possible meniscus tear. Medial pain is elicited on lateral rotation, and lateral pain is elicited on medial rotation.

Plica Tests

Because an abnormal plica can mimic meniscus pathology, it is essential that the plica tests be performed as well as the meniscus tests if one suspects a meniscus injury.

Mediopatellar Plica Test. The patient lies supine and the examiner flexes the affected knee to 30° (Fig. 11–49). If the examiner then moves the patella medially, the patient will complain of pain. This pain, indicating a positive test, is caused by the edge of the plica being pinched between the medial femoral condyle and the patella. The pain is possibly indicative of a mediopatellar plica.[30]

Plica "Stutter" Test. The patient is seated on the edge of the examining table with both knees flexed to 90°. The examiner places a finger over one patella to palpate during movement. The

patient is then instructed to slowly extend the knee. If the test is positive, the patella will stutter or jump somewhere between 60° and 45° of flexion (0° is straight leg) during an otherwise smooth movement. The test will work only if there is no joint swelling.

Hughston Plica Test. The patient lies in a supine position and the examiner flexes the knee and medially rotates the tibia with one arm and hand while pressing the patella medially with the heel of the other hand and palpating the medial femoral condyle with the fingers of the same hand (Fig. 11–50). The patient's knee is passively flexed and extended while the examiner feels for "popping" of the plical band under the fingers. The popping indicates a positive test.[24]

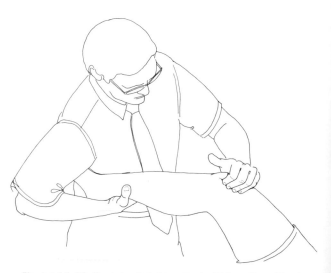

Figure 11–50. Examination for suprapatellar plica. The foot and tibia are held in internal rotation. The patella is displaced slightly medially with the fingers over the course of the plica. The knee is passively flexed and extended, eliciting "pop" of the plica and associated tenderness. (From Hughston, J. C., et al.: Patellar Subluxation and Dislocation. Philadelphia, W. B. Saunders Co., 1984, p. 29.)

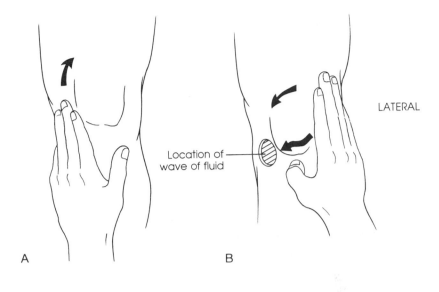

Figure 11–51. Brush test for swelling. (*A*) Hand strokes up. (*B*) Hand strokes down.

MEDIAL

LATERAL

Location of wave of fluid

A

B

Tests for Swelling

When looking at swelling, the examiner must determine the type and amount of swelling that is present. Although the tests for swelling are listed under special tests, the examiner should always be testing for swelling when examining the knee. As well, the examiner must differentiate between swelling and synovial thickening. With swelling, the knee will assume its resting position of 15 to 25° of flexion, which allows the synovial cavity the maximum capacity for holding fluid. If the injury is sufficiently severe, the fluid extravasates into the soft tissue surrounding the joint as a result of torn structures (i.e., ligaments, capsule, synovium). Thus, lack of effusion should not lull the examiner into thinking the injury is a minor one.

If the swelling is due to blood that results in a hemarthrosis, it may be due to a ligament tear, osteochondral fracture, or peripheral meniscus tear. The swelling will come on very quickly (within 1 to 2 hours), and the skin will become very tense. On palpation, it has a "doughy" feeling and is relatively hard to the touch. The joint surface will feel warm. Generally, excessive blood should be aspirated, or osteoarthritis may result from the irritation of the cartilage.

Normally, synovial fluid from joint irritation occurs in 8 to 24 hours. The feeling within the joint is a fluctuating or "boggy" feeling. The joint surface will feel warm and tender. Swelling usually occurs with activity and disappears after a few days of inactivity.

The third type of swelling is purulent or pus swelling, in which the joint surface is hot to the touch. It will often be red and the patient will have general signs of infection or pyrexia.

Brush or Stroke Test. Also called the *wipe test*, this test assesses minimal effusion. The examiner commences just below the joint line on the medial side of the patella, stroking proximally toward the patient's hip as far as the suprapatellar pouch two or three times with the palm and fingers (Fig. 11–51). With the opposite hand, the examiner strokes down the lateral side of the patella. A wave of fluid, if present, will pass to the medial side of the joint and bulge just below the medial distal portion or border of the patella. The wave of fluid may take up to 2 seconds to appear. Normally, the knee contains 5 to 7 ml of synovial fluid. This test will show as little as 4 to 8 ml of extra fluid within the knee.

Fluctuation Test. The examiner places the palm of one hand over the suprapatellar pouch and the palm of the other hand anterior to the joint with the thumb and index finger just beyond the margins of the patella (Fig. 11–52). By pressing down with one hand and then the other, the examiner may feel the synovial fluid fluctuate under the hands, moving from one hand to the other, indicating significant effusion.

Patellar Tap Test ("Ballotable Patella"). With the patient's knee extended or flexed to discomfort, the examiner applies a slight tap or pressure over the patella. When doing so, a floating of the

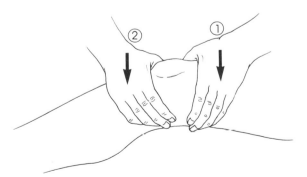

Figure 11–52. Hand positioning for fluctuation test. First one hand is pushed down (arrow 1) and then the other hand (arrow 2) and each hand is alternated. The examiner will feel fluid shifting back and forth.

patella should be felt. This test can detect a large amount of swelling in the knee.

Other Special Tests

Only those tests that the examiner feels are necessary need to be performed.

Q-Angle or the Patellofemoral Angle. The Q-angle is defined as the angle between the quadriceps muscles (primarily the rectus femoris) and the patellar tendon (Fig. 11–53). The angle is obtained by first ensuring the lower limbs are at a right angle to the line joining each anterior superior iliac spine (ASIS). A line is then drawn from the ASIS to the midpoint of the patella and from the tibial tubercle to the midpoint of the patella. The angle formed by the crossing of these two lines is called the Q-angle. The foot should be placed in a neutral position relative to supination and pronation and the hip in neutral relative to medial and lateral rotation, as it has been found that different foot and hip positions alter the Q-angle.[31] Normally, the Q-angle (quadriceps angle or patellofemoral angle) is 13 to 18° (13° for males, 18° for females) when the knee is straight. Any angle less than 13° may be associated with chondromalacia patellae or patella alta. Any angle greater than 18° is often associated with chondromalacia patellae, subluxing patella, increased

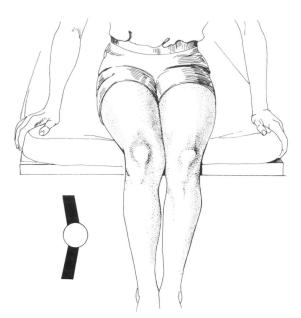

Figure 11–54. Q-angle in flexed position. Exaggerated Q-angle in the patient's right knee is seen as residual positive Q-angle with the knee flexed. Normally, the Q-angle in flexion should be 0°. (From Hughston, J. C., et al.: Patellar Subluxation and Dislocation. Philadelphia, W. B. Saunders Co., 1984, p. 24.)

femoral anteversion, genu valgum, or increased lateral tibial torsion. During the test, which may be done either with radiographs or physically on the patient, the quadriceps should be relaxed. If measured in the sitting position, the Q-angle should be 0° (Fig. 11–54). While in a sitting position, the presence of the "bayonet" sign, which indicates an abnormal alignment of the quadriceps musculature, patellar tendon, and tibial shaft, should be noted (Fig. 11–55).

Hughston advocates doing the test with the quadriceps contracted.[24] If performed with the quadriceps contracted and knee fully extended, the Q-angle should be 8 to 10°. Anything greater than 10° would be considered abnormal.

Clarke's Sign. This test assesses the presence of chondromalacia patellae. The examiner presses down slightly proximal to the upper pole or base of the patella with the web of the hand as the patient lies relaxed with the knee extended (Fig. 11–56). The patient is then asked to contract the quadriceps muscles while the examiner pushes down. If the patient can complete and maintain the contraction without pain, the test is negative. If the test causes retropatellar pain and the patient can not hold a contraction, the test is considered positive. It should be pointed out that a positive test can result in any individual if sufficient pressure is applied to the patella when the patient is asked to contract the quadriceps. Thus the amount of pressure applied must be controlled. The best way to do this is to repeat the procedure several times, increasing the pressure each time

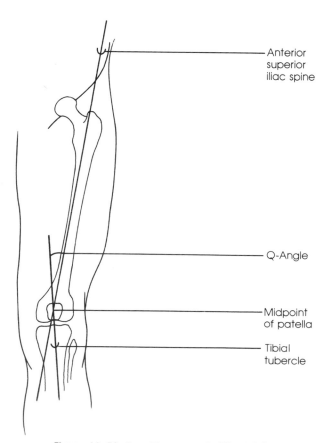

Anterior superior iliac spine

Q-Angle

Midpoint of patella

Tibial tubercle

Figure 11–53. Quadriceps angle (Q-angle).

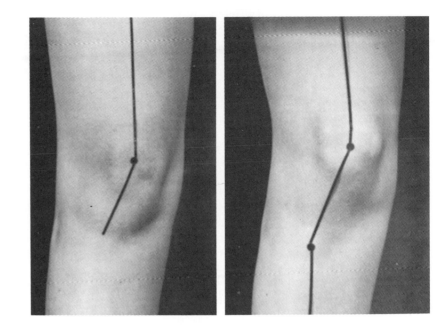

Figure 11–55. Increased Q-angle.
(*A*) Bayonet sign. Tibia vara of proximal third causes a markedly increased Q-angle. Alignment of the quadriceps, patellar tendon, and tibial shaft resembles a French bayonet. (From Hughston, J. C., et al.: Patellar Subluxation and Dislocation. Philadelphia, W. B. Saunders Co., 1984, p. 26.)
(*B*) Q-angle with the knee in full extension is only slightly increased over normal. However, with the knee flexed at 30°, there is failure of the tibia to derotate normally and the patellar tendon to line up with the anterior crest of the tibia. This is not an infrequent finding in patients with patello-femoral arthralgia. (From Ficat, R. P., and D. S. Hungerford: Disorders of the Patello-Femoral Joint. Baltimore, The Williams and Wilkins Co., 1977, p. 117.)

and comparing with the unaffected side. For testing different parts of the patella, the knee should be tested in 30°, 60°, and 90° of flexion as well as in full extension.

Waldron Test. This test also assesses the presence of chondromalacia patellae.[8] The examiner palpates the patella while the patient does several slow deep knee bends. As the patient goes through the range of motion, the examiner should note the amount of crepitus (significant only if accompanied by pain), where it occurs in the range of motion, the amount of pain, and whether there is "catching" or poor tracking of the patella throughout the movement. If pain and crepitus

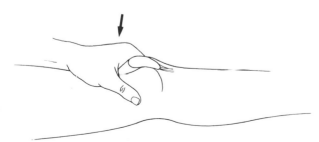

Figure 11–56. Clarke sign.

occur together during the movement, it is a sign of chondromalacia patellae.[8]

Wilson Test. This is a test for osteochondritis dissecans. The patient sits with the knee flexed over the examining table. The knee is then actively extended with the tibia medially rotated. At about 30° of flexion (0° being straight leg), the pain in the knee increases and the patient is asked to stop the flexion movement. The patient is then asked to rotate the tibia laterally, and the pain will disappear. This finding indicates a positive test, which is indicative of osteochondritis dissecans of the femur. The test would be positive only if the lesion is at the classic site for osteochondritis dissecans of the knee, namely, the medial femoral condyle near the intercondylar notch (Fig. 11–57).

Apprehension Test. This is a test for dislocation of the patella.[24] The patient lies supine with the quadriceps muscles relaxed and knee flexed to 30° while the examiner carefully and slowly pushes the patella laterally (Fig. 11–58). If the patella feels as if it is going to dislocate, the patient will contract the quadriceps muscles to bring the patella back "into line." This action indicates a positive test. The patient will also have an apprehensive look on the face.

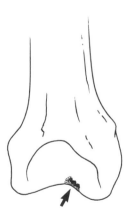

Figure 11–57. Classic site of osteochondritis dissecans.

Noble Compression Test. This is a test for iliotibial band friction syndrome.[32] The patient lies in a supine position, and the examiner flexes the patient's knee to 90°, accompanied by hip flexion (Fig. 11–59). Pressure is then applied to the lateral femoral epicondyle or 1 to 2 cm prox-

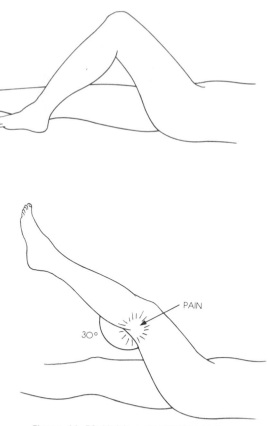

Figure 11–59. Noble compression test.

imal to it with the thumb. While the pressure is maintained, the patient's knee is passively extended. At about 30° of flexion (0° being straight leg), the patient will complain of severe pain over the lateral femoral condyle. This indicates a positive test. The patient will state that it is the same pain which occurs with activity.

Functional Test for Quadriceps Contusion. The patient lies prone while the examiner passively flexes the knee as much as possible. If passive knee flexion is 90° or more, it is only a <u>mild contusion</u>. If the passive knee flexion is less than 90°, the contusion is <u>moderate to severe</u> and the patient should not be allowed to bear weight.

Measurement of Leg Length. The patient lies supine with legs at a right angle to a line joining each ASIS. The patient's feet should face straight up as well (Fig. 11–60). With a tape measure, the examiner obtains the distance from one ASIS to the lateral malleolus on that side, placing the metal end of the tape measure immediately distal to and pushed up against the ASIS. The tape is stretched so that the other hand pushes the tape against the distal aspect of the lateral malleolus, and the reading on the tape measure is noted. The other side is tested similarly. A difference of up to 1.0 to 1.5 cm is considered normal. However, the examiner must remember that even this

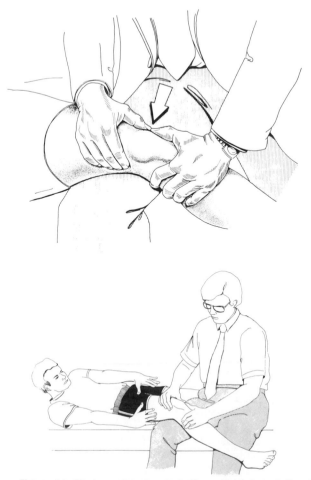

Figure 11–58. Apprehension test. (From Hughston, J. C., et al.: Patellar Subluxation and Dislocation. Philadelphia, W. B. Saunders Co., 1984, p. 31.)

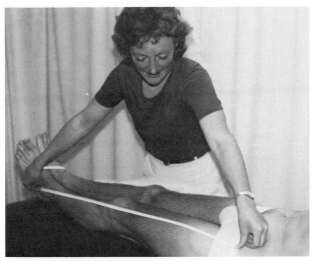

Figure 11–60. Measuring leg length (to the lateral malleolus).

Measurement of Muscle Bulk (Anthropometric Measurements for Effusion and Atrophy). The examiner selects areas where muscle bulk or swelling is greatest and measures the circumference of the leg. It is important to note on the patient's chart how far above or below the apex or base of the patella one is measuring and whether the tape measure is placed above or below that mark. The following values are common measurement points that are often used:

- 15 cm below the apex of the patella.
- Apex of the patella or joint line.
- 5 cm above the base of patella.
- 8 cm above the base of patella.
- 15 cm above the base of patella.
- 23 cm above the base of patella.

The examiner must also note, if possible, whether swelling and/or muscle bulk is being measured and remember that there is no correlation between muscle bulk and strength.

difference may result in pathology. If there is a difference, the examiner can determine its site of occurrence by measuring from the high point in the iliac crest to the greater trochanter (for coxa vara); from the greater trochanter to the lateral knee joint line (for femoral length); and from the medial knee joint line to the medial malleolus (for tibial length). Both legs are then compared. The examiner must also recognize that torsion deformities to the femur or tibia can alter leg length.

REFLEXES AND CUTANEOUS DISTRIBUTION

Having completed the ligamentous and other tests of the knee, the examiner next determines whether the reflexes about the knee joint are normal if a scanning examination has not been carried out (Fig. 11–61). The patellar (L3 and L4) and medial hamstring (L5) reflexes should be checked for differences between the two sides.

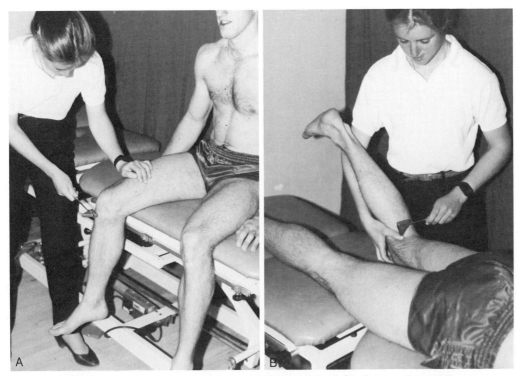

Figure 11–61. Reflexes of the knee. (*A*) Patellar (L3). (*B*) Medial hamstrings (L5).

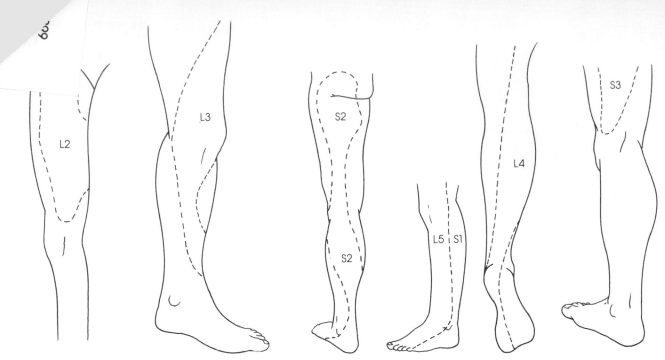

Figure 11–62. Dermatomes about the knee.

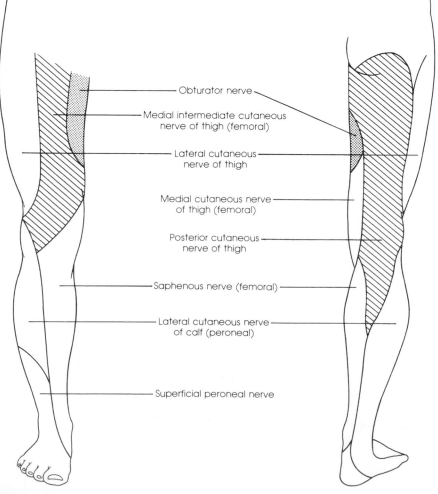

Obturator nerve

Medial intermediate cutaneous nerve of thigh (femoral)

Lateral cutaneous nerve of thigh

Medial cutaneous nerve of thigh (femoral)

Posterior cutaneous nerve of thigh

Saphenous nerve (femoral)

Lateral cutaneous nerve of calf (peroneal)

Superficial peroneal nerve

Figure 11–63. Peripheral nerve sensory distribution about the knee.

4. Anteroposterior movement of the fibula on the tibia.

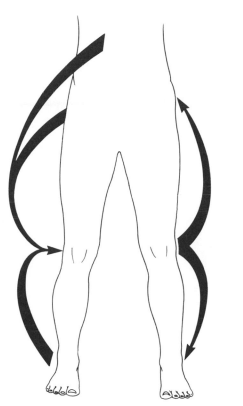

Figure 11–64. Patterns of referred pain to and from the knee.

The examiner must keep in mind the dermatomal patterns of the various nerve roots (Fig. 11–62) as well as the cutaneous distribution of the peripheral nerves (Fig. 11–63). To test for altered sensation the relaxed hands and fingers should cover all aspects of the thigh, knee, and leg. Any differences in sensation should be noted and can be further mapped out using a pinwheel, pin, cotton batten, or brush.

True knee pain tends to be localized to the knee, but it may also be referred to the hip or ankle (Fig. 11–64). In a similar fashion, pain may be referred to the knee from the lumbar spine, hip, and ankle.

JOINT PLAY MOVEMENT

For joint play movements on the knee, the patient is in a supine position. The movement on the affected side is compared with the normal side.

The following movements should be carried out at the knee (Fig. 11–65):

1. Backward and forward movement of the tibia on the femur.

2. Medial and lateral displacement of the patella.

3. Depression (distal movement) of the patella.

Backward and Forward Movement of Tibia on Femur

The patient is asked to lie supine with the test knee flexed to 90° and the hip flexed to 45°. The examiner then places the heel of the hand over the tibial tuberosity while stabilizing the patient's limb with the other hand and pushing backward with the heel of the hand. The end feel of the movement should normally be tissue stretch. To perform the forward movement, the examiner places both hands around the posterior aspect of the tibia. Prior to performing the joint play movement, the examiner must ensure the hamstrings and gastrocnemius muscles are relaxed. The tibia is then drawn forward on the femur. The examiner feels the quality of the movement, which is normally tissue stretch.

These joint play movements are similar to the anterior and posterior drawer test for ligamentous stability.

Medial and Lateral Displacement of Patella

The patient is in a supine position with the knee slightly flexed. The examiner's thumbs are placed against the medial or lateral edge of the patella and a force applied to the side of the patella, the fingers being used as a stabilizing force. The process is then repeated, with pressure applied to the other side of the patella. The other knee is tested as a comparison.

This joint play is similar to the passive movements of the patella; as in the passive test, the patella can be displaced approximately half its width medially and laterally. The examiner must do the movements slowly and carefully to ensure that the patella is not prone to dislocation.

Depression (Distal Movement) of Patella

The patient is in a supine position with the knee slightly flexed. The examiner then places one hand over the patient's patella so that the pisiform bone rests over the base of the patella. The other hand is placed so that the finger and thumb can grasp the medial and lateral edges of the patella to direct the movement of the patella. The examiner then rests the first hand over the second hand, and applies a caudal force to the base of the patella and directs the caudal move-

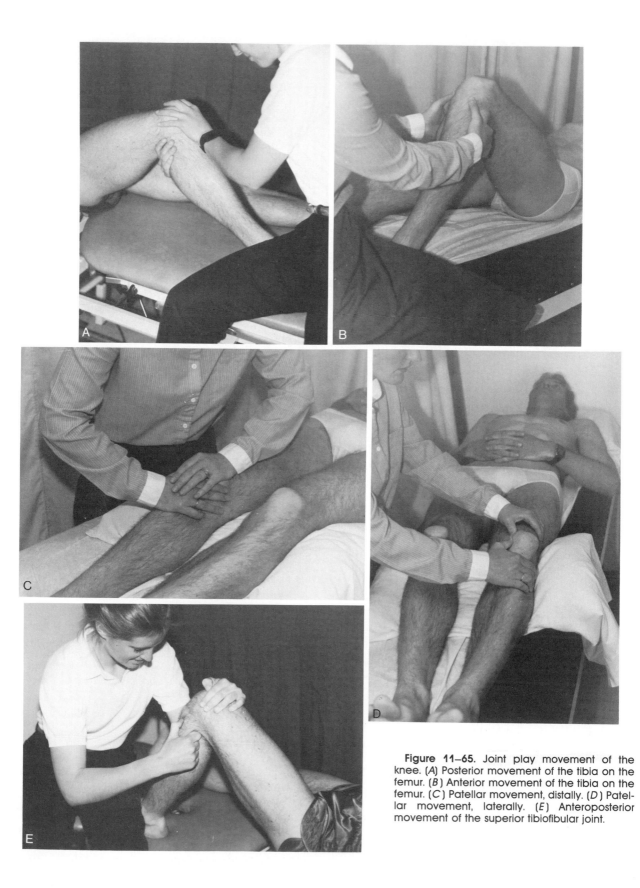

Figure 11–65. Joint play movement of the knee. (*A*) Posterior movement of the tibia on the femur. (*B*) Anterior movement of the tibia on the femur. (*C*) Patellar movement, distally. (*D*) Patellar movement, laterally. (*E*) Anteroposterior movement of the superior tibiofibular joint.

ment with the second hand so that the patella does not grind against the femoral condyles.

Anteroposterior Movement of Fibula on Tibia

The patient is in a supine position, and the knee flexed to 90° while the hip is flexed to 45°. The examiner then sits on the patient's foot and places one hand around the patient's knee to stabilize the knee and leg. The mobilizing hand is placed around the head of the fibula. The fibula is drawn forward on the tibia, and the movement and end feel are tested. The fibula will then slide back to its resting position of its own accord. The movement is tested several times and compared with the other side.

Care must be taken when performing this technique because the common peroneal nerve, which winds around the head of the fibula, may be easily compressed, causing pain. If the superior tibiofibular joint is stiff or hypomobile, the test itself will cause discomfort.

Palpation

The patient lies supine with the knee slightly flexed. In fact, it is wise to put the knee in several positions during palpation. For example, meniscal cysts are best palpated at 45°, whereas the joint line is easier to palpate at 90°. When palpating, the examiner should be looking for any abnormal tenderness, swelling, nodules, or abnormal temperature. The following structures should be palpated (Fig. 11–66):

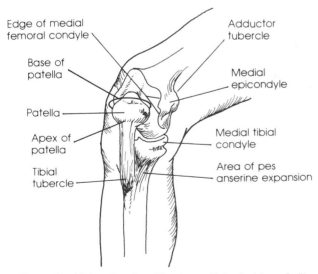

Figure 11–66. Landmarks of the knee. (Adapted from Reilly, B. M.: Practical Strategies in Outpatient Medicine. Philadelphia, W. B. Saunders Co., 1984, p. 225.)

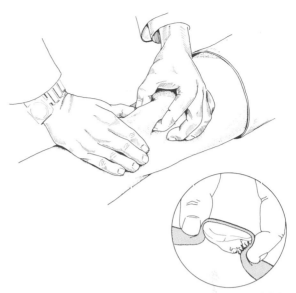

Figure 11–67. Facet tenderness. The medial and lateral facets are checked for tenderness, although this may be related to structures other than patellar surfaces beneath the examining finger. (From Hughston, J. C., et al.: Patellar Subluxation and Dislocation. Philadelphia, W. B. Saunders Co., 1984, p. 28.)

Anteriorly with Knee Extended

Patella, Patellar Tendon, Patellar Retinaculum, and Associated Bursa, Cartilaginous Surface of the Patella and Plica (If Present). The *patella* can be easily palpated overlying the anterior aspect of the knee. The base of the patella lies superiorly, the apex distally. After palpating the apex of the patella, (jumper's knee?), the examiner moves distally palpating the *patellar tendon* (tendinitis?) and overlying infrapatellar bursa (Parson's knee?) and the fat pad that lies behind the tendon. When the knee is extended, the fat pad will often extend beyond the sides of the tendon. Moving distally, the examiner will come to the tibial tuberosity, which should be palpated for enlargement (Osgood-Schlatter disease?).

Returning to the patella, the examiner can palpate the skin lying over the patella for pathology (is there prepatellar bursitis, or housemaid's knee?) and then extend medially and laterally to palpate the *patellar retinaculum* on either side of the patella. With the examiner pushing down on the lateral aspect of the patella, the medial retinaculum can be brought under tension and then palpated for tender spots. The lateral retinaculum can be palpated in a similar fashion with the examiner pushing down on the medial aspect of the patella. By stressing the retinaculum, the examiner is separating the retinaculum from the underlying tissue.

With the quadriceps muscles relaxed, the articular facets of the patella are palpated for tenderness (chondromalacia patella?) as shown in Figure 11–67. This palpation is often facilitated by

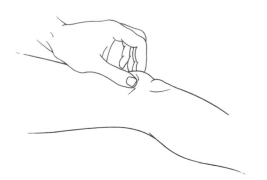

Figure 11–68. Palpation of the synovial membrane.

carefully pushing of the patella medially to palpate the medial facets and laterally to palpate the lateral facet.

As the medial edge of the patella is palpated, the examiner should carefully feel for the presence of a mediopatellar *plica*. The plica, if pathologic, may be palpated as a thickened ridge medial to the patella. To help confirm the presence of the plica, the examiner flexes the patient's knee to 30° and pushes the patella medially. If the plica is present and pathologic, this maneuver will often cause pain.

Suprapatellar Pouch. Returning to the anterior surface of the patella and moving proximally beyond the base of the patella, the fingers will lie over the suprapatellar pouch. The examiner then lifts the skin and underlying tissue between the thumb and fingers (Fig. 11–68). In this way, synovial membrane of the suprapatellar pouch, which is continuous with that of the knee joint, can be palpated. The examiner should feel for any thickness, tenderness, or nodules, the presence of which may indicate pathology.

Quadriceps Muscles (Vastus Medialis, Vastus Intermedius, Vastus Lateralis, and Rectus Femoris) and Sartorius. After palpating the suprapatellar pouch, the examiner palpates the quadriceps muscles for tenderness (first- or second-degree strain?), defects (third-degree strain?), or hard masses (myositis ossificans?).

Medial Collateral Ligament. If the examiner moves medially from the patella so the fingers lie over the medial aspect of the tibiofemoral joint, the fingers will lie over the medial collateral ligament, which should be palpated along its entire length for tenderness (sprain?) or other pathology (e.g., Pellegrini-Stieda disease).

Pes Anserinus. Medial and slightly distal to the tibial tuberosity, the examiner may palpate the pes anserinus or the common aponeurosis of the tendons of gracilis, semitendinosus, and sartorius muscles for tenderness. Any associated swelling may indicate pes anserine bursitis.

Tensor Fasciae Latae (Iliotibial Band and Head of Fibula). As the examiner moves laterally from the tibial tuberosity, the head of the fibula

can be palpated. Medially and slightly superior to the fibula, the examiner palpates the insertion of the iliotibial band into the lateral condyle of the tibia. When the knee is extended, it stands out as a strong, visible ridge anterolateral to the knee joint. As the examiner moves proximally, the iliotibial band is palpated along its length.

Anteriorly with Knee Flexed

Flexion at 45°—Tibiofemoral Joint Line and Meniscal Cysts. The examiner palpates the joint line, especially on the lateral aspect for any evidence of swelling (a meniscal cyst?), tenderness, or other pathology.

Flexion at 90°—Tibiofemoral Joint Line, Tibial Plateau, Femoral Condyles, and Adductor Muscles. If the examiner returns to the patella, palpates the apex of the patella, and moves medially or laterally, the fingers will lie on the tibiofemoral joint line, which should be palpated along its length. As the joint line is palpated, the examiner should also palpate the tibial plateau (coronary ligament sprain?) medially and laterally and the femoral condyles.

Both condyles should be carefully palpated for any tenderness (e.g., osteochondritis dissecans?). Beginning at the superior aspect of the femoral condyles, the examiner should note that the lat-

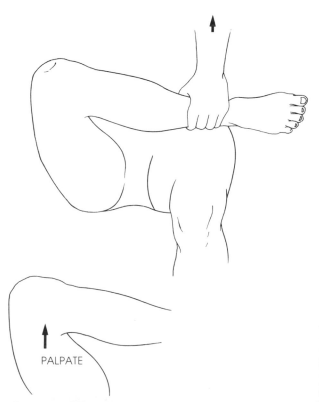

PALPATE

Figure 11–69. Palpation of the lateral (fibular) collateral ligament.

eral condyle extends further anteriorly (i.e., it is higher) than the medial condyle. The trochlear groove between the two condyles can then be palpated. As the medial condyle is palpated, a sharp edge appears on the condyle medially. If the edge is followed posteriorly, the adductor tubercle will be palpated on the posteromedial portion of the medial femoral condyle. After palpating the adductor tubercle, the examiner moves proximally, palpating the adductor muscles of the hip for tenderness or other signs of pathology.

Anteriorly with Foot of Test Leg Resting on Opposite Knee—Lateral Collateral Ligament

Kennedy has advocated palpating the lateral collateral ligament by having the patient in a sitting or lying position (Fig. 11–69).[15] The patient's knee is flexed to 90° and the hip is laterally rotated so that the ankle of the test leg rests on the knee of the other leg. The examiner then takes the knee into a varus position, and the rope-like ligament stands out if the ligament is intact.

Posteriorly with the Knee Slightly Flexed

Posterior Aspect of Knee Joint. The soft tissue on the posterior aspect of the knee should be palpated for tenderness or swelling (e.g., Baker's cyst?). In some individuals, the popliteal artery may be palpated running down the center of the posterior knee.

Posterolateral Aspect of Knee Joint. The posterolateral corner of the knee is sometimes called the *popliteus corner*. The examiner should at-

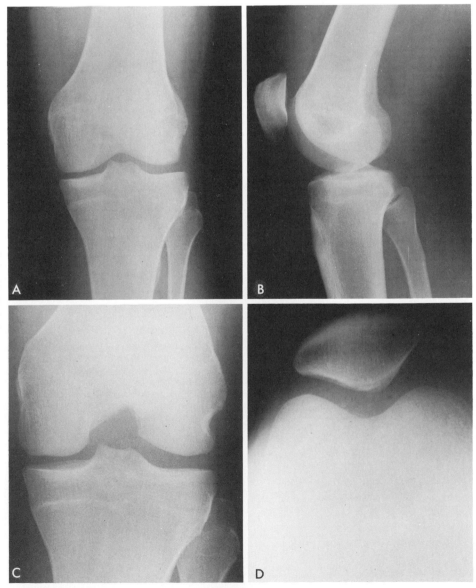

Figure 11–70. Normal radiographs of the knee. (*A*) Anteroposterior view. (*B*) Lateral view. (*C*) "Tunnel" view. (*D*) "Skyline" view. (From Reilly, B. M.: Practical Strategies in Outpatient Medicine. Philadelphia, W. B. Saunders Co., 1984, p. 242.)

VIEW	KNEE FLEXION	PATIENT POSITION	MEASUREMENT		MISCELLANEOUS

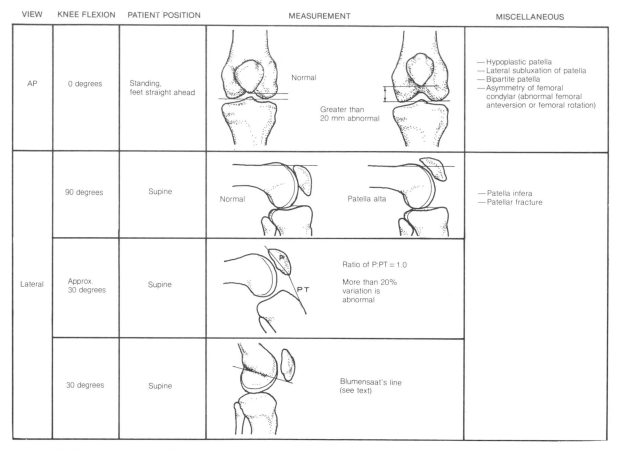

AP	0 degrees	Standing, feet straight ahead	Normal / Greater than 20 mm abnormal	— Hypoplastic patella / — Lateral subluxation of patella / — Bipartite patella / — Asymmetry of femoral condylar (abnormal femoral anteversion or femoral rotation)
Lateral	90 degrees	Supine	Normal / Patella alta	— Patella infera / — Patellar fracture
	Approx. 30 degrees	Supine	Ratio of P:PT = 1.0 / More than 20% variation is abnormal	
	30 degrees	Supine	Blumensaat's line (see text)	

Figure 11–71. Summary of radiographic findings in patella alta. (From Carson, W. A., et al.: Clin. Orthop. Relat. Res. *185*:179, 1984.)

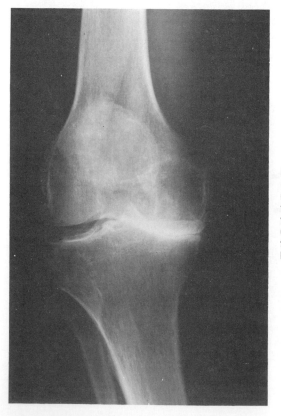

Figure 11–72. Degenerative arthritis of the knee in a 63-year-old man. He complained of chronic pain, stiffness, and swelling of both knees. The radiograph demonstrates extensive degenerative arthritis with marked narrowing of the medial joint space and hypertrophic bony changes throughout the joint. Joint fluid contained 45 white blood cells. There is a valgus deformity of the knee as a result of the osteoarthritis. This patient ultimately required a total knee replacement for amelioration of symptoms. (From Reilly, B. M.: Practical Strategies in Outpatient Medicine. Philadelphia, W. B. Saunders Co., 1984, p. 260.)

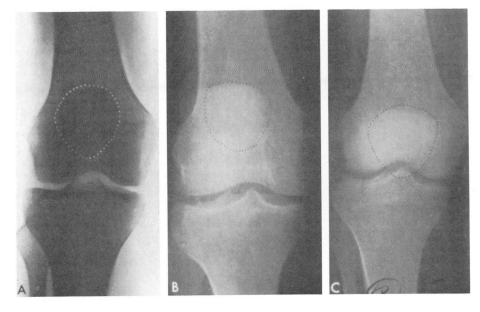

Figure 11–73. Anteroposterior view of the knee. (A) Normal patellar position. (B) Patella alta. (C) Patella baja. (From Hughston, J. C., et al.: Patellar Subluxation and Dislocation. Philadelphia, W. B. Saunders Co., 1984, p. 50.)

tempt to palpate the arcuate-popliteus complex, lateral gastrocnemius muscle, biceps femoris muscle, and possibly the lateral meniscus in this area. A sesamoid bone is sometimes found inserted in the tendon of the lateral head of the gastrocnemius muscle. This bone, referred to as the *fabella*, may be interpreted as a loose body in the posterolateral aspect of the knee by an unwary examiner.

Posteromedial Aspect of Knee Joint. The posteromedial corner of the knee joint is sometimes referred to as the *semimembranosus corner*. The examiner should attempt to palpate the following structures in the area for tenderness or pathology: the posterior oblique ligament, the semimembranosus muscle, and possibly the medial meniscus.

Hamstring and Gastrocnemius Muscles. After the various parts of the posterior aspect of the knee have been palpated, the tendons and muscle bellies of the hamstring muscle group (biceps femoris, semitendinosus, and semimembranosus) proximally and gastrocnemius muscle distally should be palpated for tenderness, swelling, or other signs of pathology.

X-RAYS (RADIOGRAPHY) OF THE KNEE JOINTS

Anteroposterior View. When looking at radiographs of the knee (Fig. 11–70), the examiner should note any possible fractures (e.g., osteochondral), diminished joint space (osteoarthritis—Figure 11–72), epiphyseal damage, lipping, loose bodies, alterations in bone texture, abnormal calcification, or tumors, accessory ossification centers, varus/valgus deformity, patella alta (Fig. 11–71 and 11–73) or baja, and asymmetry of femoral condyles.[33] Stress radiographs of this

view will illustrate excessive gapping medially or laterally, indicating ligamentous instability (Fig. 11–74). The examiner should also remember the possible presence of the fabella, which is seen in 20 per cent of the population. Epiphyseal fractures (Fig. 11–75) and osteochondritis dissecans (Fig. 11–76) may also be seen in this view.

Text continued on page 311

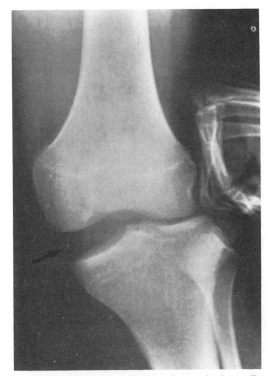

Figure 11–74. This valgus stress radiograph shows the patient's knee in full extension. Note the gapping on the medial side (arrow). (From Mital, M. A., and L. I. Karlin: Orthop. Clin. North Am. *11*:775, 1980.)

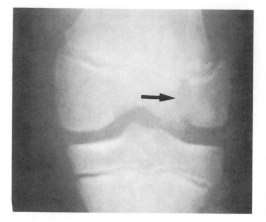

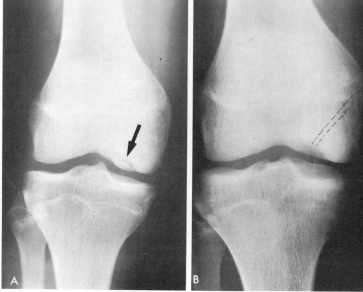

Figure 11–75. A Salter-Harris type III injury (arrow) of the growth plate and the epiphysis. Main attention should be directed toward restitution of the joint surface. (From Ehrlich, M. G., and R. E. Strain: Orthop. Clin. North Am. *10*:93, 1979.)

Figure 11–76. (*A*) Osteochondritis dissecans (actually an osteochondral fracture [arrow] of the femoral condyle), with almost the entire femoral attachment of the posterior cruciate ligament remaining attached to the fragment. (*B*) Three months following repair of posterior cruciate to femur. Excellent function is restored. Complete filling in of this defect is unlikely at this age. (From O'Donoghue, D. H.: Treatment of Injuries to Athletes, 4th ed. Philadelphia, W. B. Saunders Co., 1984, p. 575.)

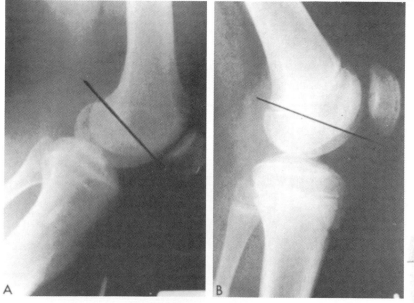

Figure 11–77. Lateral view of the patella at 45°. (*A*) Normal patellar position in relation to the intercondylar notch. (*B*) Patella alta. (From Hughston, J. C., et al.: Patellar Subluxation and Dislocation. Philadelphia, W. B. Saunders Co., 1984, p. 52.)

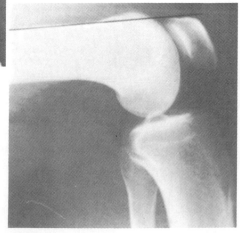

Figure 11–78. Lateral view at 90° shows the normal position of the patella. (From Hughston, J. C., et al.: Patellar Subluxation and Dislocation. Philadelphia, W. B. Saunders Co., 1984, p. 52.)

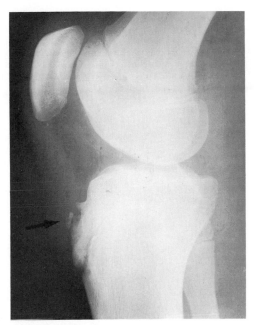

Figure 11-79. Osgood-Schlatter "disease," showing epiphysitis of the entire epiphysis (arrow), with irregularity of the epiphyseal line. Since this epiphyseal cartilage is continuous with that of the upper tibia, it should not be disturbed. If surgery is utilized, exposure should be superficial to the epiphyseal cartilage. (From O'Donoghue, D. H.: Treatment of Injuries to Athletes, 4th ed. Philadelphia, W. B. Saunders Co. 1984, p. 574.)

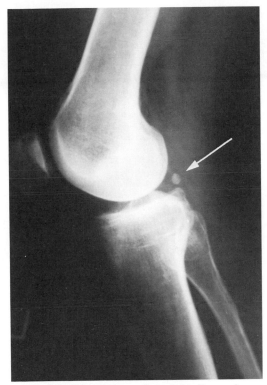

Figure 11-80. Sesamoid bone (fabella) in the gastrocnemius muscle.

TANGENTIAL VIEW	KNEE FLEXION	TECHNIQUE AND POSITION	MEASUREMENTS	MISCELLANEOUS
Hughston	55 degrees	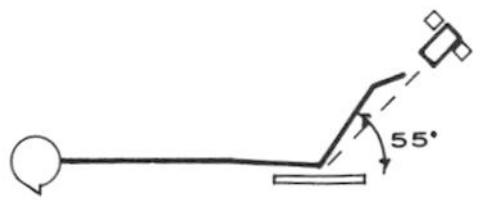 Prone position. Beam directed cephalad and inferior, 45 degrees from vertical.	1) Sulcus angle: 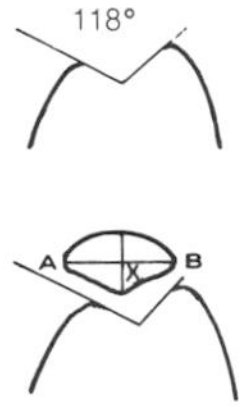 118° 2) Patella index: $\dfrac{AB}{XB-XA}$ NL: Male 15, Female 17	—Patellar dislocation —Osteochondral fracture —Soft tissue calcification (old dislocated patella or fracture) —Patellar subluxation Patellar tilt Increased medial joint space Apex of patella lateral to apex of femoral sulcus Lateral patella edge lateral to femoral condyle Hypoplastic lateral femoral condyle (usually proximal) —Patellofemoral osteophytes —Subchondral trabeculae orientation (increase or decrease) —Patellar configuration (Wiberg-Baugartl) 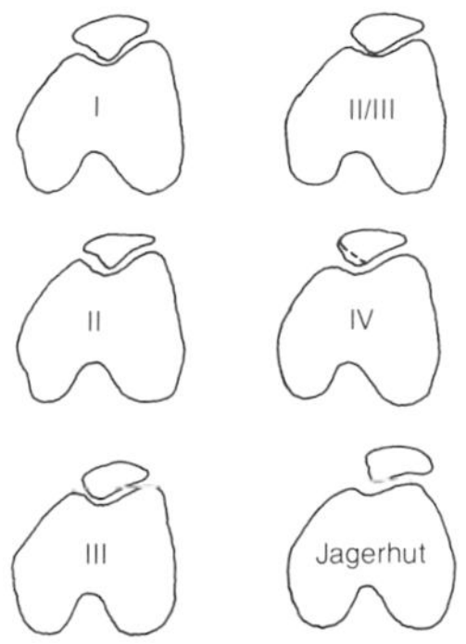
Merchant	45 degrees	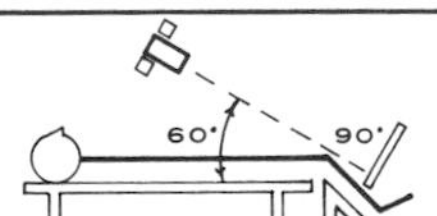 Supine position. Beam directed caudal and inferior, 30 degrees from vertical.	1) Sulcus angle: 138° 2) Congruence angle: 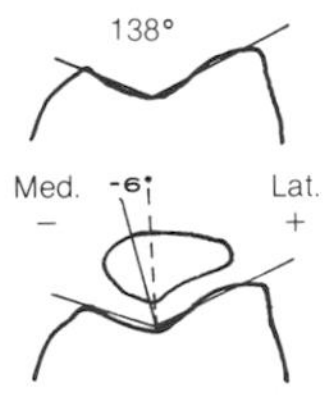 Med. -6 − / Lat. +	
Laurin	20 degrees	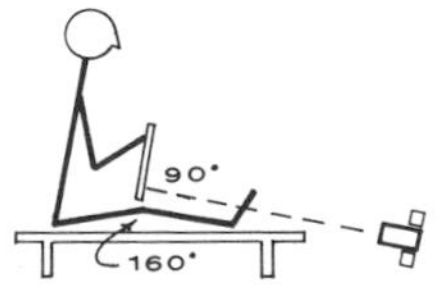 Sitting position. Beam directed cephaled and superior, 160 degrees from vertical.	1) Lateral patellofemoral angle: LAT. NL: ABNL: ABNL: 2) Patellofemoral index: Ratio A/B Normal = 1.6 or less 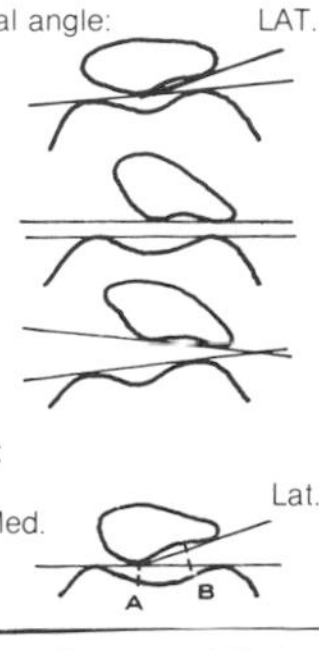	

Figure 11-81. Summary of radiographic findings, tangential view. (From Carson, W. A., et al.: Clin. Orthop. Relat. Res. 185:182, 1984.)

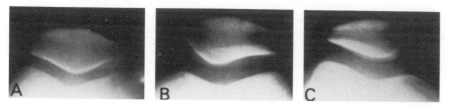

Figure 11–82. Examples of patellar variations. (*A*) Wiberg type I. (*B*) Wiberg type II. (*C*) Wiberg type III. (From Ficat, R. P., and D. S. Hungerford. Disorders of the Patello-Femoral Joint. Baltimore, The Williams and Wilkins Co., 1977, p. 53.)

Figure 11–83. Variations in patellar form that are considered dysplastic. (From Ficat, R. P., and D. S. Hungerford: Disorders of the Patello-Femoral Joint. Baltimore, The Williams and Wilkins Co., 1977, p. 55.)

Baumgartl Wiberg III Alpine hunter's cap

Pebble Half-moon Patella magna Patella parva

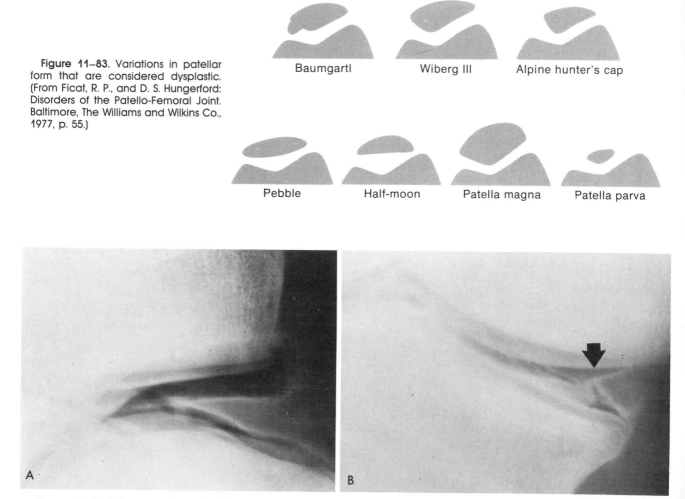

Figure 11–84. Arthrogram demonstrating a torn meniscus. The normal meniscus on the lateral side (*A*) is compared here with the easily demonstrated tear in the medial meniscus in the same patient (*B*) (arrow). (From Reilly, B. M.: Practical Strategies in Outpatient Medicine. Philadelphia, W. B. Saunders Co., 1984, p. 253.)

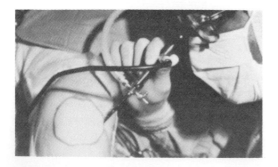

Figure 11–85. Arthroscopy of the knee. (From Patel, D.: Orthop. Clin. North Am. *13*:301, 1982.)

Lateral View. With this view,[24, 33] the examiner should note the same structures as with the anteroposterior view (Figs. 11–77 and 11–78). In addition, several patellar measurements, if desired, can be made, as shown in Figure 11–71. This view also illustrates Osgood-Schlatter disease (Fig. 11–79) and the presence of the fabella (Fig. 11–80).

Intercondylar Notch (Tunnel View X-ray). With this view (the knee flexed to 90°), the tibia and intercondylar attachments of the cruciate ligaments can be examined. Also any loose bodies or possibility of osteochondritis dissecans, subluxation, patellar tilt (lateral or medial) or dislocation should be noted.

Skyline View. This 30° tangential view is used primarily for suspected patellar problems.[34] It may be taken at different angles, as shown in Figure 11–81, or may be used to determine the type of patella present, as shown in Figure 11–82. Figure 11–83 illustrates abnormal patellar forms.

Arthrogram. Arthrograms are used in the knee primarily to diagnose tears in the menisci (Fig. 11–84).

Arthroscope. The arthroscope is being used more and more frequently to diagnose lesions of the knee as well as to repair many of them surgically.[35–37] By using various approaches to the knee, the surgeon is able to view all the structures to see if they have been injured (Fig. 11–85).

Précis of the Knee Assessment*

History
Observation
Examination
  Active movements
    Knee flexion
    Knee extension
    Medial rotation of the tibia on the femur
    Lateral rotation of the tibia on the femur
  Functional tests
  Passive movements (as in Active movements)
  Resisted isometric movements
    Knee flexion
    Knee extension
    Ankle plantar flexion
    Ankle dorsiflexion

---

*Although examination of the knee may be carried out with the patient in a supine position, some of the tests may require the patient to move to other positions (e.g., standing, lying, prone, sitting, and so on). When these tests are used, the examination should be planned in such a way that the movement, and therefore discomfort, of the patient is kept to a minimum. Thus the sequence should be from standing to sitting, to supine lying, to side lying, and, finally, to prone lying.

Tests for ligament stability
  Test for one-plane medial instability
  Test for one-plane lateral instability
  Tests for one-plane anterior and posterior instability
  Tests for anteromedial and anterolateral rotary instability
  Tests for posteromedial and posterolateral rotary instability
Special tests
  Tests for meniscus injury
  Plica tests
  Tests for swelling
  Other special tests
Reflexes and cutaneous distribution
Joint play movements
  Backward and forward movement of the tibia on the femur
  Medial and lateral displacement of the patella
  Depression of the patella
  Anteroposterior movement of the fibula on the tibia
Palpation
X-ray viewing

Following any examination, the patient should always be warned of the possibility of exacerbation of symptoms as a result of the assessment.

REFERENCES

CITED REFERENCES

1. Kaltenborn, F. M.: Mobilization of the Extremity Joints. Oslo, Olaf Norles Bokhandel, 1980.
2. Arnoczsky, S. P.: The blood supply of the meniscus and its role in healing and repair. American Association of Orthopedic Surgeons, Symposium on Sports Medicine: The Knee. St. Louis, C. V. Mosby, 1985.
3. Radin, E. L., F. de Lamotte, and P. Maquet: Role of the menisci in the distribution of stress in the knee. Clin. Orthop. Relat. Res. 185:290, 1984.
4. Seedhom, B. B.: Loadbearing function of the menisci. Physiotherapy 62:223, 1976.
5. Ficat, R. P., and D. S. Hungerford: The Patello-Femoral Joint. Baltimore, Williams and Wilkins Co., 1977.
6. Goodfellow, J., D. S. Hungerford, and M. Zindel: Patellofemoral joint mechanics and pathology: Functional anatomy of the patellofemoral joint. J. Bone Joint Surg. 58B:287, 1976.
7. Staheli, L. T., and G. M. Engel: Tibial torsion. Clin. Orthop. Relat. Res. 86:183, 1972.
8. Waldron, V. D.: A test for chondromalacia patellae. Orthop. Rev. 12:103, 1983.
9. Segal, P., and M. Jacob: The Knee. Chicago, Year Book Medical Publishers, 1983.
10. Muller, W.: The Knee: Form, Function and Ligament Reconstruction. New York, Springer-Verlag, 1983.
11. Detenbeck, L. C.: Function of the cruciate ligaments in knee stability. Am. J. Sports Med. 2:217, 1974.
12. Furman, W., J. L. Marshall, and F. G. Girgis: The anterior cruciate ligament: A functional analysis based on postmortem studies. J. Bone Joint Surg. 58A:179, 1976.
13. Girgis, F. G., J. L. Marshall, and A. R. S. Al Monajem: The cruciate ligaments of the knee joint: Anatomical, functional and experimental analysis. Clin. Orthop. Relat. Res. 106:216, 1975.
14. Baker, C. L., L. A. Norwood, and J. C. Hughston: Acute combined posterior and posterolateral instability of the knee. Am. J. Sports Med. 12:204, 1984.
15. Kennedy, J. C.: The Injured Adolescent Knee. Baltimore, Williams and Wilkins Co., 1979.

16. Jonsson, T., B. Althoff, L. Peterson, and P. Renstrom: Clinical diagnosis of ruptures of the anterior cruciate ligament: A comparative study of the Lachman test and the anterior drawer sign. Am. J. Sports Med. 10:100, 1982.

17. Butler, D. L., F. R. Noyes, and E. S. Grood: Ligamentous restraints to anterior-posterior drawer in the human knee. J. Bone Joint Surg. 622A:259, 1980.

18. Slocum, D. B., and R. L. Larson: Rotary instability of the knee. J. Bone Joint Surg., 50A:211, 1968.

19. Slocum, D. B., S. L. James, R. L. Larson, and K. M. Singer: A clinical test for anterolateral rotary instability of the knee. Clin. Orthop. Relat. Res. 118:63, 1976.

20. Fetto, J. F., and J. L. Marshall: Injury to the anterior cruciate ligament producing the pivot shift sign: An experimental study on cadaver specimens. J. Bone Joint Surg. 61A:710, 1979.

21. Galway, H. R., and D. L. MacIntosh: The lateral pivot shift: A symptom and sign of anterior cruciate ligament insufficiency. Clin. Orthop. Relat. Res. 147:45, 1980.

22. Tamea, C. D., and C. E. Henning: Pathomechanics of the pivot shift maneuver. Am. J. Sports Med. 9:31, 1981.

23. Losee, R. E., T. R. J. Ennis, and W. O. Southwick: Anterior subluxation of the lateral tibial plateau: A diagnostic test and operative review. J. Bone Joint Surg. 60A:1015, 1978.

24. Hughston, J. C., W. M. Walsh, and G. Puddu: Patellar Subluxation and Dislocation. Philadelphia, W. B. Saunders Co., 1984.

25. Noyes, F. R., D. L. Butler, E. S. Grood, et al.: Clinical paradoxes of anterior cruciate instability and a new test to detect its instability. Orthop. Trans. 2:36, 1978.

26. Hughston, J. C., and L. A. Norwood: The posterolateral drawer test and external rotational recurvatum test for posterolateral rotary instability of the knee. Clin. Orthop. Relat. Res. 147:82, 1980.

27. Jakob, R. P., H. Hassler, and H. U. Staeubli: Observations on rotary instability of the lateral compartment of the knee. Acta Orthop. Scand. (Suppl. 191) 52:1–32, 1981.

28. McMurray, T. P.: The semilunar cartilages. Br. J. Surg. 29:407, 1942.

29. Helfet, A.: Disorders of the Knee. Philadelphia, J. B. Lippincott Co., 1974.

30. Mital, M. A., and J. Hayden: Pain in the knee in children: The medial plica shelf syndrome. Orthop. Clin. North Am. 10:713, 1979.

31. Olerud, C., and P. Berg: The variation of the Q angle with different positions of the foot. Clin. Orthop. Relat. Res. 191:162, 1984.

32. Noble, H. B., M. R. Hajek, and M. Porter: Diagnosis and treatment of iliotibial band tightness in runners. Physician Sportsmed. 10:67, 1984.

33. Carson, W. G., Jr., S. L. James, R. L. Larson, et al: Patellofemoral disorders: Physical and radiographic evaluation: I. Physical examination. Clin. Orthop. Relat. Res. 185:165, 1984.

34. Speakman, H. B., and J. Weisberg: The vastus medialis controversy. Physiotherapy 63:249, 1977.

35. Mital, M. A., and L. I. Karlin: Diagnostic arthroscopy in sports injuries. Orthop. Clin. North Am. 11:771, 1980.

36. McClelland, C. J.: Arthroscopy and arthroscopic surgery of the knee. Physiotherapy 70:154, 1984.

37. Noyes, F. R., R. W. Bassett, E. S. Grood, and D. L. Butler: Arthroscopy in acute traumatic hemarthrosis of the knee. J. Bone Joint Surg. 62A:687, 1980.

General References

Adams, J. C.: Outline of Orthopedics. London, E & S Livingstone, Ltd., 1968.

Ahstrom, J. P.: Reliability of history and physical examination in diagnosis of meniscus pathology. Curr. Pract. Orthop. Surg., Vol. 7, St. Louis, C. V. Mosby, 1977.

Arnold, J. A., T. P. Coker, L. M. Heaton, et al.: Natural history of anterior cruciate tears. Am. J. Sports Med. 7:305, 1979.

Beetham, W. P., H. P. Polley, C. H. Slocumb, and W. F. Weaver: Physical Extremities of the Joints. Philadelphia, W. B. Saunders Co., 1965.

Brantigan, O. C., and A. F. Voshell: The mechanics of the ligaments and menisci of the knee joint. J. Bone Joint Surg. 23:44, 1941.

Cabaud, H. E., and D. B. Slocum: The diagnosis of chronic anterolateral rotary instability of the knee. Am. J. Sports Med. 5:99, 1977.

Cailliet, R.: Knee Pain and Disability. Philadelphia, F. A. Davis Co., 1973.

Clancy, W. G.: Evaluation of acute knee injuries. American Association of Orthopedic Surgeons, Symposium on Sports Medicine: The Knee. St. Louis, C. V. Mosby, 1985.

Collins, H. R.: Anterolateral rotary instability. American Association of Orthopedic Surgeons, Symposium on the Athlete's Knee. St. Louis: C.V. Mosby, 1980.

Cyriax, J.: Textbook of Orthopaedic Medicine, vol. 1. Diagnosis of Soft Tissue Lesions. London, Bailliere Tindall, 1975.

Davies, G. J., and R. Larson: Examining the knee. Physician Sportsmed. 6:49, 1978.

Dontigny, R. L.: Terminal extension exercises for the knee. Phys. Ther. 52:45, 1972.

Doppman, J. L.: Baker's cyst and the normal gastrocnemio-semimembranosus bursa. Am. J. Roentgenol. 94:646, 1965.

Ehrlich, M. G., and R. E. Strain: Epiphyseal injuries about the knee. Orthop. Clin. North Am. 10:91, 1979.

Ellison, A. E.: The pathogenesis and treatment of anterolateral rotary instability. Clin. Orthop. Relat. Res. 147:29, 1980.

Fetto, J. F., and J. L. Marshall: The natural history and diagnosis of anterior cruciate ligament insufficiency. Clin. Orthop. Relat. Res. 147:29, 1980.

Fowler, P. J.: The classification and early diagnosis of knee joint instability. Clin. Orthop. Relat. Res. 147:15, 1980.

Francis, R. S., and D. E. Scott: Hypertrophy of the vastus medialis in knee extension. Phys. Ther. 54:1066, 1974.

Frankel, V. H., A. H. Burstein, and D. B. Brooks: Biomechanics of internal derangement of the knee. J. Bone Joint Surg. 53:945, 1971.

Fulkerson, J. P.: Awareness of the retinaculum in evaluating patellofemoral pain. Am. J. Sports Med. 10:147, 1982.

Gartland, J. J.: Fundamentals of Orthopedics. Philadelphia, W. B. Saunders Co., 1979.

Goodfellow, J., D. S. Hungerford, and M. Zindel: Patellofemoral joint mechanics and pathology: Chondromalacia patellae. J. Bone Joint Surg., 58B:291, 1976.

Gough, J. V., and G. Ladley: An investigation into the effectiveness of various forms of quadriceps exercises. Physiotherapy 57:356, 1971.

Greenhill, B. J.: The importance of the medial quadriceps expansion in medial ligament injury. Can. J. Surg. 10:312, 1967.

Hardaker, W. G., T. L. Shipple, and F. H. Bassett: Diagnosis and treatment of the plica syndrome of the knee. J. Bone Joint Surg. 62A:221, 1980.

Hollinshead, W. H., and D. B. Jenkins: Functional Anatomy of the Limbs and Back. Philadelphia, W. B. Saunders Co., 1981.

Hoppenfeld, S.: Physical Examination of the Spine and Extremities. New York, Appleton-Century-Crofts, 1976.

Hoppenfeld, S.: Physical examination of the knee joint by complaint. Orthop. Clin. North Am. 10:3, 1979.

Hughston, J. C., J. R. Andrews, M. J. Cross, and A. Moschi: Classification of knee ligament instabilities: Part I. The medial compartment and cruciate ligaments. J. Bone Joint Surg. 58A:173, 1976.

Hughston, J. C., J. A. Bowden, J. R. Andrews, and L. A. Norwood: Acute tears of the posterior cruciate ligament. J. Bone Joint Surgery 62A:438, 1980.

Insall, J., K. A. Falvo, and D. W. Wise: Chondromalacia

patellae: A prospective study. J. Bone Joint Surg. 58A:1–8, 1976.

Jackson, J. P.: Internal derangement of the knee-joint. Physiotherapy 52:229, 1966.

Kapandji, L. A.: The Physiology of the Joints, vol. 2. Lower Limb. New York, Churchill Livingstone, 1970.

Kennedy, J. C., R. Stewart, and D. M. Walker: Anterolateral rotary instability of the knee joint: An early analysis of the Ellison repair. J. Bone Joint Surg. 60A:1031, 1974.

Leib, F. J., and J. Perry: Quadriceps function. J. Bone Joint Surg. 50A:1535, 1968.

Lucie, R. S., J. D. Wiedel, and D. G. Messner: The acute pivot shift: Clinical correlation. Am. J. Sports Med. 12:189, 1984.

Major, D.: Anatomical and functional aspects of the knee joint. Physiotherapy 52:224, 1966.

Malek, M. M., and R. E. Manjini: Patellofemoral pain syndrome: A comprehensive and conservative approach. J. Orthop. Sports Phys. Ther. 2:108, 1981.

McRae, R.: Clinical Orthopaedic Examination. New York, Churchill Livingstone, 1976.

Norwood, L. A., and J. C. Hughston: Combined anterolateral-anteromedial instability of the knee. Clin. Orthop. Relat. Res. 147:62, 1980.

O'Donoghue, D. H.: Treatment of Injuries to Athletes, 4th ed. Philadelphia, W. B. Saunders Co., 1984.

Patel, D.: Superior lateral-medial approach to arthroscopic meniscectomy. Orthop. Clin. North Am. 13:299, 1982.

Perry, J.: Function of quadriceps. J. Can. Physiother. Assoc. 24:130, 1972.

Pickett, J. C., and E. L. Radin: Chondromalacia of the Patella. Baltimore, Williams and Wilkins, 1983.

Pipkin, G.: Knee injuries: The role of the suprapatellar plica and suprapatellar bursa in simulating internal derangements. Clin. Orthop. Relat. Res. 74:161, 1971.

Reid, D. C.: Functional Anatomy and Joint Mobilization. Edmonton: University of Alberta Bookstore, 1980.

Reider, B., J. L. Marshall, B. Koslin, B. Ring, and F.G. Girgis: The anterior aspect of the knee joint. J. Bone Joint Surg. 63A:351, 1981.

Reilly, B. M.: Practical Strategies in Outpatient Medicine. Philadelphia, W. B. Saunders Co., 1984.

Rovere, G. D., and D. M. Adair: Anterior cruciate-deficient knees: A review of the literature. Am. J. Sports Med. 11:412, 1983.

Smillie, I. S.: Diseases of the Knee Joint. New York, Churchill Livingstone, 1974.

Stickland, A.: Examination of the knee joint. Physiotherapy 70:144, 1984.

Tachdjian, M. O.: Pediatric Orthopedics. Philadelphia, W. B. Saunders Co., 1972.

Torg, J. S., W. Conrad, and V. Allen: Clinical diagnosis of anterior cruciate ligament instability in the athlete. Am. J. Sports Med. 4:84, 1976.

Trickey, E. L.: Injuries to the posterior cruciate ligament: Diagnosis and treatment of early injuries and reconstruction of late instability. Clin. Orthop. Relat. Res. 147:76, 1980.

Turner, J. S., and I. S. Smillie: The effect of tibial torsion on the pathology of the knee. J. Bone Joint Surg. 63B:396, 1981.

Warren, L. F., J. Marshall, and F. Girgis: The prime static stabilizer of the medial side of the knee. J. Bone Joint Surg. 56A:665, 1974.

Warren, L. F., and J. Marshall: The supporting structures and layers on the medial side of the knee. J. Bone Joint Surg. 61A:56, 1979.

Welsh, R. P.: Knee joint structure and function. Clin. Orthop. Relat. Res. 147:7, 1980.

Wiles, P., and R. Sweetnam: Essentials of Orthopedics. London, J & A Churchill, Ltd., 1965.

12

Lower Leg, Ankle, and Foot

At least 80 per cent of people today have foot problems that can often be corrected by proper assessment, treatment, and, above all, care of the feet. Lesions of the ankle and foot can alter the mechanics of gait and, as a result, the stress on other lower limb joints; this in turn may lead to pathology in these joints.

The foot and ankle combine flexibility with stability because of the many bones that are present and because of their shape. The lower leg, ankle, and foot have two principal functions—propulsion and support. For propulsion, they act like a flexible lever; for support, they act like a rigid structure that holds up the entire body. The functions of the foot include:

1. Acting as a base of support that is sufficient to provide the necessary stability for upright posture with minimal muscle effort.

2. Providing a mechanism for rotation of the tibia and fibula during the stance phase of gait.

3. Providing flexibility to adapt to uneven terrain.

4. Providing flexibility for absorption of shock by becoming a rigid structure in the pronated position.

5. Acting as a lever during "push-off."

Although the joints of the lower leg, ankle, and foot are discussed separately, these joints act as functional groups and not in isolation. The movement occurring at each individual joint is minimal. However, taken together, there is normally sufficient range of motion in all the joints to allow normal functional mobility while providing functional stability. For ease of understanding, the joints of the foot are divided into three sections—the hindfoot, midfoot, and forefoot.

Applied Anatomy

HINDFOOT

Tibiofibular Joints. The inferior (distal) tibiofibular joint is a fibrous or syndesmosis type of joint. It is supported by the anterior tibiofibular, posterior tibiofibular, and inferior transverse ligaments as well as the interosseous ligament. The movements at this joint are minimal, but do allow for a small amount of "spread" of 1 to 2 mm at the ankle joint during dorsiflexion. The joint is supplied by the deep peroneal and tibial nerves.

Talocrural Joint. The talocrural joint (ankle joint) is a uniaxial, modified hinge synovial joint located between the *talus*, the *medial malleolus* of the tibia, and the *lateral* malleolus of the fibula. The talus is shaped in such a way that in dorsiflexion it is wedged between the malleoli, allowing little or no inversion or eversion at the ankle joint. The talus is about 2.4 mm wider anteriorly than posteriorly. The medial malleolus is shorter, extending halfway down the talus, whereas the lateral malleolus extends almost to the level of the talocalcanean joint.

The talocrural joint is designed for stability, not mobility. Its close packed position is maximum dorsiflexion, and its capsular pattern is more limitation of plantar flexion than dorsiflexion. This joint is strongest in the dorsiflexed position. The resting position is 10° of plantar flexion midway between maximum inversion and eversion.

On the medial side of the joint, the major ligament is the *deltoid,* or *medial collateral ligament,* which consists of four separate ligaments: (1) the *tibionavicular,* (2) *tibiocalcanean,* and (3) *posterior tibiotalar ligaments* superficially, which resist talar abduction, and (4) the *anterior tibiotalar ligament* deep, which resists lateral translation and lateral rotation of the talus.

On the lateral aspect, the talocrural joint is supported by (1) the *anterior talofibular ligament,* which provides stability against excessive inversion of the talus; (2) the *posterior talofibular ligament,* which resists ankle dorsiflexion, adduction ("tilt"), medial rotation, and medial translation of the talus; and (3) the *calcaneofibular ligament,* which provides stability against maximum inversion at the ankle and subtalar joints. The talocrural joint has one degree of freedom, and the movements possible at this joint are dorsiflexion and plantar flexion.

Subtalar (Talocalcanean) Joint. The subtalar joint is a synovial joint having three degrees of freedom and a close packed position of supination. Supporting the subtalar joint are the lateral talocalcanean and medial talocalcanean ligaments. In addition, the interosseous talocalcanean and cervical ligaments limit eversion.

The movements possible at the subtalar joint are gliding and rotation. As well, medial rotation of the leg causes a valgus (outward) movement of the calcaneus, whereas lateral rotation of the leg produces a varus (inward) movement of the calcaneus. The axis of the joint is at an angle of 40 to 45° inclined vertically and 15 to 18° to the sagittal plane.

MIDFOOT (MIDTARSAL JOINTS)

Talocalcaneonavicular Joint. The talocalcaneonavicular joint is a "ball-and-socket" synovial joint having three degrees of freedom. Its close packed position is supination, and supporting the joint are the dorsal talonavicular ligament, the bifurcated ligament, and the plantar calcaneonavicular (spring) ligament. Movements possible at this joint are gliding and rotation.

Cuneonavicular Joint. The cuneonavicular joint is a plane synovial joint with a close packed position of supination. The movements possible at this joint are slight gliding and rotation.

Cuboideonavicular Joint. The cuboideonavicular joint is fibrous, its close packed position being supination. The movements possible at this joint are slight gliding and rotation.

Intercuneiform Joints. The intercuneiform joints are plane synovial joints with a close packed position of supination. The movements possible in these joints are slight gliding and rotation.

Cuneocuboid Joint. The cuneocuboid joint is a plane synovial joint with a close packed position of supination. The movements of slight gliding and rotation are possible at this joint.

Calcaneocuboid Joint. The calcaneocuboid joint is saddle-shaped with a close packed position of supination. Supporting this joint are the bifurcated ligament, the calcaneocuboid ligament, and the long plantar ligaments. The movement possible at this joint is gliding with conjunct rotation.

FOREFOOT

Tarsometatarsal Joints. The tarsometatarsal joints are plane synovial joints having a close packed position of supination. The movement possible at these joints is gliding.

Intermetatarsal Joints. The four intermetatarsal joints are plane synovial joints with a close packed position of supination. The movement possible at these joints is gliding.

Metatarsophalangeal Joints. The five metatarsophalangeal joints are condyloid synovial joints having two degrees of freedom. Their close packed position is full extension. Their capsular pattern is more limitation of flexion than of extension, and their resting position is 10° of extension. Movements possible at these joints are flexion, extension, abduction, and adduction.

Interphalangeal Joints. The interphalangeal joints are synovial hinge joints with one degree of freedom. The close packed position is full extension, and the capsular pattern is more limitation of extension than flexion. The resting position of the distal and proximal interphalangeal joints is slight flexion. Movements possible at these joints are flexion and extension.

Patient History

It is important to take a detailed and complete history of the individual in an assessment of the lower leg, ankle, and foot. The examiner should ascertain the following information:

1. What is the patient's usual activity or pastime? Answers to this question should give some idea of the stresses placed on the lower leg, ankle, and foot.

2. What is the patient's occupation? Whether the patient stands a great deal and on what type of surfaces may have a bearing on what is causing the problem.

3. Is there any history of previous injury or affliction? For example, poliomyelitis may lead to a pes cavus. Systemic conditions such as diabetes, gout, psoriasis, and collagen diseases may manifest themselves first in the foot.

4. What types of shoe does the patient wear? What type of heel do the shoes have? Are the shoes in good condition? Does the patient make use of orthotics? If so, are they still functional? When an appointment is being made for an assessment, the patient should be told not to wear new shoes so that the examiner can determine the individual's usual wear pattern in that shoe. The examiner should also note whether the shoe offers proper support.

5. Does walking on various terrains make a difference in regard to the foot problem? If so, which terrains cause the most obvious problem? For example, walking on grass (an uneven surface) may bother a person more than walking on a sidewalk (a relatively even surface).

6. Does activity make a difference? Pain after activity suggests overuse. Pain during the activity suggests stress on the injured structure.

7. What was the mechanism of injury? Ankle sprains most commonly occur when the foot is inverted, with injury to the anterior talofibular ligament. Achilles tendinitis often arises as the result of overuse, increased activity, or change in a high-stress training program.

8. Are symptoms improving, becoming worse, or staying the same? It is important to know the type of onset and the duration and intensity of symptoms.

9. What are the sites and boundaries of pain or abnormal sensation? The examiner should note whether the pattern is one of a dermatome, a peripheral nerve, or another painful structure.

10. Did the patient notice a transient or fixed deformity of the foot or ankle at the time of injury? Was there any transitory locking (e.g., a loose body)?

11. Was the patient able to continue the activity after the injury? If so, the injury is probably not too severe, provided there is no loss of stability.

12. Was there any swelling or bruising (ecchymosis)? How quickly and where did it develop? This question can elicit some idea of the type of swelling (e.g., blood, synovial, or purulent) and whether it is intracapsular or extracapsular.

Observation

When performing the observation, one should remember to compare the weight-bearing and non–weight-bearing posture of the foot. The weight-bearing stance of the foot shows how the

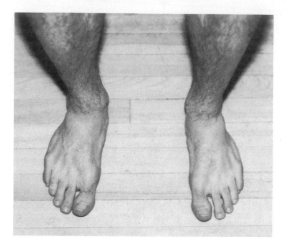

Figure 12–1. Anterosuperior view of the feet (weight-bearing position).

body compensates for structural abnormalities. The non–weight-bearing posture shows functional and structural ability without compensation. Thus, the observation includes looking at the patient from the front, from the side, and from behind in weight bearing and from the front, from the side, and from behind in sitting with the legs and feet non–weight bearing. The examiner should note the patient's willingness and ability to use the feet. The bony and soft-tissue contours of the foot should be normal and any deviation noted. Often painful callosities may be found over abnormal bony prominences. Any scars or sinuses should also be noted.

STANDING—WEIGHT BEARING (ANTERIOR VIEW)

Figure 12–1 shows the anterosuperior view of the feet in the weight-bearing stance. Is there any supination or pronation of the foot? *Supination* of the foot involves inversion of the heel, adduction of the forefoot, and plantar flexion at the subtalar joint and midtarsal joints (Fig. 12–2). As well, there is lateral rotation of the leg relative to the foot. Supination of the foot causes the proximal aspect of the tibia to move posteriorly. Supination is required during propulsion to give

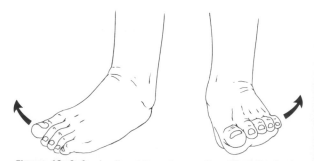

Figure 12–2. Supination (*A*) and pronation (*B*) of the foot.

rigidity to the foot and requires less muscle work than pronation.

Pronation of the foot involves eversion of the heel, abduction of the forefoot, medial rotation of the leg relative to the foot, and dorsiflexion of the subtalar and midtarsal joints (Fig. 12–2). This movement causes the proximal aspect of the tibia to move anteriorly. The pronated foot has greater subtalar motion than supination and requires more muscle work to maintain stance stability than supination. The foot is much more mobile in this position.

The definitions used in this chapter are the ones preferred by orthopedists and podiatrists. For example, anatomists and kinesiologists such as Kapandji[2] refer to _inversion_ as a combination of adduction and supination, and to _eversion_ as involving abduction and pronation. Lipscomb and Ibrahim[3] as well as Williams and Warwick[4] define _supination_ and _pronation_ as opposite to the terms just mentioned. Because of the confusion in terminology concerning the terms supination and pronation, readers of books and articles on the foot must be careful to discern exactly what each author means.

In the infant, the foot is pronated. As the child matures, the foot begins to supinate, accompanied by development of the medial longitudinal arch. The foot also appears more pronated in the infant because of the fat pad in the medial longitudinal arch.

How does the patient stand or walk? Normally, in standing, 50 to 60 per cent of the weight is taken on the heel and 40 to 50 per cent is taken by the metatarsal heads. The foot forms an angle (the Fick angle), which is approximately 12 to 18° from the sagittal axis of the body developing from 5° in children (Fig. 12–3).[5] During movement, the foot is subjected to high loading and pathology may cause the gait to be altered. The accumulative force to which each foot is subjected during the day is the equivalent of 639 metric tons in a person who weighs approximately 90 kg and is estimated to walk 13 km per day. In walking, the foot is subjected to 1.2 times the body weight; in running, two times; and in jumping from a height of 2 ft, five times.

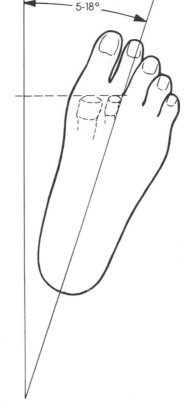

Figure 12–3. Fick angle. (From Jahss, M. H.: Disorders of the Foot. Philadelphia, W. B. Saunders Co., 1982, p. 660.)

The patient should be asked to walk on the toes, heels, and outer and inner borders of the feet. This action gives an indication of the patient's muscle power and functional range of motion. With a third-degree strain of the Achilles tendon, the patient will not be able to walk on the toes. Lack of dorsiflexion, or at least the anatomic position, will make it difficult for the individual to walk on the heels. When the patient walks on the inner or outer border of the feet, pain and difficulty will be experienced in the presence of subtalar lesion.

Does the patient use a cane or other walking aid? Using a cane in the opposite hand diminishes the stress on the ankle joint and foot by approximately one third.

Figure 12–4. Metatarsal classifications. (From Jahss, M. H.: Disorders of the Foot. Philadelphia, W. B. Saunders Co., 1982, p. 660.)

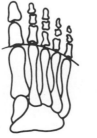

INDEX PLUS MINUS
28 %

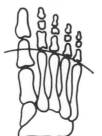

INDEX MINUS
56 %

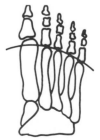

INDEX PLUS
16 %

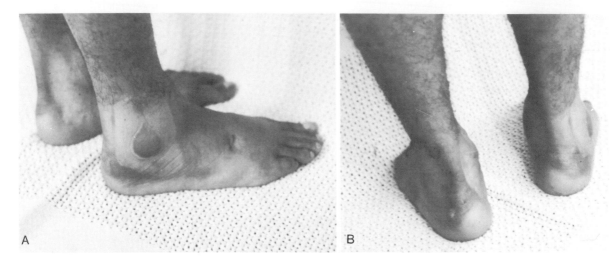

A   B

Figure 12–5. Ankle sprain. Note pattern of pitting edema on top of the right foot in *A.* The swelling is intracapsular, as indicated by swelling on both sides of the right Achilles tendon in *B.*

One should also check for the efficiency of the toes. Are the toes straight and parallel? Is the patient able to flex, extend, adduct, and abduct the toes? The toes have a primarily ambulatory function, although with training, they can develop a prehensile function. The toes extend the weight-bearing area forward and, by so doing, reduce the load on the metatarsal heads. The great toe also has a primary function of "pushing off" during gait.

Are there any prominent bumps or exostoses? Is there any splaying (widening) of the forefoot? Splaying of the forefoot and metatarsus primus varus are more evident in weight bearing. The forefoot can appear in three ways,[6] based on the length of the metatarsal bones (Fig. 12–4):

1. *Index plus type.* The first metatarsal (1) is longer than the second (2), with the others (3, 4, and 5) in progressively decreasing length so that 1 > 2 > 3 > 4 > 5.

2. *Index plus-minus type.* The first metatarsal is equal in length to the second metatarsal, with the others progressively diminishing in length so that 1 = 2 > 3 > 4 > 5.

3. *Index minus type.* The second metatarsal is

longer than the first and third metatarsal. The fourth and fifth metatarsals are progressively shorter than the third so that 1 < 2 > 3 > 4 > 5. Figure 12–4 illustrates this concept and shows the proportional representation of each in the population.

Do the toenails appear normal? The examiner should look for warts, calluses, and corns. Warts are especially tender to the pinch (but not to direct pressure), but calluses are not. Plantar warts also tend to separate from the surrounding tissues, but calluses do not.

Is there any swelling or pitting edema within the ankle (Fig. 12–5)? If there is any swelling, is it intracapsular or extracapsular? The examiner should also check the patient's gait for the position of the foot at heel strike, at foot flat, and at "toe-off." The gait cycle is described in greater detail in Chapter 13.

One should look at the tibia as well, to note any local or general bone swelling (Fig. 12–6). Does the tibia have a normal shape, or is it bowed? Is there any torsional deformity? The medial malleolus usually lies anterior to the lateral malleolus. "Pigeon toes" are due to a medial tibial

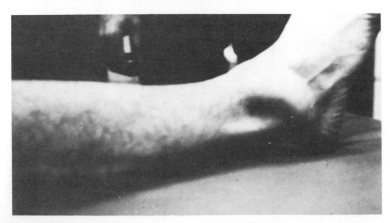

Figure 12–6. Swelling within the talocrural and subtalar joint capsule.

torsion deformity; they do not constitute a foot deformity (Table 12–1).

With the patient in a standing position, the examiner should observe whether the patient's hips are in normal position. Excessive lateral rotation of the hip elevates the medial longitudinal arch of the foot, whereas medial rotation of the hip tends to flatten the arch. Medial rotation of the hip can also cause pigeon toes. If the iliotibial band is tight, the tightness may cause eversion and lateral rotation of the foot.

Any vasomotor changes should be recorded, including loss of hair on the foot, toenail changes, osteoporosis as seen on radiographs, and possible differences in temperature between the limbs. Systemic diseases such as diabetes can also lead to foot problems as a result of altered sensation, thus allowing for easier injury.

The examiner should look for any circulatory impairment or presence of varicose veins. Brick-red color or cyanosis should be looked for when the limb is dependent as an indication of impairment. Does this condition change to rapid blanching, or does it stay normal on elevation of the limbs?

STANDING—WEIGHT BEARING (POSTERIOR VIEW)

From behind, the examiner compares the bulk of the calf muscles and notes any differences.

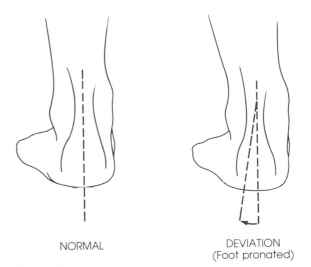

NORMAL   DEVIATION
                  (Foot pronated)

Figure 12–7. Normal and deviated Achilles tendon. The deviation is often seen with pes planus (flatfoot) and when the medial longitudinal arch is lower or has "dropped."

Variation may be due to peripheral nerve lesions, nerve root problems, or atrophy caused by disuse following injury. The Achilles tendon on both sides should be compared. If the tendon appears to curve out (Fig. 12–7), it may be caused by a fallen medial longitudinal arch, resulting in a pes planus (flatfoot condition).

The examiner notes the calcaneus for normality of shape and position. Runners often build up bone and a callus on the heel, resulting in a "pump bump" as a result of pressure on the heel (Figs. 12–8 and 12–9).

Table 12–1. Etiology of Toeing-In and Toeing-Out in Children*

Level of Affection	Toe-In	Toe-Out
Feet-ankles	Pronated feet (protective toeing-in) Metatarsus varus Talipes varus and equinovarus	Pes valgus due to contracture of triceps surae muscle Talipes calcaneovalgus Congenital convex pes planovalgus
Leg-knee	Tibia vara (Blount's disease) and developmental genu varum	External tibial torsion
	Abnormal internal tibial torsion	Congenital absence of hypoplasia of the fibula
	Genu valgum—developmental (protective toeing-in to shift body center of gravity medially)	
Femur-hip	Abnormal femoral antetorsion	Abnormal femoral retroversion
	Spasticity of internal rotators of hip (cerebral palsy)	Flaccid paralysis of internal rotators of hip
Acetabulum	Maldirected—facing anteriorly	Maldirected—facing posteriorly

*From Tachdjian, M. O.: Pediatric Orthopedics, Vol. 2. Philadelphia, W. B. Saunders Co., 1972, p. 1460.

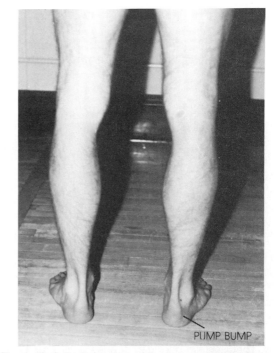

PUMP BUMP

Figure 12–8. Posterior view of the leg and foot. Note "pump bumps."

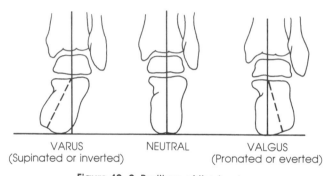

VARUS
(Supinated or inverted) NEUTRAL VALGUS
(Pronated or everted)

Figure 12–9. Positions of the heel.

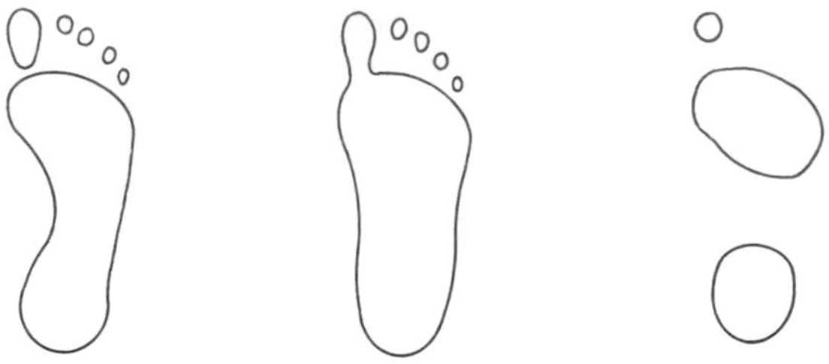

NORMAL PES PLANUS PES CAVUS

Figure 12–11. Footprint patterns.

The malleoli are compared for positioning. Normally, the lateral malleolus extends further distally than the medial malleolus; however, the medial malleolus extends further anteriorly.

STANDING—WEIGHT BEARING (LATERAL VIEW)

With the side view, the examiner is primarily observing the longitudinal arches of the foot (Fig. 12–10). The examiner should note whether the medial arch is higher than the lateral arch (as would be expected). One can often determine any differences in the arches by looking at the footprint patterns (Fig. 12–11). The footprint pattern can be established by putting a light film of baby oil, then powder, on the patient's foot and asking the patient to step down on a piece of colored paper. The footprint pattern will then become evident.

The arches of the feet (Fig. 12–12) are maintained by three mechanisms[7]: (1) Wedging of the interlocking tarsal and metatarsal bones takes place; (2) the ligaments on the plantar aspect of

the foot play a significant role; and (3) the intrinsic and the extrinsic muscles of the foot and their tendons help to support the arches. The longitudinal arches form a cone as a result of the angle formed by the metatarsal bones with the floor. With the medial longitudinal arch being more evident, this angle is greater on the medial side. The angle formed by each of the metatarsals with the floor is shown in Figure 12–13.

The *medial longitudinal arch* consists of the calcaneal tuberosity, the talus, the navicular bone, three cuneiforms, and the first, second, and third metatarsal bones (Fig. 12–14). This arch is maintained by the tibialis anterior, tibialis posterior, flexor digitorum longus, flexor hallucis longus, abductor hallucis, and flexor digitorum brevis muscles; the plantar fascia; and the plantar calcaneonavicular ligament (Fig. 12–15).[7]

The calcaneus, cuboid, and fourth and fifth metatarsal bones make up the *lateral longitudinal arch* (Fig. 12–16). This arch is more stable and less adjustable than the medial longitudinal arch. The arch is maintained by the peroneus longus, peroneus brevis, peroneus tertius, abductor digiti minimi, and flexor digitorum brevis muscles; the

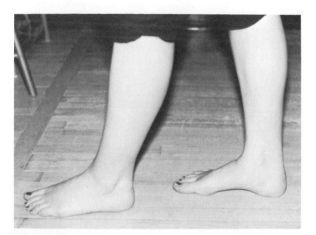

Figure 12–10. Lateral and medial views of the feet showing longitudinal arches.

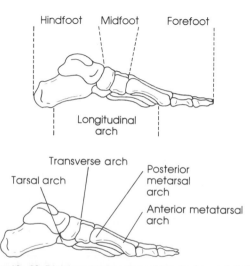

Hindfoot Midfoot Forefoot

Longitudinal arch

Transverse arch

Tarsal arch

Posterior metarsal arch

Anterior metatarsal arch

Figure 12–12. Divisions and arches of the foot (medial view).

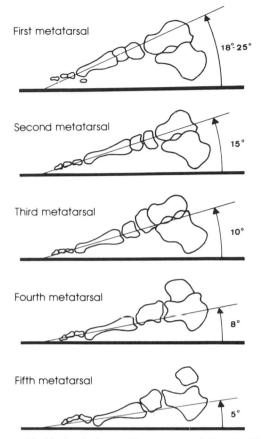

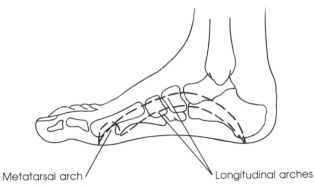

Figure 12–14. Arches of the foot (medial view).

Figure 12–13. Angle formed by each metatarsal with the floor. (Modified from Jahss, M. H.: Disorders of the foot. Philadelphia, W. B. Saunders Co., 1982, p. 661.)

plantar fascia; the long plantar ligament; and the short plantar ligament.[7]

The *transverse arch* is maintained by the tibialis posterior, tibialis anterior, and peroneus longus muscles and the plantar fascia (Fig. 12–17). This arch consists of the navicular bone, cuneiforms, and cuboid and metatarsal bones. The arch is sometimes divided into three parts: tarsal, posterior metatarsal, and anterior metatarsal. A loss of the anterior metatarsal arch results in callus formation under the heads of the metatarsal bones. The examiner will also note that the metatarsophalangeal joints are slightly extended in the normal standing position because the longitudinal arches of the foot curve down toward the toes.[7]

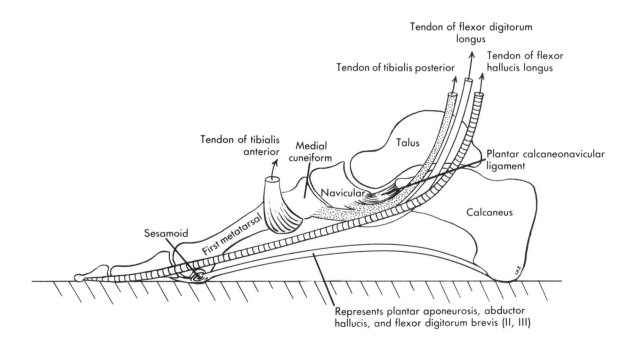

Figure 12–15. Supports of the medial longitudinal arch of the foot. (From Hamilton, J. J., and L. K. Ziemer: Functional Anatomy of the Human Ankle and Foot. AAOS Symposium on the Foot and Ankle. St. Louis, C. V. Mosby, 1983, p. 12.)

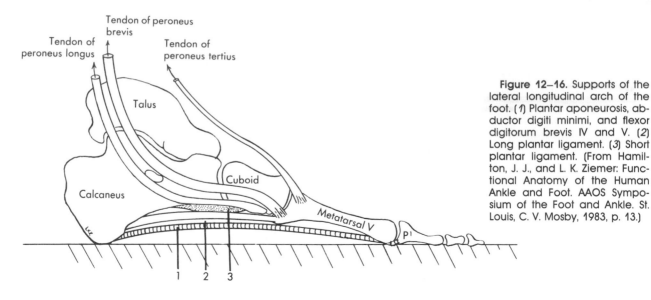

Tendon of peroneus longus

Tendon of peroneus brevis

Tendon of peroneus tertius

Talus

Calcaneus

Cuboid

Metatarsal V

P¹

1 2 3

Figure 12–16. Supports of the lateral longitudinal arch of the foot. (*1*) Plantar aponeurosis, abductor digiti minimi, and flexor digitorum brevis IV and V. (*2*) Long plantar ligament. (*3*) Short plantar ligament. (From Hamilton, J. J., and L. K. Ziemer: Functional Anatomy of the Human Ankle and Foot. AAOS Symposium of the Foot and Ankle. St. Louis, C. V. Mosby, 1983, p. 13.)

Figure 12–17. Supports of the transverse arch of the foot. Stippled tube represents tendon of tibialis posterior; black areas represent oblique head of adductor hallucis. (From Hamilton, J. J., and L. K. Ziemer: Functional Anatomy of the Human Ankle and Foot. AAOS Symposium on the Foot and Ankle. St. Louis, C. V. Mosby, 1983, p. 13.)

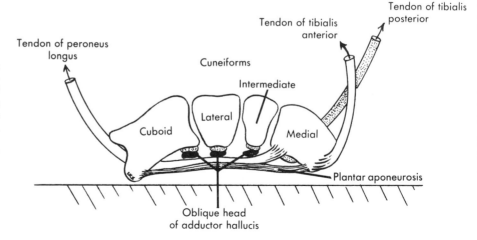

Tendon of peroneus longus

Cuneiforms

Intermediate

Tendon of tibialis anterior

Tendon of tibialis posterior

Cuboid

Lateral

Medial

Plantar aponeurosis

Oblique head of adductor hallucis

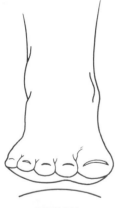
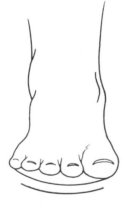

NORMAL

FALLEN ARCH

Figure 12–18. Fallen metatarsal arch.

NON–WEIGHT BEARING

With the patient non–weight bearing and in a supine position, the examiner should look for abnormal callosities, plantar warts, scars, sinuses, and so forth, on the sole of the foot. As well, by looking at the foot from above (i.e., toes to heel as shown in Figure 12–18), the examiner can note whether the patient has a "fallen" metatarsal arch. Normally, in non–weight bearing the arch can be seen. If it falls, callosities will often be found over the metatarsal heads. The arch may be reversed or may fall because of an equinus forefoot, pes cavus, rheumatoid arthritis, short heel cord, or hammertoes.

Young children should be assessed for clubfoot deformities, the most common of which is *talipes equinovarus* (Figs. 12–19 and 12–20). These types of deformities are often associated with other anomalies such as spina bifida.

SHOES

The examiner looks at the patient's shoes from the inside and outside for weight-bearing and wear patterns (Figs. 12–21 and 12–22). With the normal foot, the greatest wear on the shoe is beneath the ball of the foot and slightly to the lateral side. If shoes are too small or too narrow, they pinch the feet, causing deformities and affecting normal growth. If shoes are worn out, they offer little support. If shoes are stiff, they limit proper movement of the foot.

"Platform"-type shoes often cause painful knees because the patient, when wearing these shoes, usually walks with the knees flexed, which may increase the stress on the patella. As well, these shoes increase the potential for ankle sprains and fractures because a raised center of gravity puts one "off balance."

High heels and pointed shoes often contribute to hallux valgus, bunions, march fractures, and Morton's metatarsalgia as a result of the toes being pushed together. Continuous wearing of high-heeled shoes may also lead to contracture of the calf muscles as well as sore knees and a painful back because the lumbar spine goes into increased lordotic posture to maintain the center of gravity in its normal position.

Shoes with a negative heel (i.e., "earth" shoes) may lead to hyperextension of the knees and chondromalacia patellae. High-cut shoes that cover the medial and lateral malleolus offer more support than low-cut shoes or those that do not cover the malleoli.

Excessive bulging on the medial side of the shoe suggests a valgus or everted foot, whereas excessive bulging on the lateral side suggests an inverted foot. Drop foot resulting from musculature weakness scuffs the toe of the shoe. Oblique forefoot creases in the shoe indicate possible hallux rigidus; absence of forefoot creases indicates no toe-off action during gait.

DEFORMITIES OF THE FOOT AND TOES

Claw Toes

A claw toe deformity results in hyperextension of the metatarsophalangeal joints and flexion of

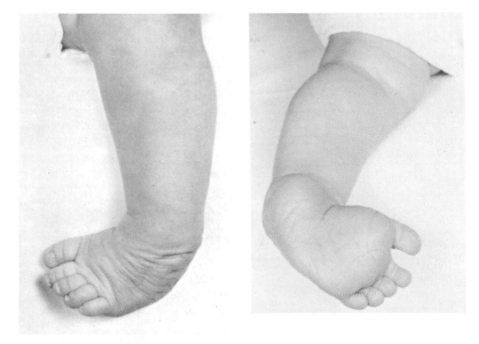

Figure 12–19. Talipes equinovarus (club foot) in a child aged 4 months. (A) Anterior view. (B) Posterior view. (From Klenerman, L.: The Foot and Its Disorders. Boston, Blackwell Scientific Publications, 1982, p. 64.)

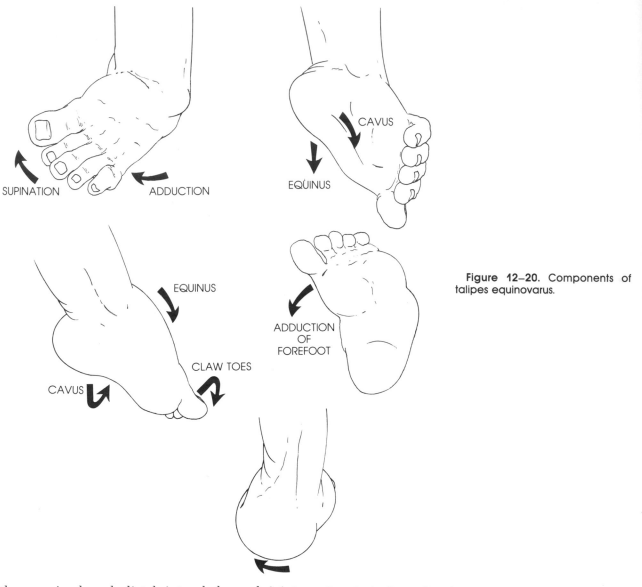

SUPINATION   ADDUCTION

CAVUS

EQUINUS

EQUINUS

CAVUS   CLAW TOES

ADDUCTION
OF
FOREFOOT

Figure 12–20. Components of talipes equinovarus.

the proximal and distal interphalangeal joints (Fig. 12–23C). Claw toes are usually due to the defective action of lumbrical and interosseus muscles so that the toes become functionless. This condition may be unilateral or bilateral and is often associated with pes cavus, spina bifida, or other neurologic problems.

Exostosis (Bony Spur)

Exostosis is an abnormal bony outgrowth extending from the surface of the bone (Fig. 12–24). It is actually an increase in the bone mass at the site of an irritative lesion in response to overuse, trauma, or pressure. The common areas of occur-

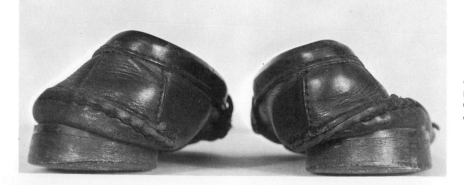

Figure 12–21. Misshapen shoes caused by severely pronated feet. (From Gartland, J. J.: Fundamentals of Orthopedics. Philadelphia, W. B. Saunders Co., 1979, p. 442.)

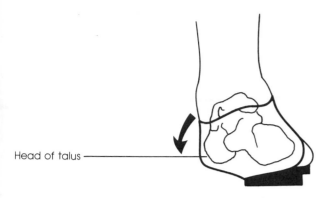

Head of talus

Figure 12–22. Pes planus ("flat" foot) or calcaneus in valgus can lead to misshapen shoes. Note the prominence of the talar head.

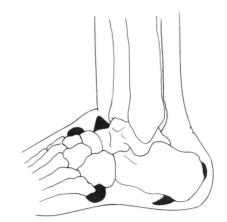

Figure 12–24. Common areas of exostosis formation in the foot.

rence in the foot are on the dorsal aspect of the tarsometatarsal joint, the head of the fifth metatarsal bone, the calcaneus (where it is often called a pump bump or runner's bump), insertion of the plantar fascia, and the superior aspect of the navicular bone.

Hallux Rigidus

Hallux rigidus is a condition in which dorsiflexion or extension of the big toe is limited because of osteoarthritis of the first metatarsophalangeal joint.[8] There are two types: acute and chronic.

The acute, or adolescent, type is seen primarily in young people with long, narrow, pronated feet and more frequently occurs in boys than in girls. Pain and stiffness in the big toe come on quickly; pain is described as constant, burning, throbbing, or aching. Tenderness may be palpated over the

metatarsophalangeal joint, and the toe is initially held stiff because of muscle spasm. The first metatarsal head may be elevated, large, and tender. The weight distribution pattern in gait is shown in Figure 12–25.

The second (chronic) type of hallux rigidus is much more common and is seen primarily in adults, again men more frequently than women. It is frequently bilateral and is usually due to repeated minor trauma, resulting in osteoarthritic changes to the metatarsophalangeal joint of the big toe. The toe stiffens gradually, and the pain, once established, persists. The patient primarily complains of pain at the base of the great toe on walking.

Hallux rigidus may also be due to an anatomic abnormality of the foot, an abnormally long first metatarsal bone (index plus type forefoot), pronation of the forefoot, or trauma.

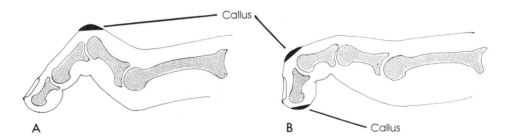

Callus

A

Callus

B

Callus

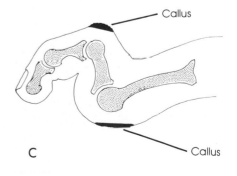

Callus

Callus

C

Figure 12–23. Toe deformities. (*A*) *Hammer toe.* Note the flexion deformity of the proximal interphalangeal joints. The distal interphalangeal joint is in neutral position or slight flexion. (*B*) *Mallet toe.* There is flexion contracture of the distal interphalangeal joint. The proximal interphalangeal and metatarsophalangeal joints are in neutral position. (*C*) *Claw toe.* Note that the proximal and distal interphalangeal joints are hyperflexed and the metatarsophalangeal joint is dorsally subluxated. (From Jahss, M. H.: Disorders of the Foot. Philadelphia, W. B. Saunders Co., 1982, p. 212.)

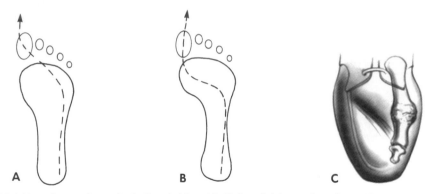

Figure 12–25. Weight-bearing patterns in hallux rigidus. (*A*) Hallux rigidus gait pattern. (*B*) Normal gait pattern. (*C*) Shoe develops oblique creases with hallux rigidus. *C* is from Jahss, M. H.: Disorders of the Foot. Philadelphia, W. B. Saunders Co., 1982, p. 112.)

Hammertoes

A hammertoe deformity consists of an extension contracture at the metatarsophalangeal joint and flexion contracture at the proximal interphalangeal joint; the distal interphalangeal joint may be flexed, straight, or hyperextended (Fig. 12–23A). The interosseus muscles are unable to hold the proximal phalanx in the neutral position,

thus losing their flexion effect; this results in the long flexors and extensors clawing the toe, leading to and accentuating the deformity. The causes of hammertoe may be an imbalance of the synergic muscles, hereditary factors, or mechanical factors such as poorly fitting shoes or hallux valgus. It is usually seen only in one toe, the second toe. Often there is a callus or a corn over the dorsum of the flexed joint. The condition is often asymp-

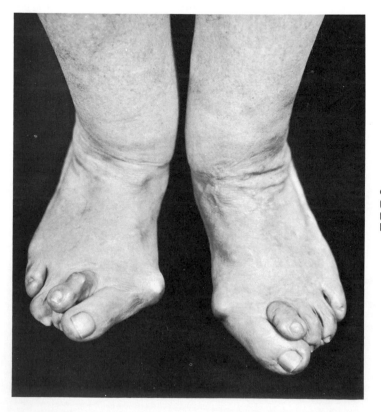

Figure 12–26. Hallux valgus with bilateral bunions and overlapped toes. Note how the deviating big toe (hallux) rotates and pushes under the second toe. (From Gartland, J. J.: Fundamentals of Orthopedics. Philadelphia, W. B. Saunders Co., 1979, p. 446.)

tomatic, especially if the hammertoe is flexible or semiflexible. The rigid type of hammertoe is likely to cause the greatest problems.

Mallet Toe

Mallet toe is associated with a flexion deformity of the distal interphalangeal joint (Fig. 12–23B). It can occur on any of the four lateral toes. Often a corn or callus is present over the dorsum of the affected joint. The condition is usually asymptomatic.

Hallux Valgus

Medial deviation of the head of the first metatarsal bone occurs in relation to the center of the body, or lateral deviation of the head in relation to the center of the foot (Fig. 12–26). As the metatarsal bone moves medially, the base of the proximal phalanx is carried with it and the phalanx pivots around the adductor hallucis muscle that inserts into it, causing the distal end along with the distal phalanx to deviate laterally. The long flexor and extensor muscles then have a "bowstring" effect as they displace to the lateral side of the joint.

A callus develops over the medial side of the head of the metatarsal bone, and the bursa becomes thickened and inflamed; excessive bone (exostosis) forms, resulting in a *bunion* (Fig. 12–27). These three changes—callus, thickened bursa, and exostosis—make up the bunion, a condition completely separate from hallux valgus, although it is the result of hallux valgus.

In normal individuals, the intermetatarsal angle (the angle between the longitudinal axis of the metatarsal bone and the proximal phalanx) is 8 to 20° (Fig. 12–28). This angle is increased in hallux valgus, depending on the type of hallux valgus present.

The first type (*congruous*) is a simple exaggeration of the normal foot. The deformity does not progress, and the valgus deformity is between 20 and 30°. The opposing joint surfaces in this case are congruent.

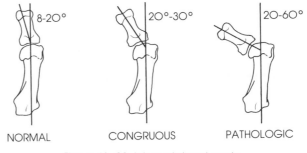

Figure 12–28. Intermetatarsal angle.

The second type (*pathologic*) is a potentially progressive deformity, increasing from 20 to 60°. The joint surfaces are no longer congruent, and some may even go to subluxation. This type may occur in *deviated* (early) and *subluxed* (later) stages.

When looking at the foot, the examiner may find that there is a widening gap between the first and second metatarsal bones and a lateral deflection of the phalanx at the metatarsophalangeal joint. The joint capsule lengthens on the medial aspect and is contracted on the lateral aspect. The toes rotate on a long axis so that the toenail faces medially because of the pull of the adductor hallucis muscle. Sometimes, the big toe will deviate so far that it lies over or under the second toe.

The etiology of hallux valgus is varied. It may be due to a hereditary factor and is often familial. Women tend to be affected more than men. Trying to keep up with fashion may be a contributing factor if the person wears tight or pointed shoes or tight stockings. Of all hallux valgus cases, 80 per cent are caused by *metatarsus primus varus*, in which the metatarsal angle is increased to greater than 15° (Fig. 12–29).[9, 10] Metatarsus primus varus is an abduction deformity of the first

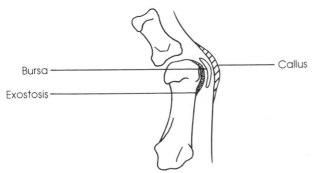

Figure 12–27. Bunion.

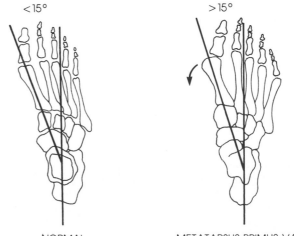

Figure 12–29. Normal foot and metatarsus primus varus.

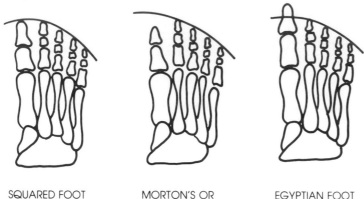

SQUARED FOOT
9%

MORTON'S OR
GREEK FOOT
22%

EGYPTIAN FOOT
69%

Figure 12–30. Types of feet seen in the population. (Modified from Jahss, M. H.: Disorders of the Foot. Philadelphia, W. B. Saunders Co., 1982, p. 660.)

metatarsal bone in relation to the other metatarsal bones, so that the medial border of the forefoot is curved. Normally, this angle is between 0 and 15°.

Morton's (Atavistic or Grecian) Foot

In Morton's foot, the second toe is longer than the first. Increased stress is put on this longer toe, and the big toe tends to be hypomobile. There is often hypertrophy of the second metatarsal bone because there is more stress put through the second toe. The different types of feet and their proportional representation in the population are shown in Figure 12–30.

Morton's Metatarsalgia (Interdigital Neuroma)

In Morton's neuroma, a digital nerve is affected, usually the one between the third and fourth toes (Fig. 12–31). While walking, the patient is suddenly seized with an agonizing pain on the outer border of the forefoot. The pain is often intermittent, as in a cramp, shooting up the side of and to the tip of the toe or the adjacent two toes. If the metatarsal bones are squeezed together, pain will be elicited because of the pressure on the digital nerve. The condition tends to be more frequent in women than in men.

Pes Cavus ("Hollow Foot")

A pes cavus may be due to a congenital problem; a neurogenic problem such as spina bifida, poliomyelitis or Charcot-Marie-Tooth disease; talipes equinovarus; or muscle imbalance. There may also be a genetic factor, since it tends to run in families.

The longitudinal arches are accentuated and the metatarsal heads are lower in relation to the

hindfoot, so that there is a "dropping" of the forefoot. The soft tissues of the sole are abnormally short, which gives the foot a shortened appearance. If the deformity persists, eventually the bones will alter shape, perpetuating the deformity. The heel is normal, at least initially. Claw toes are often associated with the condition. The examiner will often find painful callosities beneath the metatarsal heads and tenderness

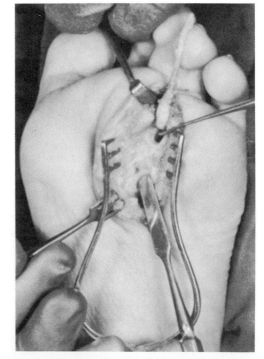

Figure 12–31. The applied anatomy of Morton's metatarsalgia. The interdigital nerve to the 3–4 space has been divided 2 cm above the "neuroma" and is reflected downward. The plantar digital vessels are seen entering the neuroma. The end of the flat dissector is on the upper margin of the transverse ligament. The end of the probe points to the intermetatarsophalangeal bursa. (From Klenerman, L.: The Foot and Its Disorders. Boston, Blackwell Scientific Publications, 1982, p. 143.)

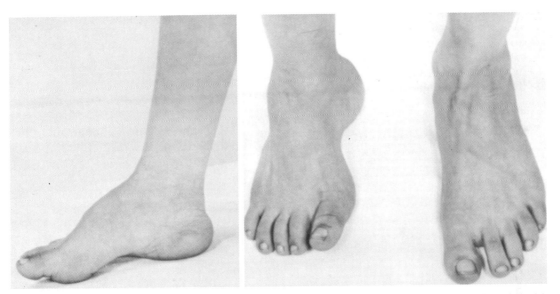

Figure 12–32. Pes cavus ("hollow foot"). Note the high medial longitudinal arch, early clawing of the big toe, and the heel in varus. (From Klenerman, L.: The Foot and Its Disorders. Boston, Blackwell Scientific Publications, 1982, p. 72.)

along the deformed toes. There is pain in the tarsal region after a period of time because of osteoarthritic changes in these joints.

The longitudinal arches are high, both on the medial and lateral aspect, and the forefoot is thickened and splayed (spread out). The metatarsal heads are prominent on the sole of the foot and the toes do not touch the ground even on active or passive movement. Individuals with pes cavus have difficulty tolerating prolonged activities, such as long-distance running and ballet.

Pes Planus (Flatfoot)

Flatfoot may be congenital or due to muscle weakness, ligament laxity or "dropping" of the talar head, paralysis, or a pronated foot. Pes planus may also be due to trauma. For example, a traumatic case of flatfoot may follow the fracture of the calcaneus. It may be due to a postural deformity, such as medial rotation of the hips or medial tibial torsion.

It must be remembered that all infants have flat feet initially up to about 2 years of age. This appearance is partly due to the fat pad in the longitudinal arch and partly due to the incomplete formation of the arches. The medial longitudinal arch is reduced, so that on standing its borders are close to or in contact with the ground. If the condition persists into adulthood, it becomes a permanent structural deformity, leading to a defect or alteration of the tarsal bones as well as the talonavicular joints.

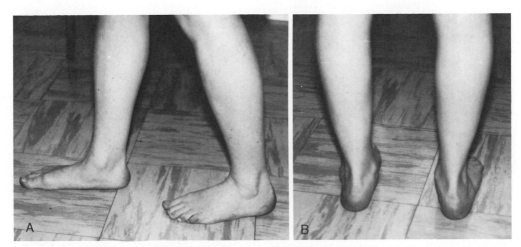

Figure 12–33. Pes planus (flatfoot). (*A*) Side view. (*B*) Posterior view. Note how the foot is pronated.

There are two types of flatfoot. The first type (*rigid* or *congenital*) is relatively rare. The calcaneus is found in a valgus position while the midtarsal region is in pronation. The talus faces medially and downward, and the navicular is displaced dorsally and laterally on the talus. There are accompanying soft-tissue contractures. The second type is *acquired* or *flexible*. In this case, the deformity is similar to the rigid flat foot but the foot is mobile. It is usually due to hereditary factors and is sometimes called a *hypermobile flatfoot*. Flexible flatfoot may be due to tibial or femoral torsion, coxa vara, or a defect in the subtalar joint. If the patient is asked to stand on tiptoes and the arch appears, it is an indication that the patient has a mobile flat foot.

"Rocker Bottom" Foot

In the rocker bottom foot deformity, the forefoot is dorsiflexed on the hindfoot; this results in a "broken midfoot," so that the medial and longitudinal arches are absent.

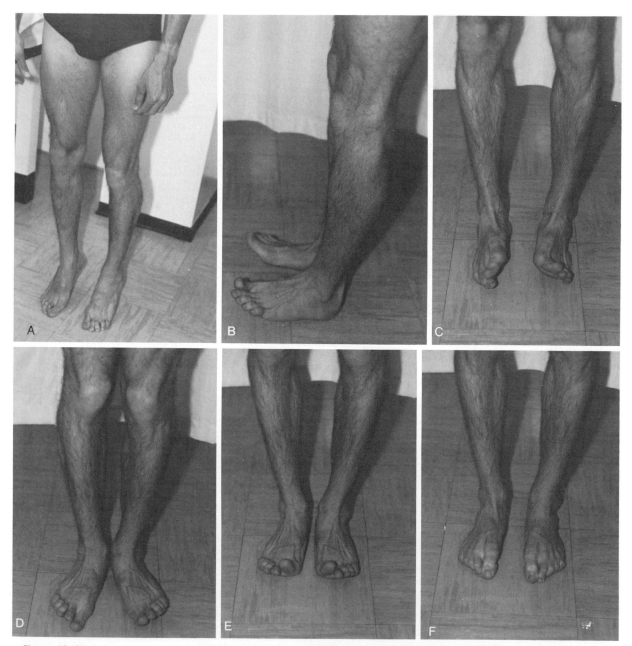

Figure 12–34. Active movements (weight-bearing posture). (*A*) Plantar flexion. (*B*) Dorsiflexion. (*C*) Supination. (*D*) Pronation. (*E*) Toe extension. (*F*) Toe flexion.

Examination

As with any assessment, the examiner must compare one side with the other and note any differences. This comparison is necessary because of the individual differences among normal people.

ACTIVE MOVEMENTS

The first movements are active, painful movements being done last. As well, the movements should be done non–weight bearing (long leg sitting or supine lying) and weight bearing, and any differences should be noted. The movements that should be carried out actively in the lower leg, ankle, and foot region are as follows:

Weight Bearing (Figs. 12–34 and 12–35)
1. Plantar flexion (flexion) (standing on the toes).
2. Dorsiflexion (extension) (standing on the heels).
3. Supination (standing on the lateral edge of the foot).
4. Pronation (standing on the medial edge of the foot).
5. Toe extension.
6. Toe flexion.

Non–Weight Bearing (Fig. 12–36)
1. Plantar flexion (flexion) (50°).
2. Dorsiflexion (extension) (20°).
3. Supination (45 to 60°).
4. Pronation (15 to 30°).
5. Toe extension (lateral four toes: MTP:40°; PIP:0°; DIP:30°/great toe: MTP:70°; IP:0°)
6. Toe flexion (lateral four toes: MTP:40°; PIP:35°; DIP:60°/great toe: MTP:45°; IP:90°)
7. Toe abduction.
8. Toe adduction.

Flexion

Plantar flexion of the ankle is approximately 50° (Fig. 12–36A), and it should be noted that the patient's heel will normally invert when the movement is performed in weight bearing (Fig. 12–37). If heel inversion does not occur, the foot will be unstable.

Dorsiflexion

Dorsiflexion of the ankle is usually 20° past the anatomic position (foot at 90° to bones of the leg) (Fig. 12–36B). For normal locomotion, 10° of dorsiflexion and 20° of plantar flexion at the ankle are required. In a baby or young child, there will be greater mobility and flexibility than in an adult. For example, in the newborn, the foot can readily be dorsiflexed so that the toes and dorsum of the foot can touch the skin over the tibia.

Supination and Pronation

Supination is 45 to 60° and pronation is 15 to 30°, although there is variability between individuals (Fig. 12–36C and D). It is more important to compare the movement with the normal side (Figs. 12–38 and 12–39). Supination combines the movements of inversion, adduction, and plantar flexion; pronation combines the movements of eversion, abduction, and dorsiflexion of the foot and ankle. As the patient does the movement, the examiner should watch for the possibility of subluxation of various tendons. The peroneal tendons are especially prone to subluxation, and their subluxation will be evident on eversion (Fig. 12–40).

Toe Extension and Flexion

Movement of the toes occurs at the metatarsophalangeal (MTP) joints and the proximal (PIP) and distal interphalangeal (DIP) joints (Fig.

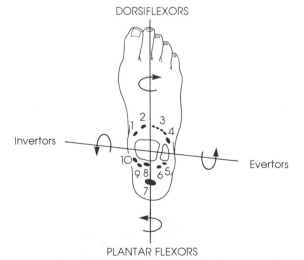

Figure 12–35. Motion diagram of the ankle. (*1*) Tibialis anterior. (*2*) Extensor hallucis longus. (*3*) Extensor digitorum longus. (*4*) Peroneus tertius. (*5*) Peroneus brevis. (*6*) Peroneus longus. (*7*) Achilles tendon (soleus and gastrocnemius). (*8*) Flexor hallucis longus. (*9*) Flexor digitorum longus. (*10*) Tibialis posterior.

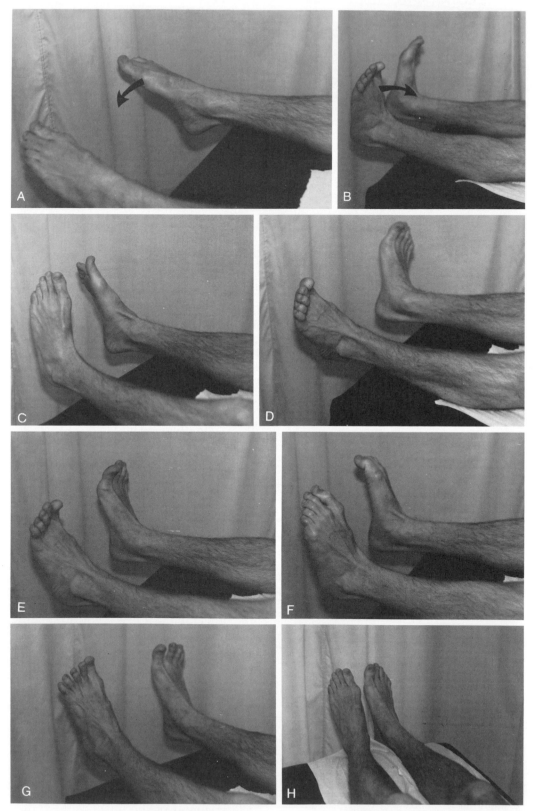

Figure 12–36. Active movements (Non–weight-bearing posture). (*A*) Plantar flexion. (*B*) Dorsiflexion. (*C*) Supination. (*D*) Pronation. (*E*) Toe extension. (*F*) Toe flexion. (*G*) Toe abduction. (*H*) Toe adduction.

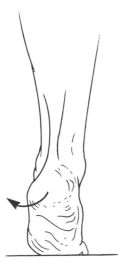

Figure 12–37. Inversion of heel while standing on toes (plantar flexion of ankle).

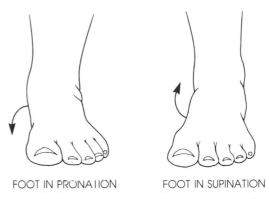

FOOT IN PRONATION   FOOT IN SUPINATION

Figure 12–39. Anterior view of the foot in pronation and supination (weight-bearing stance).

12–36*E* and *F*). For the lateral four toes, 40° flexion occurs at the metatarsophalangeal joints, 35° occurs at the proximal interphalangeal joints, and 60° occurs at the distal interphalangeal joints. For the great toe, 45° flexion occurs at the metatarsophalangeal joint and 90° occurs at the interphalangeal joint.

Extension of the great toe occurs primarily at the metatarsophalangeal joint (70°) with minimal or no extension at the interphalangeal joint. For the lateral four toes, extension occurs primarily at the metatarsophalangeal (40°) and distal interphalangeal joints (30°). Extension at the proximal interphalangeal joints is negligible.

Toe Abduction and Adduction

Abduction and adduction of the toes are measured with the second toe as midline. Although the range of motion of abduction can be measured, it is not usually done. The common practice is to ask the patient to spread the toes and then bring them back together (Fig. 12–36*G* and *H*). The amount and quality of movement are compared with the unaffected side.

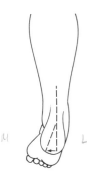
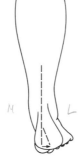

SUPINATION   PRONOATION
(Non-weight-bearing)   (Non-weight-bearing)

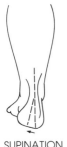
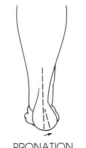

SUPINATION   PRONATION
(Weight-bearing)   (Weight-bearing)

Figure 12–38. Supination and pronation of the foot in weight-bearing and non–weight-bearing postures (posterior view of the right limb).

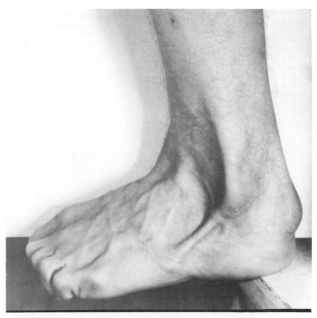

Figure 12–40. Habitual subluxation of the peroneal tendons. The peroneal tendons pass anterior to the retrofibular sulcus but not anterior to the distal fibula, in contradistinction to traumatic subluxation. (From Kelikian, H., and A. S. Kelikian: Disorders of the Ankle. Philadelphia, W. B. Saunders Co., 1985, p. 765.)

Functional Tests

If the patient is able to do the preceding activities with little difficulty, functional tests may be performed to see whether these sequential activities produce pain or other symptoms. The functional activities in order of sequence are:

1. Squatting (both ankles should dorsiflex symmetrically).
2. Standing on toes (both ankles should plantar flex symmetrically).
3. Squatting and bouncing at the end of a squat.
4. Standing on one foot at a time.
5. Standing on the toes of one foot at a time.
6. Going up and down stairs.
7. Walking on the toes.
8. Running straight ahead.
9. Running and twisting.
10. Jumping.
11. Jumping and going to a full squat.

These activities, which are examples only, must be geared to the individual patient. Older patients should not be expected to do some of the activities unless they have, in the recent past, been doing these or similar ones. Because the functional tests place a stress on the other lower limb joints, the examiner must ensure that these joints exhibit no pathology before all the tests are completed. As the patient completes the activities, the examiner must assess whether any symptoms occur at a specific time, e.g., intermittent claudication or anterior compartment syndrome.[14, 15]

Nerve Injury

When assessing the active movements, the examiner must remember that peripheral nerve injuries may alter the pattern of movement. For example, the superficial peroneal nerve may be injured as it winds around the head of the fibula, resulting in altered nerve conduction to the peroneus longus and brevis muscles.[16] Thus, the movements controlled by these muscles will be altered. As well, there will be sensory alterations. Similarly, the tibial nerve may be compressed as it passes through the tarsal tunnel on the medial aspect of the ankle (Fig. 12–41).[17] The borders of the tunnel are the tibiocalcaneal portion of the medial collateral ligament, the medial malleolus, and the calcaneus and talus. All the intrinsic foot muscles supplied by the tibial nerve and its branches will be affected, as will the sensory distribution.

PASSIVE MOVEMENTS

The passive movements of the lower leg, ankle, and foot are performed in the non–weight-bearing posture (Fig. 12–42). As with other joints, if the active range of motion was complete, overpressure could be applied during the active non–weight-bearing movements. The end feel of plantar flexion, dorsiflexion, supination, pronation, toe flexion, and extension is tissue stretch. If the active movements were not full, the following passive movements should be performed:

1. Plantar flexion at the talocrural joint.
2. Dorsiflexion at the talocrural joint.
3. Inversion at the subtalar joint.
4. Eversion at the subtalar joint.
5. Adduction at the midtarsal joints.
6. Abduction at the midtarsal joints.
7. Flexion of the toes.
8. Extension of the toes.
9. Adduction of the toes.
10. Abduction of the toes.

During the passive movements of the ankle and foot, any capsular patterns should be noted. The capsular pattern of the talocrural joint is more limitation of plantar flexion than of dorsiflexion; the subtalar joint capsular pattern shows more limitation of varus range than valgus range of motion. The midtarsal joint capsular pattern is dorsiflexion most limited, followed by plantar flexion, adduction, and medial rotation. The first metatarsophalangeal joint has a capsular pattern of extension most limited, followed by flexion.

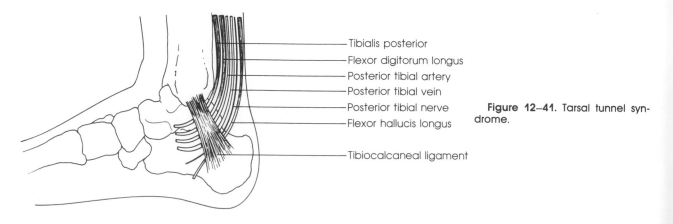

- Tibialis posterior
- Flexor digitorum longus
- Posterior tibial artery
- Posterior tibial vein
- Posterior tibial nerve
- Flexor hallucis longus
- Tibiocalcaneal ligament

Figure 12–41. Tarsal tunnel syndrome.

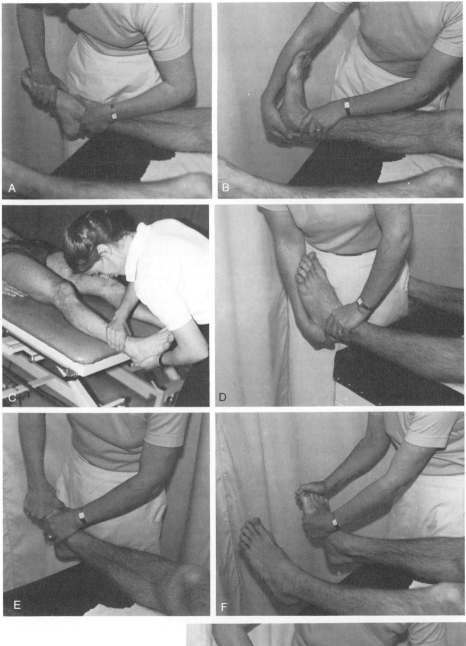

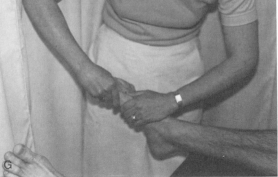

Figure 12–42. Passive movements of the ankle. (*A*) Plantar flexion. (*B*) Dorsiflexion. (*C*) Inversion. (*D*) Eversion. (*E*) Abduction/adduction. (*F*) Toe flexion. (*G*) Toe abduction.

Table 12–2. Muscles of the Lower Limb, Ankle, and Foot: Their Action, Innervation, and Nerve Root Deviation of the Peripheral Nerves

Action	Muscles Involved	Innervation	Nerve Root Deviation
Plantar flexion (flexion) of ankle	1. Gastrocnemius*	Tibial	S1, S2
	2. Soleus*	Tibial	S1, S2
	3. Plantaris	Tibial	S1, S2
	4. Flexor digitorum longus	Tibial	S2, S3
	5. Peroneus longus	Superficial peroneal	L5, S1, S2
	6. Peroneus brevis	Superficial peroneal	L5, S1, S2
	7. Flexor hallucis longus	Tibial	S2, S3
	8. Tibialis posterior	Tibial	L4, L5
Dorsiflexion (extension) of ankle	1. Tibialis anterior	Deep peroneal	L4, L5
	2. Extensor digitorum longus	Deep peroneal	L5, S1
	3. Extensor hallucis longus	Deep peroneal	L5, S1
	4. Peroneus tertius	Deep peroneal	L5, S1
Inversion	1. Tibialis posterior	Tibial	L4, L5
	2. Flexor digitorum longus	Tibial	S2, S3
	3. Flexor hallucis longus	Tibial	S2, S3
	4. Tibialis anterior	Deep peroneal	L4, L5
	5. Extensor hallucis longus	Deep peroneal	L5, S1
Eversion	1. Peroneus longus	Superficial peroneal	L5, S1, S2
	2. Peroneus brevis	Superficial peroneal	L5, S1, S2
	3. Peroneus tertius	Deep peroneal	L5, S1
	4. Extensor digitorum longus	Deep peroneal	L5, S1
Flexion of toes	1. Flexor digitorum longus	Tibial	S2, S3
	2. Flexor hallucis longus	Tibial	S2, S3
	3. Flexor digitorum brevis	Tibial (medial plantar branch)	S2, S3
	4. Flexor hallucis brevis	Tibial (medial plantar branch)	S2, S3
	5. Flexor accessorius	Tibial (lateral plantar branch)	S2, S3
	6. Interossei	Tibial (lateral plantar branch)	S2, S3
	7. Flexor digiti minimi brevis	Tibial (lateral plantar branch)	S2, S3
	8. Lumbricals (metatarsophalangeal joints)	Tibial (1st by medial plantar branch; 2nd–4th by lateral plantar branch)	S2, S3
Extension of toes	1. Extensor digitorum longus	Deep peroneal	L5, S1
	2. Extensor hallucis longus	Deep peroneal	L5, S1
	3. Extensor digitorum brevis	Deep peroneal (lateral terminal branch)	S1, S2
	4. Lumbricals (interphalangeal joints)	Tibial (1st by medial plantar branch; 2nd–4th by lateral plantar branch)	S2, S3
Abduction of toes	1. Abductor hallucis	Tibial (medial plantar branch)	S2, S3
	2. Abductor digiti minimi	Tibial (lateral plantar branch)	S2, S3
	3. Dorsal interossei	Tibial (lateral plantar branch)	S2, S3
Adduction of toes	1. Adductor hallucis	Tibial (lateral plantar branch)	S2, S3
	2. Plantar interossei	Tibial (lateral plantar branch)	S2, S3

*The gastrocnemius and soleus muscles are sometimes grouped together as the triceps surae muscles.

The pattern for the second to fifth metatarsophalangeal joints is variable. The capsular pattern of the interphalangeal joints is extension most limited, followed by flexion.

RESISTED ISOMETRIC MOVEMENTS

The resisted isometric movements are done in the sitting or supine lying position (Fig. 12–43). They are performed to test the contractile tissue around the foot. The patient's foot is placed in the anatomic position. Refer to Table 12–2 for the muscles acting over the foot and ankle. The movements tested isometrically are as follows:

1. Knee flexion.
2. Plantar flexion.
3. Dorsiflexion.
4. Supination.
5. Pronation.
6. Toe extension.
7. Toe flexion.

Plantar flexion and dorsiflexion are often tested with the patient's hip flexed to 45° and the knee flexed to 90°, as illustrated in Figure 12–43A and B. Testing with the patient in this position enables the examiner to exert a greater isometric force.

Resisted isometric knee flexion must be performed because the triceps surae (gastrocnemius and soleus muscles together) act on the knee as well as the ankle and foot.

SPECIAL TESTS

Only those special tests which the examiner feels have relevance need to be done.

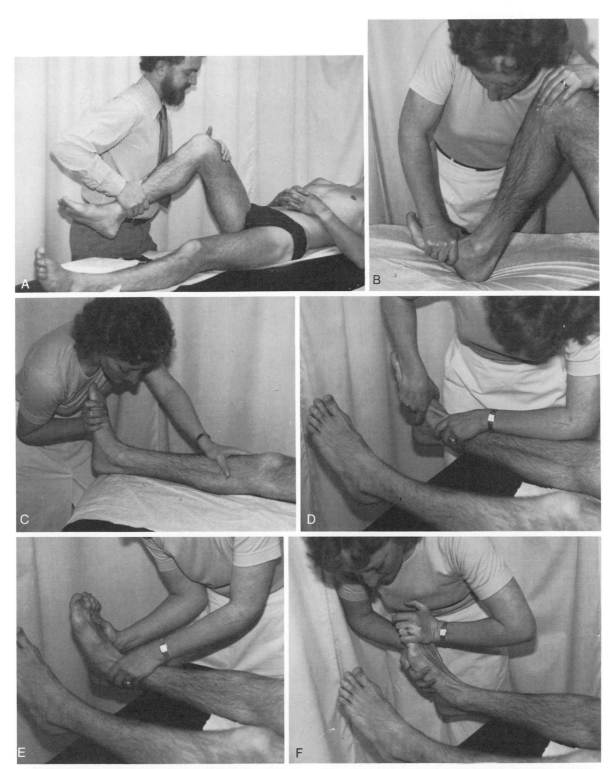

Figure 12–43. Resisted isometric movements of the lower leg, ankle, and foot. (*A*) Knee flexion. (*B*) Plantar flexion. (*C*) Dorsiflexion. (*D*) Supination. (*E*) Pronation. (*F*) Toe extension.

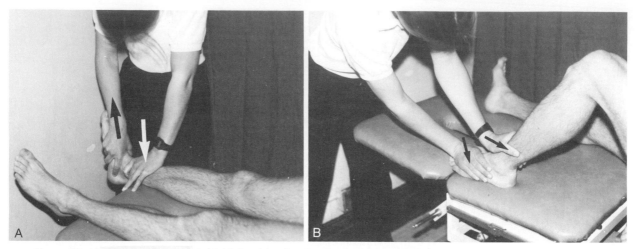

Figure 12–44. Anterior drawer test. (*A*) Method 1—drawing the foot forward. (*B*) Method 2—pushing the leg back.

Anterior Drawer Sign of the Ankle

The patient lies in the supine position with the foot relaxed. The examiner stabilizes the tibia and fibula, holds the patient's foot in 20° plantar flexion, and draws the talus forward in the ankle mortise (Fig. 12–44). In the plantar flexed position, the anterior talofibular ligament is perpendicular to the long axis of the tibia. By adding inversion, which gives an anterolateral stress, the examiner can increase the stress on the anterior talofibular ligament. If straight anterior movement or translation occurs, the test indicates both medial and lateral ligament insufficiency. This bilateral finding, which is often more evident in dorsiflexion, means that the superficial and deep deltoid ligaments, as well as the anterior talofibular ligament and anterolateral capsule, have been torn. If the tear is on one side only (e.g., the lateral side), only the one side (lateral in this case) would translate forward, causing internal rotation of the talus; the result would be anterolateral rotary instability (Fig. 12–45), which is more evident the more the foot is plantar flexed.[5, 6, 18–20]

Ideally, the knee should be placed in 90° of flexion to alleviate tension on the Achilles tendon. The test should be performed in plantar flexion and dorsiflexion to test for the straight and rotational instability.

The test may also be performed by stabilization of the foot and talus and pushing of the tibia and fibula posteriorly on the talus. In this case, excessive posterior movement of the tibia and fibula indicates a positive test.

Talar Tilt

The patient lies in a supine or side lying position with the foot relaxed (Fig. 12–46).[5, 21] The

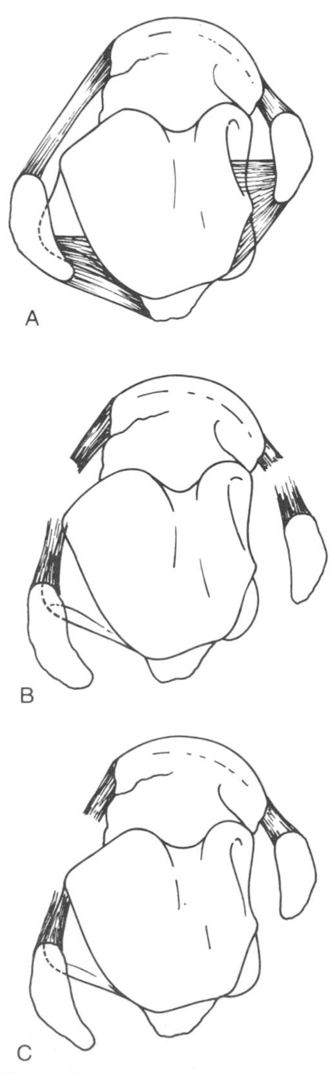

Figure 12–45. Anterior drawer test. (*A*) Normal talar-malleolar relationship. (*B*) Straight anterior translation (one plane anterior instability). (*C*) Lateral rotary translation (anterolateral rotary instability).

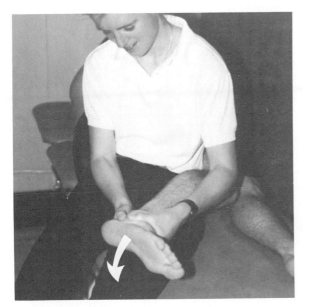

Figure 12–46. Talar tilt test.

patient's gastrocnemius muscle may be relaxed by flexion of the knee to 90°. This test is used to determine whether the calcaneofibular ligament is torn. The foot is held in the anatomic position, which brings the calcaneofibular ligament perpendicular to the long axis of the talus. The talus is then tilted from side to side into adduction and abduction. Adduction tests the calcaneofibular ligament by increasing the stress on the ligament. On a radiograph, this angle may be measured by obtaining the distance of the angle between the distal aspect of the tibia and the proximal surface of the talus (see Figure 12–72). The normal side is tested first for comparison.

Thompson Test (Sign for Achilles Tendon Rupture)

The patient lies in a prone position or kneels on a chair with the feet over the edge of the table or chair (Fig. 12–47). While the patient is relaxed, the examiner squeezes the calf muscles. A positive test is indicated by the absence of plantar flexion when the muscle is squeezed and is indicative of a ruptured Achilles tendon.[22]

One should be careful not to assume that the Achilles tendon is not ruptured if the patient is able to plantar flex the foot while non–weight bearing. The long extensor muscles can perform this function in the non–weight-bearing stance even with a rupture (third-degree strain) of the Achilles tendon.

Homans' Sign

The patient's foot is passively dorsiflexed with the knee extended. Pain in the calf indicates a positive Homans' sign for deep vein thrombophlebitis (Fig. 12–48). Tenderness will also be elicited on palpation of the calf. In addition to these findings, the examiner may find pallor and swelling in the leg, along with a loss of the dorsalis pedis pulse.

Kleiger Test

The patient sits with the knee flexed to 90° and the foot relaxed and non–weight bearing. The examiner gently grasps the foot and rotates it laterally (Fig. 12–49).[1, 6] If the Kleiger test is

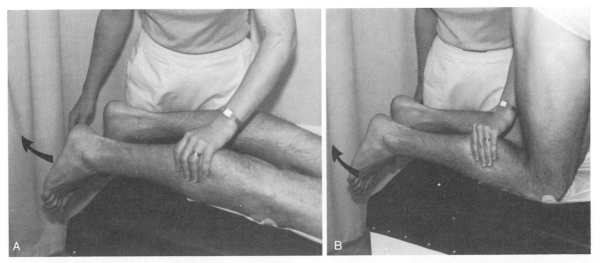

Figure 12–47. Thompson test for Achilles tendon rupture. (A) Prone lying position. (B) Kneeling position. Foot will plantar flex (arrow) if test result is negative.

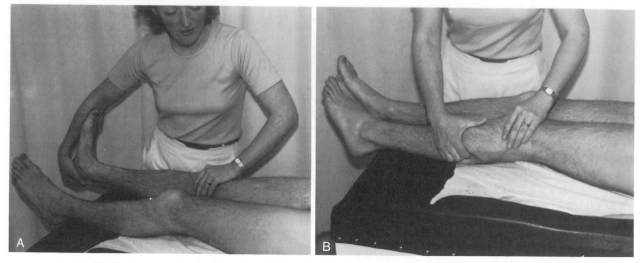

Figure 12–48. Homans' sign for thrombophlebitis. (*A*) Test. (*B*) Palpation for tenderness in thrombophlebitis.

positive, the patient will complain of pain medially and laterally and the examiner may feel the talus displace from the medial malleolus, indicating a tear of the deltoid ligament. On a radiograph, the medial clear space will be increased, suggesting rupture of the ligament (see Figure 12–72).

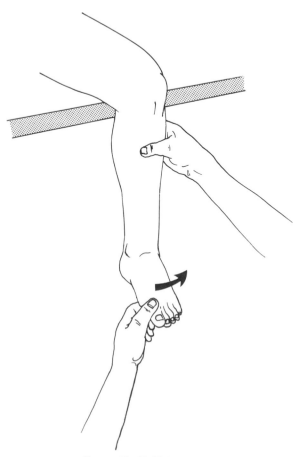

Figure 12–49. Kleiger test.

REFLEXES AND CUTANEOUS DISTRIBUTION

One must be aware of the sensory distribution of the various peripheral nerves in the foot (especially the superficial peroneal, deep peroneal, and saphenous) and the branches of the tibial nerve (sural, medial plantar, medial calcaneal, and lateral plantar) (Fig. 12–50).

The examiner must also differentiate between the peripheral nerve sensory distribution and the sensory nerve root distribution or dermatomes (Fig. 12–51). Although dermatomes vary from one individual to the next, their pattern will never be identical to the peripheral nerve distribution, which tends to be more consistent from patient to patient.

The patient's sensation should be tested by the examiner running the hands over the anterior, lateral, medial, and posterior surfaces of the patient's leg below the knee, foot, and toes. Any difference in sensation should be noted and can be mapped out more exactly with a pinwheel, pin, cotton batten, and/or brush.

The examiner must test the patient's reflexes. Commonly checked in this region is the Achilles reflex, which is derived from the S1 nerve root (Fig. 12–52). In addition to the S1 nerve root reflex, the examiner should test for pyramidal tract (upper motor neuron) disease. There are various methods for testing the reflexes, including Babinski, Chaddock, Oppenheim, and Gordon reflexes (Fig. 12–53). A positive sign in all of these tests is extension of the big toe. The Babinski reflex also causes fanning of the second to fifth toes. The most common and reliable test is the Babinski test.

One must always remember that pain may be referred to the lower leg, ankle, or foot from the lumbar spine, sacrum, hip, or knee (Fig. 12–54). Conversely, the pain from a lesion in the lower

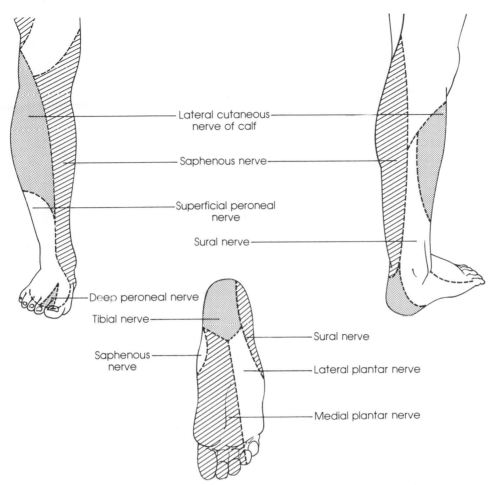

Figure 12–50. Peripheral nerve distribution in the lower leg, ankle, and foot.

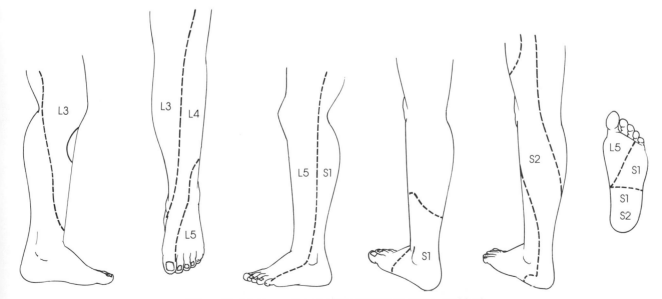

Figure 12–51. Dermatomes of the lower leg, ankle, and foot.

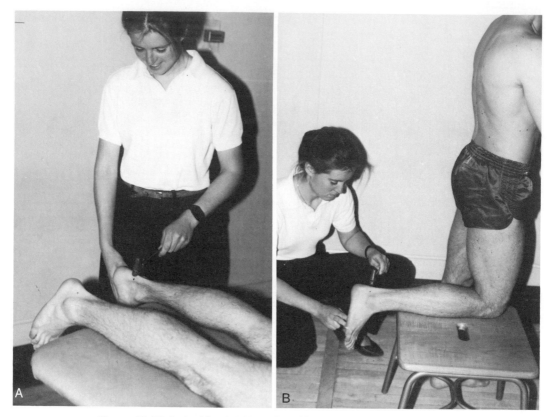

Figure 12–52. Test of the Achilles reflex (S1). (*A*) Method 1. (*B*) Method 2.

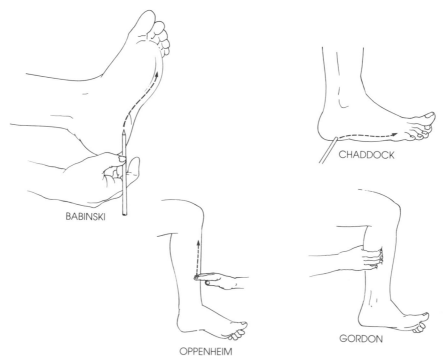

Figure 12–53. Reflexes for pyramidal tract disease.

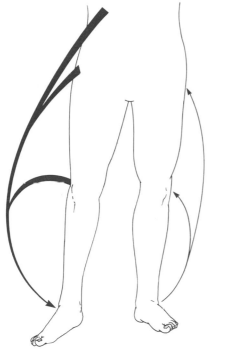

Figure 12–54. Pattern of referred pain to and from the ankle.

leg, ankle, or foot may be transmitted to the hip or knee.

JOINT PLAY MOVEMENTS

The joint play movements are done with the patient in a supine or side lying position, depending on which movement is being performed. A comparison of movement between the normal

or unaffected side and the injured side made.

The following movements should be p.. (Figs. 12–55 through 12–58):

1. At the talocrural (ankle) joint.
   a. Long axis extension (traction).
   b. Anteroposterior glide.
2. At the subtalar joint.
   a. Talar rock.
   b. Side tilt medially and laterally.
3. At the midtarsal joints.
   a. Anteroposterior glide.
   b. Rotation.
4. At the tarsometatarsal joints.
   a. Anteroposterior glide.
   b. Rotation.
5. At the metatarsophalangeal and interphalangeal joints.
   a. Long axis extension (traction).
   b. Anteroposterior glide.
   c. Lateral or side glide.
   d. Rotation.

Long Axis Extension

Long axis extension is performed by stabilizing the proximal segment and applying traction to the distal segment. For example, at the ankle, the examiner stabilizes the tibia and fibula by using a strap or may just allow the leg to relax. Both hands are then placed around the ankle, distal to the malleoli, and a distractive force is applied. At the metatarsophalangeal and interphalangeal joints, the examiner stabilizes the metatarsal bone or proximal phalanx and applies a distractive force to the proximal or distal phalanx, respectively.

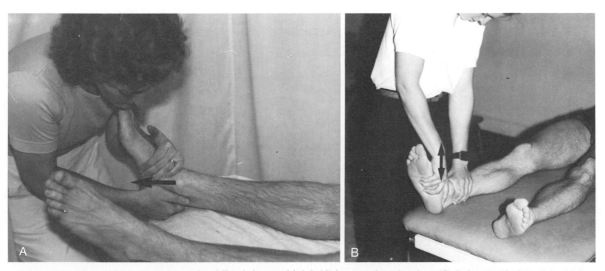

Figure 12–55. Joint play movements at the talocrural joint. (A) Long axis extension. (B) Anteroposterior glide at the talocrual joint.

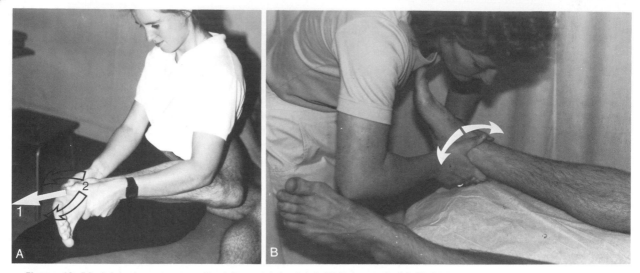

Figure 12–56. Joint play movements at the subtalar joint. (*A*) Talar rock. (*1*) Slight traction applied. (*2*) Talus is rocked medially and laterally. (*B*) Side tilt.

Anteroposterior Glide

Anteroposterior glide at the *ankle joint* is performed by stabilizing the tibia and fibula and drawing the talus and foot forward. To test the posterior movement, the examiner pushes the talus and foot back on the tibia and fibula. There is a difference in the arc of movement between the two actions in tests of joint play. During the anterior movement, the foot should move in an arc into dorsiflexion; during the posterior movement, the foot should move in an arc into plantar flexion.

Anteroposterior glide at the *midtarsal* and *tarsometatarsal joints* is performed in a fashion similar to that of the carpal bones at the wrist. For the midtarsal joints, one stabilizes the navicular, talus, and calcaneus with one hand. The other hand is placed around the distal row of tarsal bones (cuneiforms and cuboid). If the hands are positioned properly, they should touch each other, as in Figure 12–57. An anteroposterior gliding movement of the distal row of *tarsal bones* is applied while the proximal row of tarsal bones is stabilized. The examiner's hands are then moved distally so that the stabilizing hand rests over the distal row of tarsal bones, and the mobilizing hand rests over the proximal aspect of the metatarsal bones. Again, the hands should be positioned so that they touch each other. An anteroposterior gliding movement of the metatarsal bones is applied while stabilizing the distal row of tarsal bones.

Anteroposterior glide at the *metatarsophalangeal and interphalangeal joints* is performed by stabilization of the proximal bone (metatarsal or

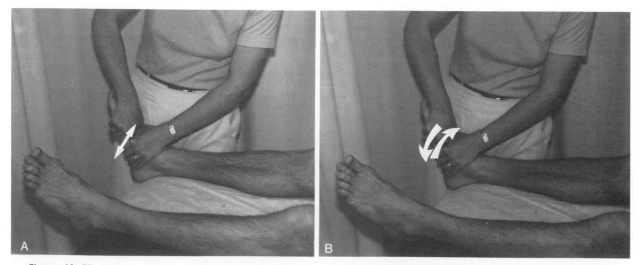

Figure 12–57. Joint play movements in the midtarsal and tarsometatarsal joints. (*A*) Anteroposterior glide. (*B*) Rotation.

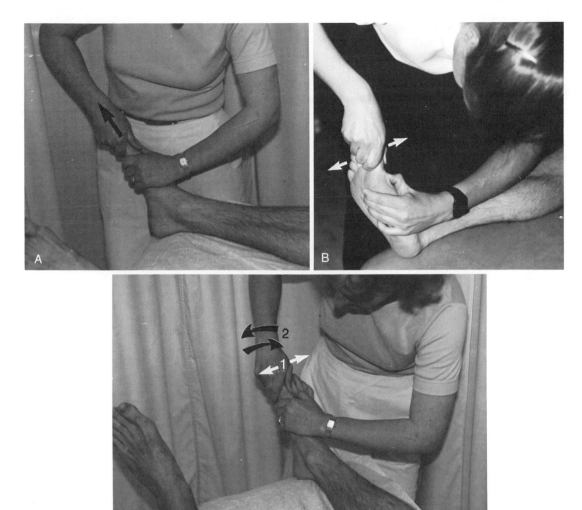

Figure 12–58. Joint play movements at the metatarsophalangeal and interphalangeal joints. (*A*) Long axis extension. (*B*) Anteroposterior glide. (*C*) Side glide (*1*) and/or rotation (*2*).

phalanx) and moving of the distal bone (phalanx) in an anteroposterior gliding motion in relation to the stabilized bone.

Talar Rock

Talar rock is the only joint play movement performed in the side lying position.[21] Both hips and knees are flexed. The examiner sits with the back to the patient as illustrated (Fig. 12–56) and places both hands around the ankle just distal to the malleoli. A slight distractive force is applied to the ankle (Fig. 12–56A, 1), and a rocking movement forward and backward is applied to the foot (Fig. 12–56A, 2). Normally, the examiner should feel a "clunk" at the extreme of each movement. As with all joint play movements, the movement is compared with the unaffected side.

Side Tilt

Side tilt at the *subtalar joint* is performed by placing both hands around the calcaneus (Fig. 12–56B). The wrists are flexed and extended, side tilting the calcaneus medially and laterally on the talus. The examiner keeps the patient's foot in the anatomic position while performing the movement. The movement is identical to that used to test the calcaneofibular ligament in the talar tilt test.

Rotation

Rotation at the *midtarsal joints* is performed in a similar fashion to the anteroposterior glide at these joints. The proximal row of tarsal bones (navicular, calcaneus, and talus) is stabilized and the mobilizing hand is placed around the distal tarsal bones (cuneiforms and cuboid). The distal row of bones is then rotated on the proximal row of bones. Rotation at the *tarsometatarsal joints* is performed in a similar fashion.

Rotation at the *metatarsophalangeal and interphalangeal joints* is performed by stabilizing the proximal bone with one hand and applying slight traction and rotating the distal bone with the other hand.

Side Glide

Side glide at the *metatarsophalangeal* and *interphalangeal joints* is performed by stabilizing the proximal bone with one hand. The other hand applies slight traction to the distal bone and then moves the distal bone sideways to the right and left in relation to the stabilized bone without causing torsion motion at the joint.

Tests for Tarsal Bone Mobility

Kaltenborn advocates "ten tests" to determine the mobility of the tarsal bones.[24] The sequential movement of the tarsal bones is as follows:

1. Fixate the second and third cuneiforms and mobilize the second metatarsal bone.
2. Fixate the second and third cuneiform bones and mobilize the third metatarsal bone.
3. Fixate the first cuneiform bone and mobilize the first metatarsal bone.
4. Fixate the navicular bone and mobilize the first, second, and third cuneiform bones.
5. Fixate the talus and mobilize the navicular bone.
6. Fixate the cuboid bone and mobilize the fourth and fifth metatarsal bones.
7. Fixate the navicular and third cuneiform bones and mobilize the cuboid bone.
8. Fixate the calcaneus and mobilize the cuboid bone.
9. Fixate the talus and mobilize the calcaneus.
10. Fixate the talus and mobilize the tibia and fibula.

PALPATION

The examiner palpates for any swelling, noting whether it is intracapsular or extracapsular. For example, extracapsular swelling around the ankle is indicated by swelling on only one side of the Achilles tendon, whereas intracapsular swelling is indicated by swelling on both sides (Fig. 12–5). Pitting edema may be present and should be noted. If swelling is present at the end of the day and absent after a night of recumbency, venous

insufficiency can possibly be implied owing to a weakening or insufficiency of the action of the muscle pump of the lower leg muscle. Swelling in the ankle may persist for many weeks after the injury as a result of this insufficiency.

One should also notice the texture of the skin and nails. It must be remembered that the skin of an ischemic foot shows a loss of hair and becomes thin and very inelastic. In addition, the nails become coarse, thickened, and irregular. Many of the nail changes seen in the hand in the presence of systemic disease will also be seen in the foot (see Chapter 6). With poor circulation, the foot will also feel colder. The foot is palpated in the non–weight-bearing and long leg sitting or supine position. The following structures, including the joints between them, should be palpated.

Anteriorly and Anteromedially

Toes and Metatarsal, Cuneiform, and Navicular Bones. Starting on the medial side, the examiner can easily palpate the great toe and its two phalanges. Moving proximally, one will come to the first metatarsal bone (Fig. 12–59). The head of the first metatarsal should be palpated carefully. On the lateral aspect, the examiner palpates for any evidence of a bunion (exostosis, callus, and inflamed bursa), which is often associated with hallux valgus. On the plantar aspect, the two sesamoid bones just proximal to the head of the first metatarsal may be palpated. The examiner then palpates the first metatarsal bone along its length to the first cuneiform bone and notes any tenderness, swelling, or signs of pathology. As the examiner moves proximally past the first cuneiform on its medial aspect, a bony prominence will be felt—the tubercle of the navicular bone. The examiner then returns to the first cuneiform bone and moves laterally on the dorsal and plantar surface, palpating the second and third cuneiforms (Fig. 12–60). Like the first cuneiform, the navicular and second and third cuneiform bones should be palpated on their dorsal and plantar aspects for signs of pathology (e.g., fracture, exostosis, or *Köhler's disease*—osteochondritis of the navicular bone).

Moving laterally, one palpates the three phalanges of each of the lateral four toes. Each of the lateral four metatarsals is palpated proximally to check for such conditions as Freiberg's disease (osteochondrosis of the second metatarsal head). Under the heads of the second and third metatarsals on the plantar aspect, one should feel for any evidence of a callus, which may indicate a fallen metatarsal arch. Care must be taken to palpate the base of the fifth metatarsal (styloid process) and adjacent cuboid bone for signs of pathology. Also, the lateral aspect of the head of the fifth metatarsal

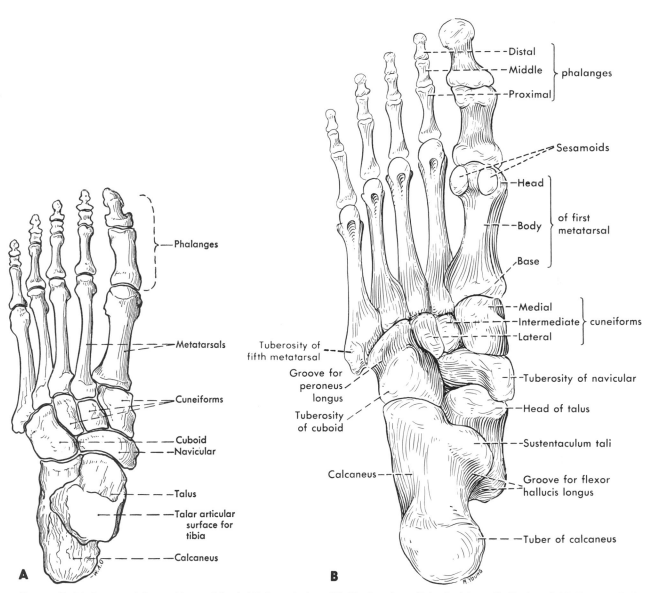

Figure 12–59. Bones of the ankle and foot. (A) Dorsal view. (B) Plantar view. (Adapted from Hollinshead, W. H., and D. B. Jenkins: Functional Anatomy of the Limbs and Back. Philadelphia, W. B. Saunders Co., 1981, pp. 194, 317.)

may demonstrate a bunion similar to that seen on the first toe; this is called a "tailor's bunion."

In addition to palpating the metatarsal bones, the examiner palpates between the bones for evidence of pathology (e.g., Morton's or interdigital neuroma) and also the intrinsic muscles of the foot.

Medial Malleolus, Medial Tarsal Bones, and Posterior Tibial Artery. The examiner then stabilizes the heel by holding the calcaneus stable with one hand, and using the other hand, palpates the distal edges of the medial malleolus for tenderness or swelling. Palpating along the medial malleolus, one will come to its distal extent. Moving from that point along a line joining the navicular tubercle, the examiner moves along the talus until the head of the talus is reached. As

the head of the talus is palpated, the examiner may evert and invert the foot, feeling the movement between the talar head and navicular bone. Eversion causes the head to become more prominent, as does the deformity pes planus. At the same time, the insertion of the tibialis posterior tendon may be palpated as it inserts into the navicular and cuneiform bones. Rupture (third-degree strain) of this tendon leads to a valgus foot. The four ligaments that make up the deltoid ligament (tibionavicular, tibiocalcanean, and anterior and posterior tibiotalar) may also be palpated for signs of pathology.

Returning to the medial malleolus at its distal extent, the examiner moves further distally (about one finger width) until another bony prominence—the sustentaculum tali of the calca-

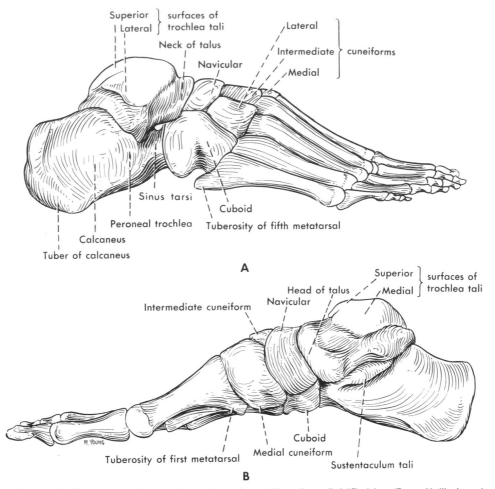

Superior ⎫ surfaces of
Lateral ⎰ trochlea tali

Neck of talus

Navicular

Lateral
Intermediate ⎱ cuneiforms
Medial

Sinus tarsi

Peroneal trochlea

Calcaneus

Tuber of calcaneus

Cuboid

Tuberosity of fifth metatarsal

A

Superior ⎫ surfaces of
Medial ⎰ trochlea tali

Head of talus

Navicular

Intermediate cuneiform

Tuberosity of first metatarsal

Medial cuneiform

Cuboid

Sustentaculum tali

F. YOUNG

B

Figure 12–60. Bones of the foot from the lateral (*A*) and medial (*B*) sides. (From Hollinshead, W. H., and D. B. Jenkins: Functional Anatomy of the Limbs and Back. Philadelphia, W. B. Saunders Co., 1981, p. 319.)

neus—is felt. This bony prominence is often small and difficult to palpate. Moving further posteriorly, one palpates the medial aspect of the calcaneus for signs of pathology (e.g., sprain, fracture, or tarsal tunnel syndrome). As the examiner moves to the plantar aspect of the calcaneus, the heel fat pad, intrinsic foot muscles, and plantar fascia are palpated for signs of pathology (e.g., heel bruise, plantar fasciitis, or bone spur).

The examiner then returns to the medial malleolus and palpates along its posterior surface, noting the movement of the tibialis posterior and long flexor tendons (and checking for tendinitis) during plantar flexion and dorsiflexion and noting any swelling or crepitus. At the same time, the posterior tibial artery, which supplies blood to 75 per cent of the foot, may be palpated as it runs posterior to the medial malleolus. This pulse is often difficult to palpate in individuals with "fat" ankles and in the presence of edema or synovial thickening.

Anterior Tibia, Neck of Talus, and Dorsalis Pedis Artery. The examiner moves to the anterior aspect of the medial malleolus following its course laterally onto the distal end of the tibia. As the examiner moves distally, the fingers will rest on the talus. If the foot is then plantar flexed and dorsiflexed, the anterior aspect of the articular surface of the talus can be palpated for signs of pathology (e.g., osteochondritis dissecans). As the examiner moves further distally, the fingers can follow the course of the neck of the talus to the talar head. Moving distally from the tibia, one should be able to palpate the long extensor tendons, tibialis anterior tendon and, with care, the extensor retinaculum (Fig. 12–61). If the examiner moves further distally over the cuneiforms or between the first and second metatarsal bones, the dorsalis pedis pulse (branch of the anterior tibial artery) may be palpated. It may be found between the tendons of extensor digitorum longus and extensor hallucis longus over the junction of the first and second cuneiform bones. If one suspects an anterior compartment syndrome, this pulse should be palpated and compared with the opposite side. It should be remembered, however, that this pulse is normally absent in 10 per cent of the population.

Anteriorly and Anterolaterally

Lateral Malleolus, Calcaneus, Sinus Tarsi, and Cuboid Bone. The lateral malleolus is palpated at the distal extent of the fibula. One should note that the lateral malleolus extends further distally and lies more posterior than the medial malleolus. The examiner then stabilizes the calcaneus with one hand and palpates with the other hand as previously. As the examiner moves distally from the lateral malleolus, the fingers lie along the lateral edge of the calcaneus, which is palpated with care. At the same time, the peroneal tendons can be palpated as they angle around the lateral malleolus to their insertion on the foot as well as to their origin in the peroneal muscles of the leg. The peroneal retinaculum, which holds the peroneal tendons in place as they angle around the lateral malleolus, is also palpated for tenderness (Fig. 12–61). While palpating the retinaculum, the examiner should ask the patient to invert and evert the foot. If the peroneal retinaculum is torn, the peroneal tendons will often slip out of their groove or dislocate on eversion (Figure 12–40).

While the lateral malleolus is being palpated, the lateral ligaments (calcaneofibular, posterior talofibular, and anterior talofibular) should be palpated for tenderness and swelling (Fig. 12–62).

Returning to the lateral malleolus, the examiner palpates its anterior surface and then moves anteriorly to the extensor digitorum muscle, the only muscle on the dorsum of the foot. If one palpates carefully and deeply through the muscle, a depression—the sinus tarsi—will be felt (Fig. 12–63). If the fingers are left in the depression and the foot inverted, the neck of the talus will be felt and the fingers will be pushed deeper into the depression. Tenderness in this area may also be indicative of a sprain to the anterior talofibular ligament (Fig. 12–63), the most frequently injured ligament in the lower leg, ankle, and foot.

The cuboid bone may be palpated in two ways. The examiner may move further distally from the sinus tarsi about one finger width and the fingers will lie over the cuboid bone or the styloid process at the base of the fifth metatarsal bone may be palpated. As the examiner moves slightly proximally, the fingers will lie over the cuboid bone. In either case, the cuboid should be palpated on its dorsal, lateral, and plantar surfaces for signs of pathology.

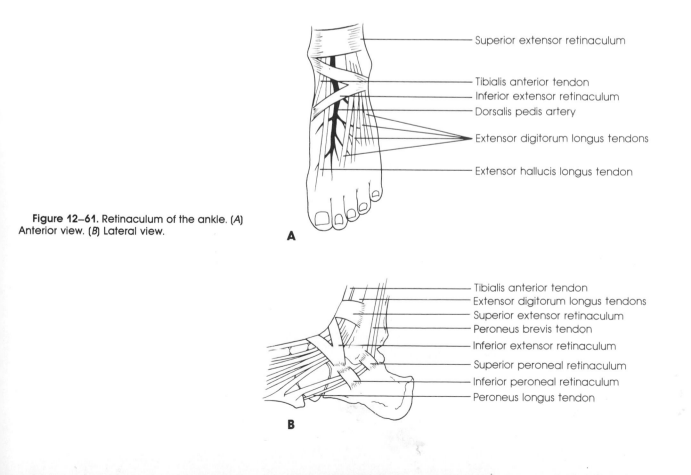

Figure 12–61. Retinaculum of the ankle. (*A*) Anterior view. (*B*) Lateral view.

Superior extensor retinaculum
Tibialis anterior tendon
Inferior extensor retinaculum
Dorsalis pedis artery
Extensor digitorum longus tendons
Extensor hallucis longus tendon

A

Tibialis anterior tendon
Extensor digitorum longus tendons
Superior extensor retinaculum
Peroneus brevis tendon
Inferior extensor retinaculum
Superior peroneal retinaculum
Inferior peroneal retinaculum
Peroneus longus tendon

B

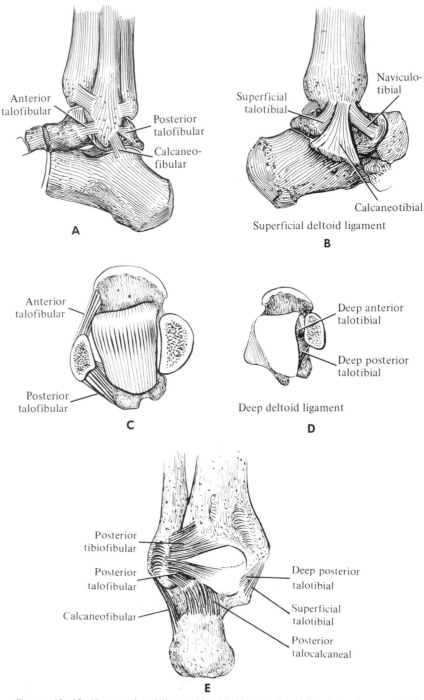

Figure 12–62. Ligaments of the ankle. (*A*) Ligaments of the lateral aspect. (*B*) Superior view of lateral ligaments. (*C*) Ligaments on the medial aspect (superficial deltoid ligaments). (*D*) Superior view of deep deltoid ligament on the medial aspect. (*E*) Posterior view of the ankle. (Adapted from Hamilton, W. C.: Anatomy: Traumatic Disorders of the Ankle. New York, Springer-Verlag, 1984, pp. 6, 7.)

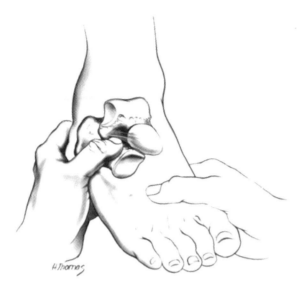

Figure 12–63. Palpation of the sinus tarsi and the anterior talofibular ligament. (From Jahss, M. H.: Disorders of the Foot. Philadelphia, W. B. Saunders Co., 1982, p. 107.)

Inferior Tibiofibular Joint, Tibia, and Muscles of the Leg. Starting at the lateral malleolus and following its anterior border, one should note any signs of pathology. The inferior tibiofibular joint is almost impossible to feel; however, it lies between the tibia and fibula and just superior to the talus. The examiner then follows the "shin" or crest of the tibia superiorly, looking for signs of pathology (e.g., shin splints, anterior tibial syndrome, or stress fracture). At the same time, the muscles of the lateral compartment (peronei) and anterior compartment (tibialis anterior and long extensors) should be carefully palpated for tenderness or swelling.

Posteriorly

The patient is then asked to lie in a prone position with the feet over the end of the examining table. The examiner palpates the following structures.

Calcaneus and Achilles Tendon. The examiner palpates the calcaneus and surrounding soft tissue for swelling (e.g., retrocalcaneal bursitis), exostosis (e.g., pump bump), or other signs of pathology. In children, one should take care palpating the calcaneal epiphysis for evidence of Sever's disease (calcaneal apophysitis) (Fig. 12–64). Moving proximally, one palpates the Achilles tendon, noting any swelling or thicken-

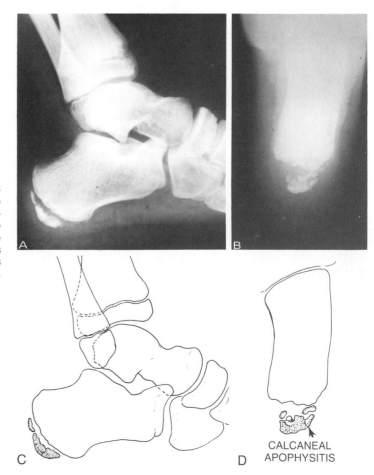

Figure 12–64. Sever's disease (calcaneal apophysitis). Fragmentation of the posterior apophysis off the calcaneus, causing achillodynia. (A) Lateral roentgenogram of a 10-year-old male with pain around the insertion of the Achilles tendon. (B) Axial view of the calcaneus. (C and D) Representations of the films above. (From Kelikian, H., and A. S. Kelikian: Disorders of the Ankle. Philadelphia, W. B. Saunders Co., 1985, p. 121.)

ing (e.g., tendonitis, retro-Achilles bursitis) or crepitation on movement. Any swelling from an intracapsular sprain of the ankle would also be evident posteriorly. Proximal to the Achilles tendon, the dome or superior surface of the calcaneus may also be palpated.

Posterior Compartment Muscles of the Leg. Moving further proximally, the examiner palpates the superficial (triceps surae) and deep (tibialis posterior and long flexors) posterior compartment muscles of the leg along their length for signs of pathology (e.g., strain or thrombosis).

RADIOGRAPHY OF THE LOWER LEG, ANKLE, AND FOOT

When viewing any radiograph, one should look for changes and differences between the right and left lower leg, ankle, and foot, such as osteoporosis or alterations in soft-tissue, joint space, and alignment. Both weight-bearing and non–weight-bearing views should be taken. To be viewed properly, individual radiographs must be made of the ankle, lower leg, and foot (Fig. 12–65).[6, 27–29]

Anteroposterior View of the Ankle. The examiner notes the shape, position (whether the medial clear space is normal), and texture of the bones and determines whether there is any fractured or new subperiosteal bone. In addition, the configuration, congruity, and inclination of the talar dome in relation to the tibial vault above it should be noted. If there are epiphyseal plates present, the examiner should note whether they appear normal. Any increase or decrease in joint space, greater reduction of the tibial overlap, widening of the interosseous space, and greater visibility of the digital fossa should be noted.

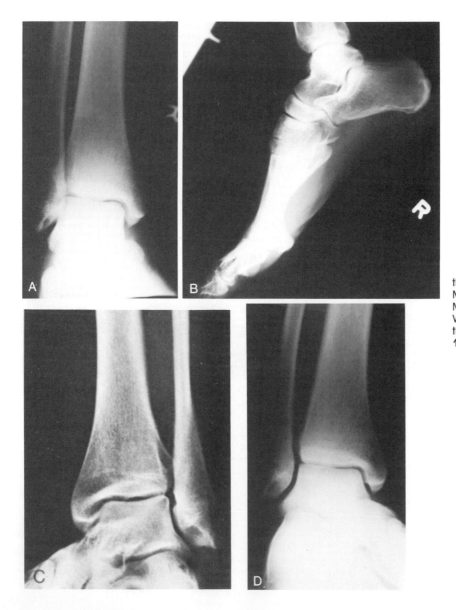

Figure 12–65. Common radiograph of the ankle. (A) Anteroposterior view. (B) Medial view of the foot and ankle. (C) Medial oblique view. (From Hamilton, W. C.: Anatomy: Traumatic Disorders of the Ankle. New York, Springer-Verlag, 1984, p. 31.) (D) Mortise view.

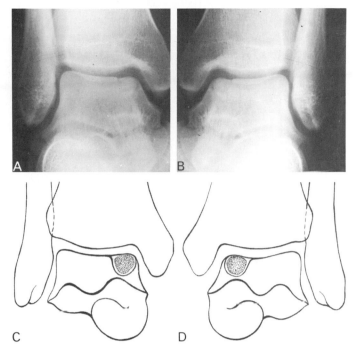

Figure 12–66. Bilateral osteochondritis dissecans of the talus. (*A* and *B*) Oblique anteroposterior films of the right and left ankles of a 29-year-old man without any antecedent trauma. (*C* and *D*) Illustrations of the roentgenograms above each. (From Kelikian, H., and A. S. Kelikian: Disorders of the Ankle. Philadelphia, W. B. Saunders Co., 1985, p. 726.)

One should also look for osteochondritis dissecans of the talus (medial side) (Fig. 12–66).[5]

Mortise View of Ankle. With this view, the ankle mortise and distal tibiofibular joint can be visualized. To obtain this view, which is a modification of the anteroposterior view, the foot and leg are medially rotated 15 to 30°.

Lateral View of Leg, Ankle, and Foot. With this view, the examiner notes the shape, position, and

texture of bones, including the tibial tubercle (Fig. 12–67).[6] Any fracture, new subperiosteal bone, or bone spurs should be noted (Fig. 12–68). One must note whether the epiphyseal lines are normal and whether there is any increase and decrease in joint space. Although this view clearly shows the talus and calcaneus, there is overlap of the midtarsal, metatarsal, and phalangeal structures. When viewing lateral films, the examiner

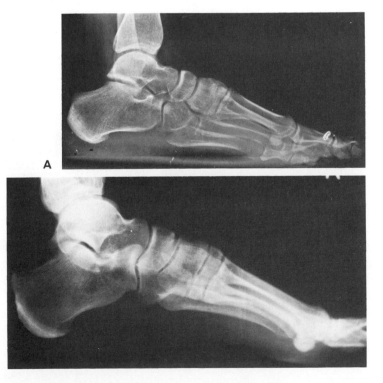

Figure 12–67. Lateral view of the foot. (*A*) Weight-bearing posture. Note the flattened soft-tissue pads beneath the heel and in the forepart of the foot and that the first metatarsal head is elevated by the sesamoids beneath it. (*B*) Non–weight-bearing posture. The bony alignment and configuration are satisfactory, but the lack of resistance from the floor to the body weight permits variations, which make such views unsatisfactory for determining foot contours. (From Jahss, M. H.: Disorders of the Foot. Philadelphia, W. B. Saunders Co., 1982, pp. 122, 126.)

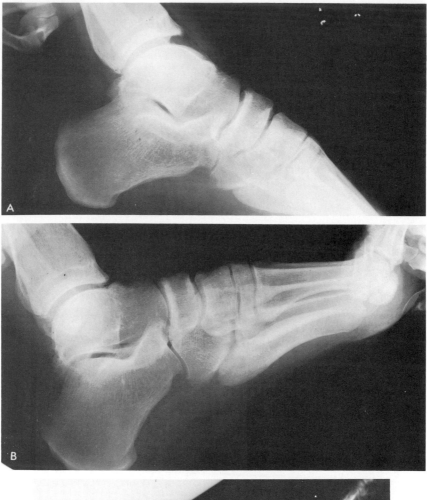

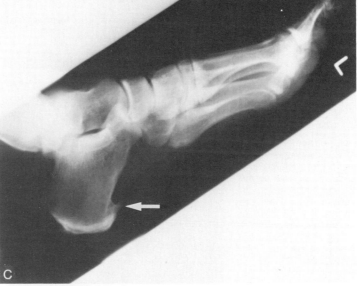

Figure 12–68. (*A*) Talotibial spurs. (*B*) Impingement occurs when the foot is dorsiflexed. (*C*) Heel spur. (*A* and *B* from O'Donoghue, D. H.: Treatment of Injuries to Athletes, 4th ed. Philadelphia, W. B Saunders Co., 1984, p. 627.)

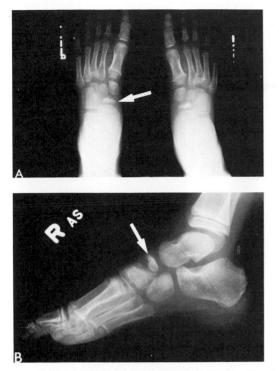

Figure 12–69. Radiographs of the foot. (*A*) Bilateral involvement with condensation in the early stage of Köhler's disease. (*B*) The same foot 2 years later shows restoration of contour on the way to completion. (From Jahss, M. H.: Disorders of the Foot. Philadelphia, W. B. Saunders Co., 1982, p. 202.)

must also be aware of Sever's disease and Köhler's disease (Fig. 12–69).

Dorsoplanar View of the Foot. As with the previous view, the examiner should note the position, shape, and texture of the bones of the foot (Fig. 12–70).[6] The presence of a metatarsus primus varus and conditions such as Köhler's disease should be noted. The dorsoplanar view is used to project primarily the forefoot.

Medial Oblique View of the Foot. This view is often taken because it gives the clearest picture of the tarsal bones and joints and the metatarsal shafts and bases (Fig. 12–71). The medial oblique view shows any pathology in the calcaneocuboid joint as well as the presence of a calcaneonavicular bar (Figs. 12–72 and 12–73).

Stress Oblique View. The examiner should note whether there is a calcaneonavicular bar or abnormality of the calcaneus or navicular bones.

Stress Film. The stress radiograph is used to compare both ankles for the integrity of the ligaments (Fig. 12–74).[17, 18, 25] With the application of an eversion or abduction stress, tilting of the talus more than 10° is considered pathologic. An increase in the medial clear space (space between medial malleolus and talus) of more than 2 to 3 mm is considered pathologic and usually indicates insufficiency of the deltoid ligament, especially the tibiotalar ligament. Instability may also

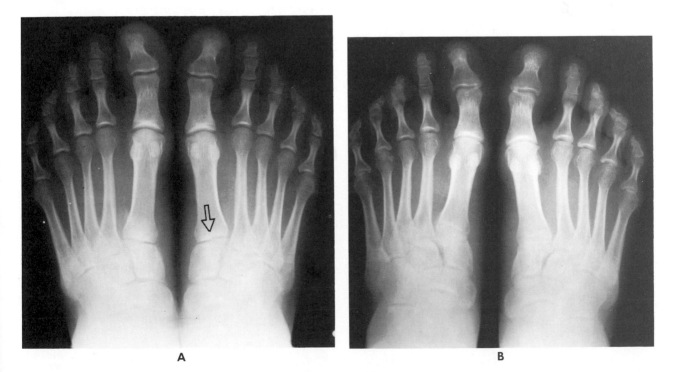

A   B

Figure 12–70. Dorsoplanar view of the foot. (*A*) Weight-bearing posture. The cuneiform–first metatarsal joint is clearly seen (arrow), as are the transverse intertarsal joints, in contrast to the non–weight-bearing roentgenograms. (*B*) Non–weight-bearing posture. The joint between the medial and middle cuneiforms is clearly seen. The other midtarsal joints are obscure. (From Jahss, M. H.: Disorders of the Foot. Philadelphia, W. B. Saunders Co., 1982.)

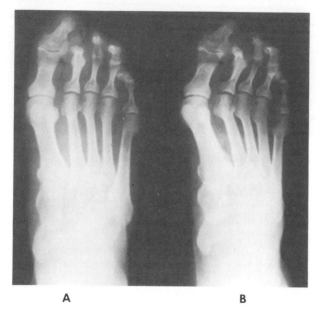

A   B

Figure 12–71. Metatarsals and phalanges. (*A*) With the beam centered directly over the foot, the metatarsal bases and adjacent tarsal bones are shown much more clearly than in *B*. (*B*) This is half of the examination of both feet with the tube centered between the feet. Marked overlap of metatarsal bases and adjacent tarsal bones is seen. The midtarsal joint can be seen as a continuous line or cyma. (From Klenerman, L.: The Foot and its Disorders. Boston, Blackwell Scientific Publications, 1982, p. 306.)

be demonstrated by widening of the syndesmosis or the mortise. An inversion or adduction stress causing 8 to 10° more movement on one side than the other is considered pathologic and is indicative of torn lateral ligaments. If the talus has not moved, or if it is fixed, but its distal end is unduly prominent, subtalar instability is suggested.

Arthrograms. Arthrograms of the ankle are indicated when there is chronic ligament laxity or indications of loose body, or osteochondritis dissecans (Fig. 12–75).[5] Leakage of the contrast medium will indicate tearing of the joint capsule or

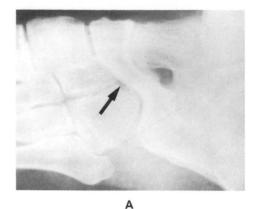

A

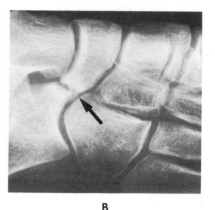

B

Figure 12–73. Calcaneonavicular coalition or bar. (*A*) Total bony union, as well as bony breaks on the upper surfaces of the navicular and talus, is demonstrated. The head of the talus may well be small. (*B*) Fibrous or cartilaginous, rather than osseous, union between the bones is seen with osteoarthritic changes of the opposing bone surfaces and an enlarged navicular. (From Klenerman, L.: The Foot and Its Disorders. Boston, Blackwell Scientific Publications, 1982, p. 340.)

capsular ligaments. Normally, the talocrural joint will admit only about 6 ml of contrast medium.

Abnormal Ossicles or Accessory Bones. Because the foot often exhibits abnormal ossicles,

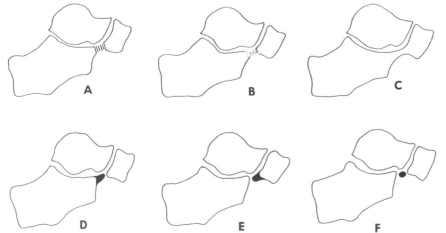

Figure 12–72. Diagrammatic representation of the types of union. (*A*) Fibrous. (*B*) Cartilaginous. (*C*) Osseous. (*D*) Prominent process of the calcaneus. (*E*) Prominent process on the navicular. (*F*) Separate calcaneonavicular ossicle (calcaneum secondarium). (From Klenerman, L.: The Foot and Its Disorder. Boston, Blackwell Scientific Publications, 1982, p. 336.)

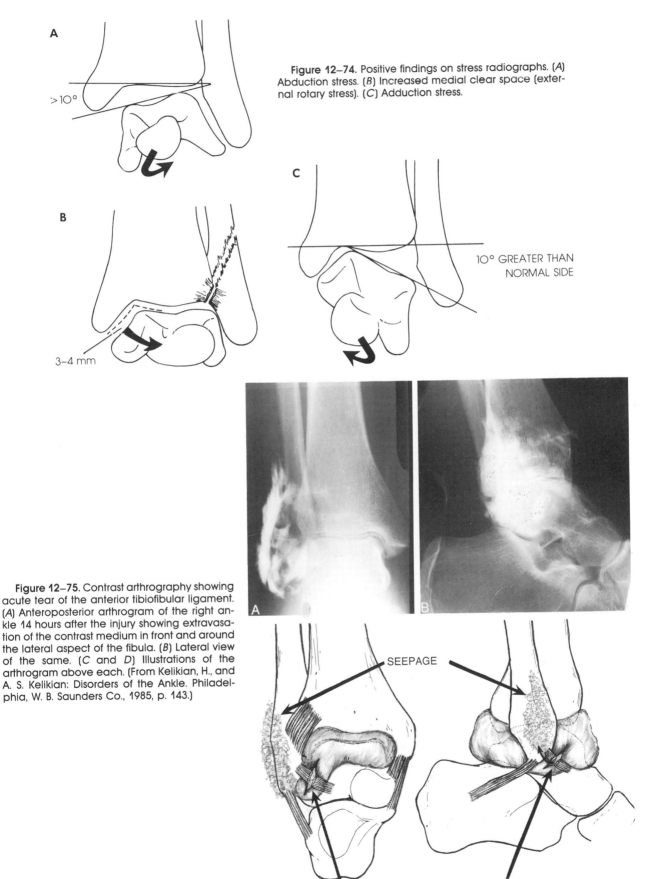

Figure 12–74. Positive findings on stress radiographs. (*A*) Abduction stress. (*B*) Increased medial clear space (external rotary stress). (*C*) Adduction stress.

Figure 12–75. Contrast arthrography showing acute tear of the anterior tibiofibular ligament. (*A*) Anteroposterior arthrogram of the right ankle 14 hours after the injury showing extravasation of the contrast medium in front and around the lateral aspect of the fibula. (*B*) Lateral view of the same. (*C* and *D*) Illustrations of the arthrogram above each. (From Kelikian, H., and A. S. Kelikian: Disorders of the Ankle. Philadelphia, W. B. Saunders Co., 1985, p. 143.)

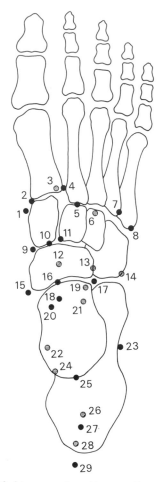

Figure 12–76. Accessory tarsal bones. (From Klenerman, L.: The Foot and Its Disorders. Boston, Blackwell Scientific Publications, 1982, p. 361.)

3. Bipartite medial cuneiform (into upper and lower halves).

4. Os vesalianum (separate tuberosity of the base of the fifth metatarsal).

5. Os sustentaculi (separate part of the sustentaculum tali).

6. Os supranaviculare (dorsum of the talonavicular joint).

Films Showing Bone Development. Like the hand, the bones of the foot form within a certain time period (Fig. 12–77). However, since the foot is subjected to greater forces and environmental effects, it is usually not used to determine skeletal age. X-rays of the foot will often show the developing bone deformities seen in club feet (Fig. 12–78). Although not all of the bones are present at birth, a series of films will show differences when compared with films of normal feet.

this may lead to incorrect interpretation of films (Fig. 12–76). These bones are parts of prominences of various tarsal bones that for some reason (e.g., fracture or a secondary ossification center) are separate from the normal bone.[26] A sesamoid bone, on the other hand, is incorporated into the substance of a tendon, with one surface articulating with the adjacent bones. A sesamoid bone moves with the tendon and is found over bony prominences or where the tendon makes a change in direction. In addition to the normal sesamoid bones under the big toe, sesamoid bones may also be found in the tendons of peroneus longus and tibialis posterior. Abnormal ossicles are more likely to occur in the foot than anywhere else in the body. Some of the more common ossicles include:

1. Os trigonium (separate posterior talar tubercle).

2. Os tibiale externum (separate navicular tuberosity).

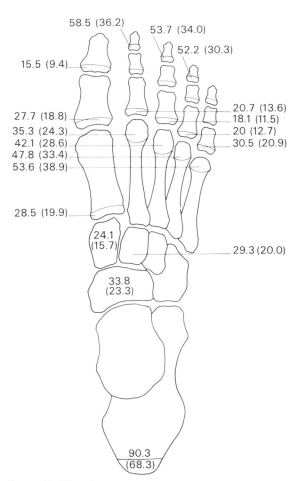

Figure 12–77. Anteroposterior diagram of the foot showing the times of appearance (in months) of the centers of ossification for boys (girls in brackets). (From Hoerr, et al. (1962), with kind permission of Charles C Thomas, Springfield, Ill.)

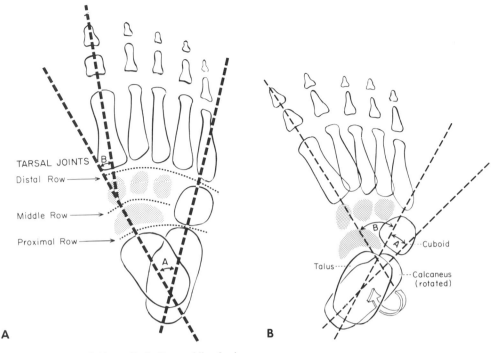

Figure 12–78. X-ray illustrations of the foot.

(*A*) Representation of the normal foot. The cuboid blocks medial movement of the foot at the midrow of tarsal joints because of its unique location. It alone occupies a position in both rows of tarsal joints. The talocalcaneal angle (angle A) is measured by drawing lines through the long axis of both these bones. One should attempt to be as accurate as possible in making these measurements. The normal range for this measurement is 20 to 40° in the young child. The talo–first metatarsal angle (angle B) is measured by drawing lines through the long axis of the talus and along the long axis of the first metatarsal. The normal range is 0 to −20°.

(*B*) Hindfoot varus, as manifest by a decreased talocalcaneal angle (angle A), and talonavicular subluxation, as manifest by a talocalcaneal angle of less than 15° and a talo–first metatarsal angle (angle B) of more than 15°. Talonavicular subluxation occurs through the medial movement of three bones, which move as a unit. The navicular, cuboid, and calcaneus move medially through the combined movements of medial translation and supination of the proximal tarsal bones, while the calcaneus inverts beneath the talus.

(From Simons, G. W.: Orthop. Clin. North Am. *9*:189, 1978.)

Précis of the Lower Leg, Ankle, and Foot Assessment

History
Observation
Examination
    Active movements (Weight bearing—standing)
        Plantar flexion
        Dorsiflexion
        Supination
        Pronation
        Toe extension
        Toe flexion

    Active movements (Non–weight bearing—sitting or supine lying)
        Plantar flexion
        Dorsiflexion
        Supination
        Pronation
        Toe extension
        Toe flexion
        Toe abduction
        Toe adduction
    Functional tests
    Passive movements (supine lying)
        Plantar flexion at the talocrural (ankle) joint
        Dorsiflexion at the talocrural joint
        Inversion at the subtalar joint

Eversion at the subtalar joint
Adduction at the midtarsal joints
Abduction at the midtarsal joints
Flexion of the toes
Extension of the toes
Adduction of the toes
Abduction of the toes
Resisted isometric movements (supine lying)
Knee flexion
Plantar flexion
Dorsiflexion
Supination
Pronation
Toe extension
Toe flexion
Special tests (supine lying)
Reflexes and cutaneous distribution (supine lying)
Joint play movements (supine and side lying)
Long axis extension
Anteroposterior glide
Talar rock
Side tilt
Rotation
Side glide
Tarsal bone mobility
Palpation (supine lying and prone lying)
X-ray viewing

Following any examination, the patient should always be warned of the possibility of exacerbation of symptoms as a result of assessment.

REFERENCES

CITED REFERENCES

1. Kleiger, B.: Mechanisms of ankle injury. Orthop. Clin. North Am. 5:127, 1974.
2. Kapandji, I. A.: The Physiology of the Joints, vol. 2. Lower Limb. New York, Churchill Livingstone, 1970.
3. Lipscomb, A. B., and A. A. Ibrahim: Acute peroneal compartment syndrome in the well conditioned athlete. Am. J. Sports Med. 5:154, 1977.
4. Williams, P. L., and R. Warwick (eds): Gray's Anatomy, 36th British ed. Philadelphia, W. B. Saunders Co., 1980.
5. Kelikian, H., and A. S. Kelikian: Disorders of the Ankle. Philadelphia, W. B. Saunders Co., 1985.
6. Jahss, M. H.: Disorders of the Foot. Philadelphia, W. B. Saunders Co., 1982.
7. Hamilton, J. J., and L. K. Ziemer: Functional Anatomy of the Human Ankle and Foot. American Association of Orthopedic Surgeons, Symposium on the Foot and Ankle. St. Louis, C. V. Mosby Co., 1983.
8. McMaster, M. J.: The pathogenesis of hallux rigidus. J. Bone Joint Surg. 60B:82, 1978.
9. Durman, D. C.: Metatarsus primus varus and hallux valgus. Arch. Surg. 74:128, 1957.
10. Price, G. F. W.: Metatarsus primus varus—including various clinicoradiologic features of the female foot. Clin. Orthop. Relat. Res. 145:217, 1979.
11. Ha' Eri, G. B., V. L. Fornasier, and J. Schatzker: Morton's neuroma: Pathogenesis and ultrastructure. Clin. Orthop. Relat. Res. 141:256, 1979.
12. Morton, D. J.: The Human Foot: Its Evolution, Physiology and Functional Disorders. Cambridge: Cambridge University Press, 1935.
13. Sweetnam, R.: Pes cavus. Physiotherapy 49:204, 1963.
14. Mubarak, S., and A. Hargens: Exertional compartment syndromes. American Association of Orthopedic Surgeons, Symposium on the Foot and Leg in Running Sports. St. Louis, C. V. Mosby Co., 1982.
15. Reneman, R. S.: The anterior and the lateral compartmental syndrome of the leg due to the intensive use of muscles. Clin. Orthop. Relat. Res. 113:69, 1975.
16. Hyslop, G. H.: Injuries of the deep and superficial peroneal nerves complicating ankle sprain. Am. J. Surg. 51:436, 1941.
17. Kaplan, P. E., and W. T. Kernahan: Tarsal tunnel syndrome: An electrodiagnostic and surgical correlation. J. Bone Joint Surg. 63A:96, 1981.
18. Colter, J. M.: Lateral ligamentous injuries of the ankle. In Hamilton, W. C. (ed.): Traumatic Disorders of the Ankle. New York, Springer-Verlag, 1984.
19. Hamilton, W. C.: Anatomy. In Hamilton, W.C. (ed.): Traumatic Disorders of the Ankle. New York, Springer-Verlag, 1984.
20. Rasmussen, O., and I. Tovberg-Jansen: Anterolateral rotational instability in the ankle joint. Acta Orthop. Scand. 52:99, 1981.
21. Mennell, J. M.: Foot Pain. Boston, Little, Brown and Co., 1969.
22. Thompson, T., and J. Doherty: Spontaneous rupture of the tendon of Achilles: A new clinical diagnostic test. Anat. Res. 158:126, 1967.
23. Gutrecht, J. A., R. E. Espinosa, and P. J. Dyck: Early descriptions of common neurological signs. Mayo Clin. Proc. 43:807, 1968.
24. Kaltenborn, F. M.: Mobilization of the Extremity Joints. Oslo, Olaf Norlis Bokhandel, 1980.
25. Rubin, G., and M. Witten: The talar-tilt angle and the fibular collateral ligaments: A method for the determination of talar-tilt. J. Bone Joint Surg. 42:311, 1960.
26. Klenerman, L.: Examination of the foot. In Klenerman, L. (ed.): The Foot and Its Disorders, 2nd ed. Boston, Blackwell Scientific Publications, 1982.
27. Black, H.: Roentgenographic considerations. Am. J. Sports Med. 5:238, 1977.
28. Hoffman, J. D.: Radiography of the ankle. In Hamilton, W. C. (ed.): Traumatic Disorders of the Ankle. New York, Springer-Verlag, 1984.
29. Renton, P., and W. J. Stripp: The radiology and radiography of the foot. In Klenerman, L. (ed.): The Foot and Its Disorders, 2nd ed. Boston, Blackwell Scientific Publications, 1982.

GENERAL REFERENCES

American Orthopaedic Association: Manual of Orthopaedic Surgery. Chicago, 1972.
Anderson, K. J., J. F. Lecocq, and E. A. Lecocq: Recurrent anterior subluxation of the ankle joint. J. Bone Joint Surg. 34A:853, 1952.
Basmajian, J. V., and G. Stecko: The role of muscles in arch support of the foot. J. Bone Joint Surg. 45A:1184, 1964.
Beetham, W. P., H. F. Polley, C. H. Slocumb, and W. F. Weaver: Physical Examination of the Joints. Philadelphia, W. B. Saunders, 1965.
Berridge, F. R., and J. G. Bonnin: The radiographic examination of the ankle joint including arthrography. J. Surg. Gynecol. Obstet. 79:383, 1944.
Bojsen-Moller, F.: Anatomy of the forefoot: Normal and pathologic. Clin. Orthoped. Relat. Res. 1422:10, 1979.
Cailliet, R.: Foot and Ankle Pain. Philadelphia, F. A. Davis Co., 1968.
Campbell, J. W., and V. T. Inman: Treatment of plantar fasciitis and calcaneal spurs with the UC-BL shoe insert. Clin. Orthop. Relat. Res. 103:57, 1974.
Carroll, N. C., R. McMurtry, and S. F. Leete: The pathoanatomy of congenital club-foot. Orthop. Clin. North Am. 9:225, 1978.

Close, J. R.: Some applications of the functional anatomy of the ankle joint. J. Bone Joint Surg. 38A:761, 1956.

Close, J. R., V. T. Inman, P. M. Poor, and F. N. Todd: The function of the subtalar joint. Clin. Orthop. Relat. Res. 50:159, 1967.

Cooper, D. L., and J. Fair: Managing the pronated foot. Physician Sportsmed. 5:131, 1979.

Cox, J. S., and R. L. Brand: Evaluation and treatment of lateral ankle sprains. Physician Sportsmed. 5:51, 1977.

Cyriax, J.: Textbook of Orthopaedic Medicine, vol. 1, 8th ed. Diagnosis of Soft Tissue Lesions. London, Bailliere Tindall, 1982.

Debrunner, H. U.: Orthopaedic Diagnosis. London, E & S Livingstone, 1970.

Ebbetts, J.: Manipulation of the foot. Physiotherapy 57:194, 1971.

Edgar, M. A.: Hallux valgus and associated conditions. In Klenerman, L. (ed.): The Foot and Its Disorders, 2nd ed. Boston, Blackwell Scientific Publications, 1982.

Fixsen, J. A.: The foot in childhood. In Klenerman, L. (ed.): The Foot and Its Disorders, 2nd ed. Boston, Blackwell Scientific Publications, 1982.

Gartland, J. J.: Fundamentals of Orthopedics. Philadelphia, W.B. Saunders Co., 1979.

Garrick, J. G.: The injured ankle: A sports medicine nemesis. Sports Med. Bull. 10:8, 1975.

Holfct, A. J., and D. M. Gruebel-Lee: Disorders of the Foot. Philadelphia, J. B. Lippincott Co., 1979.

Hlavac, H. F.: The Foot Book: Advice to Athletes. Mountain View, Calif., World Publications, 1977.

Holden, C. E. A.: Compartment syndromes following trauma. Clinical Orthop. Relat. Res. 113:8, 1975.

Hollinshead, W. H., and D. B. Jenkins: Functional Anatomy of the Limbs and Back. Philadelphia, W. B. Saunders Co., 1981.

Hoppenfeld, S.: Physical Examination of the Spine and Extremities. New York, Appleton-Century-Crofts, 1976.

Hutton, W. C., J. R. R. Stott, and I. A. F. Stokes: The mechanics of the foot. In Klenerman, L. (ed.): The Foot and Its Disorders, 2nd ed. Boston, Blackwell Scientific Publications, 1982.

Inman, V. T.: The Joints of the Ankle. Baltimore, Williams and Wilkins Co., 1976.

Judge, R. D., G. D. Zuidema, and F. T. Fitzgerald: Clinical Diagnosis: A Physiological Approach. Boston, Little, Brown and Co., 1982.

Kaumeyer, G., and T. Malone: Ankle injuries: Anatomical and biomechanical considerations necessary for the development of an injury prevention program. J. Orthop. Sports Phys. Ther. 1:171, 1980.

Kiruchi, S., M. Hasue, and M. Watanabe: Ischemic contracture in the lower limb. Clin. Orthop. Relat. Res. 134:185, 1978.

Kleiger, B.: The mechanism of ankle injuries. J. Bone Joint Surg. 38A:59, 1956.

Klenerman, L.: Functional anatomy. In Klenerman, L. (ed.): The Foot and Its Disorders, 2nd ed. Boston, Blackwell Scientific Publications, 1982.

Landeros, O., H. M. Frost, and C. C. Higgins: Post-traumatic anterior ankle instability. Clin. Orthop. Relat. Res. 56:169, 1968.

Leach, R. E.: Achilles tendinitis. Am. J. Sports Med. 9:93, 1981.

MacConaill, M. A., and J. V. Basmajian: Muscles and Movements: A Basis for Human Kinesiology. Baltimore, Williams and Wilkins Co., 1969.

Maitland, G. D.: The Peripheral Joints: Examination and Recording Guide. Adelaide, Australia, Virgo Press, 1973.

Mann, R. A.: Surgical implications of biomechanics of the foot and ankle. Clin. Orthop. Relat. Res. 146:111, 1980.

Matsen, F. A.: Compartment syndrome: A unified concept. Clin. Orthop. Relat. Res. 113:8, 1975.

McRae, R.: Clinical Orthopaedic Examination. New York, Churchill Livingstone, 1976.

Morris, J. M.: Biomechanics of the foot and ankle. Clin. Orthop. Relat. Res. 122:10, 1977.

Mubarak, S. J., and A. R. Hargens: Compartment Syndrome and Volkmann's Contracture. Philadelphia, W. B. Saunders Co., 1981.

Norfray, J. F., L. Schlachter, W. T. Kernaham, et al.: Early confirmation of stress fractures in joggers. J.A.M.A. 243:1647, 1980.

O'Donoghue, D. H.: Treatment of Injuries to Athletes, 4th ed. Philadelphia, W. B. Saunders Co., 1984.

Root, M. L., W. P. Orien, and H. J. Weed: Normal and Abnormal Function of the Foot. Los Angeles, Clinical Biomechanics Corporation, 1977.

Rorabeck, C. H., and I. Macnab: The pathophysiology of the anterior tibial compartment syndrome. Clin. Orthop. Relat. Res. 113:52, 1975.

Samuelson, K. M.: Functional anatomy. Traumatic Disorders of the Ankle. New York, Springer-Verlag, 1984.

Scheller, A. D., J. R. Kasser, and T. B. Quigley: Tendon injuries about the ankle. Orthop. Clin. North Am. 11:801, 1980.

Seligson, D., J. Gassman, and M. Pope: Ankle Instability: Evaluation of the lateral ligaments. Am. J. Sports Med. 8:39, 1980.

Sheehan, G.: Medical Advice for Runners. Mountain View, Calif., World Publications, 1978.

Sidey, J. D.: Weak ankles: A study of common peroneal entrapment neuropathy. Br. Med. J. 3:623, 1969.

Simons, G. W.: Analytical radiography and the progressive approach in talipes equinovarus. Orthop. Clin. North Am. 9:187, 1978.

Spring, J. M., and G. W. Hyatt: Treatment of sprained ankles. General Practitioner 36:78, 1967.

Subotnick, S. I.: Podiatric Sports Medicine. Mount Kisco, N. Y., Futura Publishing Co., 1975.

Subotnick, S. I.: The Running Foot Doctor. Mountain View, Calif., World Publications, 1977.

Walter, N. E., and M. D. Wolf: Stress fractures in young athletes. Am. J. Sports Med. 5:165, 1977.

Yvars, M. F.: Osteochondral fractures of the dome of the talus. Clin. Orthop. Relat. Res. 114:185, 1976.

13

Gait Assessment

Walking is the simple act of falling forward and catching oneself. With walking, one foot is always in contact with the ground, and within a cycle there are two periods of single-limb support and two periods of double-limb support. When one runs, there is a period of time during which one foot is not always in contact with the ground and there is a period called "double float."

The locomotion pattern tends to be variable and irregular until about the age of 7 years. There are several functional tasks involved in gait, including forward progression, which is executed in a stepping movement in a wide range of rapid and comfortable walking speeds. Second, one must alternately balance the body on one limb, then the other; this is accompanied by repeated adjustments of limb length. Finally, there is support of the upright body.

This chapter gives a basic overview of normal gait, but does not go into a detailed description. This task is left to other authors.[1-4] The various terms commonly used to describe gait, the normal pattern of gait, the assessment of gait, and common abnormal gaits are reviewed.

Definitions[1-4]

Gait Cycle

The gait cycle is the time interval or sequence of motions occurring between two consecutive initial contacts for the same foot (Fig. 13–1). For

example, if heel strike is the initial contact, the gait cycle for the right leg is from one heel strike to the next heel strike on the same foot. The gait cycle consists of two phases for each foot: *stance phase* and *swing phase*. As well, there are two periods of *double support* and one period of *single-leg stance* during the gait cycle.

Stance Phase

The stance phase of gait occurs when the foot is on the ground and bearing weight (Fig. 13–2). It allows the lower leg to support the weight of the body and allows for the advancement of the body over the supporting limb. Normally, this makes up 60 per cent of the gait cycle and consists of five subphases, or *instants*:

1. Initial contact (heel strike).
2. Load response (foot flat).
3. Midstance (single-leg stance).
4. Terminal stance (heel-off).
5. Preswing (toe-off).

The initial contact instant is the *weight-loading* or *weight acceptance period* of the stance leg, which accounts for the first 10 per cent of the gait cycle. During this period, one foot is coming off the floor while the other foot is accepting body weight and absorbing the shock of initial contact so that both feet are in contact with the floor; it is thus a period of *double support* or *double stance*.

The load response and midstance instants make up the *single-leg stance* or *single-leg support*

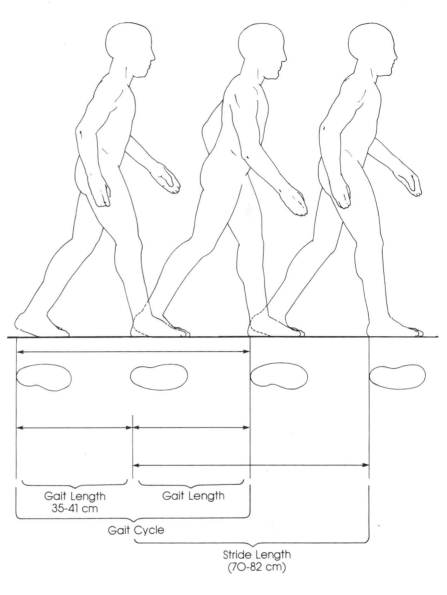

Figure 13–1. Gait cycle, stride length, and gait length.

Gait Length
35-41 cm

Gait Length

Gait Cycle

Stride Length
(70-82 cm)

period, which accounts for the next 40 per cent of the gait cycle. During this period, one leg alone carries the body weight while the other leg goes through its swing phase. The stance leg must be able to hold the weight of the body and the body must be able to balance on the one stance leg. As well, lateral hip stability must be exhibited to maintain the balance and the tibia of the stance leg must advance over the stationary foot.

The terminal stance and pre-swing instants make up the *weight-unloading period*, which accounts for the next 10 per cent of the gait cycle. During this period, the stance leg is unloading the body weight to the contralateral limb and prepares the leg for the swing phases. As with the first two instants, both feet are in contact so that double support occurs for the second time during the gait cycle.

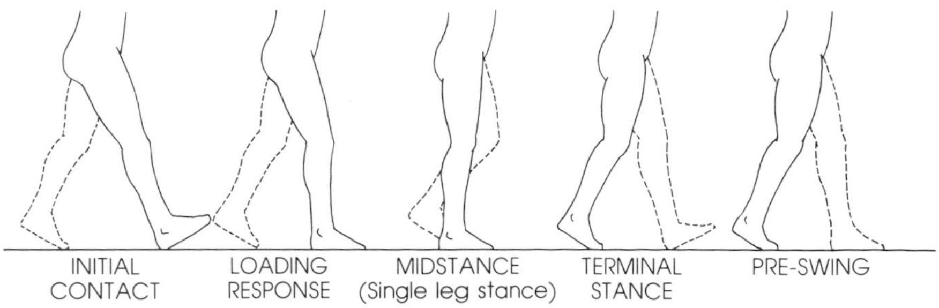

Figure 13–2. Stance phase of gait.

INITIAL CONTACT   LOADING RESPONSE   MIDSTANCE (Single leg stance)   TERMINAL STANCE   PRE-SWING

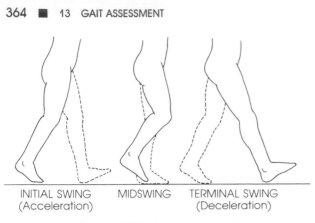

INITIAL SWING   MIDSWING   TERMINAL SWING
(Acceleration)   (Deceleration)

Figure 13–3. Swing phase of gait.

Swing Phase

The swing phase of gait occurs when the foot is non–weight bearing and moving forward (Fig. 13–3). The swing phase allows the toes to clear the floor on the swing leg and allows for leg length adjustments. In addition, it allows for the swing leg to advance forward. It makes up approximately 40 per cent of the gait cycle. It consists of three subphases:

1. Initial swing (acceleration).
2. Midswing.
3. Terminal swing (deceleration).

Acceleration occurs when the foot is lifted off the floor. During normal gait, rapid knee flexion and ankle dorsiflexion occur to allow the swing limb to accelerate forward. In some pathologic conditions, loss or alteration of the knee flexion and ankle dorsiflexion can lead to problems.

The midswing instant occurs when the swing leg is adjacent to the weight-bearing leg, which is in midstance.

During the final instant (terminal swing, or deceleration), the swinging leg slows down in preparation for initial contact with the floor. With normal gait, active quadriceps and hamstring muscle action is required. The quadriceps muscles control knee extension, and the hamstrings control hip flexion.

Double Stance

Double stance is that phase of gait in which parts of both feet are on the ground. In normal gait, it occurs twice during the gait cycle and represents about 25 per cent of the cycle. This percentage increases the more slowly one walks, and it disappears in running or becomes shorter as walking speed increases (Fig. 13–4).

Single-Leg Stance

The single-leg stance phase of gait occurs when only one leg is on the ground; this occurs twice during the normal gait cycle. It takes up approximately 30 per cent of the cycle.

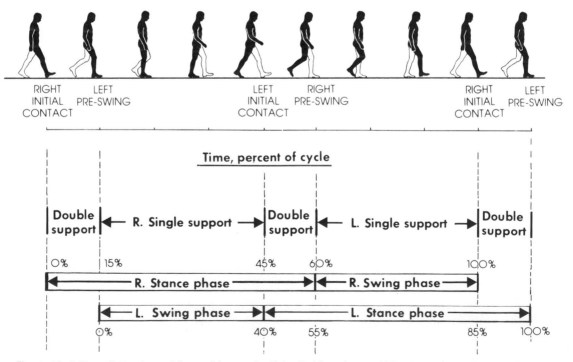

Figure 13–4. Time dimensions of the walking cycle. (Adapted from Inman, V. T., et al.: Human Walking. Baltimore, The Williams and Wilkins Co., 1981, p. 26.)

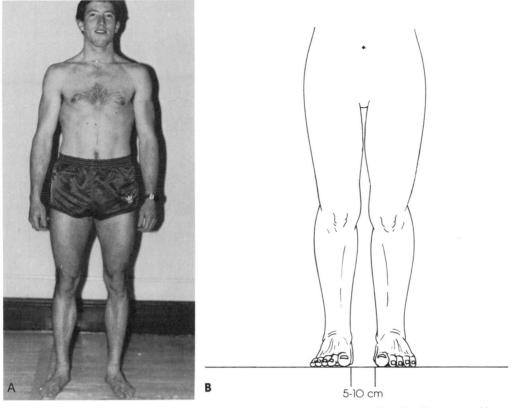

Figure 13–5. Normal base width. Photograph shows individual standing with wider than normal base width.

Normal Parameters of Gait[2–5]

Base Width

The normal base width, which is the distance between the two feet, is 5 to 10 cm (Fig. 13–5). If the base is wider than this amount, one may suspect some pathology, such as cerebellar or inner ear problems, which results in the balance being poor, or diabetes or peripheral neuropathy, which may indicate a loss of sensation. In either case, the patient tends to have a wider base in order to maintain balance.

Gait (Step) Length

Gait length is the distance between successive contact points on opposite feet. Normally, this distance is 35 to 41 cm and should be equal for both legs. It varies with age and sex, children taking smaller steps than adults and females taking smaller steps than males. Height also has an effect, a taller person taking larger steps. Step length tends to decrease with age, fatigue, pain, and disease. If gait length is normal for both legs, the rhythm of walking will be smooth. If there is pain in one limb, the patient will attempt to "get

off" the limb as quickly as possible, altering the rhythm.

Stride Length

Stride length is the linear distance in the plane of progression between successive points of foot-to-floor contact of the same foot. The stride length is normally about 70 to 82 cm in length and in reality is one gait cycle.

Lateral Pelvic Shift (Pelvic List)

Lateral pelvic shift is the side-to-side movement of the pelvis during walking and is necessary to center the weight of the body over the stance leg for balance (Fig. 13–6). The lateral pelvic shift is normally 2.5 to 5 cm. It increases if the feet are farther apart.

Vertical Pelvic Shift (Pelvic Tilt)

Vertical pelvic shift keeps the center of gravity from moving up and down more than 5 cm during normal gait. By means of a vertical pelvic tilt, the high point occurs during midstance and the low

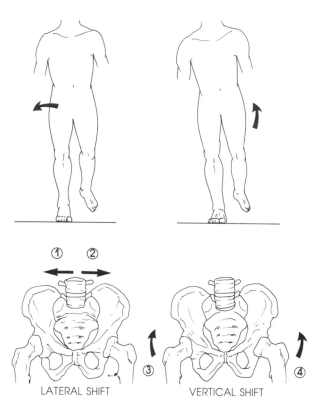

Figure 13–6. Pelvic shift. Numbers indicate that one lateral or vertical shift occurs and then the other; they do not occur at the same time. (*1*) Right lateral shift. (*2*) Left lateral shift. (*3*) Right vertical shift. (*4*) Left vertical shift.

point occurs during initial contact, although the height of these points may increase during the swing phase if the knee is fused. On the swing phase, the hip is lower on the swing side and the patient must flex the knee and dorsiflex the foot to clear the toe. This action shortens the extremity length at midstance and decreases the center of gravity rise.

Pelvic Rotation

Pelvic rotation is necessary to lessen the angle of the femur with the floor, and in so doing it lengthens the femur (Fig. 13–7). It decreases the center of gravity path amplitude of displacement and thus decreases the center of gravity dip. There is a total of 8° pelvic rotation, with 4° forward on the swing leg and 4° posteriorly on the stance leg. For balance to be maintained, the thorax rotates in the opposite direction of the pelvis. Thus, when the pelvis rotates clockwise, the thorax rotates counterclockwise and vice versa. These concurrent rotations provide counterrotation forces and help regulate the individual's speed of walking.

Center of Gravity

Normally, in the standing position, the center of gravity is 5 cm anterior to the second sacral vertebra; it tends to be slightly higher in males than in females because males tend to have greater body mass in the shoulder area. The vertical and horizontal displacement of the center of gravity describes a "figure-8" occupying a 5-cm square within the pelvis during walking. The vertical displacement can be observed from the side. The patient's head will descend during weight-loading and weight-unloading periods and will rise during single-leg stance.

Normal Cadence

The normal cadence is between 90 and 120 steps per minute. Figure 13–8 illustrates the cadence of normal gait from heel strike to toe-off. With pathology or deformity (e.g., a cavus foot), this pattern may be altered.

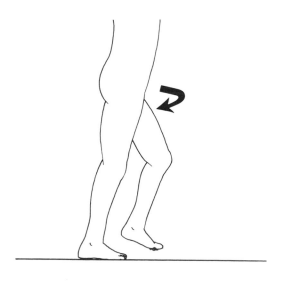

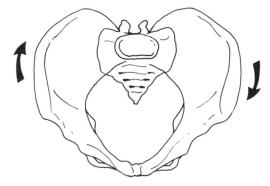

Figure 13–7. Pelvic rotation. Left forward pelvic rotation is illustrated.

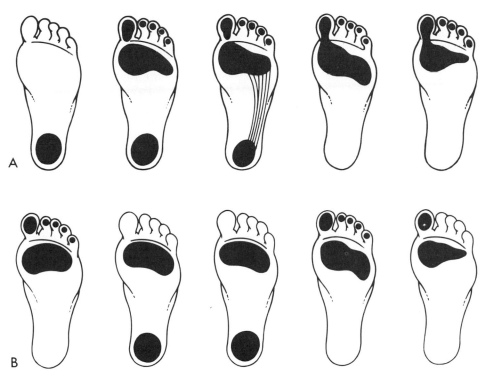

Figure 13–8. The cadence of gait. (A) Normal foot. (B) Cavus foot. (From Viladot, A.: Patología del Antepié. Barcelona, Ediciones Toray, S.A., 1975.)

Normal Pattern of Gait[1–4, 6]

Stance Phase

As previously mentioned, there are five instants involved during the stance phase of gait. These are now described in order of occurrence.

Initial Contact

During the initial contact, the hip is flexed 30 to 49° and is medially rotated; the knee is slightly flexed, or extended; the ankle is at 90° with the foot supinated; and the hindfoot is everted. The pelvis is level and medially rotated on the initial contact side while the trunk is aligned between the two lower limbs. At this instant, there is little force going through the limb. If pain occurs in the heel at this time, it may be due to a heel spur, bone bruise, bruising of the heel fat pad, or a bursitis. If the knee is weak, the patient may extend the knee by using the hand or may hit the heel hard on the ground to "whip" the knee into extension. A patient may do this because of weakness of the muscles, e.g., a reflex inhibition, poliomyelitis, or other condition; an internal derangement of the knee; a nerve root lesion (L2,

L3, or L4); or femoral neuropathy. In the past, this instant was referred to as "heel strike"; however, with some pathologic gaits, heel strike may not be the first instant. Instead, the toes, the forefoot, or the whole foot may initially contact the ground. If the dorsiflexor muscles are weak, instead of heel contact, the foot "slaps" or "flops" down. The weakness may be due to a peroneal neuropathy or nerve root lesion (L4).

Load Response

Load response is a critical event in that the person subconsciously decides whether or not the limb will be able to take the weight of the body. The forefoot is pronated to enable it to absorb the shock more effectively, and the plantar aspect is in contact with the floor. The ankle is plantar flexed, and the hindfoot is inverted. The foot is pronated, since this position unlocks the foot and enables it to adapt to different terrains and postures. The flexed and laterally rotated hip begins going into extension while the knee flexes 15 to 25°. The pelvis drops slightly on the swing leg side and medially rotates on the same side. The trunk is aligned with the stance leg. The tibia will begin to move forward over the fixed foot, and the body swings over the foot.

Midstance

The midstance instant is a period of stationary foot support. Normally, the weight of the foot is evenly distributed over the whole foot. The trunk is aligned over the stance leg while the pelvis shows a slight drop to the swing leg side.

During this stage, there is maximum extension of the hip (10 to 15°) with lateral rotation and the greatest force is on the hip. The knee begins to flex, and the ankle is locked at 5 to 8° of dorsi-flexion rolling forward on the forefoot (roll-off). The foot is in contact with the floor with the forefoot pronated and the hindfoot inverted. This instant is another critical event for the ankle. If the pain is elicited during this period, it may be due to arthritis, rigid pes planus, fallen metatarsal or longitudinal arches, plantar fasciitis, or Morton's metatarsalgia, for example. If the gluteus medius (L5 nerve root) is weak, the Trendelenburg sign will be positive.

NORMAL GAIT

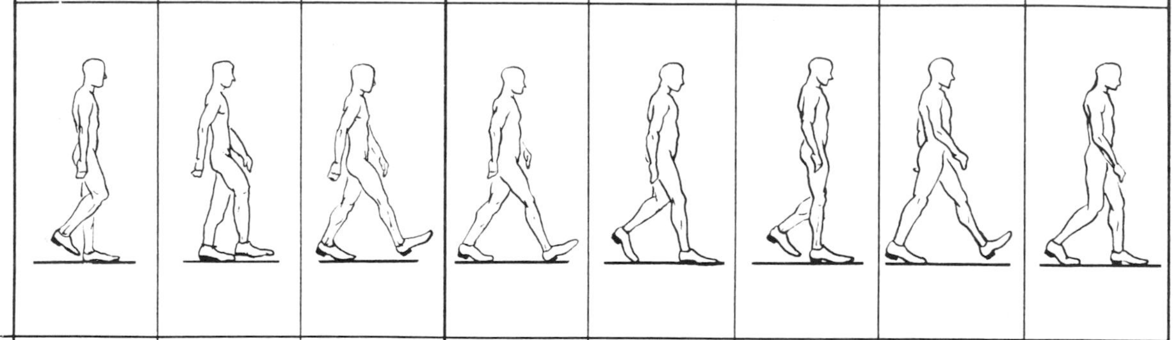

	SWING 40%			STANCE 60%				
	INITIAL SWING	MID-SWING	TERMINAL SWING	INITIAL CONTACT	LOADING RESPONSE	MID-STANCE	TERMINAL STANCE	PRE-SWING
TRUNK	ERECT NEUTRAL	ERECT NEUTRAL	ERECT NEUTRAL	ERECT NEUTRAL	ERECT NEUTRAL	ERECT NEUTRAL	ERECT NEUTRAL	ERECT NEUTRAL
PELVIS	LEVEL; BACKWARD ROTATION 5°	LEVEL; NEUTRAL ROTATION	LEVEL; FORWARD ROTATION 5°	LEVEL; MAINTAINS FORWARD ROTATION	LEVEL; LESS FORWARD ROTATION	LEVEL; NEUTRAL ROTATION	LEVEL; BACKWARD ROTATION 5°	LEVEL; BACKWARD ROTATION 5°
HIP	FLEXION 20° NEUTRAL ROTATION ABDUCTION ADDUCTION	FLEXION 20°→30° NEUTRAL ROTATION ABDUCTION ADDUCTION	FLEXION 30° NEUTRAL ROTATION ABDUCTION ADDUCTION	FLEXION 30° NEUTRAL ROTATION ABDUCTION ADDUCTION	FLEXION 30° NEUTRAL ROTATION ABDUCTION ADDUCTION	EXTENDING TO NEUTRAL NEUTRAL ROTATION ABDUCTION ADDUCTION	APPARENT HYPEREXT 10° NEUTRAL ROTATION ABDUCTION ADDUCTION	NEUTRAL EXTENSION NEUTRAL ROTATION ABDUCTION ADDUCTION
KNEE	FLEXION 60°	FROM 60° TO 30° FLEXION	EXTENSION TO 0°	FULL EXTENSION	FLEXION 15°	EXTENDING TO NEUTRAL	FULL EXTENSION	FLEXION 35°
ANKLE	PLANTAR FLEXION 10°	NEUTRAL	NEUTRAL	NEUTRAL HEEL FIRST	PLANTAR FLEXION 15°	FROM PLANTAR FLEXION TO 10° DORSIFLEXION	NEUTRAL WITH TIBIA STABLE AND HEEL OFF PRIOR TO INITIAL CONTACT OPPOSITE FOOT	PLANTAR FLEXION 20°
TOES	NEUTRAL	NEUTRAL	NEUTRAL	NEUTRAL	NEUTRAL	NEUTRAL	NEUTRAL IP EXTENDED MP	NEUTRAL IP EXTENDED MP

Figure 13–9. Normal gait cycle. (Courtesy of Ranchos Los Amigos Hospital, Downey, Calif.)

Terminal Stance and Pre-swing

In the final stages, the hip begins to flex and moves from lateral rotation to medial rotation while the knee is flexed to 50 to 60°. At the ankle, there is plantar flexion. This action helps to smooth the center of gravity pathway. The forefoot is initially in contact with the floor, and the foot progresses so that only the big toe is in contact with the floor. The forefoot begins to move from inversion to eversion.

The pelvis is initially level and laterally rotated and then dips to the swing leg side, remaining laterally rotated. The trunk is initially aligned over the lower limbs and moves toward the stance leg. If pain is elicited during these instants, it may be due to a hallux rigidus. With hallux rigidus, the patient is unable to push off on the medial aspect of the foot; instead, the patient pushes off on the lateral aspect of the foot to compensate for the painful metatarsal arch resulting from increased pressure on the metatarsal heads. If the plantar flexors are weak (e.g., S1-S2 nerve root), push-off may be absent. The foot pronates so that there is a rigid lever for better push-off.

Swing Phase

As previously mentioned, there are three instants involved during the swing phase of gait. These are now described in order of occurrence.

Initial Swing

During the first subphase of acceleration (Fig. 13–9), flexion and medial rotation of the hip and flexion of the knee occur. The pelvis medially rotates and dips the swing leg side. The trunk is aligned with the stance leg. As well, the ankle continues to plantar flex. The foot is not in contact with the floor. The forefoot continues supinating while the hindfoot continues everting. The dorsiflexor muscles contract to allow the foot to clear the ground, and the knee exhibits its maximum flexion of about 60°. If the quadriceps muscles are weak, the pelvis is thrust forward to provide forward momentum to the leg.

Midswing

During the midswing instant, the hip continues to flex and medially rotate and the knee continues to flex. The ankle is in the anatomic position for the first 25 per cent of the stance phase to permit the foot and midtarsal joints to unlock for the foot to adapt to uneven terrain on weight bearing.

The forefoot is supinated, and the hindfoot is everted. The pelvis and trunk are in the same position as during the previous stage. If the dorsiflexor muscles are weak, the patient will demonstrate a high steppage gait. In such a gait, the hip flexes excessively so that the toes can clear the ground.

Terminal Swing

During the final subphase, also called deceleration, the hip continues to flex and medially rotate while the knee reaches its maximum extension. At the ankle, dorsiflexion has occurred. The forefoot is supinated, and the hindfoot is everted. The trunk and pelvis maintain the same position as previously. The hamstring muscles are contracting during the terminal phase to slow the swing; if the hamstrings are weak (e.g., S1-S2 nerve root lesion), heel strike may be excessively harsh.

Other Patterns in Gait

Hip. The function of the hip is to extend the leg in the stance phase and to flex the leg during the swing phase. The ligaments of the hip help to stabilize it in extension. If there is loss of movement of the hip, the compensatory mechanisms are increased mobility of the knee on the same side and increased mobility of the contralateral hip. As well, the lumbar spine shows increased mobility. The hip extensors help to initiate movement, as do the hip flexors; therefore, both groups of muscles work phasically. The hip flexors (primarily the iliopsoas muscle) fire to slow extension; the hip extensors (primarily hamstring muscles) fire to slow flexion. In this way, they work eccentrically. The abductor muscles provide stability during single-leg support, another critical event for the hip.

Knee. The knee, when it is in flexion during the first three instants of the stance phase of gait, acts as a shock absorber. Painful knees are not able to do this. One of the critical events of the knee is extension. The function of the knee during gait is to bear weight, absorb shock, extend the stride length, and allow the foot to move through its swing. The quadriceps muscles use only 4 to 5 per cent of their maximum voluntary contraction to extend the knee, but in so doing they help to control weight acceptance. The hamstring muscles flex the knee and slow the leg down in the swing phase, working eccentrically. If the knee has a flexion deformity, the hip is flexed and therefore loses its extension power, which is a critical event for the hip. By observing the knee anteriorly, the examiner can usually see the rotation occurring.

Gastrocnemius and Soleus. The gastrocnemius and soleus muscles are important in gait. They use 85 per cent of their maximum voluntary contraction in normal walking. It is these muscles that help to restrain the body's own forward momentum during gait.

Observation and Examination

Overview and Patient History

The observation of an individual's gait should be included in any assessment of the lower limb. As well, one must keep in mind that the posture of the head, neck, thorax, and lumbar spine can affect gait when no pathology is evident in the lower limb. The examiner must be able to identify the action of each body segment and note any deviation from normal during the individual phases of gait. For this reason, it is important to understand the normal parameters of gait and the mechanism of gait as it occurs. If one understands these normal events and how, when, and why they occur, it will be more beneficial when attempting to determine how the gait is altered in pathologic conditions.

The examiner should first perform a general overview of the patient's gait, looking at stride length, step frequency, time of swing, speed of walking, and duration of the complete walking cycle. Once this overview is completed, the examiner can look at the more specific parts of gait in terms of its phases and what happens at each joint during these phases.

With gait constantly changing as one stops and starts, hurries, dawdles, and walks with others, it is important to remember whether the movements the patient is capable of are normal and whether the speeds, phases, strides, and duration of the cycles occur in normal combinations. Thus, in addition to the patient walking at a normal speed, slow and fast gait speeds should be examined to see if these changes affect the gait. The examiner must be able to see the lumbar spine, pelvis, hips, knees, feet, and ankles. Female patients should be in a bra and briefs and male patients in shorts. The patient should walk barefoot. In this way the motions of the toes, feet, legs, pelvis, and trunk can be properly observed.

It is important that one read the patient's charts and take a history from the patient regarding any disease or injury, past or present, that may be causing gait problems. The examiner should ask the patient to walk in the usual manner, using any aids necessary, for example, parallel bars, crutches, walker, or canes. While the patient is doing this, an initial general observation of any obvious limp or deformity should be made.

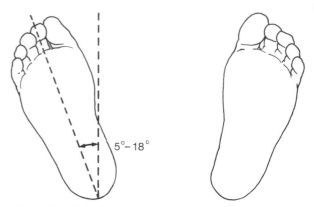

Figure 13–10. During stance and gait, the toes angle out 5 to 18° (Fick angle).

Sequential Observation

The examiner should observe the gait from the front, behind, and the side, in each instance observing from proximal to distal and watching the pelvis and lumbar spine down to the ankle and foot. This method will provide a sequential manner to the assessment and will prevent an aspect from being missed.

Anterior View

When observing from the front as the patient walks, one should note whether any lateral tilt to the pelvis occurs, whether there is any sideways swaying of the trunk, whether the pelvis rotates on a horizontal plane, or whether the trunk and upper extremity rotate in the opposite direction to the pelvis. Usually, the trunk and upper extremity rotation is approximately 180° out of phase with the pelvis; i.e., as the pelvis and lower limb rotate one way, the trunk and upper limb rotate in the opposite direction. This action helps provide a balancing effect and smoothes the forward progression of the body. One should note any bowing of the femur or the tibia; any medial or lateral rotation of the hips; and the position of the feet as the patient goes through the gait cycle (Fig. 13–10). This view is best used to examine the weight-loading period of the gait cycle. It should also be noted whether there is any abduction or circumduction of the swing leg; atrophy of the musculature of the anterior thigh and leg; and a normal base width.

Lateral View

From the side during the gait cycle, the examiner should observe any lumbar lordosis, hip movement, or limitation of flexion or extension of the hip. This view enables one to examine the interaction between the walking surface and the various body parts.

As the patient moves from initial contact to loading response, the foot flexes immediately while the knee flexes until the foot is flat on the floor. During this period, the hip is also flexed.

During midstance, the ankle dorsiflexes as the body pivots in an arc over the stationary foot. At the same time, the hip and knee extend, lengthening the leg.

As the patient moves from terminal stance to pre-swing, the ankle plantar flexes to raise the heel and the hip and knee flex as the weight is transferred to the opposite leg.

During initial swing, the ankle is plantar flexed and the hip and knee maximally flexed. As the leg progresses to midswing, the ankle dorsiflexes while the hip and knee begin to extend. As the patient moves from midswing to terminal swing, the ankle remains in the neutral position while the hip and knee continue extending. As the leg moves from terminal swing to initial contact, the knee reaches maximum extension while the ankle remains in neutral. No further hip extension occurs at this stage.

One must remember that there may be some compensation for limitation of movement of the hip by the lumbar spine. The patient should be observed to determine whether there is (1) sufficient knee extension at initial contact, followed almost immediately by slight flexion until the foot makes contact with the floor; (2) control of the slightly flexed knee during load response and midstance; and (3) sufficient flexion during pre-swing and initial swing. Also, any hyperextension of the knee during the gait cycle should be noted.

When looking at the ankle, the examiner should observe immediate plantar flexion at initial contact. The foot then dorsiflexes through midstance or single-leg stance, with maximum dorsiflexion being reached just before heel-off. It should be noted whether there is sufficient plantar flexion during push-off.

Finally, the examiner should note whether there is (1) coordination of movement between hip, knee, and ankle; (2) even or uneven gait length; and (3) equal or uneven duration of steps.

Posterior View

When observing the gait cycle from behind, one should notice the same structures as viewed from the front. Any abnormal abduction or adduction movements, as well as lateral displacement of the different body segments, should be noted. This view is best to examine the weight-unloading period of the gait cycle. The examiner can note whether heel rise is equal for both feet and whether the heels turn in or out. The observation

should also include lateral movement of the spine and the musculature of the back, buttocks, posterior thigh, and calf.

Footwear

The patient should be asked to walk in normal footwear as well as in bare feet. The examiner should take time to observe the patient's footwear and observe any wearing down of the heels and/or socks, condition of the shoe uppers, creases, and so on. The feet should also be examined for callus formation, blisters, corns, and bunions.

Compensatory Mechanisms

The examiner must try to ascertain the primary cause of gait faults and the compensatory factors used to maintain an energy-saving gait. An individual tries to use the most energy-saving gait possible. By assessing in this way, one will be able to set appropriate goals and to plan a logical approach to treatment.

Abnormal Gait

Illustrated next are some of the more common gait abnormalities. The list is by no means all-inclusive.

Antalgic Gait

The antalgic gait is self-protective and is the result of pain caused by injury to the hip, knee, ankle, or foot. The stance phase on the affected leg is shorter than on the non-affected leg as the patient attempts to "get off" the affected leg as quickly as possible. In addition, the painful region is often supported by one hand, if it is within reach, while the other arm, acting as a counterbalance, is outstretched.

Arthrogenic Gait

The arthrogenic gait is due to stiffness, laxity, or deformity, and it may be painful or pain-free. If the knee or hip is fused, or if the knee has recently been removed from a cylinder cast, the pelvis must be elevated by exaggerated plantar flexion of the opposite ankle and circumduction of the stiff leg to provide toe clearance. This movement compensates for the lack of flexion in the hip or knee.

Ataxic Gait

If the patient has poor sensation or lack of muscle coordination, there is a tendency toward poor balance and a broad base (Fig. 13–11). With cerebellar ataxia, the gait is a lurch or stagger and all movements are exaggerated. With sensory ataxia, the feet slap the ground because they cannot be felt. The patient also watches the feet while walking. The gait is irregular, jerky, and weaving.

Gluteus Maximus Gait

If the gluteus maximus muscle is weak, the patient will thrust the thorax posteriorly at initial contact to maintain hip extension of the stance leg. The resulting gait has a lurch to it (Fig. 13–12).

Gluteus Medius (Trendelenburg) Gait

If the gluteus medius muscle is weak, the patient will exhibit an excessive lateral list, thrust-

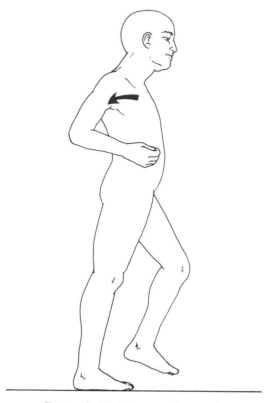

Figure 13–12. Gluteus maximus gait.

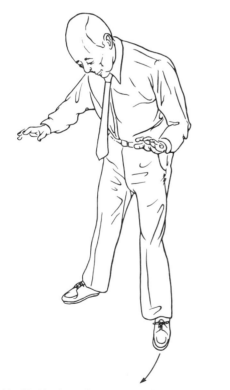

Figure 13–11. Ataxic gait. In *cerebellar ataxia* the patient has poor balance and a broad base; therefore he lurches, staggers, and exaggerates all movements. In *sensory ataxia* the patient has a broad-based gait; since he cannot feel his feet, he slaps them against the ground and looks down at them as he walks. In both types of ataxias the gait is irregular, jerky, and weaving. (From Judge, R. D., et al.: Clinical Diagnosis—A Physiological Approach. Little, Brown & Co., 1982, p. 438.)

ing the thorax laterally to keep the center of gravity over the stance leg (Fig. 13–13). A positive Trendelenburg sign will also be exhibited. If there is bilateral weakness of the gluteus medius muscles, the gait will show accentuated side-to-side movement, resulting in a "wobbling" gait or "chorus girl swing." This gait may also be seen in congenital dislocation of the hip and coxa vara.

Hemiplegic or Hemiparetic Gait

The patient swings the paraplegic leg outward and ahead in a circle (circumduction) or pushes it ahead (Fig. 13–14). In addition, the affected upper limb is carried across the trunk for balance. This is sometimes referred to as a neurogenic or *flaccid gait*.

Parkinsonian Gait

The patient's neck, trunk, and knees are flexed. The gait is shuffling or characterized by short rapid steps (marche á petits pas) at times. The arms are held stiffly and do not have their normal associative movement (Fig. 13–15). During the gait, the patient may lean forward and walk progressively faster as though unable to stop (festination).

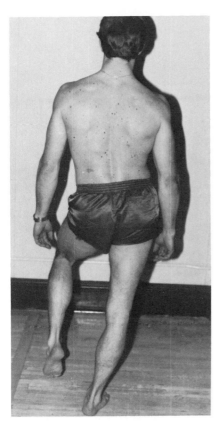

Figure 13–13. Gluteus medius (Trendelenburg) gait.

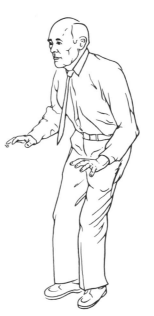

Figure 13–15. Parkinsonism. The head, trunk, and knees are flexed; the arms are held rather stiffly with poor associative movement. The gait is shuffling or characterized at times by short, rapid steps (marche á petits pas). The patient may lean forward and walk progressively faster, seemingly unable to stop himself (festination). (From Judge, R. D., et al.: Clinical Diagnosis—A Physiological Approach. Little, Brown & Co., 1982, p. 439.)

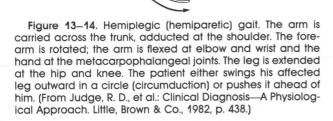

Figure 13–14. Hemiplegic (hemiparetic) gait. The arm is carried across the trunk, adducted at the shoulder. The forearm is rotated; the arm is flexed at elbow and wrist and the hand at the metacarpophalangeal joints. The leg is extended at the hip and knee. The patient either swings his affected leg outward in a circle (circumduction) or pushes it ahead of him. (From Judge, R. D., et al.: Clinical Diagnosis—A Physiological Approach. Little, Brown & Co., 1982, p. 438.)

Psoatic Limp

The psoatic limp is seen in conditions affecting the hip, such as Legg-Calvé-Perthes disease. The limp may be due to weakness or reflex inhibition of the psoas major muscle. The limp shows classically as lateral rotation, flexion, and adduction of the hip (Fig. 13–16). The patient will exaggerate movement of the pelvis and trunk to help move the thigh into flexion.

Scissors Gait

This gait, the result of spastic paralysis of the hip adductor muscles, causes the knees to be drawn together so that the legs can only be swung forward by swinging the hips forward with great effort (Fig. 13–17). This is seen in spastic paraplegics and may be referred to as a neurogenic or *spastic gait*.

Short Leg Gait

If one leg is shorter than the other, or if there is a deformity in one of the bones of the leg, the patient will demonstrate a lateral shift to the affected side and the pelvis will tilt down on the affected side, creating a limp (Fig. 13–18). The

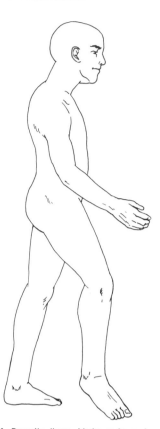

Figure 13-16. Psoatic limp. Note external rotation, flexion, and abduction of affected hip.

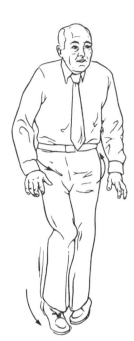

Figure 13-17. Scissors gait. Spasticity of thigh adduction, seen in spastic paraplegics, draws the knees together. The legs are advanced (with great effort) by swinging the hips. (From Judge, R. D., et al.: Clinical Diagnosis—A Physiological Approach. Little, Brown & Co., 1982, p. 439.)

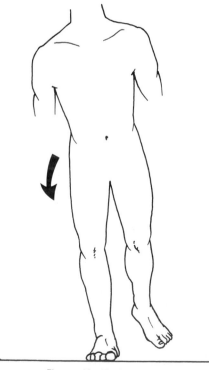

Figure 13-18. Short leg gait.

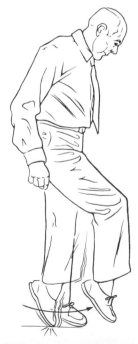

Figure 13-19. Steppage or footdrop gait. To avoid dragging his toes against the ground (since he cannot dorsiflex the foot), the patient lifts his knee high and slaps the foot to the ground on advancing. (From Judge, R. D., et al.: Clinical Diagnosis—A Physiological Approach. Little, Brown & Co., 1982, p. 438.)

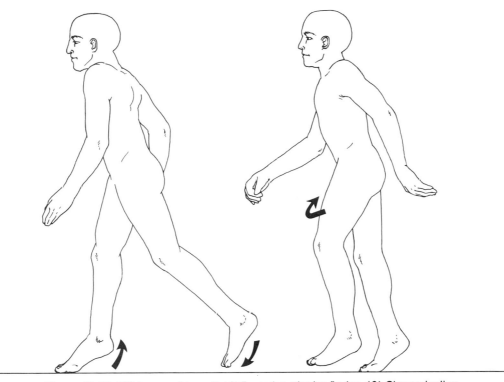

Figure 13–20. Stiff knee or hip gait. (*1*) Excessive plantar flexion. (*2*) Circumduction.

weight-bearing period may be the same for both legs. With proper footwear, the gait may appear normal. This may also be termed *painless osteogenic gait.*

Steppage or Footdrop Gait

The patient has weak or paralyzed dorsiflexor muscles, resulting in a foot drop. To compensate and to avoid dragging the toes against the ground, the patient lifts the knee higher than normal; this results in a high steppage gait (Fig. 13–19). At initial contact, the foot slaps on the ground because of loss of the control of the dorsiflexor muscles.

Stiff Knee or Hip Gait

Because of a stiff hip or knee, the entire leg is lifted higher than normal to clear the ground. To do this, excessive plantar flexing of the other foot occurs and the affected leg swings through an arc moving the leg anteriorly (Fig. 13–20). The arc of movements helps to decrease the elevation needed to "clear" the affected leg. Because of the loss of flexibility in the hip or knee or both, the gait length will be different for both legs. When the stiff limb is weight bearing, the gait length will usually be smaller.

REFERENCES

CITED REFERENCES

1. Bowker, J. H., and C. B. Hall: Normal human gait. *In* Atlas of Orthotics: Biomechanical Principles and Applications. St. Louis, C. V. Mosby Co., 1975.
2. Inman, V. T., H. J. Ralston, and F. Todd: Human Walking. Baltimore, Williams and Wilkins Co., 1981.
3. Koerner, I. B.: Normal Human Locomotion and the Gait of the Amputee. Edmonton, University of Alberta Bookstore, 1979.
4. Koerner, I.: Observation of Human Gait. Videotapes produced by the Health Sciences Audiovisual Education, University of Alberta, 1984.
5. Hoppenfeld, S.: Physical Examination of the Spine and Extremities. New York, Appleton-Century-Crofts, 1976.
6. Perry, J., and H. J. Hislop: The mechanics of walking: A clinical interpretation. *In* Principles of Lower-Extremity Bracing. New York, American Physical Therapy Association, 1970.

GENERAL REFERENCES

Chondera, J. D.: Analysis of gait from footprints. Physiotherapy *60*:179, 1974.
Eberhart, H. D., V. T. Inman, and B. Bresler: Principal elements in human locomotion. *In* Human Limbs and Their Substitutes. New York, McGraw-Hill Co., 1954.
Grieve, D. W.: The assessment of gait. Physiotherapy *55*:452, 1969.
Finley, F. R., K. A. Cody, and R. V. Finizie: Locomotion patterns in elderly women. Arch. Phys. Med. Rehabil. *50*:140, 1969.

Gruebel-Lee, D. M.: Disorders of Hip. Philadelphia, J. B. Lippincott Co., 1983.

Inman, V. T.: The Joints of the Ankle. Baltimore, Williams and Wilkins Co., 1976.

Inman, V. T.: Functional aspects of the abductor muscles of the hip. J. Bone Joint Surg. 29:607, 1947.

Judge, R. D., G. D. Zuidema, and F. T. Fitzgerald: Clinical Diagnosis: A Physiological Approach. Boston, Little, Brown and Co., 1982.

Macleod, J.: Clinical Examination. New York, Churchill Livingstone, 1976.

Murray, M. P., A. B. Brought, and R. C. Kory: Walking patterns of normal men. J. Bone Joint Surg. 46A:335, 1964.

Murray, M. P.: Gait as a total pattern of movement. Am. J. Phys. Med. 46:290, 1967.

Murray, M. P., D. R. Gore, and B. H. Clarkson: Walking patterns of patients with unilateral pain due to osteoarthritis and avascular necrosis. J. Bone Joint Surg. 53A:259, 1971.

Normal Gait Chart. Rancho Los Amigos Hospital, Downey, Calif., 1981.

Perry, J.: Pathologic gait. In Atlas of Orthotics: Biomechanical Principles and Applications. St. Louis, C. V. Mosby Co., 1975.

Root, M. L., W. P. Orien, and J. H. Weed: Normal and Abnormal Function of the Foot. Los Angeles, Clinical Biomechanics Corporation, 1977.

Saunders, J. B. M., V. T. Inman, and H. O. Eberhart: The major determinants in normal and pathological gait. J. Bone Joint Surg. 35A:543, 1953.

Simon, S. R., R. A. Mann, J. L. Hogy, and L. J. Larsen: Role of the posterior calf muscles in a normal gait. J. Bone Joint Surg. 60A:465, 1978.

14

Assessment of Posture

Posture Development

Posture, which is the relative disposition of the body at any one moment, is a composite of the positions of the different joints of the body at that time. Thus, the position of one joint has an effect on the position of the other joints. *Correct posture* is the position in which minimum stress will be applied to each joint. Any position that increases the stress to the joints may be called *faulty posture*. If the individual has strong and flexible muscles, faulty postures may not affect the joints because the individual has the ability to change position readily so that the stresses do not become excessive. If the joints are stiff or too mobile and the muscles are weak, however, the posture cannot be easily altered to the correct alignment and the result can be some form of pathology. The pathology may be due to the cumulative effects of repeated small stresses over a period of time or to constant abnormal stresses over a shorter period of time. These chronic stresses can result in the same problems that are seen when a sudden (acute) severe stress is applied to the body. The abnormal stresses cause excessive wearing of the articular surfaces of joints as well as produce osteophytes and traction spurs, which are the result of the body attempting to alter its structure to accommodate these repeated stresses. The soft tissue (such as muscles and ligaments) may become weakened, stretched, or traumatized by in-

creased stress. The application of an acute stress on the chronic stress may exacerbate the problem and may indeed produce the signs and symptoms that initially prompt the patient to seek aid.

At birth, the whole spine is concave forward or flexed (Fig. 14–1). Curves of the spine found at birth are called *primary curves*. The curves that maintain this position—the thoracic spine and sacrum—are thus classified as primary curves of the spine. As the child grows (Fig. 14–2), *secondary curves* appear and are *convexed* forward or extended. In the cervical spine, at about the age of 3 months, when the child begins to lift its head, the cervical spine becomes convexed forward, producing the cervical lordosis. In the lumbar spine, the secondary curve develops slightly later (6 to 8 months) when the child begins to sit up and walk. In old age, the secondary curves again begin to be lost as the spine starts to return to a flexed position as a result of disc degeneration, ligamentous calcification, osteoporosis, and vertebral wedging.

In the child, the center of gravity is at the level of the T12 vertebra. As the child grows older, the center of gravity drops to reach the level of the second sacral vertebra in adults, being slightly higher in males. The child will stand with a wide base to maintain balance, and the knees will be flexed. Initially, the knees will be slightly bowed (genu varum) until about 18 months of age. The child then becomes slightly knock-kneed (genu valgum) until the age of 3 years. By the age of 6 years, the legs should naturally straighten out (see

377

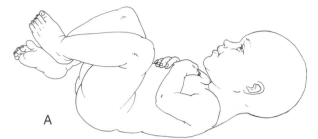

Figure 14–1. Postural development. (*A*) Flexed posture in a newborn. (*B*) Development of secondary cervical curve. (*C*) Development of secondary lumbar curve.

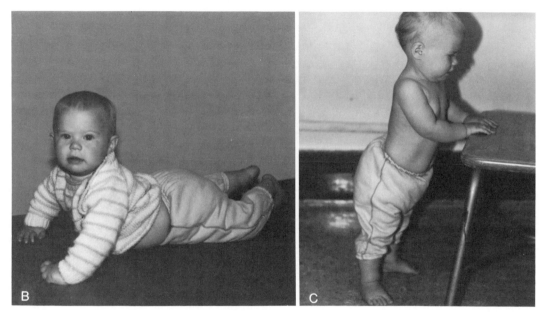

Figure 14–24). The lumbar spine in children has an exaggerated lumbar curve, or excessive lordosis. This accentuated curve is due to presence of large abdominal contents, weakness of the abdominal musculature, and the small pelvis characteristic of this age.

Initially, a child is flat-footed, or appears to be, as a result of the minimal development of the medial longitudinal arch and a fat pad that is found in the arch. As the child grows, the fat pad slowly decreases in size, making the medial arch more evident. In addition, as the foot develops and the muscles strengthen, the arches of the feet develop normally and become more evident.

The advantage of an erect posture, as seen in human beings, is that it enables the hands to be free and the eyes to be farther from the ground so that the individual can see farther ahead. The disadvantages include an increased strain on the spine and lower limbs and comparative difficulties in respiration and transport of the blood in reaching the brain.

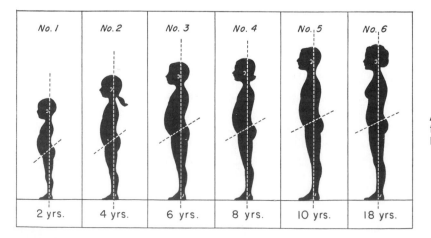

Figure 14–2. Postural changes with age. Apparent kyphosis at ages 6 and 8 is due to scapular winging. (From McMorris, R. O.: Pediatr. Clin. North Am. *8:*214, 1961.)

FACTORS AFFECTING POSTURE

Several anatomic factors may affect correct posture, including:

1. Bony contours (e.g., hemivertebra).
2. Laxity of ligamentous structures.
3. Fascial and musculotendinous tightness (e.g., hamstrings, tensor fasciae latae, pectorals, hip flexors).
4. Muscle tonus (e.g., gluteus maximus, abdominals, erector spinae).
5. Pelvic angle (normal is 30°).
6. Joint position and mobility.
7. Neurogenic outflow and inflow.

These factors may be further enhanced or cause additional problems when combined with pathologic or congenital states, such as Klippel-Feil syndrome, Scheuermann's disease (juvenile kyphosis), scoliosis, or disc disease.

CAUSES OF POOR POSTURE

There are many causes of poor posture (Fig. 14–3). Some of these causes are *postural* (positional), and some are *structural*.

Postural Factors

The most common postural problem is poor postural habit; i.e., for whatever reason, the individual does not hold a correct posture. This type of posture is often seen in the individual who stands or sits for long periods of time and begins to slouch. Maintaining a correct posture requires muscles that are strong, flexible, and easily able to adapt to environmental change. These muscles must continually work against gravity and in harmony with one another to maintain an upright posture.

Another cause of poor postural habits, especially in children, is their not wanting to appear taller than their peers. If a child has an early, rapid growth spurt, as an example, there will be a tendency to slouch in order not to appear different. Such a spurt may also result in the unequal growth of the various structures, and this may lead to altered posture; for example, the growth of muscle may not keep up with the growth of bone. This process is sometimes evident in adolescents with tight hamstrings.

Another cause of poor posture is muscle imbalance or muscle contracture. For example, a tight iliopsoas muscle increases the lumbar lordosis in the lumbar spine.

Pain may also cause poor posture. Pressure on a nerve root in the lumbar spine can lead to pain in the back and result in a scoliosis as the body unconsciously adopts a posture that decreases the pain.

Respiratory conditions (such as emphysema), general weakness, being overweight, loss of proprioception, and muscle spasm (as seen in cerebral palsy) may also lead to poor posture.

Structural Factors

Structural deformities may cause an alteration of posture. For example, a significant difference in leg length or anomalies of the spine, such as a hemivertebra may alter the posture.

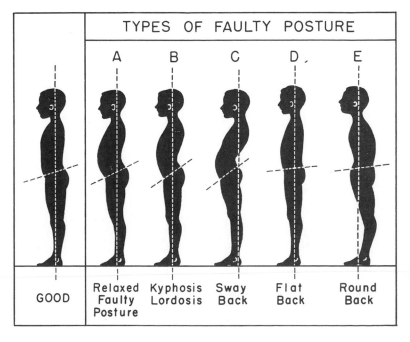

Figure 14–3. Types of faulty posture. (From McMorris, R. O.: Pediatr. Clin. North Am. *8:*217, 1961.)

Common Spinal Deformities

Lordosis

Lordosis is an excessive anterior curvature of the spine (Fig. 14–4).[1–5] Pathologically, it is an exaggeration of the normal curves found in the cervical and lumbar spines. Causes of increased lordosis include (1) postural deformity; (2) lax muscles, especially the abdominal muscles; (3) a heavy abdomen due to overweight or pregnancy; (4) compensatory mechanisms that are due to another deformity, such as kyphosis (Fig. 14–5); (5) hip flexion contracture; (6) spondylolisthesis; (7) congenital problems, such as congenital dislocation of the hip; (8) failure of segmentation of the neural arch of a facet joint segment; or (9) fashion. For example, wearing high heels will increase the lordotic curve.

Associated with the lordosis, one may often observe sagging shoulders, medial rotation of the legs, and poking forward of the head so that it is in front of the center of gravity. This posture is adopted by the individual in an attempt to keep the center of gravity where it should be. Deviation in one part of the body often leads to deviation in another part of the body in an attempt to maintain the correct center of gravity and the correct visual plane.

With lordosis, the pelvic angle, normally approximately 30°, is increased. With excessive lor-

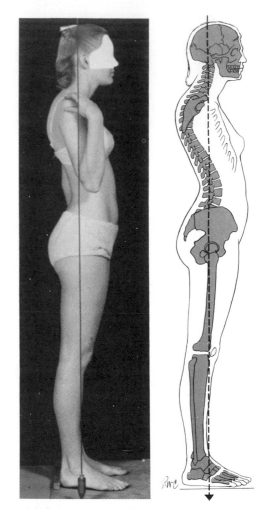

Figure 14–5. Faulty posture illustrating exaggerated lordosis and kyphosis. (From Kendall, F. P., and E. K. McCreary: Muscles—Testing and Function. Baltimore, The Williams and Wilkins Co., 1983, p. 281.)

dosis, there is an increase in the pelvic angle to about 40°, accompanied by a mobile spine and an anterior pelvic tilt. With *swayback*, there is increased pelvic inclination to approximately 40° and the thoracolumbar spine exhibits a kyphosis (Fig. 14–6). A swayback deformity results in the spine bending back rather sharply at the lumbosacral angle.

Kyphosis

Kyphosis is an excessive posterior curvature of the spine (Figs. 14–7 and 14–8).[3, 5–10] Pathologically, it is an exaggeration of the normal curve found in the thoracic spine. There are several causes of kyphosis. The etiology includes tuberculosis, vertebral compression fractures, Scheuermann's disease, ankylosing spondylitis, senile osteoporosis, tumors, compensation in conjunction with lordosis, or congenital anomalies.[6] Some of

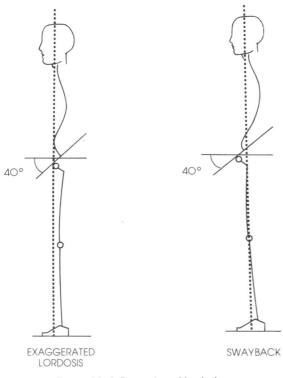

40°   40°

EXAGGERATED LORDOSIS   SWAYBACK

Figure 14–4. Examples of lordosis.

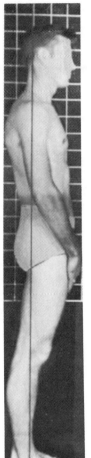

Figure 14–6. Faulty posture illustrating a sway back. (From Kendall, F. P., and E. K. McCreary: Muscle—Testing and Function. Baltimore, The Williams and Wilkins Co., 1983, p. 284.)

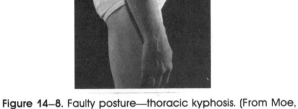

Figure 14–8. Faulty posture—thoracic kyphosis. (From Moe, J. H., et al.: Scoliosis and Other Spinal Deformities. Philadelphia, W. B. Saunders Co., 1978, p. 152.)

these congenital anomalies include a partial segmental defect, as is seen in osseous metaplasia, or centrum hypoplasia and aplasia.[9,11,12] In addition, paralysis may lead to a kyphosis because of the loss of muscle action needed to maintain the

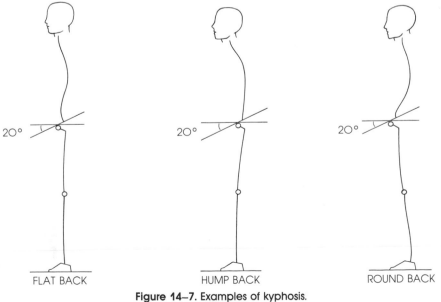

Figure 14–7. Examples of kyphosis.

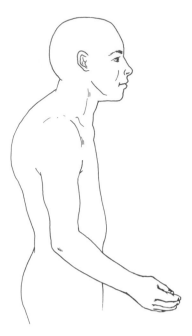

Figure 14–9. Humpback or gibbus deformity.

Figure 14–10. Faulty posture—flat back. (From Kendall, F. P., and E. K. McCreary: Muscles—Testing and Function. Baltimore, The Williams and Wilkins Co., 1983, p. 285.)

Figure 14–11. Loss of height resulting from osteoporosis, leading to "dowager's hump." Note the flexed head and protruding abdomen, which occur partially to maintain the center of gravity in its normal position.

Figure 14–9

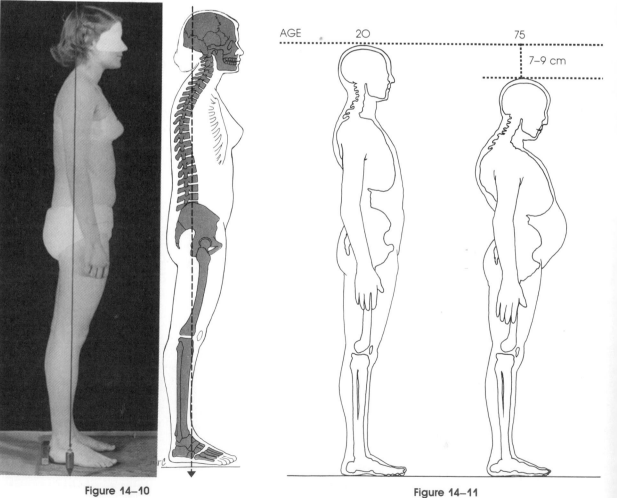

Figure 14–10

Figure 14–11

correct posture combined with the forces of gravity.

There are four types of kyphosis:

1. *Round back*. The individual with a round back has a long rounded curve with decreased pelvic inclination (less than 30°) and thoracolumbar kyphosis. The patient will often present with the trunk flexed forward and a decreased lumbar curve.

2. *Humpback or gibbus*. There is a localized sharp posterior angulation in the thoracic spine (Fig. 14–9).

3. *Flat back*. There is decreased pelvic inclination to 20° and a mobile lumbar spine (Fig. 14–10).

4. *Dowager's hump*. This is often seen in older individuals, especially women. The deformity is due to osteoporosis in which the thoracic vertebral bodies begin to degenerate and wedge in an anterior direction resulting in a kyphosis (Fig. 14–11).

Pathologic conditions such as Scheuermann's vertebral osteochondritis may also result in a structural kyphosis (Fig. 14–12). In this condition,

inflammation of the bone and cartilage around the ring epiphysis of the vertebral body occurs. The condition often leads to an anterior wedging of the vertebra. It is a growth disorder that affects about 10 per cent of the population, and usually several vertebra are affected. The most common area for the disease to occur is between T10 and L2.

Scoliosis

Scoliosis is a lateral curvature of the spine.[6, 8, 13–99] In the cervical spine, a scoliosis is called a *torticollis* (Fig. 14–13). There are several types of scoliosis, some of which are nonstructural (Fig. 14–13) and some which are structural. *Nonstructural scoliosis* may be due to postural problems, hysteria, nerve root irritation, inflammation, or compensation caused by leg length discrepancy or contracture (in the lumbar spine).[18] *Structural scoliosis* may be congenital and due to wedge vertebra, hemivertebra (Fig. 14–14), or failure of segmentation; idiopathic (genetic) (Fig. 14–15) or neuromuscular because of upper or lower motor neuron lesion; myopathic in cases of muscular dystrophy; or arthrogryposis (persistent joint flexure or contracture).[12] In addition, scoliosis may result from conditions such as neurofibromatosis, mesenchymal disorders, or trauma. It is also seen in infection, tumors, and inflammatory conditions and in conjunction with malocclusion and ear problems.

With regard to nonstructural scoliosis, there is no bony deformity and it is not progressive. The spine will show segmental limitation, and side bending is usually symmetric. The scoliotic curve will disappear on forward flexion. This type of scoliosis is usually found in the cervical, lumbar, or thoracolumbar area.

In structural scoliosis the patient lacks normal flexibility, and side bending becomes asymmetric. This type of scoliosis may be progressive, and the curve will not disappear on forward flexion.

Idiopathic scoliosis accounts for 75 to 85 per cent of all cases of (structural) scoliosis. The vertebral bodies rotate into the convexity of the curve, with the spinous processes going toward the concavity of the curve. There is a fixed rotational prominence on the convex side, which is best seen on forward flexion from the "skyline" view. This prominence is sometimes called a "razorback spine." This disc spaces are narrowed on the concave side and widened on the convex side. There is distortion of the vertebral body, and vital capacity is considerably lowered when the lateral curvature exceeds 60°; compression and malposition of the organs within the rib cage also occur. Examples of scoliotic curves are shown in Figure 14–16.

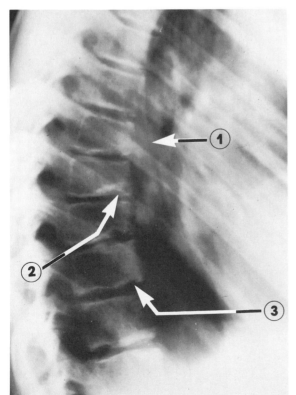

Figure 14–12. A classical x-ray appearance of the spine in a patient with Scheuermann's disease. Note the wedged vertebra (1), Schmorl's nodules (2), and marked irregularity of the vertebral endplates (3). (From Moe, J. H., et al.: Scoliosis and Other Spinal Deformities. Philadelphia, W. B. Saunders Co., 1978, p. 332.)

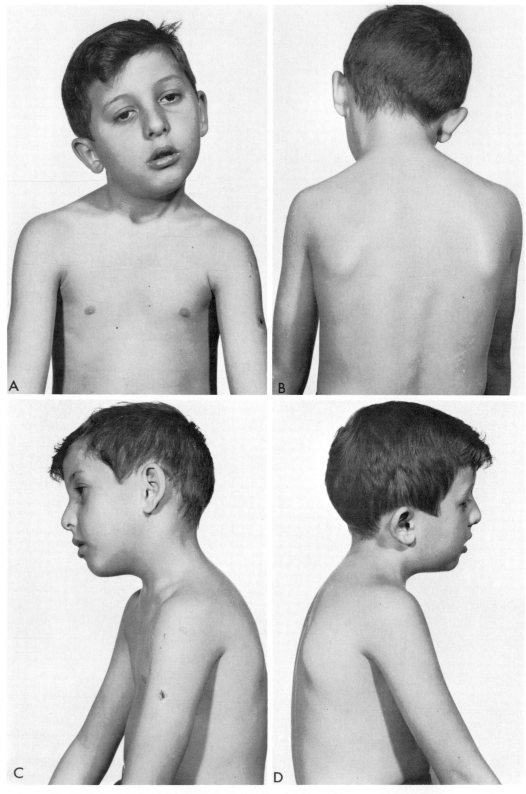

Figure 14–13. Congenital muscular torticollis on the right in a 10-year-old boy. Note the contracted sternocleidomastoid muscle. (From Tachdjian, M. O.: Pediatric Orthopedics. Philadelphia, W. B. Saunders Co., 1972, p. 74.)

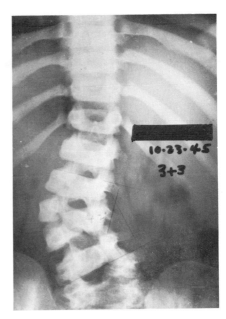

Figure 14–14. Scoliosis caused by hemivertebra. (From Moe, J. H., et al.: Scoliosis and Other Spinal Deformities. Philadelphia, W. B. Saunders, 1978, p. 134.)

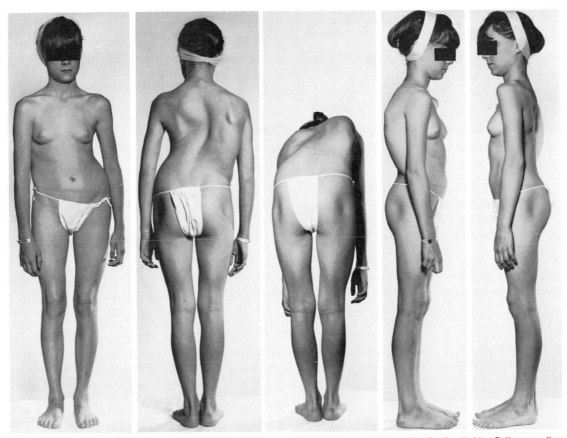

Figure 14–15. Idiopathic structural right thoracic scoliosis. (From Tachdjian, M. O.: Pediatric Orthopaedics. Philadelphia, W. B. Saunders Co., 1972, p. 1200.)

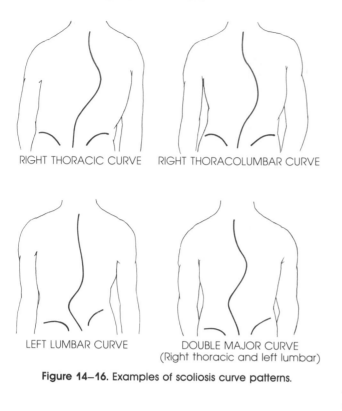

RIGHT THORACIC CURVE   RIGHT THORACOLUMBAR CURVE

LEFT LUMBAR CURVE   DOUBLE MAJOR CURVE
(Right thoracic and left lumbar)

Figure 14–16. Examples of scoliosis curve patterns.

Postural History

As with any history, one must ensure that the information obtained is as complete as possible. Often by listening to the patient, the examiner will develop a comprehension of the problem. The information should include a history of the problem, the patient's general condition and health, and family history. If a child is being examined, the examiner must obtain a prenatal and postnatal history as well, including the health of the mother during pregnancy, any complications during pregnancy or delivery, and drugs taken by the mother during that period, especially the first trimester.

It should be remembered that it is unusual for an individual to present with just a postural problem. It is the symptoms produced by pathology caused by or causing the postural abnormality that initiate the consultation. Thus, the examiner must be cognizant of various underlying pathologic conditions when assessing posture. The following questions should be asked:

1. Does the family have any history of back problems or special problems? Conditions such as hemivertebra, scoliosis, and Klippel-Feil syndrome may be congenital.

2. Has the patient had any previous illnesses, operations, or severe injuries?

3. Is there any history of other conditions, such as connective tissue diseases, which have a high incidence of associated spinal problems?

4. Has there been any previous treatment? If so, what was it?

5. How old is the patient? Many spinal problems begin in childhood or may be the result of degeneration.

6. In the child, has there been a growth spurt? If so, when did it begin?

7. For females, when did menarche begin? Does back pain seem to be associated with menses? Menarche indicates the point at which approximately two thirds of adolescent growth spurt has been completed.

8. For males, has there been a voice change? If so, when?

9. For children, is there difficulty in fitting clothes? For example, with scoliosis, the hem of a dress is usually uneven because of the spinal curvature.

10. If a deformity is present, is it progressive or stationary?

11. Does the patient have any difficulty breathing?

12. Which hand is the dominant one? Often, the dominant side will show a lower shoulder with the hip slightly deviated to that side (Fig. 14–17). The spine may deviate slightly to the opposite side, and the opposite foot will be pronated slightly more.[3] The gluteus medius on the dominant side may also be weaker.

13. Does the patient experience any neurologic symptoms (e.g., "pins and needles" or numbness)?

14. What is the nature, extent, type, and duration of the pain?

15. What positions or activities increase the pain or discomfort?

16. What positions or activities decrease the pain or discomfort?

Observation

To assess posture correctly, the patient must be adequately undressed. Male patients should be in shorts and female patients in bra and shorts. Ideally, the patient should not wear shoes or stockings. However, if the patient is using walking aids, braces, collars, or orthotics, they should be noted and may be used after the patient has been assessed in the "natural" state to assess the effect of the appliances.

The patient should be examined in the habitual, relaxed posture that is usually adopted. Often, it may take some time for the patient to adopt the usual posture because of tenseness or uncertainty.

In the standing and sitting positions, the assessment is the same as the observation for the

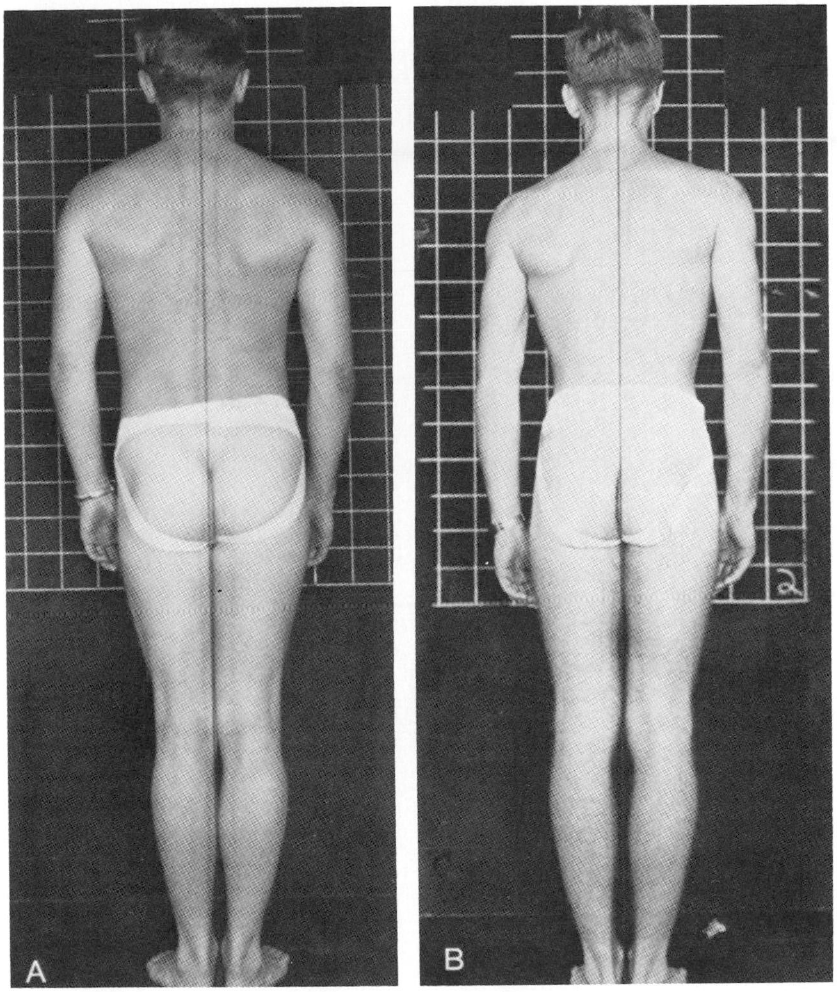

Figure 14–17. Effect of handedness on posture. (*A*) Right hand dominant. (*B*) Left hand dominant. (From Kendall, F. P., and E. K. McCreary: Muscles—Testing and Function. Baltimore, The Williams and Wilkins Company, 1983, p. 294.)

upper and lower limb scanning examinations of the cervical and lumbar spines. Assessment of posture should be carried out with the patient in the standing, sitting, and lying (supine and prone) positions. Once the patient has been examined in these positions, the examiner may decide to include other habitual postures assumed by the patient to see whether these postures increase or alter symptoms. The patient may also be assessed wearing different footwear to determine the effects on the posture and symptoms.

STANDING

The examiner should first determine body type (Fig. 14–18).[19] There are three body types: ectomorphic, mesomorphic, and endomorphic. The ectomorph is a person who has a thin body build characterized by a relative prominence of structures developed from the embryonic ectoderm. The mesomorph has a muscular or sturdy body build characterized by relative prominence of structures developed by the embryonic mesoderm. The endomorph has a heavy (fat) body

build characterized by relative prominence of structures developed from the embryonic endoderm.

In addition to body type, one should note the emotional attitude of the patient. Is the patient tense, bored, or lethargic? What is the appearance? Does the patient appear healthy-looking, emaciated, or overweight? Answers to these questions can help the examiner determine how much will have to be done to correct any problems. For example, if the patient is lethargic, it may take longer to correct the problem than if the individual appears truly interested in correcting the problem. The examiner must remember that posture is an expression of one's personality, sense of well-being, and self-esteem.

Anterior View

When observing the patient from the front (Fig. 14–19), the examiner should ensure that the following conditions hold true:

1. The head is straight on the shoulders (in midline). The examiner should note whether the

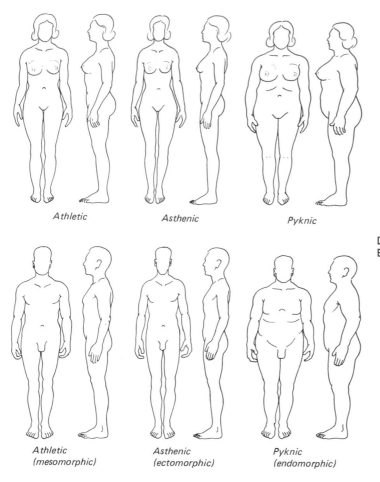

Athletic   Asthenic   Pyknic

Figure 14–18. Male and female body types. (From Debrunner, H. U.: Orthopaedic Diagnosis. London, E & S Livingstone, 1970, P. 86.)

Athletic (mesomorphic)   Asthenic (ectomorphic)   Pyknic (endomorphic)

head is tilted to one side or rotated habitually (Fig. 14–20). The cause of altered head position must be established. For example, it may be due to weak muscles, trauma, a hearing loss, temporomandibular joint problems, or the wearing of bifocal glasses.

2. The posture of the jaw is normal. In the resting position, the normal jaw posture is lips gently together, teeth slightly apart (freeway space), with the tip of the tongue behind the upper teeth in the roof of the mouth. This position maintains the mandible in a good posture; i.e., slight negative pressure in the mouth reduces work of the muscles. It also enables respiration through the nose and diaphragmatic breathing.

3. The tip of the nose is in line with the manubrium sternum, xiphisternum, and umbilicus. This line is the anterior line of reference used to divide the body into right and left halves. If the umbilicus is used as a reference point, the examiner should remember that the umbilicus is almost always slightly off-center.

4. The trapezius neck line is equal on both sides. The muscle bulk of the trapezius muscles should be equal, and the slope of the muscles should be close to equal. Since the dominant arm usually shows greater laxity by being slightly

lower, the slope on the dominant side may be slightly greater.

5. The shoulders are level. In most cases, the dominant side will be slightly lower.

6. The clavicles and acromioclavicular joints are level and equal. They should be symmetric. Any deviation should be noted. Deviations may be due to subluxations or dislocations of the acromioclavicular or sternoclavicular joints, fractures, or clavicular rotation.

7. There is no protrusion, depression, or lateralization of the sternum, ribs, or costocartilage. If there are changes, they should be noted.

8. The waist angles are equal, and the arms are equidistant from the waist. If a scoliosis is present, one arm will hang closer to the body than the other arm. The examiner should also note whether the arms are equally rotated medially or laterally.

9. The carrying angle at each elbow is equal. Any deviation should be noted. The normal carrying angle varies from 5 to 15°.

10. The palms of both hands face the body in relaxed standing. Any differences should be noted and may give an indication of rotation in the upper limb.

11. The high points of the iliac crest are the

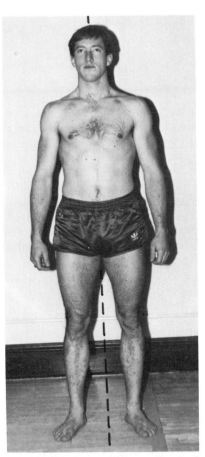

Figure 14–19. Posture in the standing position (anterior view).

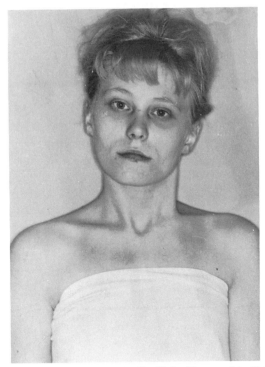

Figure 14–20. Congenital torticollis in 18-year-old girl. Note the asymmetry of the face. (From Tachdjian, M. O.: Pediatric Orthopedics. Philadelphia, W. B. Saunders Co., 1972, p. 68.)

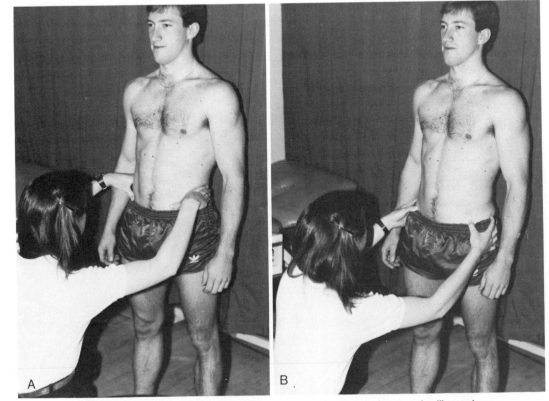

Figure 14–21. Viewing height equality. (A) Iliac crests. (B) Anterior superior iliac spines.

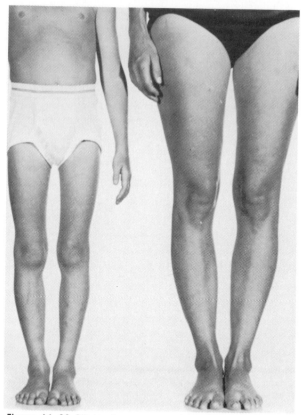

Figure 14–22. Bilateral genu varum in mother and son. Note the associated internal tibial torsion. (From Tachdjian, M. O.: Pediatric Orthopedics. Philadelphia, W. B. Saunders Co., 1972, p. 1462.)

same height on both sides (Fig. 14–21). With a scoliosis, the patient may feel that one hip is "higher" than the other. This apparent high pelvis is due to the lateral shift of the trunk. The pelvis will usually be level. The same condition can cause the patient to feel that one leg is shorter than the other.

12. The anterior superior iliac spines (ASIS) are level. If one ASIS is higher than the other, there is a possibility that one leg will be shorter than the other or that the pelvis may be rotated more or shifted up or down more on one side relative to the other side.

13. The pubic bones are level at the symphysis pubis. Any deviation should be noted.

14. The patellae of the knees point straight ahead. Sometimes the patellae face outward ("frog's eye" patella) or inward ("squinting" patella). The position of the patella may be altered by torsion of the femur or tibia.

15. The knees are straight. The knees may be in genu varum or genu valgum. The examiner should note whether the deformity results from the femur, tibia, or both bones. In children the knees go through a progression of being straight, going into genu varum (Fig. 14–22), to straight, to genu valgum (Fig. 14–23), and finally straight again in the first 6 years of life (Fig. 14–24).[8]

16. The heads of the fibula are level.

17. The medial and lateral malleoli of the ankles are level. Normally, the medial malleoli are

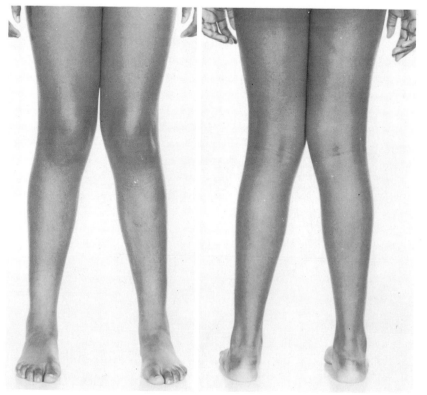

Figure 14–23. Bilateral genu valgum in an adolescent. (From Tachdjian, M. O.: Pediatric Orthopedics. Philadelphia, W. B. Saunders Co., 1972, p. 1467.)

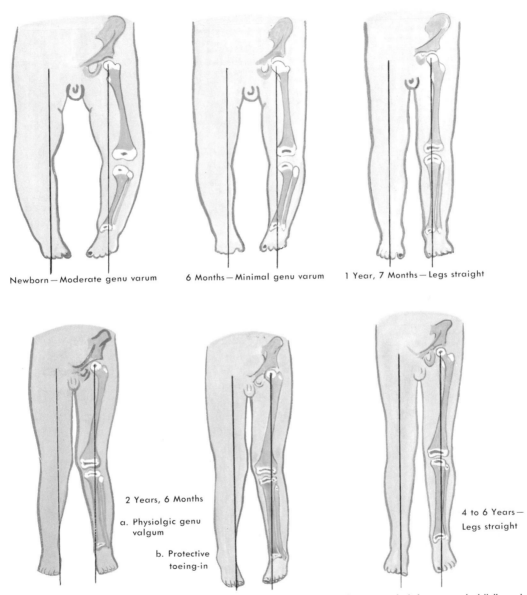

Newborn—Moderate genu varum

6 Months—Minimal genu varum

1 Year, 7 Months—Legs straight

2 Years, 6 Months

a. Physiolgic genu valgum

b. Protective toeing-in

4 to 6 Years— Legs straight

Figure 14–24. Physiologic evolution of lower limb alignment at various ages in infancy and childhood. (From Tachdjian, M. O.: Pediatric Orthopedics. Philadelphia, W. B. Saunders Co., 1972, p. 1463.)

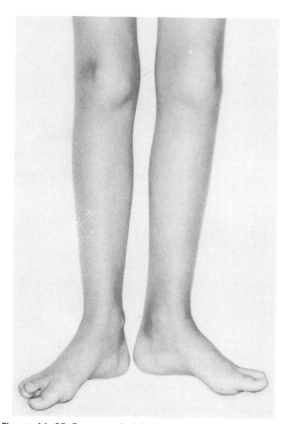

Figure 14–25. Exaggerated tibial torsion. In stance, with the patellae facing straight forward, the feet point outward. (From Tachdjian, M. O.: Pediatric Orthopedics. Philadelphia, W. B. Saunders Co., 1972, p. 1461.)

longitudinal arch will be visible. The examiner should note any pes planus (flatfoot), pes cavus ("hollow" foot), or other deformities.

19. The feet angle out equally (usually 10°) (Fig. 14–25). This finding means that the tibia are normally slightly laterally rotated. The presence of "pigeon toes" usually indicates medial rotation of the tibia.

20. There is no bowing of bone. Any bowing may indicate diseases such as osteomalacia or osteoporosis.

21. The bony and soft-tissue contours are equal on both halves of the body.

The patient's skin is observed for abnormalities such as hairy patches (e.g., from diastematomyelia), pigmented lesions (e.g., from café au lait or neurofibromatosis), subcutaneous tumors, and scars (e.g., Ehlers-Danlos syndrome), all of which may lead to or contribute to postural problems (Fig. 14–26).

Lateral View

From the side, the examiner should look to ensure that:

1. The ear lobe is in line with the tip of the shoulder (acromion process) and the high point of the iliac crest. This line is the lateral line of reference dividing the body into front and back halves (Fig. 14–27). If the chin pokes forward, an excessive lumbar lordosis may be present as well. This compensatory change is due to the body's attempt to maintain the center of gravity in the normal position.

2. Each spinal segment has a normal curve (Fig. 14–28). Large gluteus maximus muscles or exces-

slightly anterior to the lateral malleoli, but the lateral malleoli extend further distally.

18. The arches are present in the feet and equal on both sides. In this position, only the medial

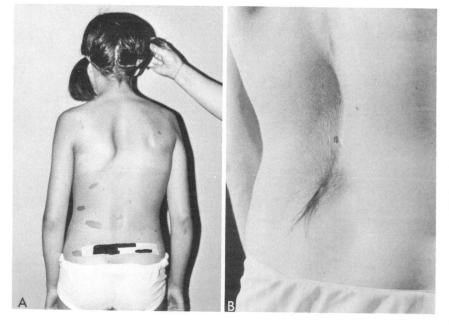

Figure 14–26. Abnormal skin markings. (A) Café-au-lait areas of pigmentation seen in neurofibromatosis. (B) Lumbar hair patch seen in diastematomyelia. (From Moe, J. H., et al.: Scoliosis and Other Spinal Deformities. Philadelphia, W. B. Saunders Co., 1978, p. 20.)

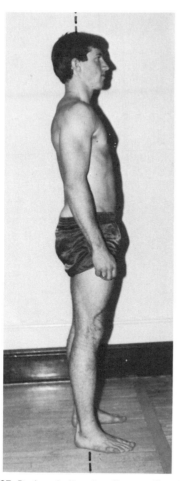

Figure 14–27. Posture in the standing position (side view).

Figure 14–30 illustrates the normal and some of the abnormal deviations seen when viewing the patient from the side.

Posterior View

From behind (Fig. 14–31), the examiner should note whether:

1. The shoulders are level and the head is in midline. These findings should be compared with those from the anterior view.

2. The spines of the scapula and inferior angles of the scapula are level (Fig. 14–32). Defects such as Sprengel's deformity should be noted (Fig. 14–33).

3. The spine is straight or curved laterally, indicating scoliosis. A plumbline may be dropped from the spinous process of the seventh cervical vertebra (Fig. 14–34). The distance from the ver-

sive fat may give the appearance of an exaggerated lordosis. One should look at the spine in relation to the sacrum. Likewise, the scapulae may give the optical illusion of an increased kyphosis in the thoracic spine.

3. The shoulders are in proper alignment. If the shoulders droop forward, "rounded shoulders" are indicated. This improper alignment may be due to habit or tight pectoral muscles.

4. The chest, abdominal, and back muscles have proper tone. Weakness or spasm of any of these muscles can lead to postural alterations.

5. There are no chest deformities, such as pectus carinatum (undue prominence of the sternum) or pectus excavatum (undue depression of the sternum).

6. The pelvic angle is normal, or 30° (Fig. 14–29).

7. The knees are straight, flexed, or in recurvatum (hyperextended). Usually, in the normal standing position, the knees are slightly flexed (0 to 5°). Hyperextension of the knees may cause an increase in lordosis in the lumbar spine. As well, tight hamstrings can cause knee flexion.

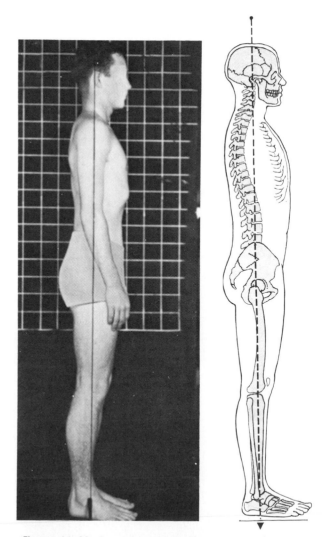

Figure 14–28. Correct postural alignment. (From Kendall, F. P., and E. K. McCreary: Muscles—Testing and Function. Baltimore, Williams and Wilkins Co., 1983, p. 280.)

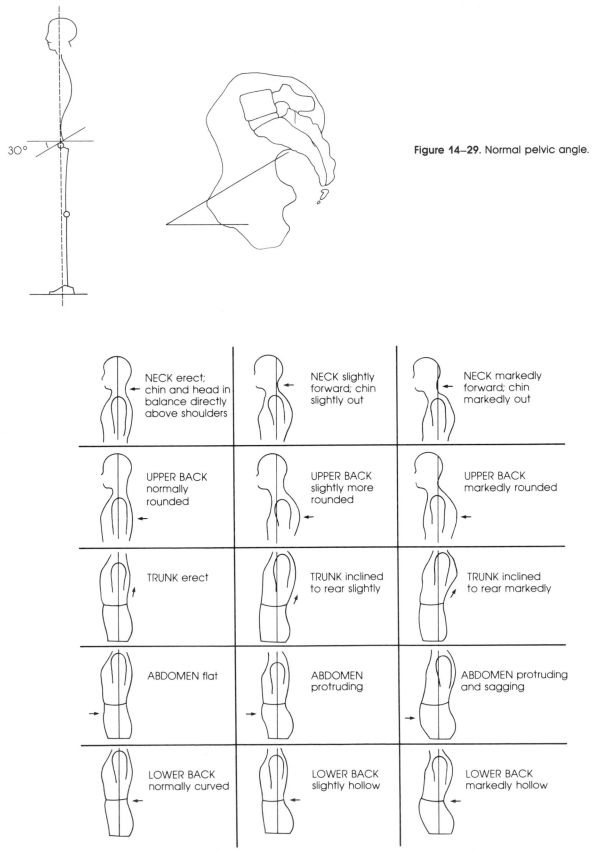

30°

Figure 14–29. Normal pelvic angle.

NECK erect; chin and head in balance directly above shoulders	NECK slightly forward; chin slightly out	NECK markedly forward; chin markedly out
UPPER BACK normally rounded	UPPER BACK slightly more rounded	UPPER BACK markedly rounded
TRUNK erect	TRUNK inclined to rear slightly	TRUNK inclined to rear markedly
ABDOMEN flat	ABDOMEN protruding	ABDOMEN protruding and sagging
LOWER BACK normally curved	LOWER BACK slightly hollow	LOWER BACK markedly hollow

Figure 14–30. Postural deviations obvious from the side view. (Redrawn from Reedes, Inc., Aubuin, N.Y.)

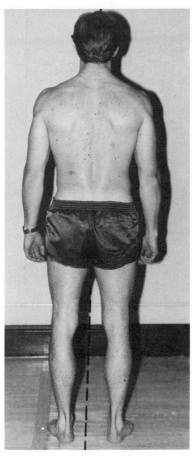

Figure 14–31. Posture in the standing position (posterior view).

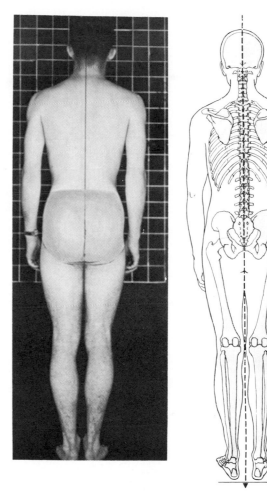

Figure 14–32. Correct postural alignment. (From Kendall, F. P., and E. K. McCreary: Muscles—Testing and Function. Baltimore, Williams and Wilkins Co., 1983, p. 290.)

Figure 14–33. Sprengel's deformity. Note the small, high scapula on the right. (From Tachdjian, M. O.: Pediatric Orthopedics. Philadelphia, W. B. Saunders Co., 1972, p. 82.)

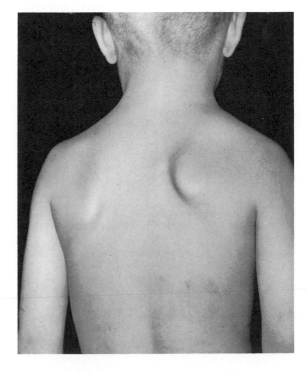

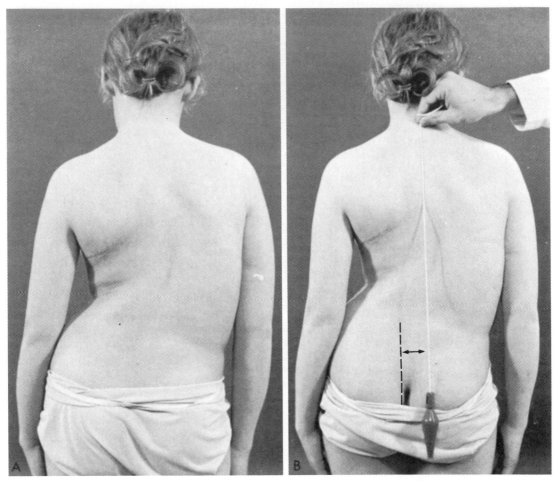

Figure 14–34. The patient is viewed from the back to evaluate the spine deformity.

(A) A typical right thoracic curve is shown. The left shoulder is lower and the right scapula more prominent. Note the decreased distance between the right arm and the thorax, with the shift of the thorax to the right. The left iliac crest appears higher, but this is due to the shift of the thorax with fullness on the right and elimination of the waistline. The "high" hip is thus only apparent, not real.

(B) Plumbline dropped from the prominent vertebra of C7 (vertebra prominens) measures the decompensation of the upper thorax over the pelvis. The distance from the vertical plumbline to the gluteal cleft is measured in centimeters and is recorded noting the direction of fall from the occipital protuberance (inion).

(From Moe, J. H., et al.: Scoliosis and Other Spinal Deformities. Philadelphia, W. B. Saunders Co., 1978, p. 14.)

tical string to the gluteal cleft can be measured. This distance is sometimes used as a measurement of spinal imbalance, and it is noted whether the deviation is to the left or right. If a torticollis or cervicothoracic scoliosis is present, the plumbline should be dropped from the occipital protuberance.[6]

4. The ribs protrude.

5. The waist angles are level.

6. The arms are equidistant from the body and equally rotated.

7. The posterior superior iliac spines (PSIS) are level (Fig. 14–35). If one is higher than the other, one leg may become shorter or it may be due to rotation of the pelvis. The examiner should note how the PSIS relate to the ASIS. If the ASIS on one side is higher and the PSIS on the same

side lower than the ASIS and PSIS on the other side, there is a torsion deformity at the sacroiliac joint. If the ASIS and PSIS on one side are higher than the ASIS and PSIS on the other side, there may be an upslip at the sacroiliac joint on the high side.

8. The gluteal folds are level. Muscle weakness, nerve root problems, or nerve palsy may lead to asymmetry.

9. The knee joints are level. If they are not, it may indicate that one leg is shorter than the other (Fig. 14–36).

10. The Achilles tendons both descend straight to the floor. If the tendons angle out, it may indicate flat feet (pes planus).

11. The heels are straight or angled in (varus) or out (valgus).

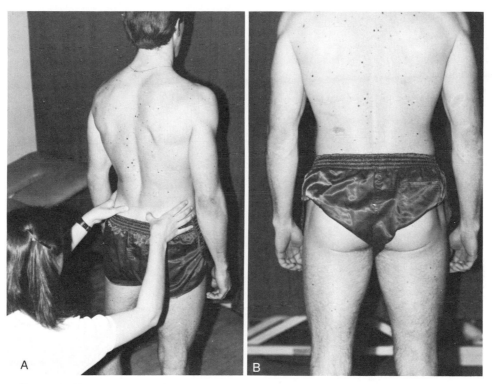

Figure 14–35. Viewing height of equality. (*A*) Posterior superior iliac spines. (*B*) Gluteal folds.

12. Bowing of bones is present.

Figure 14–37 illustrates the normal and some of the abnormal deviations seen when viewing from behind.

When viewing posture, the examiner should remember that the pelvis is usually the key to proper back posture. The normal pelvic angle is 30° and is held or balanced in this position by

Figure 14–36. (*A* and *B*) Functional scoliosis resulting from short leg. (*C* and *D*) The spinal position with short leg is corrected. (From Tachdjian, M. O.: Pediatric Orthopedics. Philadelphia, W. B. Saunders Co., 1972, p. 1192.)

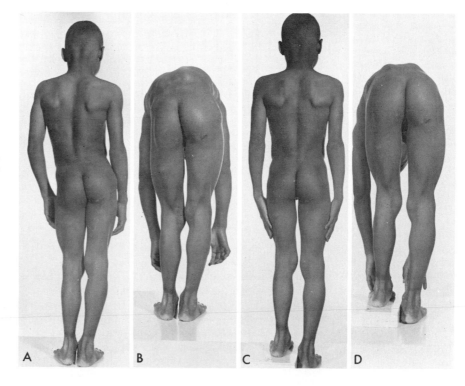

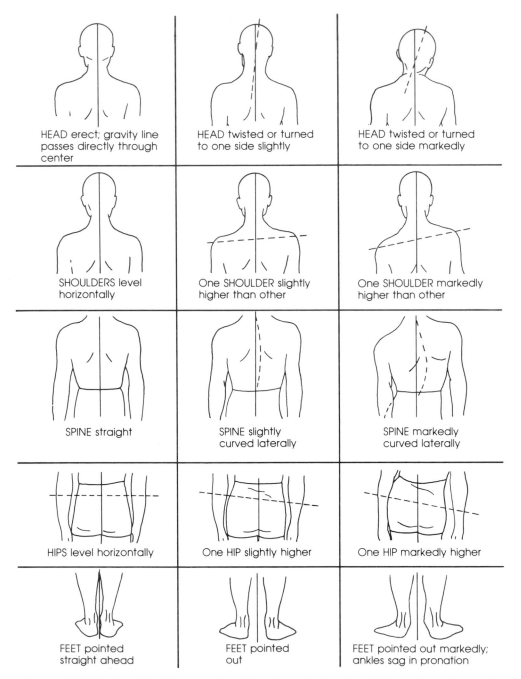

HEAD erect; gravity line passes directly through center

HEAD twisted or turned to one side slightly

HEAD twisted or turned to one side markedly

SHOULDERS level horizontally

One SHOULDER slightly higher than other

One SHOULDER markedly higher than other

SPINE straight

SPINE slightly curved laterally

SPINE markedly curved laterally

HIPS level horizontally

One HIP slightly higher

One HIP markedly higher

FEET pointed straight ahead

FEET pointed out

FEET pointed out markedly; ankles sag in pronation

Figure 14–37. Postural deviations obvious from the posterior view. (Redrawn from Reedes, Inc., Aubuin, N.Y.)

muscles. In order for the pelvis to "sit properly" on the femur, the following muscles must be strong, supple, and balanced: (1) the abdominals, (2) the hip flexors, (3) the hip extensors, (4) the back extensors, (5) the hip rotators, and (6) the hip abductors and adductors.

If the height of the patient was measured, especially a child, one could estimate the focal height of the child by using a chart such as the one shown in Table 14–1.[20]

FORWARD FLEXION

Having completed the assessment of normal standing, the examiner asks the patient to flex forward at the hips with the finger tips of both hands together so that the arms drop vertically (Fig. 14–38). The feet should be together and both knees straight. Any alteration from this posture will cause the spine to rotate, giving a false view.

Table 14–1. Percentage of Mature Height Attained at Different Ages*

Chronological Age (Years)	Percentage of Eventual Height	
	Boys	Girls
1	42.2	44.7
2	49.5	52.8
3	53.8	57.0
4	58.0	61.8
5	61.8	66.2
6	65.2	70.3
7	69.0	74.0
8	72.0	77.5
9	75.0	80.7
10	78.0	84.4
11	81.1	88.4
12	84.2	92.9
13	87.3	96.5
14	91.5	98.3
15	96.1	99.1
16	98.3	99.6
17	99.3	100.0
18	99.8	100.0

*From Bayley, N.: Modern Problems in Pediatrics 7:234–255, 1954.

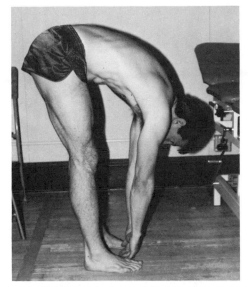

Figure 14–38. Posture in forward flexion. Note flattening or "rounding" of lumbar curve.

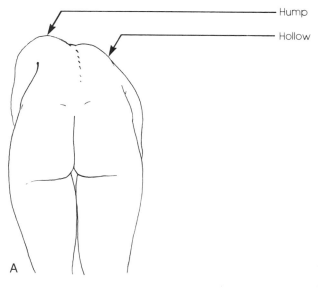

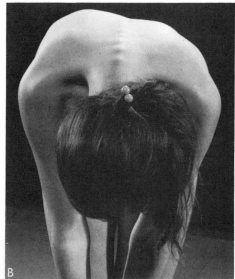

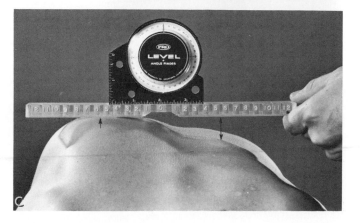

Figure 14–39. Rib hump in forward bending test.

(A) Posterior view.

(B) Anterior view. The two sides are compared. Note the presence of a right thoracic prominence.

(C) Measurement of the prominence. The spirit level is positioned with the zero mark over the palpable spinous process in the area of maximal prominence. The level is made horizontal and the distance to the apex of the deformity (5 to 6 cm) noted. The perpendicular distance from the level to the valley is measured at the same distance from the midline. A 2.4-cm right thoracic prominence is shown.

(From Moe, J. H., et al.: Scoliosis and Other Spinal Deformities. Philadelphia, W. B. Saunders Co., 1978, p. 17.)

From this position, using the anterior and posterior skyline view, the examiner can note:

1. Whether there is any asymmetry of the rib cage, e.g., rib hump. If a hump is present, a level and tape measure may be used to obtain the perpendicular distance between the hump and hollow (Fig. 14–39).[6]

2. Whether there is any asymmetry in the spinal musculature.

3. Whether a kyphosis is present.

4. Whether the lumbar spine straightens or flexes.

5. Whether there is any restriction to forward bending, such as spondylolisthesis or tight hamstrings (Figs. 14–40 and 14–41).

SITTING

With the patient seated on a stool so that the feet are on the ground and the back is unsupported, the examiner looks at the individual's posture (Fig. 14–42). This observation is carried out, as in the standing position, from the front, back, and side. If any anteroposterior or lateral deviations of the spine are observed, one should remember whether they were present when the patient was examined standing. It should be noted whether the spinal curves increase or decrease in

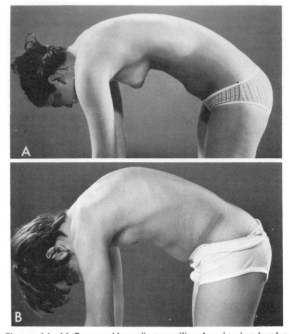

Figure 14–41. Forward bending position for viewing kyphosis (lateral view). (*A*) Normal thoracic roundness is demonstrated with a gentle curve to the whole spine. (*B*) An area of increased bending is seen in the thoracic spine, indicating structural changes—Scheuermann's disease, in this example. (From Moe, J. H., et al.: Scoliosis and Other Spinal Deformities. Philadelphia, W. B. Saunders Co., 1978, p. 18.)

the sitting position. From the front, it can be noted whether the knees are the same distance from the floor. If they are not, this may indicate a possible shortened tibia. From the side, it can be noted whether one knee protrudes further than the other. If it does, this may indicate a shortened femur.

SUPINE LYING

With the paient in the supine lying position, the examiner notes the position of the head and cervical spine as well as the shoulder girdle. The chest area is observed for any protrusion, such as pectus carinatum, or sunken areas, such as pectus excavatum.

The abdominal musculature should be observed to see whether it is strong or flabby, and the waist angles should be noted to see whether they are equal. As in the standing position, the ASIS should be viewed to see if they are level. Any extension in the lumbar spine should be noted. As well, it should be noted whether bending of the knees helps to decrease the lumbar curve. If it does, it may indicate tight hip flexors. The lower limbs should descend parallel from the pelvis. If they do not or if they cannot be aligned parallel, and at right angles to a line

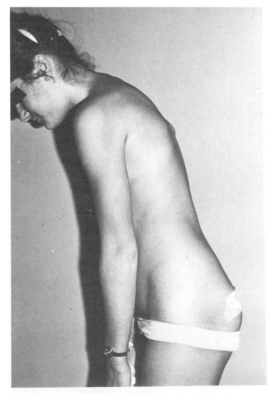

Figure 14–40. Abnormal forward bending resulting from tight hamstrings, as seen in this patient with spondylolisthesis. (From Moe, J. H., et al.: Scoliosis and Other Spinal Deformities. Philadelphia, W. B. Saunders Co., 1978, p. 19.)

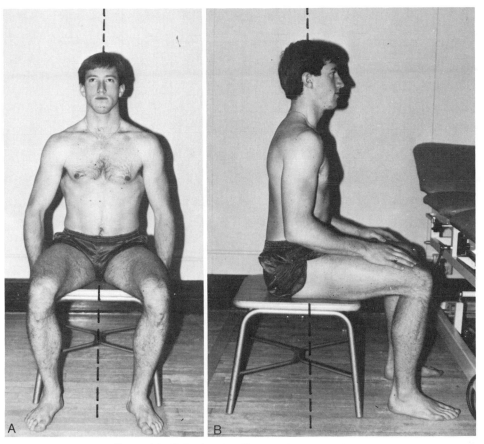

Figure 14–42. Posture in sitting positions (*A* and *B*).

joining the ASIS, it may indicate an abduction or adduction contracture at the hip.

PRONE LYING

With the patient lying prone, the examiner notes the position of the head, neck, and shoulder girdle as previously. The head should-be positioned so that it is not rotated, side flexed, or extended. Any condition such as Sprengel's deformity or rib hump should be noted, as should any spinal deviations. The examiner should determine whether the PSIS are level and should ensure that the musculature of the buttocks, posterior thigh, and calves is normal (Fig. 14–43).

Figure 14–43. Structural kyphosis does not disappear on extension. (From Moe, J. H., et al.: Scoliosis and Other Spinal Deformities. Philadelphia, W. B. Saunders Co., 1978, p. 339.)

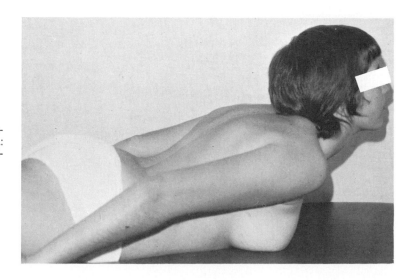

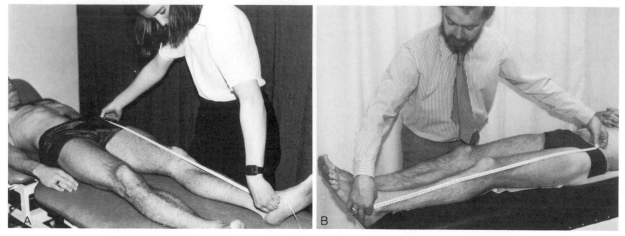

Figure 14–44. Measuring leg length. (A) To medial malleolus. (B) To lateral malleolus.

Examination

Assessment of posture, as previously mentioned, involves primarily history and observation. If, on completing the history and observation, the examiner feels that an examination is necessary, he or she should refer to other chapters of this text and follow the procedure outlined for that area of the body.

With every postural assessment, however, the examiner should always perform two tests—the leg length measurement[21–24] and the straight leg raise test.

Leg Length Measurement. The patient lies supine with the pelvis set square or "balanced" on the legs; i.e., the legs are at an angle of 90° to a line joining the ASIS. The legs should be 15 to 20 cm apart and parallel to each other (Fig. 14–44).

The examiner then places one end of the tape measure against the distal aspect of the ASIS, holding it firmly against the bone. The index finger of the other hand is placed immediately distal to the medial or lateral malleolus and pushed against it. The thumbnail is brought down

Table 14–2. Good and Faulty Posture: Summary Chart*

Good Posture	Part	Faulty Posture
Head is held erect in a position of good balance.	Head	Chin up too high. Head protruding foward. Head tilted or rotated to one side.
Arms hang relaxed at the sides with palms of the hands facing toward the body. Elbows are slightly bent, so forearms hang slightly forward. Shoulders are level and neither one is more forward or backward than the other when seen from the side. Scapulae lie flat against the rib cage. They are neither too close together nor too wide apart. In adults, a separation of about four inches is average.	Arms and shoulders	Holding the arms stiffly in any position forward, backward, or out from the body. Arms turned so that palms of hands face backward. One shoulder higher than the other. Both shoulders hiked-up. One or both shoulders drooping forward or sloping. Shoulders rotated either clockwise or counterclockwise. Scapulae pulled back too hard. Scapulae too far apart. Scapulae too prominent, standing out from the rib cage ("winged scapulae").
A good position of the chest is one in which it is slightly up and slightly forward (while the back remains in good alignment). The chest appears to be in a position about halfway between that of a full inspiration and a forced expiration.	Chest	Depressed, or "hollow-chest" position. Lifted and held up too high, brought about by arching the back. Ribs more prominent on one side than on the other. Lower ribs flaring out or protruding.
In young children up to about the age of 10 the abdomen normally protrudes somewhat. In older children and adults it should be flat.	Abdomen	Entire abdomen protrudes. Lower part of the abdomen protrudes while the upper part is pulled in.
The front of the pelvis and the thighs are in a straight line. The buttocks is not prominent in back but slopes slightly downward.	Spine and pelvis (side view)	The low back arches forward too much (lordosis). The pelvis tilts forward too much. The front of the thigh forms an angle with the pelvis when this tilt is present.

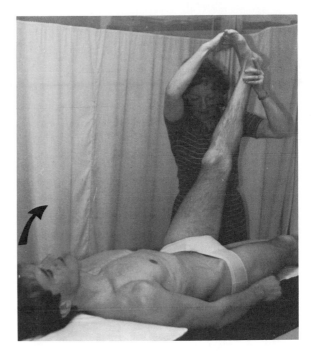

Figure 14–45. Straight leg raise test.

against the tip of the index fingers so that the tape measure is pinched between them. A reading is taken where the thumb and finger pinch together. A slight difference, up to 1.0 to 1.5 cm, is considered normal, but can still be relevant.

Further information on measuring true leg length may be found in Chapter 10, "The Hip."

Straight Leg Raise Test. The patient lies in a supine position with the knees extended and hips medially rotated (Fig. 14–45). The examiner passively flexes the patient's hip, keeping the knee extended and the hip medially rotated until the patient complains of pain or tightness in the back of the leg. The hip is then extended slightly until

Table 14–2. Good and Faulty Posture: Summary Chart* *Continued*

Good Posture	Part	Faulty Posture
The spine has four natural curves. In the neck and lower back the curve is forward, in the upper back and lowest part of the spine (sacral region) it is backward. The sacral curve is a fixed curve while the other three are flexible.	Spine and pelvis (side view) *Continued*	The normal forward curve in the low back has straightened out. The pelvis tips backward and there is a slightly backward slant to the line of the pelvis in relation to the front of the hips (flat back). Increased backward curve in the upper back (kyphosis or round upper back). Increased forward curve in the neck. Almost always accompanied by round upper back and seen as a forward head. Lateral curve of the spine (scoliosis); toward one side (C-curve), toward both sides (S-curve).
Ideally, the body weight is borne evenly on both feet and the hips are level. One side is not more prominent than the other as seen from front or back, nor is one hip more forward or backward than the other as seen from the side. The spine does not curve to the left or the right side. (A *slight* deviation to the left in right-handed individuals and to the right in left-handed individuals should not be considered abnormal, however. Also, since a tendency toward a *slightly* low right shoulder and *slightly* high right hip is frequently found in right-handed people, and vice versa for left-handed, such deviations should not be considered abnormal.)	Hips, pelvis, and spine (back view)	One hip is higher than the other (lateral pelvic tilt). Sometimes it is not really much higher but appears so because a sideways sway of the body has made it more prominent. (Tailors and dressmakers often notice a lateral tilt because the hemline of skirts or length of trousers must be adjusted to the difference.) The hips are rotated so that one is farther forward than the other (clockwise or counterclockwise rotation).

Table continued on following page

Table 14–2. Good and Faulty Posture: Summary Chart* *Continued*

Good Posture	Part	Faulty Posture
Legs are straight up and down. Patellae face straight ahead when feet are in good position. Looking at the knees from the side, the knees are straight, i.e., neither bent forward nor "locked" backward.	Knees and legs	Knees touch when feet are apart (genu valgum). Knees are apart when feet touch (genu varum). Knee curves slightly backward (hyperextended knee) (genu recurvatum). Knee bends slightly foward, that is, it is not as straight as it should be (flexed knee). Patellae face slightly toward each other (medially rotated femurs). Patellae face slightly outward (laterally rotated femurs).
Toes should be straight, that is, neither curled downward nor bent upward. They should extend forward in line with the foot and not be squeezed together or overlap.	Toes	Toes bend up at the first joint and down at middle and end joints so that the weight rests on the tips of the toes (hammer toes). This fault is often associated with wearing shoes that are too short. Big toe slants inward toward the midline of the foot (hallus valgus). This fault is often associated with wearing shoes that are too narrow and pointed at the toes.
In standing, the longitudinal arch has the shape of a half dome. Barefoot or in shoes without heels, the feet toe out slightly. In shoes with heels the feet are parallel. In walking with or without heels, the feet are parallel and the weight is transferred from the heel along the outer border to the ball of the foot. In running the feet are parallel or toe-in slightly. The weight is on the balls of the feet and toes because the heels do not come in contact with the ground.	Foot	Low longitudinal arch or flat foot. Low metatarsal arch, usually indicated by calluses under the ball of the foot. Weight borne on the inner side of the foot (pronation). "Ankle rolls in." Weight borne on the outer border of the foot (supination). "Ankle rolls out." Toeing out while walking, or while standing in shoes with heels ("outflared" or "slue-footed"). Toeing in while walking or standing ("pigeon-toed").

*Modified from Kendall, F. P., and E. K. McCreary: Muscles: Testing and Function. Baltimore, Williams and Wilkins Co., 1983.

no pain or tightness is felt. The patient is asked to flex the head so that the chin rests on the chest. If pain returns, it is an indication of a nerve root injury. If the pain does not return. it may be an indication of tight hamstrings. The other leg should be tested in a similar fashion and any differences noted.

Further information of the straight leg raise test may be found in Chapter 8, ''The Lumbar Spine.''

Additional Tests. Other tests may also be performed based on what the examiner has observed. For example, if the hip flexors appeared tight, the Thomas test should be performed (see Chapter 10).

Refer to Table 14–2 for a detailed presentation of postural problems.

Précis of Postural Assessment

History
Observation
    Standing (front, side, and behind)
    Forward flexion (front, side, and behind)
    Sitting (front, side, and behind)
    Supine lying
    Prone lying
Examination
Leg length measurement
Straight leg raise test
Examination of specific joints (see appropriate chapter)

As with any assessment, the patient must be warned that there may be some discomfort following the examination and that this discomfort is normal. Discomfort following any assessment should decrease within 24 hours. The examiner must always keep in mind that several joints may be affected at the same time, being either as the result of, or as the cause of, faulty posture. Thus, the examination of posture may be an extensive one, with observation of the posture in general but also several specific joints in detail.

REFERENCES

CITED REFERENCES

1. Fahrni, W.H.: Backache: Assessment and Treatment. Vancouver Musquean Publishers, Ltd., 1976
2. Finneson, B.E.: Low Back Pain. Philadelphia, J.B. Lippincott Co., 1981.

3. Kendall, E.P., and E.K. McCreary: Muscles: Testing and Function. Baltimore, Williams and Wilkins Co., 1983.

4. McKenzie, R.A.: The Lumbar Spine: Mechanical Diagnosis and Therapy. Waikanae, N.Z., Spinal Publications, 1981.

5. Wiles, P., and R. Sweetnam: Essentials of Orthopaedics. London, J & A Churchill Co., 1965.

6. Moe, J.H., D.S. Bradford, R.B. Winter, and J.E. Lonstein: Scoliosis and Other Spinal Deformities. Philadelphia, W.B. Saunders Co., 1978.

7. McMorris, R.O.: Faulty posture. Pediatr. Clin. North Am. 8:213, 1961.

8. Tachdjian, M.O.: Pediatric Orthopedics. Philadelphia, W.B. Saunders Co., 1972.

9. Tsou, P.M.: Embryology and congenital kyphosis. Clin. Orthop. Relat. Res. 128:18, 1977.

10. White, A.A., M.M. Panjabi, and C.C. Thomas: The clinical biomechanics of kyphotic deformities. Clin. Orthop. Relat. Res. 128:8, 1977.

11. Hensinger, R.N.: Kyphosis secondary to skeletal dysplasias and metabolic disease. Clin. Orthop. Relat. Res. 128:113, 1977.

12. Tsou, P.M., A. Yau, and A.R. Hodgson: Embryogenesis and prenatal development of congenital vertebral anomalies and their classification. Clin. Orthop. Relat. Res. 152:211, 1980.

13. Cailliet, R.: Scoliosis: Diagnosis and Management. Philadelphia, F.A. Davis Co., 1975.

14. Figueiredo, U.M., and J.I.P. Mames: Juvenile idiopathic scoliosis. J. Bone Joint Surg. 63B:61, 1981.

15. Goldstein, L.A., and T.R. Waugh: Classification and terminology of scoliosis. Clin. Orthop. Relat. Res. 93:10, 1973.

16. James, J.I.P.: The etiology of scoliosis. J. Bone Joint Surg. 52B:410, 1970.

17. White, A.A.: Kinematics of the normal spine as related to scoliosis. J. Biomec. 4:405, 1971.

18. Papaioannou, T., I. Stokes, and J. Kenwright: Scoliosis associated with limb length inequality. J. Bone Joint Surg. 64A:59, 1982.

19. Debrunner, H.U.: Orthopaedic Diagnosis. London, E & S Livingstone, 1970.

20. Bayley, N.: The accurate prediction of growth and adult height. Modern Problems in Pediatrics 7:234, 1954.

21. Clarke, G.R.: Unequal leg length: An accurate method of detection and some clinical results. Rheumatism and Physical Medicine 11:385, 1972.

22. Fisk, J.W., and M.L. Baigent: Clinical and radiological assessment of leg length. N.Z. Med. J. 81:477, 1975.

23. Nichols, P.J.R., and N.T.J. Bailey: The accuracy of measuring leg-length differences. Br. Med. J. 2:1247, 1955.

24. Woerman, A.L., and S.A. Binder-Macleod: Leg-length discrepancy assessment: Accuracy and precision in five clinical methods of evaluation. J. Orthop. Sports Phys. Ther. 5:230, 1984.

GENERAL REFERENCES

Anderson, B.J.G., R. Ortengon, A.L. Nachemson, et al.: The sitting posture: An electromyographic and discometric study. Orthop. Clin. North Am. 6:105, 1975.

Cailliet, R.: Nerve and Arm Pain. Philadelphia, F.A. Davis Co., 1964.

Cyriax, J.: Textbook of Orthopaedic Medicine, vol. 1: Diagnosis of Soft Tissue Lesions. London, Bailliere Tindall, 1982.

Kapandji, I.A.: The Physiology of the Joints, vol. 2: The Trunk and Vertebral Column. New York, Churchill Livingstone, 1974.

Littler, W.A.: Cardiorespiratory failure and scoliosis. Physiotherapy 60:69, 1974.

MacDougall, J.D., H.A. Wenger, and H.J. Green: Physiological Testing of the Elite Athlete. Ottawa, Canadian Association of Sports Sciences, 1982.

Matthews, D.K.: Measurement in Physical Education. Philadelphia, W.B. Saunders Co., 1973.

Mennell, J.: Back Pain: Diagnosis and Treatment Using Manipulative Techniques. New York, Little, Brown and Co., 1960.

Rothman, R.H., and F.A. Simeone: The Spine. Philadelphia, W.B. Saunders Co., 1982.

Torcell, G., A. Nordwall, and A. Nachemson: The changing pattern of scoliosis treatment due to effective screening. J. Bone Joint Surg. 63A:337, 1981.

Index

Page numbers in italics refer to illustrations; t indicates tables.

407